Applied Channel Theory
in Chinese Medicine

Applied Channel Theory in Chinese Medicine

Wang Ju-Yi's Lectures on Channel Therapeutics

Wang Ju-Yi

Jason D. Robertson

EASTLAND PRESS ▸ SEATTLE

Published by Eastland Press, Inc.
P.O. Box 99749
Seattle, WA 98139, USA
www.eastlandpress.com

Library of Congress Control Number: 2007941200
ISBN: 978-0-939616-62-6

    6 8 10 9 7 5

Illustrations by Bruce Wang
Cover illustration by Arne Bendik Sjur
Cover design by Patricia O'Connor

Edited by CT Holman, Dan Bensky, John O'Connor, Todd Gonzales

Book design by Gary Niemeier

ABBREVIATED CONTENTS

Chapter Contents

■ The Channel System

■ HOW TO PALPATE THE CHANNELS

■ CHOOSING THE CHANNEL FOR TREATMENT

■ THE ACUPUNCTURE POINTS

■ ACUPUNCTURE TECHNIQUE

■ Point Pairs

■ Appendices

Preface

THIS TEXT IS the result of the study and clinical application of the fascinating concepts of traditional acupuncture channel theory. The information in the following pages was generated by a process that took place over several decades. While working for thirty years in Beijing hospitals treating patients, I was always careful to keep in mind the classical texts which hold the fundamental theories of our medicine. During this process, my patients informed my understanding of the classics while my clinical understanding evolved and grew by returning to the classics.

One might ask why this text is entitled *Applied Channel Theory* rather than *Applied Acupuncture*. The title of the text serves to emphasize my realization that, in order to dramatically improve one's theoretical grasp of any of the fields of Chinese medicine, one must delve as deeply as possible into basic channel theory. Simply put, channel theory is one of the fundamental pillars of Chinese medicine, and is at the very core of acupuncture.

Looking over China's vast medical tradition, one often finds that those who developed a more rigorous understanding of channel theory were also those who made the most lasting and clinically useful contributions to the field. By contrast, a survey of modern discussions of acupuncture often reveals authors who have neglected to discuss (apart from a perfunctory mention) the deeper principles outlined in the *Inner Classic* (內經 *Nèi jīng*), *Classic of Difficulties* (難經 *Nàn jīng*), and the *Systematic Classic* (甲乙經 *Jiǎ yǐ jīng*). Most modern acupuncture literature emphasizes what might be termed 'experiential points'—dissertations on which points to use for treating specific diseases. The result is that the complex, systemic theoretical models of classical acupuncture have been reduced to a shadow medicine that searches for nothing more than points to treat specific symptoms or diseases. This approach has not only dramatically slowed the evolution of the medicine, it has also served to narrow the scope of conditions treated with acupuncture in many modern hospitals and clinics.

Having noted this trend in the field, I have spent a great deal of time and effort in recent years discussing solutions with colleagues while also striving to bring what I do know to students in both China and abroad. This text represents another step along that path. My student and friend Jason Robertson (孫傑生) has worked quite hard with me since our first meeting in 1997, finally coming to Beijing to live and work for over a year. During that time, he heard and translated many of my lectures with Chinese and non-Chinese students. He also took the time to think about my ideas, ask follow-up questions regarding difficult concepts, organize the material, and then translate the following pages into what is hopefully both a readable and enjoyable English text. My hope is that this work will serve to plant the seeds for the future growth of classical channel theory in other countries throughout the world.

For those of you reading this text, I fervently hope that you will not become trapped in the surface of acupuncture therapy, striving only to learn experiential points from your teachers and colleagues. Bring the medicine to life by incorporating the system of channel theory, expand its applications, and innovate from a place of theoretical integrity. The field of acupuncture must continue to develop and expand, treating the new diseases of the modern era while always keeping a firm grasp on the basics.

— *Wang Ju-Yi*

Acknowledgments

I would like to thank students and friends who have helped with this and other projects, including Nyssa Tang, L.Ac., Yefim Gamgoneishvili, L.Ac., CT Holman, L.Ac., Amos Ziv, L.Ac., and Sandra Chiu, L.Ac. There are many, many others who have been a part of this growing community as well, and I thank you all.

— Dr. Wang Ju-Yi

I would like to thank a few people without whom this project would not have succeeded. Most importantly of course, I thank Dr. Wang for the generosity of spirit which has allowed for a true meeting of minds across generations and cultures. Without his patience and determination to have me 'get it,' this book would have been but a translation and not a transmission. Also, to CT Holman who meticulously read, criticized, debated and rehashed nearly every word of the original draft. His crucial insight comes from having also spent quite a bit of time studying with Dr. Wang and practicing in his style. I am also indebted to CT for much of the structure and organization of the text—not a small thing given the volume of source material. I would also like to thank Stephen Brown and Yefim Gamgoneishvili for reading early versions of the text and offering much advice and needed encouragement at a relatively early stage. Thanks go to the editing team at Eastland Press (Dan Bensky and John O'Connor), and the design team (Bruce Wang, Lilian Bensky, and Gary Niemeier), all of whom have nerves of steel for the long-haul project and wondrous eyes for detail. Thanks to Todd Gonzales for his jeweler's eye in proofing the entire text. Thanks to Dave and Annie Sullivan and the Alliance Digital team for 'sponsoring' me in Beijing.

Lastly, I give my deepest thanks to my wife Tracy who has provided patience, love and support from the very beginning. You helped get me to Beijing just weeks after our marriage and, in the last few years, never wavered in your belief in me. This is for you.

—*Jason D. Robertson*

INTRODUCTION

今夫五藏之有疾也．譬猶刺也．猶污也．猶結也．猶閉也．
刺雖久．猶可拔也．污雖久．猶可雪也．結雖久．猶可解也．
閉雖久．猶可決也．或言久疾之不可取者．非其說也．
夫善用鍼者．取其疾也．猶拔刺也．猶雪污也．猶解結也．
猶決閉也．疾雖久．猶可畢也．言不可治者．未得其術也．

W<small>HEN THE FIVE</small> yin and six yang organs are diseased, it is like there is a thorn, a piece of dirt, a knot, or a blockage. Although the thorn may be long-standing, it can be removed. Although the dirt may be long-standing, it can be wiped away. Although the knot may be long-standing, it can be untied. Although the blockage may be long-standing, it can be opened up. [Those who] say that old diseases cannot be taken up speak wrongly. Those [who] use needles should look for [the cause of] disease. Then the thorn can be removed, the dirt wiped away, the knot untied, and the blockage opened up. Even though a disease is long-standing, it can be stopped. Those who say [these conditions] cannot be treated have not yet realized their skill.

—*Inner Classic, Divine Pivot,* Chapter 1

Channel Theory and Chinese Medicine

At its roots, Chinese medicine is about channel theory. The earliest comprehensive text on the subject, the *Yellow Emperor's Inner Classic* (黃帝內經 *Huáng Dì nèi jīng*),[1] is an important milestone in the history of medical thought. In that text, which was likely compiled, revised, and commented upon by numerous scholars over a five-hundred-year period between approximately 100 B.C. and 400 A.D., a true physiological system was described. Before the emergence of the *Inner Classic* as a primary medical source, much of the medicine practiced in China, like that of many other ancient cultures, linked disease to demonic entities that invaded the body. Disease was like a thorn in the skin and treatment focused primarily on removal. But in the first millennium, Chinese medicine began to take a new course. In the *Inner Classic*, a revolutionary assertion was made that disease, the body, and the practitioner formed a triumvirate, all of which were to be considered in the process of healing. No longer content to simply remove the pathological thorn, this new medicine strove to understand how disease affects the organs, and, in the process of recovery, how to reestablish healthy function.

A key element of this new approach involved a conception of the body as a system unified by a network of channels. In this conception, the channels have discrete pathways which connect the organs, and distinct processes by which the body interacts with the environment at large. Without the unifying role played by the channels, the principle of 'holism' in Chinese medicine makes little sense. The channels create a fabric that unifies organs, environment, disease, and treatment within an integrated network. A conception of the body that fails to account for the channel system may be likened to an agricultural theory that denies the importance of natural water systems.

Thus, very early on, the theorists of Chinese medicine, like theorists in other classical Chinese sciences, strove to appreciate the relationship between the microcosm and the macrocosm, between the human body and its environment. As the clinical tradition developed, the relationship of the channels to the external world continued to be an important consideration in guiding therapeutic strategy.

Unfortunately, many modern schools of Chinese medicine emphasize the organs and treatment modalities without describing the physiological system as a whole. Disease is discussed before the underlying physiological principles are explored. We might learn of 'heart-kidney not interacting' or of the 'five-phase relationships', but there is a feeling that the ideas are not part of a cohesive, functional whole (Fig. 1).

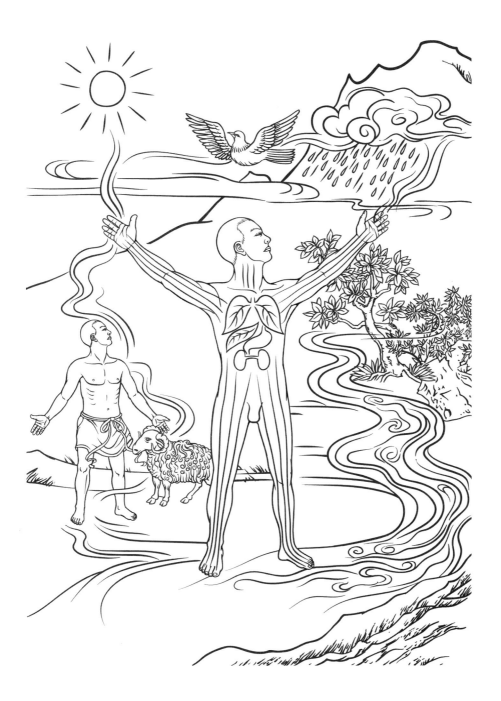

Fig. 1
The channels create a fabric that unifies organs,
environment, disease, and treatment.

In this book, the term 'channel system' refers to a larger idea than the familiar lines seen in acupuncture charts and textbooks. The channels are about physiology. Understanding the channels helps bring the modern mind closer to the classical understanding of how the body works. By appreciating the details of function, a more subtle understanding can be brought to bear on diagnosis. Diagnosis, in turn, involves more than the common techniques of asking, looking, palpating the pulse, and observing the tongue. It also means developing skills for placing the hands on the body to feel the channels themselves. Because the channels pass along the body surface, they can be felt. This isn't about feeling something that is mysteriously subtle, as the 'movement of qi' is often portrayed. Rather, the techniques that will be described in the following pages are easy to understand and can be applied immediately by anyone. Once one begins to feel the nodules, tightness, softness, and other irregularities described here, the next critical step is to categorize those findings, and then use them to refine treatment. The general outline of the book will reflect these goals.

Wang Ju-Yi

This book is both by and about Dr. Wang Ju-Yi. The layout of the text is designed to present not only Dr. Wang's ideas but also to explore his life. It is a life that has included some of the classic signs of success as judged by the standards of modern China. He has been a professor of Chinese medicine at the China Academy of Traditional Chinese Medicine in Beijing and a guest lecturer at other schools in China and around the world. He has served as president of one of Beijing's largest hospitals and as the editor of an international journal of Chinese medicine. And yet, despite all the trappings of achievement in his field, Dr. Wang describes himself today as a clinician. This is due both to his natural humility, and to a very real sense that clinical work is his greatest strength. In discussions, he always points out that he is happiest when bathed in the exciting chaos of a busy clinic.

Dr. Wang truly enjoys being with patients, and that alone may account for the careful thoroughness that characterizes his initial patient intakes. Like a host on a talk show, Dr. Wang literally 'interviews' his patients. He hears their stories and asks about their lives. Of course, while this is going on, he is also carefully palpating the course of the patient's channels with his hands. For those who have studied with Dr. Wang, the most familiar image is of him speaking amiably with a patient while his eyes follow his fingers from one channel to the next.

Dr. Wang represents a rare intersection of diligence, open-minded intelligence, and luck. Since elementary school he had been interested in

Chinese philosophy and history and pursued these subjects with tenacity. His intelligence is immediately evident to students who hear him speak or observe the careful precision of his clinical diagnoses. Dr. Wang's luck can be found in the fact that he happened to receive his training in Chinese medicine from a remarkable group of teachers. During the late 1950s, the Beijing University of Chinese Medicine was staffed with very experienced doctors. Having just been established in the nation's capital as one of the five official universities of Chinese medicine, the school served as a magnet for some of the best clinicians of the older generation. Dr. Wang, a member of the first graduating class from the newly-established school, studied fundamental theory with internationally famous teachers such as Qin Bo-Wei and Wang Le-Ting. He of course also studied with many others who are less well known outside of China. Now, after forty years of clinical experience, he has incorporated the training of a generation now passed and developed a unique understanding of his own.

Dr. Wang is an appropriate teacher for the current generation because of his ability to render his understanding of Chinese medicine in plain language, with the goal of using these ideas in the modern clinic. Although he draws much of his understanding from classical sources, he is able to present those concepts in a modern light by tapping into his clinical experience and skill as a storyteller. Also, unlike some clinicians of his generation in China, Dr. Wang is excited about sharing his accumulated experience with anyone willing to devote the time.

The Role of the Apprentice

Throughout the history of Chinese medicine there have always been physicians and their apprentices. The apprentice was usually a member of the physician's family or a chosen student. By contrast, modern Chinese medicine, like medicine in the West, proceeds from a different premise. Instead of an individual physician passing his or her knowledge directly to a student, modern medical traditions strive for open, standard practices accessible to all. Each method has its strengths. The structure of this text represents an attempt to re-create some of the experience of the former method while acknowledging the importance of the latter. To that end, dialogues between physician and apprentice are interwoven with theory and application to create a different type of modern textbook. The result is not only a picture of the ideas of a living master practitioner, but also insight into the thought process and experience that brought those ideas about. An attempt is made to reproduce not only a *way of thinking*, but also a particular *way of seeing*. The way that one sees is obviously influenced by the place where one lives and the rhythm of one's daily activities.

To prepare for writing this text, fourteen months were spent with Dr. Wang in Beijing, where I experienced the rhythm of his life and of his city. Raw material for the dialogues and narratives was gleaned from clinic shifts, time spent in tea houses or driving around the chaotic streets of Beijing, moments between patients or in translating for visiting practitioners, and meals eaten in crowded restaurants. Following the initial fourteen months, three years were spent writing and revising the text through an active dialogue that involved many return trips to Beijing. This is the process through which the system of Chinese medicine is passed from one generation to the next through the important venue of personal transmission. In the end, what is being passed on is the living thread of one of humanity's oldest medical traditions. It is alive in the minds of those who practice and not in books. The material must come alive in the mind of the student in order to be truly transmitted.

What is presented here is not just another tome to be added to the library of Chinese medicine. Although we do explore fundamental concepts from classical Chinese texts, this book does not focus excessively on presenting the views of the past. Instead, in accordance with a long tradition in China, this book represents a reevaluation of ideas from the past in a contemporary light. Specifically, the information presented is the result of over forty years of sifting through the staggering wealth of Chinese medical literature along with rigorous clinical application. Dr. Wang often emphasizes that "theory cannot be used to create reality; it can only attempt to explain it." By this he means that even the most revered theories of classical Chinese medicine must be judged by their performance. If the theories cannot improve the physician's understanding of a patient, they should be left to the important work of historians.

A unique issue that has affected the role of the apprentice described in these pages involves the thorny question of translation. Whenever possible, this book translates ideas originally expressed by Dr. Wang in contemporary colloquial Chinese into contemporary English. The importance of conveying his ideas in clear, modern English influenced Dr. Wang's choice of a native English speaker to oversee this project. Because the overriding goal was to create readable English, occasional liberties were taken by the translator with respect to rendering turns of phrase or organizational style. Where relevant, the original Chinese characters and pinyin are provided for technical terms. Sometimes, historical or theoretical context has been added, and the Chinese language is itself discussed. Nevertheless, an important aspect of this book has been to avoid presenting ideas that never passed between teacher and student. Difficulties regarding the direct translation of Chinese into English were addressed by repeated discussion of concepts over many cups of tea.

The Chapter Format

In addition to describing the system that guides a modern master of Chinese medicine in the clinic, a secondary goal of this book is to provide context for the information. While many appreciate the role of context in Chinese medical diagnosis (e.g., asking about a patient's living environment), the role of context in learning is less often discussed. In traditional approaches to the transmission of medical knowledge, it is important to consider where information comes from and how it is passed along.

For nearly two-thousand years, the practice of Chinese medicine has been both a vocation and a way of life. In modern China this continues to be true, although it is quite different from the mythical lives of the 'scholar physicians' of the past. One thing that certainly hasn't changed is that even a modern physician of Chinese medicine never removes his or her medical hat. The diagnostic approach, and the organic nature of the medical system, means that a practitioner of Chinese medicine sees medical theories reflected in the interactions of people, in the rhythms of nature, and even the construction of cities. To better convey the context of a practicing physician in modern China, three vehicles have been used in this book: the dialogue, the narrative, and the case study.

Dialogues

Unlike most contemporary translations of Chinese source material, this book represents an *oral transmission*. Although much of the raw material is preserved in digital recordings, its essence is to be found in our oral conversations. The nature of conversation, of course, is that it is usually less formal than a written narrative. Whenever possible, we have therefore tried to go beyond the standard textbook approach in order to preserve, within a general structure, the more informal nature of the oral dialogue.

Most chapters take their shape from the structure of Dr. Wang's lectures to visiting students, Chinese practitioners, or to the co-author. During these lectures, or during discussions in the clinic, questions would inevitably arise. Often, the questions would stimulate Dr. Wang to explain his point from a different angle, or to use metaphor to clarify a theoretical concept. In order to preserve some of the spontaneity of these discussions, the main text in many chapters is followed (or sometimes interrupted) by questions asked either by the co-author or by visiting students during the course of a lecture or clinical discussion. It is hoped that these questions will be representative of those that the typical advanced student of Chinese medicine might raise in response to some of Dr. Wang's ideas. While Dr. Wang comes from the same intellectual tradition that has given rise to standard 'TCM', he is by no means a strict adherent of every assertion made in modern Chinese medical textbooks. Sometimes he disagrees with the conventional view, and other times he simply understands and explains concepts at a level of greater complexity. Consequently, questions often arose. These differences are reflected throughout the book.

The use of dialogue in this text follows a long and ancient tradition in Chinese medicine. Beginning with questions posed and answered in the *Inner Classic*, the role of the questioning student has always been a crucial part of academic transmission. The use of dialogue in the earliest classics also reflects a didactic approach to clinical training. Long before there were written texts on the subject of healing, there were healers and their apprentices. Hopefully, by bringing the reader into the dialogue of a modern apprenticeship, some of the spirit and flavor of that approach can be revived.

Narratives

As noted earlier, not only his ideas, but also elements of Dr. Wang's life are described throughout the book. A series of short topical narratives are presented that bring the more 'textbook' style of information to life. Many chapters are followed by a story that relates or expands upon the information presented in that chapter. This is also a reflection of Dr. Wang's teaching style. When lecturing to students, he would often pause after a particularly complex theoretical presentation to tell a story. What would seem at first to be a digression would often end up clarifying a point just made. Not only did this approach serve to keep students awake and interested in the subject matter, it also deepened and broadened our understanding by showing how the concepts work in flesh and blood.

The narratives help illuminate the important role that Chinese culture plays in the practice of Chinese medicine. Additionally, for the non-Chinese reader, the narratives provide a glimpse of how Chinese medicine is practiced in modern China. Because Dr. Wang has been practicing for well over forty years, there is also historical relevance to his musings about how medicine (and daily life) has evolved in China.

Case studies

Like many textbooks of both Chinese and Western medicine, this book makes use of clinical case studies to illustrate practical applications of the information presented. Some of the case studies are relatively brief, while others provide greater detail about the thought processes that guide treatment. The shorter case studies provide concise demonstrations of how theory looks in the clinic, while the longer ones delve into the mental process that an experienced practitioner engages in when refining a diagnosis or treating a case that evolves over time.

Within the flow of a typical chapter there are three speakers. The first (and most loquacious) speaker is the 'textbook' itself. This is comprised of selected translations and reworkings of more formal lectures and case studies from Dr. Wang. The second speaker is the translator/co-author (Jason Robertson). As might be expected, this is the voice of a student asking questions. The third speaker is Dr. Wang himself with his more off-the-cuff commentary and stories.

Dr. Wang's wish

Students studying with Dr. Wang are often asked to take the information he provides and make it grow in their own work. On the final day of a series of lectures, he would always close with a familiar series of statements. He would remind students that his work is not finished and that there is still a great deal that is not understood. In many cases, he would also encourage the students to keep up their interest in the medicine by revisiting the core concepts. These so-called basics, in his mind, continue to evolve and grow in the mind with passing decades and clinical experience. He would then remind students of the importance of being focused in the clinic, and of treating patients with respect. An oft-quoted analogy is that of the channel system as a "finely-tuned instrument on which the acupuncturist plays like a musician." He would then close with the hope that those who studied with him would start palpating channels right away and report back with the new insights they experienced. The main point was that the information he presented should improve diagnosis and patient results in a way that can be communicated to others. He also asked that readers of this book keep the same admonitions in mind—wherever you may be.

■ Narrative: The Ancient City

A STUDENT SURVEYS A NEW HOME

Ask anyone about a year spent in north China and responses often involve the weather, the pollution, the dust, the magnificence, the pettiness. It is also a fascinating city to see on foot. The city center is a staggering amalgam of ancient glories and the contrasts of people living the remnants of a third-world existence in the shadows of first-world aspirations. Vast swaths of the ancient city and its famous maze-like alleys, the *hutongs* (衚衕 *hú tòng*—the word comes from the Mongolian *hottog*, which means 'well'), are disappearing under a wave of frenetic construction. 'Progress,' the oft-cited rallying cry of modern China, continues to demand sacrifices. New maps are now made by the Beijing city government every six months so that the citizens of 'New China' don't become hopelessly lost in their capital. Still, most Chinese don't complain. While a visiting tourist may become preoccupied with the loss of architecture, a Beijinger is more likely to point to running water in every apartment and the views from their place at the top of one of countless new high-rises.

In the cacophony of nine-million voices, there are those who talk of the need for people to live close to the ground so that they can feel the 'breath of the earth' (地氣 *dì qì*). The loss of the small alleys of the city is more than the loss of buildings; it is the loss of a way of life. Already, so early in the process of transformation, one sees re-created pieces of 'old Beijing.' There is the ironic presence of amusement park versions of a life still existing in reality only two blocks away. Wax figures of old men selling fresh noodles are perused by children wearing Nike shoes while grandparents a mile away shuffle past food stalls virtually unchanged for centuries.

I lived in the heart of this city, ten minutes by foot from the lakes and playgrounds of emperors. Traveling each morning through an alley built in the Ming dynasty to a bus with digital ticker tape, I was part of the contrast of the new Beijing. I was noticed but not stared at as I traveled wearing sunglasses and a backpack to the very center of China's new capitalist heart. The *Wáng Fǔ Jǐng* (王府井) shopping corridor is lined with lights and the clean lines of international commerce. Shoppers here, too sophisticated to gawk at the wares of Europe and the Americas, juggle coffee and cell phones. I once even stopped to watch a bungee jumping platform right in the middle of this huge open-air shopping complex where the faces of young voyeurs were temporarily rippled with g-shock as they bounced up and down in front of windows filled with fashion-wear. Here, in a twelve-story building next to the curved glass modernity of the Beijing Hyatt is the Cui Yue-Li Ping Xin Tang Clinic of Traditional Chinese Medicine.

Founded by the eponymous Cui Yue-Li, the clinic is a unique blend of the traditional elements of Chinese medicine with modern management style. Mr. Cui (now deceased) was a member of the upper echelon of the Chinese government in his post as director of the Department of Health during the 1960s and 70s. To older doctors of Chinese medicine, he is remembered for his efforts to preserve traditional medicine in times of chaos and 'reform.' When other officials in Mao Zedong's government, trained in Western sciences in Moscow, clamored for the banishment of medical 'superstitions,' Mr. Cui quietly pointed out that the traditional methods worked. Even before he rose to the highest post in his department, Cui Yue-Li had been helpful in the organization and support of the first government sanctioned schools of traditional medicine in Beijing, Nanjing, Guangzhou, Shanghai, and Chengdu.

Today, the clinic that bears his name is run by his son as a for-profit private clinic. Capitalizing on the good will that his father's name provides, he has recruited some of the best doctors in the country. The Ping Xin Tang Clinic is staffed by thirty very experienced doctors, now in semi-retirement, who see patients in a modern clinic decorated with reproductions of antique Chinese furniture. A plasma flat-screen television with American cartoons provides entertainment for waiting children. The doctors themselves move about the clinic with the studied grace that one sees in certain members of Beijing's older generation. Many of them grew up in the city and have participated, in one way or another, in the evolution of China from an imperial backwater to the host of a continental war, then to a communist power-player, and now...to something different. It's difficult to define what China has become in the midst of so much change and contradiction. In any case, the doctors of the Ping Xin Tang Clinic now enjoy the revered status afforded to older medical practitioners throughout Chinese history. The slow maturation of forty years (or more) is considered essential for a doctor to have 'ripe (熟 *shú*) experience.' Classical medical texts often point out that only after the age of sixty can a doctor begin to add to the corpus of medical literature that has amassed over two-thousand years. Apparently, one requires forty years of rumination before an idea of what all that literature is actually saying begins to take shape.

When I was studying there, Dr. Wang Ju-Yi worked in the largest of the treatment rooms at Ping Xin Tang. As the only acupuncturist among herbalists, more room was needed for the four treatment tables he constantly kept filled. Unlike most acupuncture clinics in Western countries, treatment in China is generally a communal experience. It isn't unusual to see patients who are lying on tables talking with each other about the course of their illness or the news of the day. There are thin curtains between treatment tables, but they create only a semblance of privacy. In the medical clinic, as with many other aspects of life in modern China, the individual is subordinated to the pressing demands of a large population. The room was always very clean and well lit with paper sheets for each patient. Disposable needles were used. This is a private clinic where patients at the time paid top-dollar (US$15 per treatment). It should be remembered that acupuncture treatments in the public hospitals funded by the state continue to be dramatically cheaper than in the private clinics (usually about 50 cents). Two years earlier, I had helped treat patients in the hospital of the Chengdu University of TCM. Doctors worked in that hospital in large old rooms with 20 beds, using needles sterilized by autoclave. The needles had often been re-sterilized so many times that the handles had become rusty. That was acupuncture on the front lines. Dr. Wang also worked in a similar environment for over 30 years at two of Beijing's largest hospitals. By comparison, the Ping Xin Tang Clinic was a five-star hotel moving at a glacial pace. Nevertheless, as Dr. Wang often points out, it was those days of seeing fifty patients in a single morning that stimulated him to think about the roots of channel theory.

It is to the mind of Dr. Wang that we now turn. The experience of being an apprentice to a practitioner of Chinese medicine is often about learning how another person thinks. This may sound obvious at first, but it bears mentioning given that many of us who go to China for advanced study become focused on the collection of helpful formulas or acupuncture prescriptions for particular conditions and complaints. This is only part of the transmission of a healing art. Although it is absolutely imperative that one become adept at formulas and point prescriptions, memorization can only bring the student so far along the path to developing the best-possible clinical results. As many of the best non-Chinese practitioners have already found, further growth as a clinician requires that one tackle the difficult task of learning how to see the patient through an entirely different cultural/ theoretical lens. Much of the so-called 'art' of Chinese medicine is to be found in the appreciation of the cultural and historical context that provides classical Chinese science with its unique understanding of human physiology.

In short, the process of understanding how a traditional Chinese physician might approach treatment involves cultivating an appreciation for how that doctor actually sees the patient from the moment they walk in the door. When developing treatment strategies, the physician draws not only from clinical experience, but also from considerations involving the culture and language from which their art derives. This aspect of Chinese medicine is difficult, but not impossible, for the non-Chinese practitioner to appreciate.

In order to promote the adaptation of Chinese medicine in different cultural environments, one goal of this book is to provide a few answers to a single meta-question: How can an understanding of channel theory and the unique concepts of classical Chinese physiology contribute to clinical results in a modern, non-Chinese setting? The short answer is that we, as students of Chinese medicine, must become as familiar as possible with the practice of this healing art by those who have inherited it. Only then will we be qualified to adapt it to the different cultures in which we practice. Otherwise, we're going to waste a lot of time 'discovering' concepts that were already right before us.

A vital part of practice is the art of diagnosis. As many of us who trained in Western countries know (especially those who have treated patients for a few years), the greatest challenge in practicing Chinese medicine arises from problems in refining this fundamental skill. Even the most elegantly constructed formulas lead to less than satisfactory results when applied to a foggy diagnosis. Of course, the meaning of the term 'diagnosis' itself is one of the crucial differences between

Chinese and Western medicine. Training in Chinese medicine puts a great deal of emphasis on cultivating the doctor's ability to correctly interpret the structure of symptom-patterns (徵候結構 *zhēng hòu jié gòu*). Instead of focusing on determining proper diagnostic testing, as is often the case for Western doctors, Chinese medicine puts the diagnostic tests in the doctor's own mind and hands. Diagnosis is often very complex while treatment can appear simple by comparison. Much of the literature available in Western countries about channel theory is focused on the application of treatment. While acknowledging that treatment is the obvious goal of any medical practice, there is a need to expand our understanding of the integral role which channel theory plays in diagnosis.

Dr. Wang often says that channel theory is the web that provides the linkages suggested in eight-principle (or parameter) organ (臟腑 *zàng fǔ*) theory. This idea represents the core of Dr. Wang's vision. The channels bring organ theory to life; they allow it to live dynamically in the doctor's mind. The ideas he presents regarding physiology are not exactly his own, but are instead his own reading and interpretation of the classics based on decades of mining the texts. This process of careful review of classical works, followed by rigorous clinical application and modification, is at the heart of the living tradition of Chinese medicine. The result is a unique way of thinking for each practitioner based on the particular texts, teachers, and experiences that make up their lives. It is the job of the apprentice to integrate this way of thinking as faithfully as possible, and then to carry that tradition ahead through another lifetime of careful study, clinical observation, and reevaluation. In trying to integrate a lifetime of experience for the next generation, the apprentice must try to enter the teacher's mind.

In the Beijing clinic, the mind of Dr. Wang was most often encased in a white cotton cap. Older doctors in China often wear this symbol of their position. Whenever he was working or teaching, Dr. Wang would wear his cap. The first thing that many patients note upon entering the treatment room is that Dr. Wang is a big man by Chinese standards. At over six feet tall, he is often the tallest man in the room. Although he may laugh and tell jokes in the clinic, his demeanor becomes quite serious when he begins to interview a patient. I myself quickly learned that it is best not to interrupt him when he is going through the process of asking questions. Patients begin their treatment with an interview at Dr. Wang's large wooden desk. He would sit behind the desk in a comfortable wooden chair while I sat across from him on a metal stool. The patient sat on a stool between us.

Usually, after five minutes of questioning, Dr. Wang would ask for the patient's hand. He would then hold the patient's arm firmly with his right hand and begin palpating along each of the six channels of the arm, one at a time, with the left. During this process he would often stop at certain points to ask more questions, or simply freeze to think for a moment. After checking both arms in a similar fashion, the patient would be directed to a treatment table where Dr. Wang would continue palpating the six channels of the leg, interspersed with more questions. Finally, after about 20 minutes, Dr. Wang would stop for a long moment to think through his treatment principle. He would then begin treatment with acupuncture, which might be followed by the writing of an herbal formula.

What are the mental steps that Dr. Wang takes in this process? Before discussing process, it is important to explore context. To that end, the first chapter will trace the concept of channel theory back to the roots of the medicine. We will see that the idea of what we call a channel (經 *jīng*) ultimately derives from observations of nature described first by the compilers of the *Inner Classic,* and later expanded upon in the *Classic of Difficulties* (難經 *Nàn jīng*). The chapter begins with a brief revisiting of the concepts of yin-yang, the five phases, and the organs. Then the discussion turns to human physiology and the idea that there are six 'levels' in the body, each designed to metabolize one of the 'six external qi' as they interact with the internal environment. The notion will be introduced that each of these levels has a way of being, a way of moving—toward the outside, swirling as a pivot, or closing inward. In the eight chapters which follow Chapter 3, we will proceed from this brief review of context to Dr. Wang's understanding of physiology, and, in the final chapters of the book, to the moment of treatment through the eyes of a modern classical practitioner. But first, to the "pillars" of the medicine…

CHANNEL THEORY AND
THE PILLARS OF CHINESE MEDICINE

BEFORE EXPLORING THE theoretical pillars of Chinese medicine, a few historical considerations should be addressed. The early history of what we now call Chinese medicine continues to be somewhat imprecise. In general, the picture painted by scholars is one of great intellectual ferment followed by gradual synthesis during the late Warring States to early Han dynasty periods (200 B.C.–220 A.D.). An important aspect of this new synthesis was a heightened appreciation of the role that the channels played in integrating the body with the larger environment. This appreciation grew largely from efforts by natural philosophers, physicians, and politicians to develop a world view that placed human beings and their social structures within the context of nature and the wider universe.

Context, in this case, involved building bridges between what might be called political and natural philosophy. At least in theory, the goal was to create a government that was in harmony with the movements of heaven and earth. A major driving force in this effort was the desire of the nascent Han dynasty to legitimize itself. The early emperors believed that supporting efforts to categorize and standardize the inherited culture could reinforce their legitimacy. For students of Chinese medicine, the most important outcome of this effort to collect the wisdom of the past is the *Inner Classic*.

In the centuries during which the *Inner Classic* was likely compiled, standardization also seems to have led to innovation. In this text, a network is described in which qi and blood circulates within a channel system that integrates the organs with the external environment. The idea of a channel system, so important to the physiology as conceived by the *Inner Classic*, was described in a language quite different from any spoken in the modern era, including that of modern China. Notably, the language and culture of early China placed particular emphasis on relationships—placing the individual within the context of the whole. In fact, intellectual thought at this time might be said to have been more contextual than linear. Consequently, for those of us trying to understand channel theory, it is particularly important to consider how this theory fits into the larger picture of classical Chinese medicine.

The Three Concepts[1]

In the *Inner Classic*, three fundamental concepts are described which form the foundational pillars of the medicine. These concepts, which were probably brought together into one system during the Han dynasty (they had likely existed in China for quite some time), form the basic organizing principles of Chinese medicine. They are:

- yin-yang and five-phase theory
  (陰陽五行理論 *yīn yáng wǔ xíng lǐ lùn*)
- internal organ theory (臟腑理論 *zàng fǔ lǐ lùn*)
- channel theory (經絡理論 *jīng luò lǐ lùn*)

These three concepts should be regarded as broad categories. The theory of yin-yang and the five phases represents the basic language of traditional Chinese medicine. With this language, the parts of the body, disease, and basic treatment principles can be categorized. Next, organ theory categorizes physiology and pathology. It is especially important for conceptualizing treatment. Finally, channel theory in Chinese medicine describes the network that brings the other theories to life. It integrates the organs and links the body to the world at large (Table 1.1).

Many contemporary students of Chinese medicine find that their training emphasizes organ theory and devotes less time to yin-yang and the five phases. On the other hand, students trained in modern five-phase style acupuncture might learn less about organ theory and its pivotal role in Chinese herbal medicine in particular. And for both of these dominant styles of modern 'oriental' medicine, channel theory is often a second-tier subject. A notable exception is the modern field of 'meridian style acupuncture' that has developed from living traditions in 20th century Japan.[2]

In a typically Chinese fashion, these three foundational concepts are interdependent; each supports and influences the others. This is especially true of the theories of yin-yang and the five phases, which shaped the scientific language of the Han dynasty and beyond.

I. Yin-yang and the five phases: the language	II. Organ (臟腑 *zàng fǔ*) theory: the categories of physiology and pathology	III. Channel theory: the living process

Table 1.1
The three pillars of Chinese medicine

The First Pillar: Yin-Yang and the Five Phases

Largely due to the influence of the *Inner Classic*, the concept of yin-yang and the five phases has become the fundamental language of medical dialogue in China. In order to understand the meaning of the *Inner Classic* and other texts that explain reality in terms of this concept, a helpful starting place would be the different roles they played in classical scientific thought. Both yin-yang and the five phases describe ways of categorizing qi. In this text, qi is defined as the smallest functional unit in any environment, in living creatures and in the organs. It is the prime mover, the spark, not only of life, but also of movement in the universe. However, qi is also a substance, or more precisely, it is the potential for change within a physical substance. The theory of yin-yang and the five phases is a tool for conceptualizing the otherwise unwieldy subject of qi. Specifically, yin-yang theory is generally concerned with analysis of the various aspects of a substance or condition while five-phase theory focuses on both categorization and unification within a whole[3] (Table 1.2).

Yin-yang theory looks analytically at the general nature of a particular subject. For example, something that is expanding, opening, moving, growing, or warm would be characterized as yang, while if it is contracting, closing, nourishing, shrinking, or cool it would be characterized as yin. Yin-yang analysis also takes into account the tendency of things to change. The nature of change can be summarized by the concepts of counterbalance, interdependence, mutual convertibility, and waxing-waning.[4] In any given moment, the tendency of any phenomenon—be it a thing, event, or illness—to change can be understood by considering these guiding principles.

When looking at something through the lens of yin-yang, one is not trying to categorize so much as to quantify in a relative sense. All things have some degree of both yin and yang within their nature; the key is to analyze where along the continuum a particular subject falls and what factors

Qi (氣) The smallest functional unit in any environment, in living creatures and in the organs	
Yin-yang and the five phases conceptualize qi	YIN-YANG: analyzes FIVE PHASES: categorize and unify

Table 1.2

Classical concepts of qi

might influence it to change. Because of the tendency of Chinese thought to consider parts as aspects of a whole (holism), the relative 'yin nature' or 'yang nature' of a subject depends on what it is being compared with. For example, when compared with the feet, the top of the head is considered to be more yang, but when compared with the heavens, the entire body is decidedly yin-natured. On the other hand, the human body is yang in relation to the ultimate yin of the earth itself (Fig. 1.1).

Five-phase theory is about categorization and unification. Categorization using the five phases is different from the classification often pursued by Western sciences. Chinese categorization strives to maintain an understanding of the relationship of each piece to the others within a whole at every step along the way. It thus unifies while categorizing. This can be contrasted with categorization in Western science, with its careful separation of a subject into its constituent parts. For example, when talking about the five phases within the human body, an appreciation of the way that each phase interacts with the others is paramount to a complete understanding. The 'wood' phase and the liver, for example, cannot be considered on their own. Each of the five phases is always understood in relation to the other four, and is difficult to define without reference to the others. The same is true of the five colors, the five sounds, the five tastes, or any of the myriad aspects of existence that Chinese scholars have categorized using this system.

The unifying aspect of five-phase theory means that each phase enables/ expands one phase while, at the same time, limits/contracts another. Enabling/expanding means that each phase depends on another for support. Limiting/contracting can be likened to the actions of a policeman directing traffic—limiting full freedom but not exactly holding back. The entire sys-

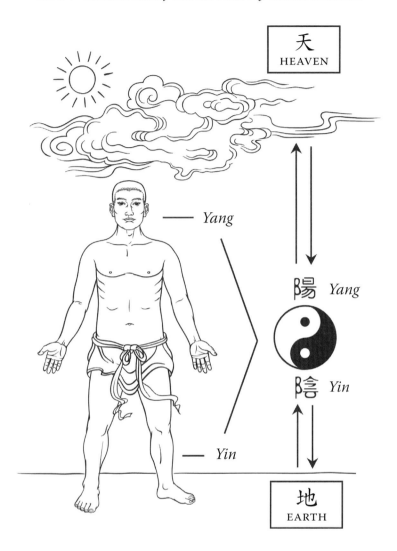

Fig. 1.1
Yin-yang theory looks analytically at the general nature of a given subject
while taking into account the constant tendency to change.

tem is always in a state of dynamic balance. One can also look to ecosystems for an understanding. If a particular species is withdrawn from a complex biosphere, both the species that depend on it in some way for food (called the 'generating cycle' in Chinese medicine) and those whose population was controlled by its appetites (termed the 'controlling cycle' in Chinese medicine) will be affected. In fact, the organs of the body are perceived to be working within a complex biosphere of their own. While one organ might enable the functions of another, it is at the same time being held in check by complementary functions of a third organ (Fig. 1.2).

Consider the spleen in classical physiology. The function of the spleen often revolves around the creation of nutrition and the transformation of fluids. It 'generates' lung-metal. Functionally, this means that the upward movement of the spleen qi dynamic balances and activates the downward movement of the lung in respiration. At the same time, the spleen is 'controlled' by the liver. In this case, the dredging and draining (qi-moving) function of the liver regulates the rate and efficiency of spleen metabolism—slowing and accelerating as necessary (Fig. 1.3).

An important thing to keep in mind about five-phase theory is that it represents an attempt to explain an otherwise unknowable whole. That unknowable whole is the more general concept of qi. A mistake that has been made historically in many fields of Chinese science is a tendency to force things into the mold of five-phase categorization. There are instances, for example, of entire armies rushing to change the colors of their shields before battle so as to carry the 'conquering' phase against a competing army of

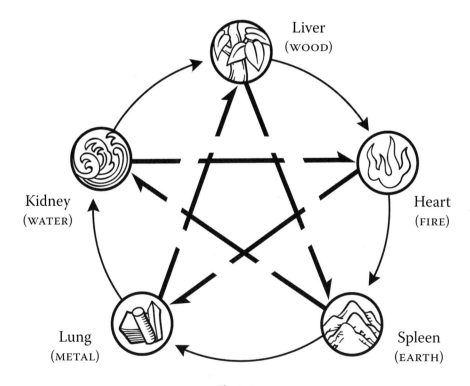

Fig. 1.2
Five-phase theory divides into categories while also
maintaining a unified and interrelated whole.

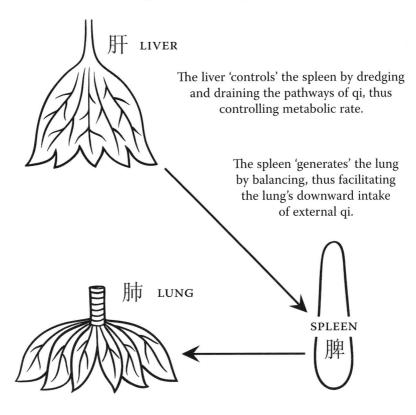

肝 LIVER

The liver 'controls' the spleen by dredging and draining the pathways of qi, thus controlling metabolic rate.

The spleen 'generates' the lung by balancing, thus facilitating the lung's downward intake of external qi.

肺 LUNG

SPLEEN
脾

Fig. 1.3
The generating and controlling relationships of the spleen
help categorize metabolic functions within the larger, unified system.

a different color. For purposes of Chinese medicine, the important thing to remember about five-phase categorization is that aspects of the body (and the natural world) can be placed in categories to facilitate understanding, and that these categories are always interrelated.

To summarize, the theory of yin-yang and the five phases was very important not only to medical dialogue, but also to the political and philosophical discussions of the Han dynasty. In general, yin-yang theory is used to analyze the nature of a substance or situation, while five-phase theory characterizes concepts within a unified whole. Unlike the precise definitions of modern science, these theoretical structures are malleable and can thus be applied to different fields. Also, the terminology may take on a different meaning in a different context, depending on which 'unified whole' one is looking at. For example, in the animal kingdom, fish in general may have a water nature when compared with the fire nature of birds, but among fish themselves, some types may be relatively fire-natured when compared with other types. The debates about five-phase categorization are many and are not the subject of this book. For our purposes as modern clinicians, the important thing to remember is that these theories provide a framework for beginning to understand the subtle movement of qi.

Yin-yang and the five phases also help to shape channel theory. As students of Chinese medicine should know, each of the twelve channels has a nature (yin-yang) and a category (five-phase) that guides understanding and treatment. Much more will be said later about how these characterizations reflect the classical understanding of physiology.

THE SECOND PILLAR: ORGAN THEORY

While yin-yang and the five phases provide the language of classical medical discourse, the organs are the main subject of discussion. Throughout most of Chinese medical history, health and disease are described within the framework of the major organs, which are the recipients of both stimulus and substance from the external world. It is also from the organs that substances within the body are created. When discussing physiology, the organs are the primary players. Contemporary students of Chinese medicine are likely to be familiar with the theory of the organs and the role that they play in shaping treatment with modern Chinese herbal medicine and acupuncture. The organs also play a major role in the physiological system described in this book. To the more common understanding of organ theory will be added their network of interaction, which involves the channel system.

THE THIRD PILLAR: CHANNEL THEORY

The third pillar constitutes the major subject of this text. A careful reading of early classical works indicates that channel theory is in fact the living web from which the concepts of the other two pillars is woven. As mentioned earlier, channel theory provides structure to the concept of 'holism' in Chinese medicine. Yin-yang and the five phases assume a physical form in the body as channels and organs with unique natures. The channels link organs to organs and the body to qi in the external environment. In fact, in classical Chinese medicine, the channels are an integral part of the organs themselves. In that respect, organ theory and channel theory are inseparable. The channels are not hollow pathways carrying substances among the various organs, but instead are active participants in the actual process of physiology. This is a complex concept that will be explained in chapters to come (Fig. 1.4).

While the idea that the body contains a system of channels is one of the most ancient in Chinese medicine, in the modern era the physiological role of the channel system has been underemphasized. The reasons for this are complex but seem to stem from an increased emphasis on organ theory by court physicians in the later imperial dynasties. Nevertheless, until the 20th century, a lively tradition of channel-based physiology and treatment likely continued to exist throughout China. Only during the second half of the 20th century did the understanding of channel theory truly begin to decline. This was largely a function of the practice of placing acupuncture theory strictly within the organ (臟腑 *zàng fǔ*) framework that characterizes modern Chinese herbal medicine.

Consider, for example, the acupuncture point functions listed in many modern textbooks. The functions of the points in these texts sound strikingly similar to the functions of herbs. This is no accident. During the

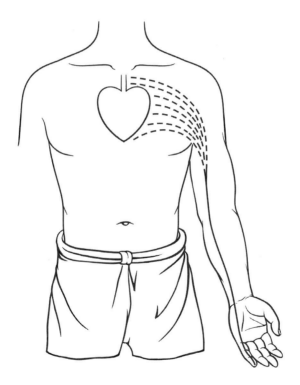

Fig. 1.4

The channels are not hollow passageways carrying mysterious
substances but are active participants in the actual *process* of physiology.
The heart organ and its channel, for example, are part of a functional whole.

process of standardization that took place in China from the 1940s to the 1970s, there was a movement to streamline terminology and theory among the various branches of traditional Chinese healing. For acupuncture, this meant abandoning, in many ways, the theoretical framework within which it had been practiced for millennia. Consequently, in recent decades, acupuncture in China has actually lost some of its effectiveness because of the diminished understanding of its classical mechanisms. In short, in some modern Chinese hospitals, acupuncture is used for treating far fewer conditions than it is capable of treating. Already, practitioners outside of China are quite aware of the fact that acupuncture can actually be used for a wide range of conditions. In China, too, there are still many practitioners who understand this, based on their clinical experience, and the tide seems to be moving once again toward a renewed interest in the classical roots of acupuncture therapy.[5]

In addition, it is a mistake to believe that channel theory is only about acupuncture, or that organ theory only describes herbal medicine. The two are actually interwoven and both acupuncture and herbal therapies have much to gain from the more complete physiology that their union describes. The goal of reviving classical channel theory is not meant to advocate an absolute return to a premodern medical system. Rather, the modern clinician has much to gain by developing a deeper understanding of classical concepts. Lessons learned from nearly two-thousand years of experience with the human organism should not be set aside lightly—especially not before the core of that experience is more fully understood.

For those interested in further exploration of the historical and theoretical roots of channel theory, the corpus of Chinese medicine remains relatively intact. This is because the Chinese have kept meticulous records. The cumulative clinical experience of generations has repeatedly been analyzed, critiqued, and modified. This process continues today. In the modern era, as in times past, innovative modification depends on first establishing deep roots in the theoretical underpinnings of the medicine. Otherwise, modern practitioners are doomed to constantly reinvent concepts that were always right under their noses. In addition, there is still quite a bit of truly innovative thinking that could come about by carefully reading the opinions of practitioners in ages past and reflecting on them in the light of what we know in the 21st century. The three pillars described above, enlivened and unified by a better understanding of the channel system, may represent one way that not only Chinese medicine, but medicine in general, can get back to the roots of these interrelationships.

Q: *I can understand your assertion that channel theory is one of the core concepts of Chinese medicine. There is still a lot to learn about exactly how the channels work in the body. For now, though, I'm curious to hear your personal understanding of the roots of channel theory. Where do you think these ideas came from?*

DR. WANG: As you can imagine, I've thought about this question quite a bit. To me, there are five basic sources from which classical channel theory likely draws:

- historical autopsy
- historical surgery and imperial punishments
- esoteric *qì gōng* techniques
- classical clinical experience
- classical Chinese philosophy

Historical autopsy Classical Chinese medicine, like many traditional medical systems, has a tradition of observing the human body after life has ended. Throughout Chinese history, physicians and students of medicine made examinations of the internal organs of former patients. Obviously, these were less detailed than the microscopic examinations made by modern physiologists. Nevertheless, through a long history of careful observation, Chinese medicine accumulated a foundation in basic anatomy. For example, the *Classic of Difficulties* (難經 *Nàn jīng*) and the *Systematic Classic of Acupuncture and Moxibustion* (針灸甲乙經 *Zhēn jiǔ jiǎ yǐ jīng*) of Huang-Fu Mi (皇甫謐 215–282 A.D.) both contain many references to the location, physical connections, size, and average weight of the major organs.[6] I have read many of these texts and am often impressed with their detail. Although much has been learned since, it indicates that they were thinking in the right direction.

Historical surgery and imperial punishments Despite an unclear understanding of sepsis, classical Chinese physicians conducted rudimentary surgical procedures in cases where no other option was available. For example, the famous Han-dynasty physician Hua Tuo (華佗) is reported to have conducted simple surgery within the abdominal cavity. Although such techniques were arguably rare and often led to infection, they provided valuable insight. A more grisly example of how China's physicians were able to observe living human tissue was by observing imperial punishments. One such punishment involved the slow dismemberment of the condemned. Court physicians were sometimes allowed to be present at these executions. They could therefore observe first-hand the physical changes that took place along the path from life to death. Later generations have these unfortunate prisoners to thank for information that likely saved the lives of many.

Esoteric *qì gōng* techniques The study of *qì gōng* (氣功 lit. 'working with qi') has a very long history in China. Rooted in the soil of prehistoric shamanistic techniques, *qì gōng* has developed over the millennia into a kind of scientific field of its own. Practitioners follow rigorous programs designed to improve the body's ability to heal itself. The history of *qì gōng* also abounds with stories of practitioners who, having practiced for many years or having been born with special talents, are able to sense the movement of qi. Some were reportedly able to sense movement with their hands, while others claimed to be able to actually "see" qi as a physical phenomenon. In any case, some of the earliest diagrams of channel pathways through which qi is said to move involve reference to *qì gōng* in the form of breathing techniques. Because all physicians are also scientists, it is helpful to avoid dogmatic dismissal of that which is not understood. In the case of *qì gōng*, it has been helpful throughout Chinese history to take its presence seriously because of direct benefits to patients. As to whether or not adepts throughout history (and even today) are able to "see qi," it is difficult to say.

Classical clinical experience Observation of actual effects has always held a very prominent place in Chinese medicine. No matter how esoteric the theory or unusual the procedure, if results were not obtained, it eventually fell out of use. To me, this is probably the most important source for channel theory. As the use of needles as a treatment modality grew through the centuries, physicians were able to observe patient response. The understanding of channel pathways was surely improved by the reports of patients who felt sensations far away from the point of insertion. Needles placed in the foot or leg, for example, caused changes in sensation on the face. Furthermore, meticulous historical records identifying those points which were able to treat particular internal or external conditions provided a treasure of information from which channel theory has drawn.

Classical Chinese philosophy Encompassing not only philosophy in the traditional sense of the word but also the larger topic of culture itself, channel theory is drawn from the Chinese way of life. Most students of Chinese medicine are familiar with the theory of yin-yang and the five phases. As I mentioned earlier, the philosophical language of yin-yang and the five phases was used to describe the human body. In this way, the philosophical undercurrents of Daoism, Confucianism, Buddhism, and even Mohism all contributed to the way that we describe and understand the channels.

Q: *Could you provide a basic definition of the term 'channel' (經絡 jīng luò)? To which physical structure do you understand this term to refer in the body?*

DR. WANG: There are two answers to this question. Narrowly speaking, one might say that the channels are 'spaces' (間隙 jiàn xì) in the body. In other words, in this definition the channels are pathways and might be thought of as the spaces within the fibrous connective tissues of the body.

In a larger sense, the concept of channel refers not only to the spaces but also to everything wrapped within them. In this definition, the concept broadens to include not only the spaces within the connective tissues, but also the structures (and fluids) held and brought together by these connective tissues. A channel is then like a river in that it includes the riverbanks and also the complexity of life within the water itself held by those banks. In the body, the channels are then groupings of connective tissue that bring together the blood vessels, bones, lymphatic vessels, nerves, tissues, and interstitial fluids within their purview.

This is a starting place for understanding. The difficulty is to unify these physical concepts with the classical understanding of qi transformation (氣化 qì huà). In other words, what does Chinese medicine have to say about what is actually happening in these spaces? The answer to that question will take some explaining...[7]

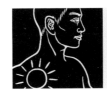

CHAPTER 2

FUNDAMENTALS OF CHANNEL THEORY

THE FIRST CHAPTER described the role of channel theory within the context of Chinese medicine as a whole. It identified channel theory as the web that unifies the organs and brings to life the principle of holism. In this chapter we will begin to describe the structure of classical channel theory.

For many who study the fascinating (and sometimes mystifying) field of classical Chinese medicine, channel theory is the missing link. On the other hand, some modern practitioners believe that the channel system described in ancient texts is little more than a proto-scientific attempt to map the pathways of nerves, blood vessels, and/or lymphatic circulation. While the architects of channel theory likely took basic anatomical structures into account, they were actually describing a broader concept. Channel theory is about human physiology, the evolution of disease, and mechanisms for the treatment of disease. There are three basic concepts within channel theory that can help clarify how Chinese physicians understand this system to work.

Fundamental Concepts of Channel Theory

The channels are an interwoven network (網絡 wǎng luò)

The channel system connects the internal organs to one another, to the surface of the body, and to the environment at large. The channel network unifies the other systems of the body—digestive, lymphatic, nervous, reproductive, and others—into a coherent and responsive whole. It is through this network that living organisms adapt to changes in the external environment. Through the prism of channel theory, the human body is viewed as being essentially inseparable from its environment and woven into the larger network of the biosphere. Again, it is important to remember that the network of channels is itself an integral part of physiology in classical Chinese medicine. In other words, the channels are 'alive' in the same way that one might consider the heart or lung to be alive.

The channels are pathways (通道 *tōng dào*)

The channel network is a system of pathways through which the vital energy and nutrition of the body move. The channels can be thought of as conduits within which one might find nerves, blood vessels, and lymphatic circulation. In this respect, they serve to unify or integrate the anatomical structures associated with particular internal organs. They act as pathways not only for the flow of substances like interstitial fluids *around* these anatomical structures, but also for the flow *within* the structures. For example, the pathway known as the lung channel includes certain muscles, nerves, arteries, and lymphatic vessels on the forearm. Healthy circulation within and around these structures falls within the purview of the lung 'channel'.

As one might surmise, not only do these pathways conduct the elements of a healthy physiology, they also serve as conduits for disease. The channels conduct externally-generated pathologies because of their location exterior to the internal yin and yang organs. When an external pathogen invades the body, it often travels first through the channels. Sometimes disease moves very quickly from the channels to the internal organs, and at other times more slowly. In addition, because of their role as integrators, when organ or emotional dysfunction leads to internally-generated disease, the channel pathways also become involved. Thus, the channels are affected by the presence of either externally- or internally-generated disease, which may cause palpable changes on the body surface along the course of the channels. This tendency to manifest palpable change is precisely due to the role of channels as pathways for both physiology and pathology. The specific changes associated with each of the channels will be discussed in later chapters.

The channels are a communication system (途徑 *tú jìng*)

The concept of the channels as pathways is one aspect of the channel network. Another is as a system of communication. In classical physiology, the channels are viewed as conveyors of information about the external environment to the internal organs. They also convey information among the internal organs themselves. The concept of qi in the channels is related to this function. The 'pathway' function of the channels refers more to the conveyance of material substances, while the 'system' function is associated more with the conveyance of qi. The two functions are interwoven and sometimes difficult to separate. The progression of disease in the channels, for example, involves 'material' changes brought about by relatively 'non-material' changes in the flow of qi.

The system function of the channels is also similar to, but not the same as, the nervous system, as understood by modern physiology. The concept of the channel network implies a kind of 'body intelligence' in which information about the condition of the organs moves through the connective tissues. This idea will be developed in later chapters.

In general, if the channel system is unable to properly respond to or integrate changes in the internal and external environments—which may include changes in air pressure and temperature, as well as changes in organ metabolism or even social conditions—disease or discomfort will ensue. Simply put, when the organs are not functioning properly, it is the channel system that helps to restore normal metabolism. In a healthy body, organ dysfunction may resolve fairly quickly because of the functions of the channels. This is an important concept and, frankly, one that is sometimes ignored altogether in modern Chinese medical education (Fig. 2.1).

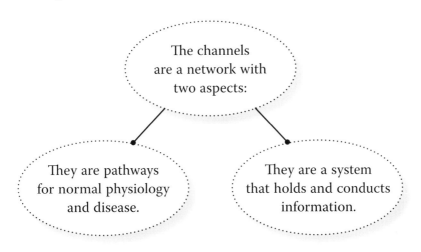

Fig. 2.1
The three principles of the channel system

Naming the Channels

Having outlined the basic functions of the channel system, the next step is to look at how the channels are described and understood. When looking at the acupuncture channels, the first thing that should be noted is how they are named. The system of names helps to classify the various parts of the channel network. Each channel is associated with an area on the surface of the body, an internal organ, and a level (or depth) within the body. Thus the classical names for each of the twelve primary channels have three distinct parts (Table 2.1).

Location of Channel	Nature of Channel	Associated Organ
Arm	*Tài yáng*	Small intestine
Leg		Bladder
Arm	*Shào yáng*	Triple burner
Leg		Gallbladder
Arm	*Yáng míng*	Large intestine
Leg		Stomach
Arm	*Tài yīn*	Lung
Leg		Spleen
Arm	*Shào yīn*	Heart
Leg		Kidney
Arm	*Jué yīn*	Pericardium
Leg		Liver

Table 2.1

The twelve primary channels

Location (arm or leg) of the external pathway of the channel

In Chinese, the first part of any channel's name includes the character for arm or leg. Each of the six channel levels (more on this in a moment) has an arm and a leg aspect. For example, the arm *tài yīn* channel is that of the lung while the leg *tài yīn* channel is associated with the spleen. Whether a particular channel is found on the arm or leg is dictated by the location of the yin (臟 *zàng*) organ with which it is associated (Fig. 2.2). For example, the heart, pericardium, and lung organs are found in the upper aspect of the body, which is reflected in their associated channel pathways on the arms. Similarly, the yin channels of the spleen, liver, and kidney are found on the legs and reflect the location of those organs in the lower part of the trunk. The six yang (腑 *fǔ*) channels follow their paired yin counterparts. The large intestine channel of the arm, for example, flows through the arm next

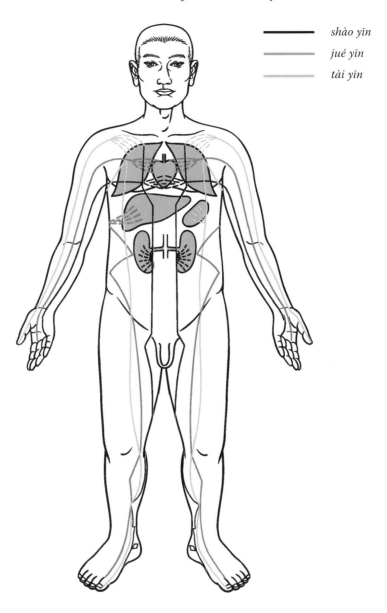

shào yīn
jué yīn
tài yīn

Fig. 2.2
The pathways of the yin channels reflect
the relative location of their associated organs.

to its paired yin channel the lung. The same is true throughout the system
(Fig. 2.3a and 2.3b). The significance of the yin-yang channel pairings is discussed later in this chapter.

[19]

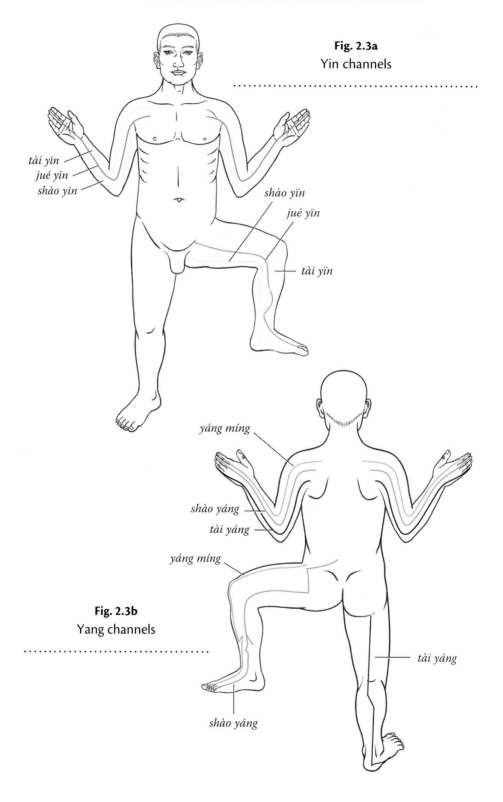

Fig. 2.3a
Yin channels

tài yīn
jué yīn
shào yīn

shào yïn
jué yïn

tài yïn

yáng míng

shào yáng
tài yáng

yáng míng

Fig. 2.3b
Yang channels

tài yáng

shào yáng

The location of the channels on the surface of the body is a reflection of their depth within the channel system. For example, the lung channel is located lateral to the pericardium and heart channels. Because the lateral portions of the arm are considered to be more yang (exterior), the fact that the lung channel traverses this area says something about the nature of lung physiology. Similar inferences can be drawn about channel depth based on the locations of the yang channels relative to each other (Fig. 2.4).

		Arm	Leg
———	*Shào yīn*	Heart	Kidney
———	*Jué yīn*	Pericardium	Liver
~~	*Tài yīn*	Lung	Spleen

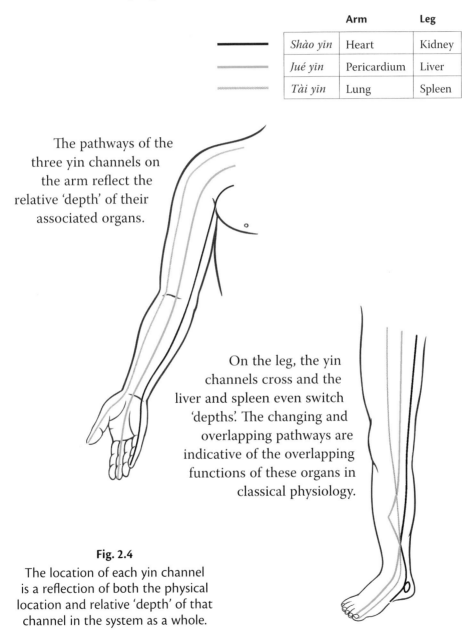

The pathways of the three yin channels on the arm reflect the relative 'depth' of their associated organs.

On the leg, the yin channels cross and the liver and spleen even switch 'depths'. The changing and overlapping pathways are indicative of the overlapping functions of these organs in classical physiology.

Fig. 2.4
The location of each yin channel is a reflection of both the physical location and relative 'depth' of that channel in the system as a whole.

When trying to conceptualize yin and yang areas of the body, the most helpful image is that of a person with their hands to their sides, thumbs outward. By picturing the body in this stance, it is possible to quickly ascertain the relative yin or yang nature of a given channel or area on the body. If the person were to face away from the sun, areas suffused with sunlight would be yang while those in the shadows would be increasingly yin, with the center line of the abdomen being most yin (Fig. 2.5 and 2.6).

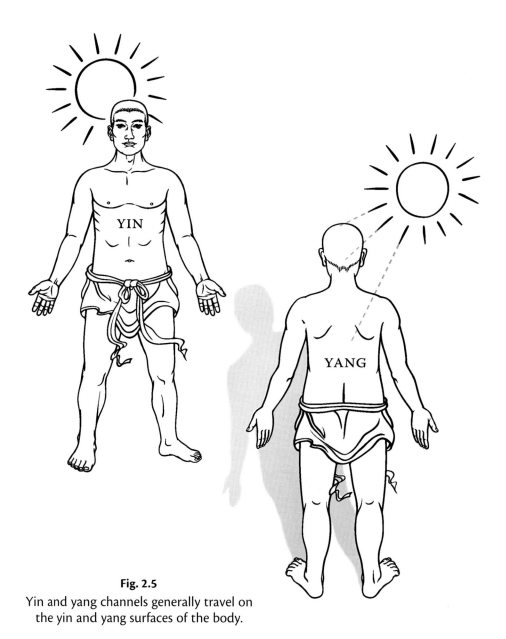

Fig. 2.5
Yin and yang channels generally travel on
the yin and yang surfaces of the body.

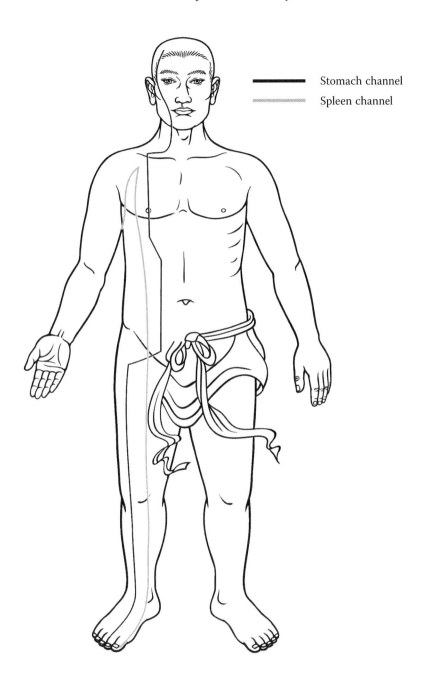

Stomach channel
Spleen channel

Fig. 2.6
The only significant exception is the stomach channel which, switching
over the spleen channel, passes through a yin area on the abdomen.
This is a reflection of the interwoven (and often inseparable) functions
of the spleen and stomach in providing nourishment.

Organ association

The second part of the name of any channel is the particular organ with which the channel is associated. This reflects the internal yin or yang organ with which the area of the body traversed by the channel has a special physiological connection. Remember, however, that the channels themselves are active parts of this physiology: they both connect the organs and are part of their living function.

The channel system is a network in which each of the organs has a place (or depth) within the whole. The place of the organ within the larger network is identified in the third part of the channel's name.

Nature of the channel

This part of the name describes the place of the channel within the overall network, using the language of yin and yang. In Chapter 1 we described how yin-yang theory was an integral part of the language of science during the era that gave birth to many of the fundamental theories of Chinese medicine. Thus when early physicians described the natures of the twelve channels, they did so using yin-yang terminology. When a subject is observed through the prism of yin-yang theory, the goal is to determine relative position. In this case, the twelve regular channels are broken down into six sub-types of yin and yang. The sub-types are not categories per se, but are descriptive of their personality and position in the body relative to the other channels along the spectrum of yin to yang. These sub-types provide even more clues to the functions of the channels (Table 2.2).

Thus a tripartite division of both yin and yang gives rise to the six basic levels that comprise the building blocks of channel theory. (For an explanation of why there are six major sub-types, refer to the question at the end of this chapter.) This means that there are six possible natures to the channels, ranging from absolute yang to absolute yin. These so-called 'six levels' are *tài yáng* (太陽 or greater yang), *shào yáng* (少陽 or lesser yang), *yáng míng* (陽明 or yang brightness), *tài yīn* (太陰 or greater yin), *shào yīn* (少陰 or lesser yin), and *jué yīn* (厥陰 or terminal or reverting yin). Each consecutive level is deeper than the one before it, with *tài yáng* at the surface of the body and *jué yīn* deep in the blood.

The Classical Understanding of the Six Levels

The concept of the six levels describes the process through which the interior of the body relates to the world at large. The concept of process is very important to keep in mind because it serves to emphasize the very fluid, active nature of the channels and organs. The 'levels' do not refer to

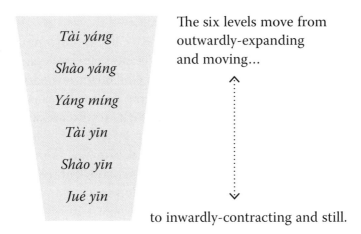

The six levels move from outwardly-expanding and moving...

to inwardly-contracting and still.

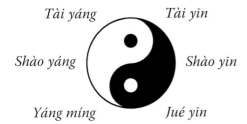

Remember, however, that all of the channels are positioned relative to one another in a moving, living system.

Table 2.2
The six levels

so many steps on a ladder, but represent six simultaneous physiological processes, each comprised of two organs. They are not separated from each other like self-sufficient systems, but are constantly engaged in processes of change and interplay. Not only does each level and its constituent organs interact with other organs, it also integrates a particular aspect of the environment at large. Before considering the relationship of the channels to the external environment (via the so-called 'six qi'), we will first take a look at their interrelationships within the internal landscape. On this subject, the *Inner Classic* has much to say.

For example, the importance of understanding the nature of the six levels is discussed in the *Divine Pivot* (靈樞 *Líng shū*) volume of the *Inner Classic*. Chapter 5, "Roots and Junctions" (根結 *gēn jié*), shows the direct clinical relevance of the channels. The first part of this chapter begins with a kind of soliloquy by the court physician Qi Bo. He asks the questions and then provides his own answers. Two questions relevant to our discussion ask how one's approach to disease might change depending on the season. Although it is not obvious at first how this will help clarify the concept of channel interactions, the connection becomes clear as the passage develops.

The first of the two questions asks how a doctor might tailor treatment in response to the climate of spring, when "yin qi is less and yang qi is abundant." Qi Bo begins his answer by stating that, "First, you consider the relative states of yin and yang." In other words, begin by analyzing whether yin or yang is predominant in the disease pattern that presents. Clear enough. He then asks himself another question: "Okay, what about in the fall when yang qi is less and yin qi is more abundant. How do you know how to tonify and drain?" In other words, how might the treatment strategy change in the fall? The answer begins like the answer to the first question, but, in an apparent burst of enthusiasm, something more is added and the result is a window into the mind of the Han dynasty:

> You must begin by considering the relative amounts of yin and yang as the situation presents in order to determine tonification and draining. Unusual qi has entered the channels and, if you can't help the organs [treat the condition], it is because you don't understand what the roots and junctions are about! You don't understand the yin and yang organs and how they move by opening, closing, and pivoting. Yin and yang might be failing and you wouldn't know where to start!

This outburst by Qi Bo is one of conviction and serves to emphasize two of the fundamental concepts of channel theory. The first involves the concept of 'roots and junctions,' which is a reference to the channels and their junctions, the acupuncture points (see discussion of 'points' in Chapter 15). In short, the ancient text asserts that, in order to approach the complexity of the human body, one must first try to understand the way that it is woven together by channels, punctuated by discrete collection points (junctions).

Next, it says that the organs open, close, and pivot (開,闔,樞 *kāi, hé, shū*). This is a statement about the way that each of the six levels—and the channels associated with those levels—'moves'. Each has a characteristic way of moving within the unified system. The more external yang levels have three parts, one opening toward the outside, a second pivoting in the middle, and a third closing and uniting inward. The three internal yin levels have a similar dynamic.[1] The organs of the body function within the larger framework of these six levels in a dynamic balancing act. Each level joins two organs in a metabolic duet dedicated to a particular aspect of classical physiology. The *Inner Classic* summarizes the nature of the channels (Table 2.3).

The natures of the six levels represent a physiological philosophy based on observation of both the human body and the natural environment that

Tài yáng	Greater yang	Governs opening (開 *kāi*) to the outside
Shào yáng	Lesser yang	Governs the yang pivot (樞 *shū*)
Yáng míng	Yang brightness	Governs uniting (闔 *hé*) to the inside
Tài yīn	Greater yin	Governs opening (開 *kāi*) to the outside
Shào yīn	Lesser yin	Governs the yin pivot (樞 *shū*)
Jué yīn	Terminal yin	Governs uniting (闔 *hé*) to the inside

Table 2.3
Nature of channels

surrounds it. Observations were made of inception, growth and decay, the changes of the seasons, disease and recovery, and countless other aspects of the process of life. These phenomena were judged to have general tendencies and rhythms which the channels of the human body are thought to replicate. Specifically, the six levels describe the transformational process from expansive, outwardly-moving yang to the closing, restful silence of absolute yin; or, reversing itself, from the material substance of yin into the pure motive force of yang. This is the constant interplay of energy and matter.

Classical Chinese medical theory breaks down this process into six generalized stages. The yang aspect involves the evolution from the absolute outward-facing and radiating state of *tài yáng* to a pivot of change in *shào yáng*, followed by a closing inward from the external levels toward the interior of the body at *yáng míng*. In the yin aspect, the outward radiation of nourishing yin substance at *tài yīn* is motivated by the fundamental pivot of ancestral life force at *shào yīn* to finally close inward for rest and storage at *jué yīn*. This process is ever continuous and cyclic. We will explore the details later.

An analogy from Chinese cooking provides a different perspective for understanding the natures of the six levels. Pictured here is a typical dumpling steamer that one might see in a Chinese restaurant. The principle is simple and involves the use of hot boiling water in a cooking pot below a sealed bamboo steamer in which dumplings are placed. As steam rises up from the boiling water, the dumplings inside are cooked while steam rises off the top of the steamer through a woven bamboo lid. Here, the steamer can be thought of as the yang levels of the body while the cooking pot is analogous to the yin levels (Fig. 2.7).

Tài yáng

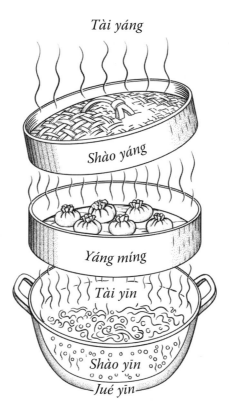

Shào yáng

Yáng míng

Tài yīn

Shào yīn

Jué yīn

Fig. 2.7
The process of steaming dumplings may likewise
be broken down into six component processes.

Taking the yang levels first, the steam radiating off the top has the out-wardly-moving nature that characterizes *tài yáng*. The ability of the bamboo lid to regulate and maintain a slow release of steam is likened to the *shào yáng* level, classically described as 'between the outside and the inside'. The warm, transforming steam and the dumplings themselves within the steamer are likened to the *yáng míng* level that holds and warms while clos-ing inward to interact with the yin levels below.

In the yin aspect, the three levels have distinctly different natures. *Tài yīn* opens outward not to the world at large, but to the 'outside of the in-side'.[2] In the steamer analogy, the *tài yīn* level can be likened to the steam coming up off the boiling water that mixes with *yáng míng* at the place where the internal and external truly meet. This is where the yin material of the water opens outward as steam. The *shào yīn* level is analogous to the upward-moving bubbles within the pot that serve as a pivot between the solid yin substance of the heating pot itself and the outward-opening above. *Jué yīn* is where yin becomes firm and begins to revert to yang. Here it is the solid iron pot that holds the yin together while also being the place from which the transformation begins from yin to the yang of radiating heat.

While this metaphor may help to put the levels in perspective, it does not fully explain the complex interactions described by classical physiology. The yin levels in particular are much more subtle than the metaphor implies. Nevertheless, the dumpling metaphor may be helpful in that it expresses the idea that the channel system involves a *process*. This process may be divided into distinct parts for the purpose of study, but those parts are never really separate from the whole. Each of the different levels influences and is influenced by the others. To extend our metaphor, the fire beneath the pot may be likened to the source qi that radiates from the kidney gate of vitality (an interesting subject that will be taken up later). If, due to source qi deficiency, the bubbles in the pot slow down, steam will radiate from the pot more slowly, the inside of the steamer will become less active, and the bamboo lid will no longer radiate steam off the top. In a similar but much more complex way, the network of internal organ metabolism is unified and interactive.

Over the course of nearly two thousand years, Chinese physicians took these basic concepts from the *Inner Classic* and built upon them in the clinic. Over time, greater and greater subtlety of understanding was achieved and results in the clinic thereby improved. The characteristics of the different levels of the channel system and their pervasive influence on organ function describe the mechanisms that underlie many classical therapeutic choices. This would include the system of herbal medicine first described in the *Discussion of Cold Damage* (傷寒論 *Shāng hán lùn*). Without this physiological model, unified by the channels, the practitioner is forced to collect a handful of 'empirical' treatments that might work for certain complaints, but will lack the flexibility of a living, breathing system. Understanding the system allows more flexibility in diagnosis and treatment.

The Six Qi

There is also a process in the world at large that mirrors the interactive process occurring inside the body. Here, too, the concept of channels as a network provides a door to understanding. The culture from which channel theory emerged believed that the body is a microcosm of the universe and that living beings are interconnected with the world. As a result, the channel system is conceived to connect with both heaven above and earth below. Humankind stands between the two—another pivot. Situated "between heaven and earth," there is a constant transfer of influences from above and below passing through the body. Over time, these influences became known as the 'six qi' (六氣 *liù qì*), described in *Basic Questions,* Chapter 66.

The concept of the six-level division described in the *Divine Pivot* was thus broadened to include influences from the natural environment. The six qi found in nature are wind, fire, summerheat, dampness, dryness, and cold (風,火,暑,濕,燥,寒 *fēng, huǒ, shǔ, shī, zào, hán*). In the atmosphere, these six meteorological tendencies were understood to constantly interact with one another to produce climate and patterns of weather. For clarity, it should be pointed out that summerheat is a type of heat that readily combines with dampness and often occurs during the summer season. Fire, on the other hand, is the more rarely occurring excessive dry heat that might flare up in spring, summer, or even fall (Table 2.4).

風	(*fēng*)	Wind
寒	(*hán*)	Cold
暑	(*shǔ*)	Summerheat
濕	(*shī*)	Dampness
燥	(*zào*)	Dryness
火	(*huǒ*)	Fire

Table 2.4
The six environmental qi

Each of the six qi has a place in normal weather patterns, and the rhythms of nature depend on their regular arrival and departure. When the six qi interact in the environment with regularity, healthy human bodies can adjust to the change and externally-contracted illness is less likely to occur. On the other hand, if the six types of environmental qi suddenly move in unusual ways or shift to new patterns to which the body has difficulty adjusting, then sickness may follow. When the six qi cause illness, they are known as the 'six pernicious influences' (六淫 *liù yín*). If the ability of a person to properly respond to the six qi is compromised, illness may ensue even in a relatively normal natural environment. Factors that might affect the ability of a person to respond include preexisting illness, unusual patterns of eating or drinking, emotional disharmony, or other aspects of lifestyle.

Each of the six environmental qi interacts with the internal landscape through the physiology of one of the six channels (Fig. 2.8). In fact, the goal of therapy in Chinese medicine is to maintain or reestablish the health of this system of integration. Integration is occurring both within the body and between the body and its external environment. While modern man has developed a number of ways for altering the environments in which we function, the ability to adjust to even small changes is still very difficult for some of us. In fact, while our home and office environments have become relatively more stable, the health of the human organisms that inhabit these environments has become increasingly chaotic. This is largely due to the irregularity of eating and drinking and the emotional complexity of life in the 21st century. Yet despite this radically changed picture, classical channel theory still offers a clear method for addressing complaints and preventing disease. This is because the human body and the principles that underlie its metabolism are still essentially the same, despite the new environment.

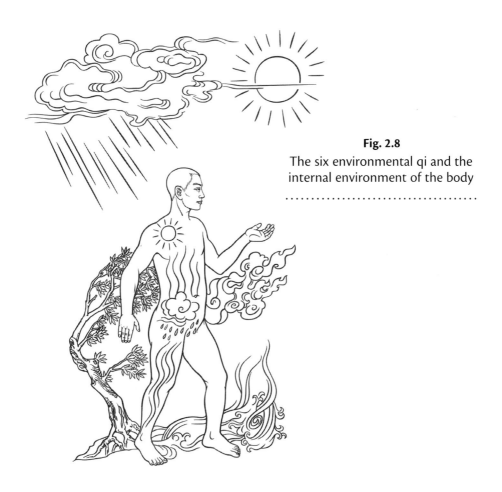

Fig. 2.8

The six environmental qi and the internal environment of the body

....

The six qi are thus a starting point for understanding metabolic processes. Specifically, each of the six levels of the body integrates a pair of organs which, in turn, are responsible for integrating and metabolizing a particular environmental qi.

Here is a list showing the associations among the six levels, the organs, and the six environmental qi (Table 2.5).

Level	Organs	Environmental qi
Tài yáng	Bladder/small intestine	Cold (寒 *hán*)
Shào yáng	Triple burner/gallbladder	Summerheat (暑 *shǔ*)
Yáng míng	Stomach/large intestine	Dryness (燥 *zào*)
Tài yīn	Lung/spleen	Dampness (濕 *shī*)
Shào yīn	Heart/kidney	Fire (火 *huǒ*)
Jué yīn	Pericardium/liver	Wind (風 *fēng*)

Table 2.5

Associations among levels, organs, and environmental qi

Table 2.5 presents a more complete picture of how the body's channel network interacts with the surrounding environment. In addition, according to traditional Chinese science, the body has particular conduits for conveying each of the six environmental qi—these are the channels. Remember that these conduits are not thought of as hollow tubes, but as functional aspects of normal physiology that are associated with certain areas of the body (the commonly-understood channels along the skin surface). The body's ability to incorporate the benefits of exposure to the surrounding environment while properly reacting to excesses or deficiencies of particular environmental factors is a function of the channel system.

It should be pointed out that while all the channels interact with the external environment, this is not true of all of the organs. The organs associated with the three yin channels are 'held on the inside', meaning that they are charged with refining, transforming, and storing within the body and do not directly interact with the external environment. The lungs are an obvious exception to this rule, and their connection to the qi of the external environment (although mediated by the throat and trachea) may explain why it is known as a 'delicate' organ that is easily damaged. Each of the organs associated with the three yang channels, however, has a direct opening to the outside world. The stomach, large intestine, small intestine, and gallbladder are all part of the digestive tract. The food passing through this tract is from the external environment. The triple burner organ opens to the outside in all three levels of the body trunk, and even in the four limbs. (The concept of the triple burner organ will be discussed at some length in Chapter 9.) The bladder opens to the external environment by passing urine out of the body.

Significance of Organ Pairings in Each of the Six Levels

At each level of the channel system is a pair of organs. These are generally functional pairings. As noted earlier, the organs at each level work together to metabolize one of the six external or environmental qi. However, the responsibilities of each pair are not limited to responding to the external environment. In another chapter we will discuss how the *tài yīn* lung-spleen pair, for example, is responsible for dealing with external dampness and for the metabolism of internal fluids. The specific functions of the spleen and lung allow them to work synergistically to this end. There are unique relationships between the organs paired at each of the other five levels as well. These relationships vary in each case, as their physiological duties differ. The same general principle of physiological balance also holds true in the pairings of interior-exterior, yin-yang organs as well. All of these relationships will be explored in upcoming chapters.

When considering the physiological implications of these functional pairs, it is important to return to the concept that each level has a relative 'depth' in the body. In the most general terms, the three yin channels are 'held on the inside' while the three yang channels 'open to the outside'. This is not the same as saying, for example, that the skeletal system is deeper in the body than the skin. The depths of each of the six levels help describe function, yet at the same time, all the levels constantly interact. A concrete example may help to clarify this. Consider the fact that, although they are yin organs 'held on the inside', the *tài yīn* lung-spleen pair plays an important role in maintaining the 'breathing' and nourishment of the skin. In other words, here are two organs 'held on the inside' which are nonetheless involved with aspects of the body at its most external surface. Similarly, each of the other levels has functions that are difficult to categorize using the normal definition of 'depth'.

In fact, the concept of depth might also be viewed as a way of dividing the body into 'systems'. In some respects, this is analogous to Western medicine's division of the body into systems—digestive, nervous, endocrine, etc. In both cases, however, the 'systems' approach risks creating a notion of the body that is neatly divided into unrelated and unconnected departments. In the case of Chinese medicine, it will be seen that the apparent gray areas in the understanding of these systems reflect a subtle appreciation of the way that the functions of one system spill over to affect others. In the end, it comes back to the idea that the six levels are aspects of an interwoven whole.

 Q: *Why are there six sub-types of yin and yang and not four or eight, for example?*

DR. WANG: This question gets us back to the very edge of prehistory in Chinese philosophy. It is reasonably easy to see how an idea like yin-yang might develop. There are so many aspects of life that manifest this dual nature: men and women, night and day, growth and decline, hot and cold. The list goes on and on. Many cultures throughout the world have come to the conclusion that there are two forces at work in the universe. It is after this fundamental observation that Chinese culture began to explore the significance of further breaking down those primary forces. Channel theory is also drawn from this seemingly simple concept.

Yin-yang theory is a system that is paradoxically both binary (composed of two parts) and tripartite (composed of three parts). Fundamentally, there is yin and yang. The two are understood as differentiated aspects of the 'supreme ultimate' (太極 *tài jí*), that is, the undifferentiated and unknowable source from which all existence flows. However, in order for yin and yang to become present and actualize, they must interact. The fruit of their interaction is qi. Qi then spreads to become the whole universe (Fig. 2.9).

So there is both the binary recognition that the universe has two primary forces (yin and yang) as well as a conception of three primary modes of existence. These primary modes might be thought of as yin, yang, and qi, or as earth, heaven, and humankind. They are also the states of birth, flowering, and decline that all animals, events, and nations experience. In order for the idea of 'six levels' to come about, the concept was proposed that both yin and yang might be broken down into these three levels. Within the large subdivision of yin, for example, there is yet another subdivision into three parts: heaven (yang within yin in this case), humankind (qi within yin), and earth (yin within yin). The yang aspect is divided in exactly the same way. As a result, much of Chinese cosmology is based on a system of two sets of tripartite images (Fig. 2.10). The trigrams of the *Book of Changes* (易經 *Yì jīng*) are the oldest examples of this breakdown.

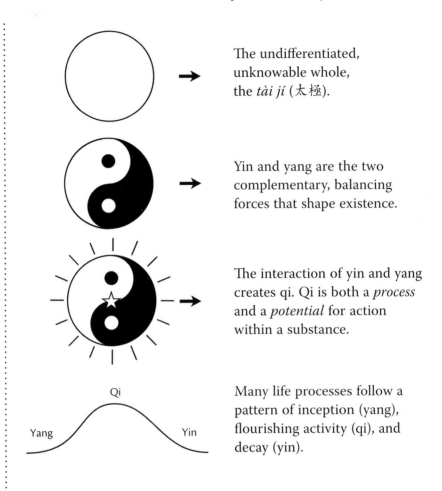

The undifferentiated, unknowable whole, the *tài jí* (太極).

Yin and yang are the two complementary, balancing forces that shape existence.

The interaction of yin and yang creates qi. Qi is both a *process* and a *potential* for action within a substance.

Many life processes follow a pattern of inception (yang), flourishing activity (qi), and decay (yin).

Fig. 2.9
Yin and yang in life

One can see the interesting interplay of yin and yang within levels of three by looking at the trigrams and noting that the broken lines represent yin while the solid lines represent yang.

I should also point out that another way that the idea of a three-part breakdown of yin-yang came about was from observations by early Chinese healers. They began to conceive of the middle stage between yin and yang as the 'pivot' or point at which yin and yang meet and comingle. So, in breaking yin and yang down into three parts, the ancient philosophers were not only accounting for the fact that yin and yang in combination create qi, but also that there is a pivot between yin and yang that is itself a state of being (Fig. 2.11).

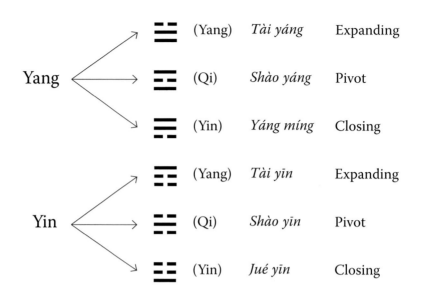

Fig. 2.10
The movement associated with the six levels

These ideas were prevalent at a time of great development in classical Chinese science (late Warring States–Han dynasty, ca. 300 B.C. to 220 A.D.) As a result, they were very influential in the development of channel theory. In other words, the understanding of the process of nature that the earliest Chinese scientists espoused involved placing nature, the channels of the body, and even the process of disease along a continuum with three main points of demarcation. In medical science, this tripartite division of existence means that there is a period where both ascent and decline of yin and yang coexist. An example would be the peak of life for human beings, between the ages of 30 and 60. This is the pivot. It is a time not necessarily associated with the absolute yang of youth or the absolute yin of old age. This analogy can be extended to many aspects of physiology, for example, the menstrual cycle or even certain periods in the feedback cycles of the endocrine system.

In the end, we in the modern era will likely never know exactly how these concepts developed. Remember that even though they are ancient, these concepts have proven over time to be helpful in achieving effective clinical results. To me, this is most important.

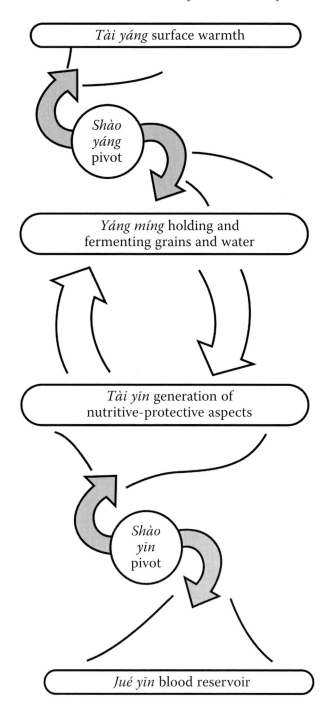

Fig. 2.11

In the classical model, there is a process of opening, pivoting, and closing inward
which helps describe the broad physiological functions of the channels and organs.

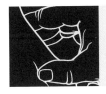

CHAPTER 3

An Introduction to Channel Diagnosis

T HE PREVIOUS CHAPTER introduced the basic concepts of channel theory. Here we will provide an overview of how theory guides diagnosis in the clinic. In the most basic sense, diagnosing the channels involves palpation. However, it is not enough to simply palpate the traditional channel pathways to locate reactive points for needling. The information gleaned from observation of the body surface reflects the state of internal physiology. In other words, the first goal of palpation is not to find points for needling, but to find clues about the state of organ function. Palpation should be thought of first as a diagnostic tool and only later as a tool for finding appropriate points for treatment. Of course, sometimes the points with tenderness, nodules, or other changes will also be those chosen for treatment—but not always. More often than not, there are too many areas of change found during palpation to treat them all. Narrowing down the choices from palpation to needle insertion involves a process, one that should occur within the larger context of what might be termed the clinical encounter, as shown in Fig. 3.1.

Each of the topics in this figure will be covered to some degree in later chapters. However, the interview process and eight-principle diagnosis are topics that are left to other texts. The individual organs will be discussed, but not in the same manner that they are covered in most 'TCM' textbooks.[1] In this book, special emphasis will be placed on the relationship of the organs to the channel system. Commonly-described Chinese medicine organ functions will then be reevaluated in this context. Fig. 3.1 describes the arc of how this book will present a treatment approach in which new interpretations of classical channel theory and organ functions can be readily

[39]

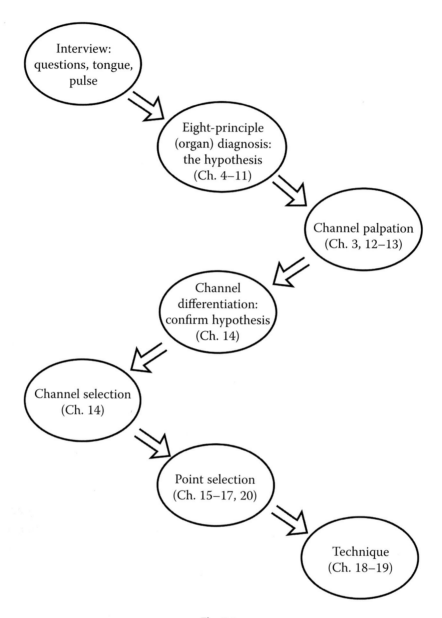

Fig. 3.1
The clinical encounter and related chapters in this book

applied in the modern clinic. It is important to emphasize, however, that the ideas introduced in these pages find their precedents in classical texts. To that end, it will be helpful to begin by taking a look at what some of those texts have to say about the subject of channel diagnosis.

Classical Channel Diagnosis

What do the classics have to say about the possibility that channels can be 'felt'? Chapters 73 and 75 of the *Divine Pivot* (靈樞 *Líng shū*) introduce two terms that are relevant to answering this question. The first, found in Chapter 73, is 切 *qiē,* meaning 'to slice'. In modern medical terminology, this character is used to describe 'pressing', meaning to separate the flesh with the tips of one's fingers. In modern texts, this character is used specifically to describe the process of examining the radial pulse. When one feels the pulse, one is carefully separating or parsing meaning from multiple levels.

Of particular interest to the discussion of channel palpation is a second character, found in Chapter 75. The word is 循 *xún,* which means 'to go along with'. This second character describes the process of going along the course of the channel with the fingers to ascertain the condition of the vessels. Thus, while *qiē* (separate) refers to pulse diagnosis, the word *xún* can be translated as 'palpating'—as in palpating the entire course of the channel with one's hands. In the discussions that follow, palpating refers to a specific technique of feeling the channels by going along their courses with the medial side of the thumb. It is important to note that, in these sections, the *Inner Classic* seems to consider channel palpation to be of equal importance to radial pulse diagnosis (Fig. 3.2).

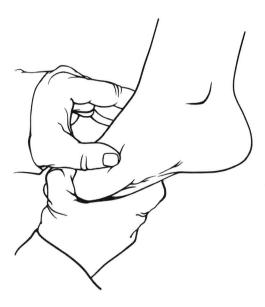

Fig. 3.2

The *Inner Classic* emphasizes the importance of palpating the pathways of the channels as part of the diagnostic process.

Besides introducing the topic of palpating the channels, Chapter 75 also describes other diagnostic techniques:

> Before using needles one must first scrutinize the channels to determine excess or deficiency. One must separate [*qiē*] and palpate [*xún*]. One must press and pluck. Observe how the channel responds and moves before continuing.

Thus the *Inner Classic* suggests quite clearly that one should not only check the pulse and palpate, but also "press and pluck" the channels with the hands. Furthermore, one should carefully observe "how the channel responds" before considering what channels or points are appropriate for treatment. The term 'pressing' (按 *àn*) refers to the technique of applying pressure to ascertain tenderness at particular points along the channel. 'Plucking' (彈 *tán*), on the other hand, can be thought of as a type of pinching technique used to test the elasticity of the skin along the course of the channel (Table 3.1).

切	*Qiē*	'Separate' the radial pulse
循	*Xún*	'Go along' the course of the channel
按	*Àn*	'Press' for spots of tenderness
弹	*Tán*	'Pluck' to check skin elasticity

Table 3.1
Manual techniques described in the *Inner Classic*

The *Inner Classic* makes another reference to channel palpation in Chapter 20 of *Basic Questions* (素問 *Sù wèn*):

> When treating disease, one must first ask about how the condition began and how it is now. Afterwards, one should press and palpate the vessels to see if the channels and collaterals are floating or submerged [浮沉 *fú chén*].

Here, one can see that the techniques of pressing (pulse taking) and palpating (going along the channel) are again described, followed by a statement about their purpose. It says that the doctor should try to determine if the "channels and collaterals are floating or submerged." Here, the concept of "floating or submerged" involves more than the usual modern meaning of a floating or submerged radial pulse. Rather, because the passage advises that both pressing and palpating be used to ascertain the condition of the channel, there is a suggestion that a broader area be observed. When using palpation to check the vessels, floating might be understood to represent a palpable puffiness or a sense of fullness along the course of whole sections of the channel (a coming upward), while submerged describes a sensation of weakness or softness (a sense of going downward).

Later, in Chapter 20, a situation is described where the practitioner discerns 'knots' (結 *jié*) along the collaterals of the vessel in the presence of a condition of 'excess above and deficiency below'. The text describes how one might bleed the channel to loosen the knot and reestablish normal movement. The important thing to note is that there is a familiarity both here and in other parts of the *Inner Classic* with the idea of palpating the channel pathways to look for irregularities. Moreover, one can see that puffiness, weakness, knots, or nodules were considered to be diagnostically significant by classical physicians.

Also likely compiled during the Han dynasty, the *Classic of Difficulties* addresses the subject of channel palpation in Chapter 13. Here, the process of checking the condition of the forearm from the elbow to the wrist is described. There is a specific reference to how the area will feel upon palpation in the presence of various organ disorders. In particular, it is suggested that changes in the vessels of the body will be mirrored by palpable change along the forearm:

> If the vessels are fast, there will also be a kind of fast feeling in the skin of the forearm. If there is urgency in the vessels, the skin of the forearm will also have urgency. If the vessels are relaxed, so too will be the skin of the forearm. If the vessels are rough, the skin of the forearm will be rough. If [flow in] the vessels is moving smoothly, then so too will the skin of the forearm.

Here, in the midst of chapters discussing radial pulse diagnosis, the *Classic of Difficulties* suggests that there are other diagnostic techniques that should also be considered. In fact, in the final lines of Chapter 13, the *Classic of Difficulties* highlights the importance of bringing all diagnostic methods to bear in the clinic: "Thus the inferior doctor knows one [diagnostic approach], the mediocre two, while the superior doctor can utilize all three." Based on references earlier in the chapter, the three diagnostic methods referred to here are likely radial pulse diagnosis, observation of the skin color (especially on the face), and palpation of the forearm. The ability to integrate all three methods will have a direct impact on the treatment outcomes: "The superior ones can cure nine out of ten illnesses, the mediocre ones help eight out of ten, while the inferior doctor only cures six out of ten."

A Modern Perspective on Classical Concepts

Having explored some of the historical descriptions of channel palpation as a diagnostic tool, the question of why and how this information is important in the modern clinic should be addressed. The short answer is that it helps improve results. The long answer will take up most of the remaining chapters of this book. Simply put, in the physiology of classical Chinese science, the channel pathways on the body surface reflect internal metabolism. In particular, the chapters on *shào yáng* physiology (Chapter 9) and the five transport points (Chapter 16) will explain how classical physicians might have understood this phenomenon. To look ahead a bit, the *shào yáng* chapter describes the role played by fluids in the spaces between the nerves, muscles, and other tissues to provide what Chinese medicine calls 'source qi' (原氣 *yuán qì*). The nature of the unique, 'formless' triple burner organ and its role in channel physiology will be explored in detail. Later, in the chapter on the five transport points, we will discuss how 'channel qi' develops from the fingers to the trunk of the body by drawing upon nutrition provided by fluids traveling within the so-called 'twelve channel circuit'. These fairly complex classical concepts should be considered slowly and repeatedly over time until they begin to take form in the mind.

In any case, the goal of these later chapters will be to describe the special role and unique nature of the areas below the elbows and knees in normal physiology. In particular, the idea that problems with internal organ metabolism are reflected as changes in fluid circulation in the distal areas of the body will be explored at some length. These irregularities in fluid circulation lead, in turn, to palpable changes along the surface of the body. Observation and palpation of these changes can then be considered in conjunction with other signs and symptoms to help guide diagnosis.

In fact, by developing the ability to refine diagnosis of symptom-patterns through channel palpation, a practitioner can gain insight not only to the development of a disease, but also to the rate of recovery. This can be gauged by palpating and taking note of patterns of change in the channels over time. This is not difficult. All that is required is that the practitioner palpate the channels and notice what feels normal and what does not.

As shown in Fig. 3.3, a logical process can be followed which also incorporates traditional organ diagnosis. For example, consider the case of a patient who presents with a chronic cough and asthma that includes symptoms of fatigue, expectoration of clear phlegm, a pale face, and dry skin. From the perspective of organ diagnosis, the interview indicates a likely pattern of lung qi deficiency. However, if one were also to consider channel theory, one might suspect involvement not only of the externally-paired large intestine channel, but also the 'same-name' *(tài yīn)* paired spleen channel. Further reflection may even lead one to consider possible involvement of other channels and patterns, such as the *shào yīn* kidney organ not 'accepting qi'.

In other words, how does one verify one's initial hypothesis that the patient is experiencing lung qi deficiency? An obvious first step would be pulse diagnosis. A thin pulse at the right distal position of the radial pulse might suggest deficiency of lung qi. But what about the involvement of other organs? There are, of course, skilled practitioners of pulse diagnosis who can quite deftly ascertain the complete pattern by palpating just the radial pulse. For many practitioners, however, the addition of other diagnostic tools will be quite helpful.

Channel palpation provides another step in the diagnostic process that can lead to more precise diagnosis. Returning to the lung qi deficiency pattern described above, if palpation of both the lung and kidney channels reveals tenderness or even a sense of weakness along the course of the channels, one might refine the diagnosis. It could then be described as involving more the *tài yīn* (lung) and *shào yīn* (kidney) instead of a purely *tài yīn* pattern (lung-spleen), or one with the internally-externally paired channels *tài yīn* and *yáng míng* (lung-large intestine). Most importantly, this refinement might occur even in the absence of clear kidney symptoms such as low back/knee pain: the channels themselves may reveal disharmony before the symptom-pattern evolves or becomes visible (Fig. 3.3).

Thus, by noting the relative intensity of the changes felt on the channels (e.g., the thickness, hardness, weakness or volume of small nodules), the practitioner can gain insight into the state of the patient's internal organs, just as in pulse diagnosis. It also provides *objective* input, given the tendency of some patients to overemphasize the intensity of their symptoms and others to underreport them. Finally, as mentioned earlier, the process of channel palpation provides a measuring stick by which patient progress can be gauged: as the patient improves, the channels will change. Thickness and hardness will soften, weakness may become more firm, and nodules may dissipate (Table 3.2).

Later chapters will describe in greater detail the process of channel palpation and provide strategies for categorizing the changes as a means for guiding treatment. First, however, it is important to explore how channel and organ physiology interrelate. As noted earlier, in order to glean the greatest amount of information from the channels, the classical conception of how the channels are working in the body must first be understood as thoroughly as possible.

Channel palpation provides:

• insight into a patient's metabolism
• an objective diagnostic tool
• a measuring stick for tracking progress

Table 3.2
Channel palpation

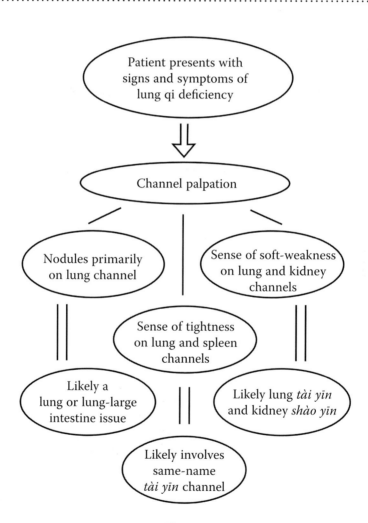

Fig. 3.3
Palpation in a case of chronic cough

Q:

> *This is a very clear description of a diagnostic approach that isn't mentioned very often by teachers in our schools nowadays. Why isn't it discussed?*

DR. WANG: In order to answer this question, you have to consider a few important trends in Chinese culture. There are two basic trends that have most affected the transmission of channel palpation as a diagnostic technique. The first has to do with the way that the medical profession evolved. The second has to do with a growing conservatism in Chinese society. Fundamentally, they are both related to life at the imperial courts.

The records of medical traditions from earlier dynasties were almost entirely written by highly literate scholar physicians. Because of their status and position in society, these doctors were very often called upon to treat the upper echelons of Chinese society. Consequently, medical traditions that had been passed down from before the current written texts later became the medicine of the more educated and well-off strata of society. Over the course of centuries, there was also an increasing conservatism in Chinese society. It became socially impossible for a person of the physician's rank to conduct an extensive physical examination due to proscriptions against physical contact. Because of the trend toward less and less physical contact between doctor and patient, the skills of careful differential diagnosis through the asking of questions became more and more important. Eventually for many doctors, their physical contact with the patient was reduced to palpation of the radial pulse. Thus pulse-taking continued, while channel palpation became less and less common in recent centuries among the elite medical traditions (i.e., those that were written down). One might speculate that channel palpation did continue among doctors of the lower classes, but there are no written records of this.

As you well know, radial pulse diagnosis is a very important and effective part of classical Chinese diagnosis. The process of differential diagnosis is also crucial. I don't mean to imply otherwise. My point is that there was another important tradition that placed a great deal of emphasis on palpating the channel pathways, especially in the area below the elbows and knees, as described in Chapter 13 of the *Classic of Difficulties*. As that chapter argues, we need to bring as many diagnostic skills to bear as possible when observing a patient so as to more fully understand how a presenting problem fits within the entire picture of organ interrelationships.

Today, acupuncturists in both China and other countries tend to have a different approach to diagnosis than that described in the *Divine Pivot* or *Classic of Difficulties*. How many times have you seen an acupuncturist ask the patient, What is your chief complaint? or What is your [Western] medical diagnosis? and then immediately begin to debate which points are most appropriate to address the symptom or medical disease? These doctors might then briefly look at the tongue and take the pulse, but will quickly send the patient to the treatment table. In fact, I strongly suspect that while they're taking the pulse, they are really just thinking through lists of 'experience points' for the most appropriate points from their teachers or textbooks! While this approach might get results some of the time, it is not classical acupuncture, and, more importantly, it is a disservice to the field. We can do much better.

If one takes the time to carefully think through how the pathodynamic (病機 *bìng jī*) of the patient has come about and which channels are affected before even allowing points to enter one's mind, much better results can be achieved. After developing a clear understanding of the pathodynamic and channel involvement, it is much easier to choose the points that will have the best effects.

I ran into this problem myself when I first began seeing patients in 1960. I would see that the patient had, for example, a clear pattern of liver-kidney yin deficiency leading to ascendant liver yang. That was the organ diagnosis and I might prescribe a modification of the herbal formula Lycium Fruit, Chrysanthemum, and Rehmannia Pill *(qǐ jú dì huáng wán)*. When it came to acupuncture treatment, however, I found that it was harder to use the organ diagnosis to help generate effective treatment approaches. For example, while some points may be said to 'tonify kidney yin' or 'quiet and descend ascendant liver yang', I would often just try to think of particular points to treat the symptoms in front of me. At that time, I knew from my basic understanding of the classics that acupuncture was not just about symptomatic treatment. I therefore began the long process that has eventually led to my personal understanding of channel theory.

I looked at acupuncture classics such as the *Systematic Classic of Acupuncture and Moxibustion* by Huang-Fu Mi (215–282 A.D.) and saw that, when these texts talked about disease, they usually discussed which channel was involved before suggesting points. As I continued my research over the decades, I found that there were many, many instances where channel diagnosis was discussed, especially before the Ming dynasty. In the current era, I don't think that the majority of practitioners of Chinese medicine think about channel qi transformation (氣化 *qì huà*) when they develop acupuncture treatments.

On a similar note, the use of channel diagnosis may have also suffered historically due to the ever-increasing emphasis on the organ style of diagnosis that is so important to Chinese herbal medicine. As I just said, organ diagnosis might be helpful for thinking about acupuncture points in a very simple way, but in order to really think in the style of classical physiology, one must reintegrate organ theory with channel theory. There are herbalists here in Beijing who are studying channel palpation and classical physiology with me as a means of improving their understanding of herbal medicine. Of course, there may have been a time when channel palpation was an important part of diagnosis not only for acupuncturists, but also for herbalists. In my own experience, I have found that palpation helps with my understanding of the pathodynamic and thus can improve my herbal formulas as well. Again, the most important thing is to use all diagnostic approaches at your disposal to get the most three-dimensional picture you can of the pattern of disharmony (徵候結構 *zhēng hòu jié gòu*) at work in your patient.

Basic Questions, CHAPTER 8

THE FIRST THREE CHAPTERS have introduced the fundamental principles of channel theory. Chapter 1 placed the channels within the context of Chinese medicine as a whole. Chapter 2 delved deeper into the fundamental principles of channel theory, and Chapter 3 introduced the concept of channel palpation as a diagnostic tool. Now we will begin to address the question of physiology. Once again, remember that considerations of physiology and metabolism, in the classical model, are vital for interpreting what the findings of palpation mean. In other words, in order to understand the implications of the nodules, thickening, weakness, tenderness, or other changes introduced in Chapter 3, the practitioner must first consider the functions of the channels in normal qi transformation. The next eight chapters will therefore turn from the discussion of channel palpation on the body surface to considerations of the way that channel and organ theories come together to describe the workings of the internal landscape. Later, in Chapter 12, armed with a more complete understanding of classical physiology, the concept of channel diagnosis will be addressed in detail.

A traditional place to begin a discussion of organ theory is *Basic Questions,* Chapter 8.[1] This oft-quoted chapter provides a concise definition of the natures of the organs in classical thought. It is also a door to the type of thinking that produced the *Inner Classic.* The chapter discusses the organs, not in the context of yin and yang or the five phases, but with a metaphorical comparison of the organs to officials in the imperial government. This might seem strange at first, but recall the description in Chapter 1 of a philosophical/political trend in the Han dynasty that emphasized the interrelationship of all things. The *Inner Classic* should be viewed in the context of a civilization searching to discover how universal forces could be perceived not only in nature and society, but within the body as well.

The motivation for this quest came from a new dynastic system that believed its own stability could be guaranteed (and legitimized) by maintaining the proper relationship with the larger forces of the universe. Many of the insights underlying the models of interrelationships developed at this time were based on careful observation of the natural world and the human body. In many ways, these models represent the collective wisdom of the centuries leading up to that time. Thus the concepts presented in the *Inner Classic* represent an attempt to define the role of medicine within this larger, interwoven system. It would therefore not seem quite so strange to natural philosophers of the early Han dynasty to look for the answers to questions about human physiology in the workings of a healthy political state.

Chapter 8 of *Basic Questions* begins with a question from the Yellow Emperor to Qi Bo: "Can you tell me how to differentiate the functions and relationships of the twelve organs?" The first words of reply express surprise at the enormity of the question: "Your query is quite comprehensive!" Then, in an interesting response, Qi Bo makes a series of metaphorical statements in which he likens each of the internal organs to one or another aspect of the political-social system of the Han dynasty. For each organ, two metaphors are provided. The first likens the organ to either a government official or an aspect of civil government while the second describes a related function. Taken together, each pair of metaphors provides a clue as to how physicians understood the human body at the time when the *Inner Classic* was compiled. For the modern reader, the answer to the Yellow Emperor's question represents an opportunity to get closer to the mindset of the creators of this important text:

- The heart holds the office of emperor and is the issuer of spirit clarity.[2] (心者. 君主之官也. 神明出焉。 *Xīn zhě, jūn zhǔ zhī guān yě, shén míng chū yān.*)

- The lung holds the office of prime minister and is the issuer of management and regulation. (肺者. 相傅之官. 治節出焉。 *Fèi zhě, xiàng fù zhī guān, zhì jié chū yān.*)

- The liver holds the office of general and is the issuer of strategies and planning. (肝者. 將軍之官. 謀慮出焉。 *Gān zhě, jiāng jūn zhī guān, mó lǜ chū yān.*)

- The gallbladder holds the office of rectifier and is the issuer of decisions.[3] (膽者. 中正之官. 決斷出焉。 *Dǎn zhě, zhōng zhèng zhī guān, jué duàn chū yān.*)

- The pericardium holds the office of governmental envoy; happiness issues from it.[4] (膻中者．臣使之官．喜樂出焉。 *Tán zhōng zhě, chén shǐ zhī guān, xǐ lè chū yān.*)

- The spleen-stomach holds the office of the granaries and issues the five flavors. (脾胃者．倉廩之官．五味出焉。 *Pí wèi zhě, cāng lǐn zhī guān, wǔ wèi chū yān.*)

- The large intestine holds the office of transport master, issuing change and transformation. （大腸者．傳道之官．變化出焉。 *Dà cháng zhě, chuán dào zhī guān, biàn huà chū yān.*)

- The small intestine holds the office of abundant reception, issuing material transformation. (小腸者．受盛之官．化物出焉。 *Xiǎo cháng zhě, shòu chéng zhī guān, huà wù chū yān.*)

- The kidney holds the office of forceful accomplishment and is the issuer of wondrous talent. (腎者．作強之官．伎巧出焉。 *Shèn zhě, zuò qiáng zhī guān, jì qiǎo chū yān.*)

- The triple burner holds the office of irrigation design; the water pathways issue from it. (三焦者．決瀆之官．水道出焉。 *Sān jiāo zhě, jué dú zhī guān, shuǐ dào chū yān.*)

- The bladder holds the office of regional rectifier, storing up fluids, and is ultimately dependent on qi transformation for release. （膀胱者．州都之官．津液藏焉．氣化則能出矣。 *Páng guāng zhě, zhōu dū zhī guān, jīn yè cáng yān, qì huà zé néng chū yǐ.*)

At first glance, certain parts of this section might seem unnecessarily general and vague, not the stuff from which a modern clinician might benefit. But one should keep in mind that these short statements are both metaphor and mnemonic device. The analogies present core ideas regarding the nature of the organs while being concise enough to remember. This is another important trait of classical Chinese. It is a language that communicates with hints of multiple meanings and the imagery of the shapes of the characters themselves. Understanding the meaning of a phrase therefore involves understanding other associations that a particular character might bring to mind in a Chinese reader well versed in classical texts. Consequently, rather than long, wordy dissertations about the minutiae of an idea, there are brief comments that strike the mind with a flash of metaphorical clarity. Literal translation is impossible, and thus each rendering into another language might look vastly different from another. The images are filtered through the mind of the translator who is trying to convey all of these permutations of meaning, always one step removed from the cultural context of the original.

The next question that might come to mind is, given the brevity of the language used, how can a modern practitioner of Chinese medicine who reads little or no Chinese begin to understand what these classical texts are talking about? The answer to this question involves a brief return to the role of the teacher in transmitting this medical art.

During the long history of Chinese medicine, written texts have been explained and interpreted for students by their teachers. While much of this explanation has been recorded as the 'commentary' to the texts, there remains a need for competent elucidation by an experienced clinician. Without the addition of contemporary clinical insight, a text like the *Inner Classic* becomes much more difficult to apply to patient treatment in the modern clinic. The learning process might be described as a triangular relationship between the teacher, the text, and the student. All three must be in place in order to truly bring the text to life. Later chapters will recreate this approach by introducing sections on each of the twelve organs with a discussion of the short descriptions provided in Chapter 8 of *Basic Questions* (Fig. 4.1).

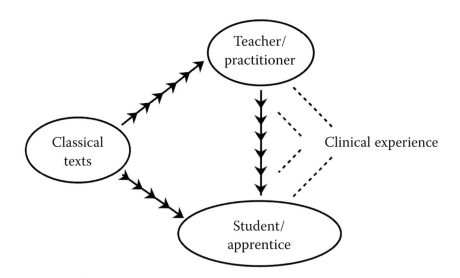

Fig. 4.1
The learning process might be described as a triangular relationship among the teacher, the text, and the student, all happening in the clinic.

The metaphors of the *Inner Classic* will thus provide a starting point for a broad evaluation of the role of each organ within the unified whole. To be clear, the unified whole, at least in the context of this book, involves an appreciation of how a thoughtful and experienced modern physician uses what they have learned from classical texts to understand how the organs function within the channel system. In the modern era, this process also necessarily includes integrating concepts that are not 'classical'. Therefore, in the pages that follow, the understanding of classical texts is shaped and informed by concepts from modern science. The goal of the next few chapters is thus to create an interaction of classical text with modern experience, to present what might otherwise be seen as the vague, stilted political imagery of a classical text in the context of the physiology of the living human body.

The Role of Metaphor in Discussions of the Organs

Before beginning our discussion of the organs, a few more aspects of the language used in the *Inner Classic* should be mentioned. In particular, the role of metaphor should always be kept in mind when evaluating classical texts.

The Chinese language abounds in metaphors. There is a clear cultural tendency in China, even in the modern era, to explain the unknown with reference to the known. While this is, of course, a necessary starting place for any culture when confronted with something new, classical Chinese writers seem particularly fond of this rhetorical device. For example, in contrast to modern English, rather than coining a completely new term when confronted with a new idea, classical Chinese would instead often modify the meaning of an old term. This may actually be a reflection of the nature of the written Chinese language, in which a single character can quite comfortably possess multiple meanings.

The written characters are, for the most part, built from 'classifiers'— pieces of the characters which are also known as 'radicals'—that can convey either the pronunciation of the character, its meaning, or both. Characters that share the same classifiers are linked in a manner unfamiliar to readers of other written languages. A shared classifier most often indicates that two characters have a similar sound or a related category of meaning. Apart from the classifier, the rest of an individual character (the 'remainder') is often called the 'phonetic'. As the name implies, the phonetic might also determine how the character is pronounced. The combinations of classifiers and phonetics join in different ways to weave together disparate but related ideas and thereby create a staggering variety of characters (Fig. 4.2).

人	(rén)	Human being
言	(yán)	Speech, written language
信	(xìn)	Trust, faith (a human by their word)

肉	(ròu)	Flesh
田	(tián)	Field
胃	(wèi)	Stomach (the 'field' from which 'flesh' comes)

Fig. 4.2
Classifiers are the building blocks of Chinese characters.

In addition, a Chinese character lacks the independent existence that English words, for example, often have. While etymology is also important for understanding a language like English, the apparent ideographic nature of the Chinese language leads to unique interrelationships. The types of relationships that characters have with one another can seem almost familial. Even in the two-character 'words' of modern Chinese, each character maintains a constant link to its same-classifier cousins, brothers, parents, and aunts. Sometimes the meaning of a particular character is barely distinguishable from that of another with the same component classifier. At other times, two characters might be pronounced the same way because of a shared phonetic, but have little similarity in meaning. Like the relationships of an extended family, there are grades of similarity along a spectrum (Fig. 4.3).

How is this relevant to the study of Chinese medicine? A few familiar examples found in Chapter 8 of *Basic Questions* will help answer this question. The 'flesh' classifier or radical (肉 or 月) is a constituent of nine of the twelve characters used in Chapter 8 (and elsewhere) to describe the organs. (The heart, pericardium, and triple burner are the exceptions.) In fact, even the characters for the yin and yang organs, 臟 *(zàng)* and 腑 *(fǔ)*, include the flesh classifier. Based on this common classifier, a reader of Chinese who looks at the written names of the various organs immediately perceives a relationship. Most obvious is the fact that the characters represent 'flesh'

昜	*Yáng*	bright
陽	*Yáng*	bright next to the side of a hill: *yáng* of yin-yang
揚	*Yáng*	bright next to a hand: to raise up, promote
煬	*Yáng*	bright next to fire: to melt metal
楊	*Yáng*	bright next to wood: the poplar tree
瘍	*Yáng*	bright under sickness: a sore or ulcer
禓	*Yáng*	bright next to 'a showing': to drive out demons

Fig. 4.3

Characters with shared classifiers (character pieces) have an almost familial relationship. All of these characters are pronounced exactly the same, while most have some commonality in meaning.

and therefore have something to do with a living organism. Generally, other characters with the flesh classifier represent parts of the body, either human or animal.

On the other hand, the fact that the characters for heart, pericardium, and triple burner do *not* contain the flesh classifier indicates that there is something inherently different about those organs. In the case of the character for heart (心 *xīn*), some say that it came about during the earliest phases of the development of the written language as a derivative of the character for fire (火 *huǒ*). In addition, as reflected in the passage from *Basic Questions* above, the heart maintains a unique and superior position as monarch of the organs, which sets it apart. In the case of the pericardium (心包 *xīn bāo*) and triple burner (三焦 *sān jiāo*), their lack of a flesh radical is a tacit acknowledgment on the part of the authors of the *Inner Classic* that these organs have a different physical presence than those which are more readily seen on dissection. The unique and interesting nature of the triple burner in particular will be explored in Chapter 9 (Fig. 4.4).

Another character that is repeatedly used in Chapter 8 of *Basic Questions* is 官 (*guān*), translated above as 'organ'. Standing alone, this term might mean either civil administrator or organ of the body. The authors of the *Inner Classic* chose this particular term instead of the more specific

Organ	Chinese Name	*Inner Classic* Political Metaphor
Yin Organ	臟 *zàng*	Organ of creation
Lung	肺 *fèi*	Prime minister
Spleen	脾 *pǐ*	Office of granaries
Heart	心 *xīn*	Emperor
Kidney	腎 *shèn*	Office of accomplishment
Pericardium	心包 *xīn bāo*	Envoy
Liver	肝 *gān*	General
Yang Organ	腑 *fǔ*	Organ of movement
Large Intestine	大腸 *dà cháng*	Transport master
Stomach	胃 *wèi*	Office of granaries
Small Intestine	小腸 *xiǎo cháng*	Office of abundant reception
Bladder	膀胱 *páng guāng*	Regional rectifier
Triple Burner	三焦 *sān jiāo*	Office of irrigation
Gallbladder	膽 *dǎn*	Rectifier

Fig. 4.4

The names of nine of the twelve primary organs, and the characters for
the *zàng* (yin organ) and *fǔ* (yang organ), contain the 'flesh' (肉) classifier.
The fact that the heart, pericardium, and triple burner do not contain
this classifier hints at the special nature of those organs.

terms 臟 *(zàng)* and 腑 *(fǔ)*, which are used elsewhere to refer to the twelve
organs. At the time that the *Inner Classic* was compiled, the term was used
to describe organic structures and, even today, the terms for both government ministers and the sensory organs of the body continue to share this
character.

The use, in the *Inner Classic*, of a term that might mean both government minister and organ is a means to an end. The goal of Chapter 8 of the
Inner Classic was not to subordinate medical science to political constraints.
Rather, it was an attempt to link the human body with the political structure—a true 'body politic'. In fact, later in Chapter 8, the balance among the

organs in the body is likened to the balance that a leader must maintain in society at large. Without an understanding of the interrelationships found among all aspects of society and physiology, "the twelve officials/organs will be in danger, the communication paths will become blocked, and there will be great damage." Or to put it another way, just as with the emperor in the empire, if there is disease or a lack of clarity in the heart, chaos will prevail in the body. It might be asked whether the authors of the *Inner Classic* are borrowing medical metaphors here to make a point about politics, or using political concepts (with which emperors are naturally familiar) to make statements about physiology. The rest of the *Inner Classic,* and clinical experience down through the millennia, would suggest that the information presented here certainly had a real effect on treating human suffering. Nevertheless, because of the interweaving of politics and the natural sciences in Chinese history, there is likely wisdom here for the political class couched in the metaphors of physiology as well.

The use of a character that carries two implicit meanings is another example of how classical Chinese is able to convey quite a bit of subtle information in a very short space. Medical Chinese is filled with other examples of characters whose meaning is best appreciated by considering the relationships implied by their component classifiers. For readers of this text, it is most important to remember that these relationships represent a kind of undertone or subtext in the language, which will be mentioned whenever it can be used to deepen our understanding of a concept. The goal is not to make unnecessary diversions into etymology, but to provide windows into a different way of thinking that is shaped by language. The mere appreciation of the fact that these differences exist brings the non-Chinese reader one step closer to the classics.

To summarize, Chapter 8 of *Basic Questions* compared the organs and their functions to readily observable political phenomena of the time in order to draw the broad brush-strokes of the roles of the organs in the landscape of human physiology. An important idea to take away from that chapter is that the culture of the time perceived both the human body and the body politic as resonating with the movements and forces of the natural world. Politics, health, and nature were inseparable. It would be a mistake, however, to think that the understanding of physicians at that time did not go far beyond these basic starting points. The remainder of the *Inner Classic* and the complex physiological models that they present should be enough to convince the reader otherwise. Having started with language, we will now begin exploring in more detail the important roles played by the organs and their channels in physiology.

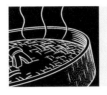

CHAPTER 5

太陰

THE *Tài Yīn* (GREATER YIN) SYSTEM

The General Nature and Function of *Tài Yīn*

BECAUSE THE YIN organs are the foundation of classical Chinese physiology, they will be discussed first. The journey through the six channels begins with the most external of the three yin channels: *tài yīn* (greater yin). Although the *tài yáng* (greater yang) level is considered to be the most external, it is in the yin levels that function begins to take physical form. The six yin organs are the generators of the fluids, flesh, and blood that comprise the physical body. By contrast, the organs associated with the yang channels are pathways, hollow conduits for substances needed and produced by the physiology of the yin organs. The yin organs are thus described by the *Inner Classic* as being "replete [with essence] but not full [of raw substances]" while the yang organs are "full [of raw substances] but not replete [with essence]."[1]

Like *tài yáng* in the yang levels, *tài yīn* is said to open outward (開 *kāi*). While *tài yáng* opens to the external environment, *tài yīn* may be thought of as opening the yin channels to the internal environment. *Tài yáng* opens to radiate warmth and defend the exterior. Postnatal qi, the ultimate product of yin organ physiology, percolates outward from *tài yīn* to nourish the body.

Tài yīn is comprised of the spleen and lung organs and channels. In fact, *tài yīn* is actually one channel with two functional parts: spleen and lung. The organ pairs associated with each of the six levels have a very close physiological relationship. In the case of *tài yīn*, there is also a particularly important relationship between the spleen and lung and their paired yang organs. Specifically, the *tài yīn* organs work with the *yáng míng* stomach and large intestine in a coordinated system of fluid and food metabolism.

The *tài yīn* channel is also associated with dampness. This affinity for dampness at *tài yīn* is balanced by a corresponding affinity for dryness at *yáng míng*. The *tài yīn* and *yáng míng* channels maintain the delicate balance of dampness and dryness required by the digestive process and in the body as a whole. Consequently, whenever one considers *tài yīn* function, the important role of the *yáng míng* organs should also be kept in mind.

The close relationship of the *tài yīn* and *yáng míng* levels can be further appreciated by understanding that *yáng míng* is the most internal of the three yang levels while *tài yīn* is the most external of the three yin levels. Nourishment, in the form of nutritive blood (營血 *yíng xuè*) and refined fluids, opens outward to the internal environment from *tài yīn*, while food and raw fluids from the external environment are transported inward through the passageways of *yáng míng*. This is where the internal (yin) meets the external (yang).

Think back to the metaphor of the boiling pot and steaming dumplings mentioned earlier. The *tài yīn* system can be likened to the steam rising off the top of the boiling kettle—just at the point where it reaches the more external level of the steamer itself. This is different from the warmth that fills the skin and hair at the *tài yáng* level. At *tài yīn*, a steam of nutrition infuses the internal organs with a nourishing bath that surrounds every cell. To be more specific, the nourishment of this cellular bath is maintained by the nutritive aspect of the blood, the final result of *tài yīn* qi transformation. (The relationship of nutritive-protective *(yíng-wèi)* to *tài yīn* is discussed more below.)

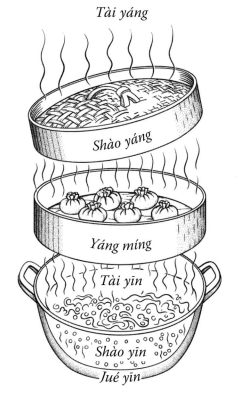

Tài yáng

Shào yáng

Yáng míng

Tài yīn

Shào yīn

Jué yīn

Tài yīn metabolism may be divided into two basic functions: the regulation of dampness and the distribution of nutrition. Although, for the sake of discussion, it is helpful to separate these two functions in the mind, they are actually interrelated. One way to conceive of this interrelationship is to remember that the body's nutrition travels through a fluid medium. *Tài yīn* metabolism involves:

Dampness   The *tài yīn* association with dampness means that it is responsible for the integration of external dampness (adjusting to humidity in the environment) while also transforming internally-generated dampness and helping to create the healthy fluids of the body. The relationship of the spleen to dampness is well known, but the lung is also important to fluid physiology because its movement of qi is vital to spleen circulation.

Nutrition   Besides providing a balance to *yáng míng* dryness, the *tài yīn* level is the source of the body's nourishing postnatal qi. The spleen transforms food and drink to create the nutritive aspect of the blood. The transformation of qi in the *tài yīn* lung, in concert with the beating of the heart, distributes the nutritive aspect throughout the body and outward to the skin. The provision of nutrition therefore also includes the lung function of 'commanding the qi' because it is the qi that provides the movement for distribution (Fig. 5.1).

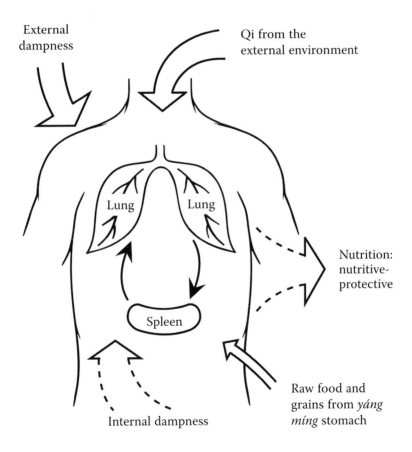

Fig. 5.1
The *tài yīn* system metabolizes dampness and produces nutrition.

The lung and spleen are thus synergistically involved in the metabolism of both fluids and nutrition. The infusion of qi from the external environment by the lung provides the driving force to distribute fluids and nutrition from the spleen to the rest of the body. A damp pathology might therefore involve dysfunction of either or both *tài yīn* organs: water metabolism by the spleen, or the qi-moving function of the lung, or both. If there is an excess of dampness in the body that cannot be effectively metabolized by the *tài yīn* system, signs of spleen qi deficiency (fatigue, low appetite, edema) might present. This is basically a condition of excess (accumulation of dampness) that presents with signs of deficiency. A lack of dampness (fluids) in the body, on the other hand, tends more often to affect the lungs and may cause symptoms of dry cough or even atrophy disorder (痿症 *wěi zhèng*), associated with weakness and muscle atrophy.

Among the three yin systems, the *tài yīn* maintains the most direct connection to the external environment. Physically, the *tài yīn* lung organ is connected via the trachea and nose to the outside world, while the spleen organ opens through the stomach and mouth. The lung is also connected to the outside through its relationship to the skin.

Spleen

"The spleen-stomach holds the office of the granaries and issues the five flavors."

(脾胃者.倉廩之官.五味出焉。 *Pí wèi zhě, cāng lǐn zhī guān, wǔ wèi chū yān.*)

—*Basic Questions*, Chapter 8

This is the first of what will eventually be twelve short discussions of the metaphors used in Chapter 8 of *Basic Questions* to describe the functions of each of the organs. It is fitting that this first passage is also one of the easiest to understand. In fact, those who have studied Chinese medicine are likely already familiar with it, as it is often mentioned in other texts.

The first thing to note in this passage is that the spleen and stomach are described together in the *Inner Classic*, rather than individually. The other ten yin and yang organs are each given lines of their own. This highlights the uniquely close functional relationship of the spleen with its paired yang organ. The importance of the balance between dampness and dryness in the *tài yīn / yáng míng* system was previously noted, as was their close relationship on the surface of the body, reflected in the relatively yin pathway traced by the *yáng míng* stomach channel on the abdomen, just next to the *tài yīn* spleen channel. While the other yang channels flow along the more yang surfaces of the body, the stomach channel traverses the yin abdomen, the storage area of food and fluids (see Fig. 2.6 in Chapter 2).

The remainder of the passage above may be less clear. The original Chinese for the phrase translated here as 'five flavors' is *wǔ wèi* (五味). The character for flavor (味) is the same one used to designate the 'taste' of herbs in the materia medica. In this case, however, the character has a different meaning. The term 'five flavors' is actually a reference to the nutritive aspect of food. In other words, when the *Inner Classic* states that the spleen-stomach "issues the five flavors," it is saying that nutrition is ultimately derived from these organs.

In the classics, the spleen organ is situated below the lungs and heart and above the kidney and liver. Its location in the center of the five yin organs facilitates the distribution of nutrition. The spleen is said to group around the eleventh thoracic vertebra,[2] and the *dū* (governing vessel) point at this level (GV-6) is thus appropriately named 'spine center' (脊中 *jǐ zhōng*). Again, this is illustrative of the spleen's place at the center of the organ system.

It is important to remember that the concept of 'organ' in Chinese physiology is both anatomical and functional. That is to say, in addition to its physical structure, each organ has a number of interrelated physiological

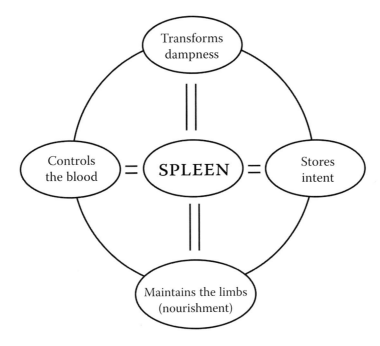

Fig. 5.2
Functions of the spleen

functions. Or to put it another way, Chinese medicine breaks down physiology into functional categories that we refer to as the yin and yang organs (臟腑 *zàng fǔ*). For example, the functions of transforming dampness, moving the qi, maintaining the limbs, and storing intent are all interrelated aspects of the spleen 'organ' (Fig. 5.2).

The entire body is made up of these functional organ groups interacting with each other. Thus Chinese physiology might be thought of as a web of functional levels or groupings (*tài yīn, shào yīn, jué yīn,* etc). Each level has a defined relationship to the others, its place within the whole. These relationships are described in different ways. One involves the familiar patterns of organ theory. Another is the relationships described by five-phase theory. The channel system, too, can be thought of as yet another way to understand the interactions of the organs. But it is also an overarching system that unifies all other approaches into a networked whole. This is the channel system in a nutshell. The largest categories in this system are the six levels themselves.[3] The smallest categories are described by the various functions of the individual organs (Fig. 5.3).

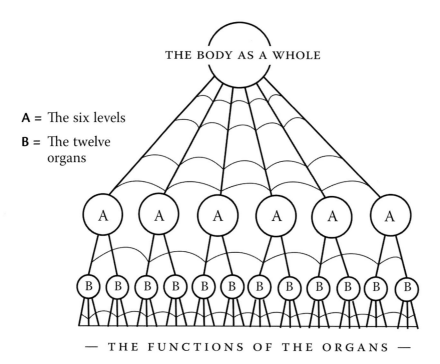

A = The six levels

B = The twelve organs

THE BODY AS A WHOLE

— THE FUNCTIONS OF THE ORGANS —

Fig. 5.3
The channel system is like a web which connects, integrates, and communicates among the various aspects of physiology.

FUNCTIONS OF THE SPLEEN

Governs blood

The spleen's relationship to blood is woven into its role as provider of nutrition. Specifically, the blood is the medium for the transportation of nutritive qi. Many modern textbooks say that the spleen is responsible for 'transformation and transportation' (化運 *huà yūn*). This refers to the spleen's transformation of food that has been stored and fermented by the dry warmth of the stomach, and its transport of the resulting nutrition into the blood.

While the heart gives movement (行 *xíng*) to the blood, sending it through the body, and the liver stores (藏 *cáng*) the blood in the deepest levels, it is the spleen which governs the nutritive blood at the point where it interacts with the 'external' environment inside the body. In modern physiological terms, this refers to those places within the internal environment where the smallest blood vessels intersect with the interstitial fluids surrounding the cells. The word 'governs' is often used as a translation of the Chinese term *tǒng* (统), but does not convey the entire meaning. Nigel Wiseman translates the term as 'manages'—a very helpful image, but also not quite broad enough. *Tǒng* refers to the process of unifying and gathering together into an interconnected system. In the case of the spleen, on one hand this organ gathers the necessary constituents to provide the nutritive aspect of the blood, and on the other, it gathers the blood at the level of microcirculation to bring it back into the vessels (Fig. 5.4).

When thinking of the role of the spleen in gathering blood into the vessels, a distinction should be made between the functions of the spleen and the liver. Specifically, when one says that the spleen 'governs' blood, this does not mean that the spleen is responsible for holding the blood in the large vessels. This is a function of the liver, which stores blood at the deepest level. Instead, the spleen's function relates to the reuptake of blood at the level of small vessel circulation. This can be likened to the activity at the point where arterial and venous capillaries meet and there is a commingling of nutrition with the interstitial fluid. The spleen therefore provides nutrition through transformation at two distinct levels: first with the transformation of food and fluids, and then, in a broader sense, at the point where the blood leaves the vessels.

One also sees that these functions are related to the fundamental *tài yīn* role in maintaining the quality of fluids. If the fluids in this cellular environment begin to lack nutritive quality, then dampness will result. Dampness, in other words, is a condition where fluids without beneficial qualities accumulate and develop pathology.

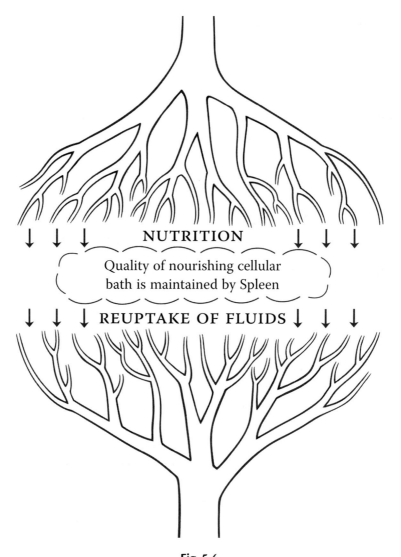

Fig. 5.4
The spleen maintains the nutritive quality of the fluids
which surround all the cells of the body.

A modern understanding of the spleen function of controlling blood might therefore include the reuptake of fluids at the capillary level. Given this association, a common symptom said to arise from an inability of the spleen to control blood can be more clearly understood. Namely, a tendency to bruise easily implies a lack of proper reuptake of substances into the blood by the spleen at the capillary level. If one bruises easily, the most external level of the internal environment is not being properly maintained. Not only bruises, but other dermatological conditions can be rooted in an inability of the spleen to nourish the skin through its 'cellular bath'. The *tài yīn* spleen channel is therefore often important in the treatment of chronic skin conditions such as eczema and psoriasis (see case study below). The nature of spleen function in controlling the blood is also helpful in understanding the role of the organ in gynecological bleeding. This will be discussed further in connection with liver function (see question in Chapter 7).

Q: *You've mentioned the relationship of the spleen to the nutritive aspect of blood. What about the relationship of nutritive and protective (yíng and wèi) that we often hear so much about?*

DR. WANG: Nutritive and protective are important aspects of *tài yīn* physiology. They represent the interplay of lung and spleen qi transformation. As we've discussed, 'nutritive' refers to the nutritive core of the blood arising from the spleen. 'Protective', on the other hand, depends on the stimulus of lung qi. It serves to move the nutritive aspect while also being nourished by it. Fundamentally, nutritive and protective both come from the same source: the combination of the subtle essence from food transformed by the spleen with the natural qi taken in by the lung. In other words, they are not separate entities but are two aspects of the product of *tài yīn* qi transformation. Relatively speaking, the spleen is more associated with the nutritive while the lung is more associated with the protective aspect.

The *Classic of Difficulties* discusses the nutritive-protective aspects in Chapter 30. There it says that, after being received by the stomach, food and water become the source of both the nutritive and protective aspects. It goes on to say that the 'clear' (清 *qīng*) becomes nutritive while the 'turbid' (濁 *zhuó*) becomes protective. The terms clear and turbid have a different meaning here than in the case of the 'separation of clear and turbid' that occurs in the small intestine. Here, 'clear' can be interpreted to mean gentle and rhythmic while 'turbid' describes a chaotic and active nature. The *Inner Classic* describes the protective qi as having a 'fierce' (悍 *hàn*) nature that allows it to accumulate quickly to repel invasion from external qi.[4]

Think once again of the blood in the vessels. The nutritive aspect is inside the vessels and is always moving at a constant, rhythmic pace to all parts of the body. The protective aspect, on the other hand, moves quickly to where it is needed, like a rescue unit during an emergency.

The protective aspect travels outside the vessels in the more superficial levels of the body where defense is needed, but always maintains a connection to the material support provided by the nutritive aspect of the blood. Another helpful analogy is that of a nation in which the economy (nutritive aspect) requires continuous and open transportation to all corners, while the country's defense (protective aspect) requires the ability to move with fierceness to wherever it is needed. There is always mutual interdependence (Fig. 5.5).

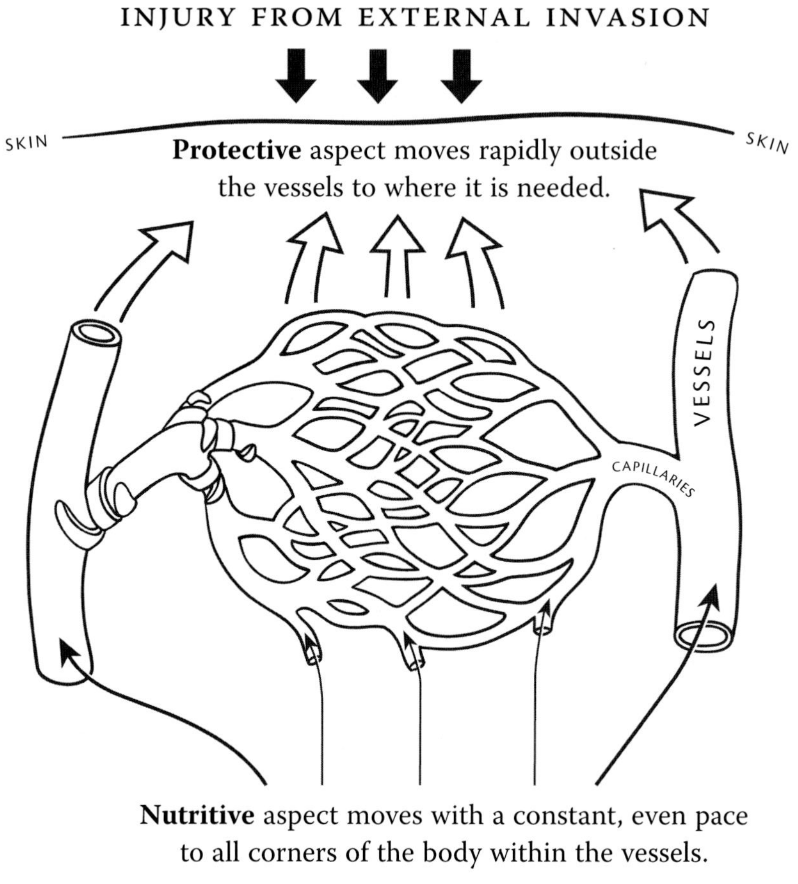

Fig. 5.5
Movement of the nutritive-protective aspects

The commonly-heard diagnosis of nutritive-protective disharmony is often a type of *tài yīn* condition. Look at the herb pair commonly used to harmonize nutritive and protective: Paeoniae Radix alba *(bái sháo)* and Cinnamomi Ramulus *(guì zhī)*. Paeoniae Radix alba *(bái sháo)* nourishes the blood and enters the spleen channel while Cinnamomi Ramulus *(guì zhī)* moves and enlivens the qi in the lung channel. This pair of herbs has a specific effect on *tài yīn* qi transformation. There are therefore many uses for Cinnamon Twig Decoction *(guì zhī tāng)* in addition to the common exterior deficiency pattern discussed in the early chapters of the *Discussion of Cold Damage* (傷寒論 *Shāng hán lùn*). Turn your mind to the role of nutrition and yang at the surface of the body. This should illuminate how Cinnamon Twig Decoction *(guì zhī tāng)* might benefit aches in the body and even certain types of allergic conditions in the skin or nose: it can be used where *tài yīn* qi transformation is compromised and there is abnormal interaction between the nutritive-protective aspects.

Moves the qi and transforms dampness

Everywhere in the internal environment, *tài yīn* is responsible for transformation of nutrition and dampness. The association of the spleen with 'moving the qi' (行氣 *xíng qì*) is rooted in the fact that the liveliness of post-natal qi depends on the nutrition provided by the transformative action of the spleen. Nourishment and the movement of qi are thus interdependent. This is an important and sometimes under-appreciated aspect of spleen function. In order to move the qi, the spleen and lung work together to combine nourishment with external qi from the environment.

The spleen relationship to dampness is more complex than is often presented in basic textbooks. One sees that the spleen 'dislikes dampness' (惡濕 *wù shī*) and 'transforms dampness' (化濕 *huà shī*) but there is also a need for a certain amount of healthy fluids for proper spleen function. This is the concept of spleen yin.

Simply put, the relationship of the spleen to dampness is reflected in the functions associated with spleen qi and those associated with spleen yin. Both are necessary. Spleen qi is involved in the transformation (removal) of pathogenic dampness while spleen yin is involved in providing nourishing fluids (津液 *jīn yè*) and the nutritive aspect of the blood. While dampness, fluids, and the nutritive aspect of blood share certain similarities, dampness is pathogenic while the others are necessary parts of normal physiology. Ultimately, dampness and healthy fluids are not of the same nature, and one does not become the other. Consequently, there are no common treatment principles whereby pathogenic dampness is transformed into beneficial fluids or blood. When dampness has become pathogenic, transformation is basically a process of removal (Table 5.1).

Dampness (濕 *shī*)	Pathogenic substance removed from the body by spleen qi
Fluids (津液 *jīn yè*)	Necessary physiological fluids provided by spleen yin

Table 5.1
Both dampness and fluids are intimately related to the spleen.

Returning to spleen qi and yin, it is helpful to look to the herbs used to 'benefit the spleen' for insight. Herbs such as Atractylodis macrocephalae Rhizoma *(bái zhú)* and Atractylodis Rhizoma *(cāng zhú)* are acrid and drying to support the qi of the spleen. On the other hand, herbs such as Dioscoreae Rhizoma *(shān yào)*, Rehmanniae Radix *(shēng dì huáng)*, and Coicis Semen *(yì yǐ rén)* can benefit the yin of the spleen. Think of the formula Tonify the Middle and Augment the Qi Decoction *(bǔ zhōng yì qì tāng)* in relation to the qi of the spleen, and part of Six-Ingredient Pill with Rehmannia *(liù wèi dì huáng wán)* in relation to benefiting spleen yin. Problems connected with spleen yin can also be a factor in atrophy syndrome (also associated with the lung) while a spleen qi pattern includes such symptoms as edema, diarrhea, and fatigue.

Often, a damp pathodynamic will not involve insufficiency of spleen yin or qi, but will be associated with qi counterflow leading to abnormal qi transformation. In these cases, herbs such as Poria *(fú líng)* and Polyporus *(zhū líng)*, which regulate spleen function, should be considered. The concept of qi transformation, of course, also applies to acupuncture treatment. For example, the point pair LU-5 *(chǐ zé)* and SP-9 *(yīn líng quán)* has a regulating effect on spleen function that can be likened to the effects of Poria *(fú líng)* and Polyporus *(zhū líng)*. On the other hand, the combination of LU-5 *(chǐ zé)* with the kidney metal point KI-7 *(fù liū)* is better for strengthening yin. Finally, combining the source points LU-9 *(tài yuān)* and SP-3 *(tài bái)* serves to benefit *tài yīn* qi.

We will explore the effects of particular point combinations on qi transformation throughout the book, and especially in Chapter 20. However, before proceeding with our discussion of spleen function, it might be helpful to consider a few basic concepts regarding point pairs. The pairs described in this book are not selected so much on the basis of individual point functions. Rather, points are considered to have particular effects on the channels with which they are associated, and, by combining points with specific channel effects, a kind of synergistic shift in qi transformation may be initiated. For example, the use described in the previous paragraph comes from considering the effects of combining LU-5 *(chǐ zé)* and SP-9 *(yīn líng quán)*, the sea (uniting) points, on the qi transformation of the *tài yīn* system. Table 5.2 is a rather simplified, but useful, model for considering how both acupuncture and herbal medicine can communicate in the language of qi transformation.

Point Pair	Herbs	Effect on Qi Transformation
LU-9 *(tài yuān)* and SP-3 *(tài bái)*	Atractylodis macrocephalae Rhizoma *(bái zhú)*, Atractylodis Rhizoma *(cāng zhú)*	Strengthens spleen qi to transform dampness
LU-5 *(chǐ zé)* and KI-7 *(fù liū)*	Dioscoreae Rhizoma *(shān yào)*, Rehmanniae Radix *(shēng dì huáng)*, Coicis Semen *(yì yǐ rén)*	Benefits fluids to support spleen yin
LU-5 *(chǐ zé)* and SP-9 *(yīn líng quán)*	Poria *(fú líng)*, Polyporus *(zhū líng)*	Regulates *tài yīn qi* dynamic

Table 5.2
Similarities between acupuncture and herbal medicine
using language of qi transformation

Turning now to the spleen function of 'moving qi', a principle often stated in modern textbooks is that the spleen 'warms the five yin organs' (溫五臟 *wēn wǔ zàng*). The creation of warmth is related to the concept of moving qi. It is another way of saying that the spleen provides nourishment to the rest of the body through its transformative action on food, and proper nourishment of the organs leads to warmth. Warming the organs gets the qi moving. This can be contrasted with the ability of the spleen's paired organ, the lung, to 'command the movement of qi', which is discussed below.

A helpful image for understanding how the spleen warms the organs can be found at the cellular level. The process of cellular respiration involves the intake of nourishment and a net release of warmth. The spleen provides the postnatal raw material for this process. This modern concept illustrates another way of understanding how the functions of what Chinese medicine calls the 'spleen' extend throughout the body, even beyond the boundaries of the digestive system.

Remember, as always, that such comparisons between Chinese medicine and modern physiology are made to provide images that facilitate understanding; they are not meant to create direct links between modern biology and classical Chinese medicine. The goal is to provide some common ground where ideas from the very different scientific traditions might overlap. Obviously, the authors of ancient texts had a very different understanding of human physiology than what is described by modern science. Nevertheless, both systems observe the same human body in an attempt to describe a basis for diagnosis, principles of treatment, and techniques to heal disease. Common truths are there to be apprehended.

Responsible for muscles and the four limbs

The third aspect of spleen function is closely related to the second. The ability of the spleen to effectively nourish the muscles is dependent on its transformation of grains and water, that is, its qi-moving function. Muscles become weak or atrophied when they lack nourishment from the spleen. Remember though that this is not always due to spleen qi deficiency. Spleen function may be compromised in other ways, both from excess and deficiency. Accumulation of dampness in either the spleen organ or in the channels can lead to muscle weakness or atrophy. This is often forgotten in the rush to 'strengthen the spleen' when there are weak or atrophied muscles. Sometimes it is better to clear than to strengthen; dampness may be in the channels and collaterals instead of the organs.

Palpation of the channels is a very helpful tool for distinguishing excess from deficiency in cases of muscle atrophy. Deficiency of spleen qi will manifest as softness of the muscle tissues along the *tài yīn* channels, while accumulation of dampness often involves tenderness and soreness and possibly nodules. It should also be remembered that long-term accumulation of dampness readily leads to the development of phlegm. If phlegm is involved, one is even more likely to find palpable nodules along the course of the channels. The most common situation is a combination of excess and deficiency, where it is advisable to regulate channel function before beginning tonification.

Stores intent (藏意 *cáng yì*)

One of the five psychic aspects (五志 *wǔ zhì*), often translated as intent, reflection, or signification, is stored and regulated by the spleen. Both intent and digestion require a composure that depends in turn on the rhythm (節律 *jié lù*) of the spleen. For intent, this rhythm represents the slow, methodical process by which random ideas gradually form into organized thought.

This is similar to the even pace of digestion, where there is a transformation of raw food into useful nutrition. Intent, like digestion, must be maintained at an even pace. Over-concentration (excessive intent) is a loss of balance that becomes obsession, while lack of intent manifests as scattered, disorganized thought.

Of course, the presence of healthy mental composure also optimizes the spleen function of providing nourishment. What is often called 'over-thinking' injures the spleen by interrupting the rhythm and composure of the subconscious mind. Of course, over-thinking also leads one to spend more time sitting and less time exercising the muscles. The importance of rhythm also includes a recognition that one must move about in order to properly distribute the nourishment of the spleen to the appendages. Therefore, the tranquility and composure of rhythmic movement provides a basis for healthy thought (Fig. 5.6).

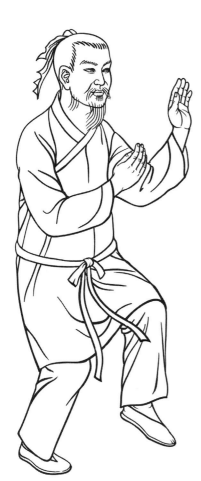

Fig. 5.6
Both digestion and intent require a healthy rhythm. The image of the slow, constant movement of *tài jí quán* provides a visual metaphor.

· ·

It should be pointed out that there is a difference between the five psychic aspects and the seven emotions (七情 *qī qíng*). In the case of the spleen, the associated psychic aspect is intent, while the associated emotion is thought or pensiveness (思 *sī*). While the two are related, the first is considered to be a fundamental aspect of the subconscious mind while the second involves a response to external stimulus. In addition, intent is a capacity while thought is an activity. The five psychic aspects are associated more with the prenatal (deep-seated) aspects of personality or character while the seven emotions are more postnatal manifestations of the interaction of the individual with the world. The five psychic aspects are with a person from birth and are considered to be inherent in the organs themselves.[5] And just as the organs have a capacity for change over time, becoming strengthened and weakened by the process of existence, so do the psychic aspects. In case of disease, either the psychic aspects or the seven emotions might be affected.

The concept of over-thinking described above provides an example of how the five psychic aspects interact with the seven emotions. A person may have an inherent ability to focus intent due to strong spleen function. This type of person would be less likely to suffer from excessive thinking (the emotion). Thus, one could say that the psychic aspect of the spleen (intent) can be affected by an excess of its emotional aspect (thought). The relationship of the psychic aspects to the emotions is unique to each of the organs and should be considered carefully by combining physical symptom-patterns with observed emotional states (Table 5.3a, b).

CLINICAL PEARLS OF WISDOM
ABOUT SPLEEN PATHOLOGY

The important rhythms of spleen function are facilitated by the even breaths of the lung. Consequently, many conditions will benefit from regulating the interaction of these two organs. In many cases, Dr. Wang will begin treatments that have a lung or spleen component with the point pair LU-5 *(chǐ zé)* and SP-9 *(yīn líng quán)*. The general regulating effects of this pair are in some ways similar to those of the four-gates (LI-4 *[hé gǔ]* and LR-3 *[tài chōng]*). For further discussion, see Chapter 20.

Lung

> The lung holds the office of prime minister and is the issuer of management and regulation. (肺者. 相傅之官. 治節出焉。 *Fèi zhě, xiàng fù zhī guān, zhì jié chū yān.*)
>
> —*Basic Questions,* Chapter 8

Emotion	Effect on Qi Transformation	Organ often Affected
Joy, elation (喜 *xǐ*)	Causes qi to slacken; moderates excessive emotions	Heart
Anger (怒 *nù*)	Causes qi to rise; moves to the head; blood follows qi in counterflow	Liver
Thought/ thinking, pensiveness (思 *sī*)	Causes qi to knot and bind; qi dynamic doesn't move	Heart, spleen, stomach
Sorrow (悲 *bēi*)	Dispels qi; prevents free flow in the upper burner by depressing the lung	Heart, lung
Melancholy, worry (憂 *yōu*)	Effects not described in *Inner Classic*; often combined with sorrow	Lung, spleen
Fear (恐 *kǒng*)	Causes qi to descend; kidney fails to hold urine, feces, or even essence	Kidney
Fright (驚 *jīng*)	Causes disorder of qi; affects the clarity of the heart; one cannot think	Heart

Table 5.3a

Seven emotions describe interaction with the external world

· ·

Mind	Associated Organ	Character Attribute
Corporeal soul (魄 *pò*)	Lung	Tenacity, physical endurance
Intent, reflection (意 *yì*)	Spleen	Organized, logical thought
Spirit (神 *shén*)	Heart	Spark of intelligence, 'recognition'
Essence (精 *jīng*)/ Will (志 *zhì*)	Kidney	Ability to finalize intended actions
Ethereal soul (魂 *hún*)	Liver	Balanced courage

Table 5.3b

Five psychic aspects describe inherent character

Unlike the passage cited earlier in *Basic Questions* describing the spleen-stomach, this one is a bit more difficult to grasp. First, it should be said that the lung is the 'prime minister' to the heart's 'emperor'. In this metaphor, just as the prime minister begins the process of shaping the emperor's commands into policy, so too is the lung woven into the function of the heart. The true qi (真氣 *zhēn qì*) brought into the body by the lung is necessary to activate heart blood. In other words, there is potential in blood that is activated by qi; the two are interdependent. Thus the lung and heart are the ultimate source of movement for both qi and blood. The two organs work together, the lung commanding the qi (主氣 *zhǔ qì*) and the heart moving the blood (行血 *xíng xuè*).

The second part of the passage—"issuer of management and regulation"—sounds very bureaucratic to the modern ear. The characters *chū yān* (出焉), translated as "is the issuer of," literally means "issue from it." Therefore, when the *Inner Classic* says that the lung is the "issuer of administration," it is saying that "administration comes out (gets its start) at this point." This implies, in the suggestive manner characteristic of classical Chinese, that 'administration' of qi begins (but does not end) with the lung. In other words, whenever this phrase is used, the substance or action that 'issues' from an organ goes on to develop and differentiate throughout the body. In this particular passage, the administration (or regulation) of qi is initiated by the movement of lung qi. This brings the reader closer to what is meant by the statement that the lung is the commander of qi. It is an assertion that all movement of qi begins with the rhythm of the breath that originates in the lung.

The paired spleen organ depends on this rhythm to support digestion, transform dampness, and maintain the focus of intent. At the same time, the clarifying and descending (肅降 *sù jiàng*) action of the lung is balanced and aided by the action of the spleen in sending clear yang upward (Fig. 5.7).

The lung is said to hang from the third thoracic vertebrae. Changes palpated along the spine in this area often indicate not only lung pathology, but also digestive disorders that are rooted in a lack of the rhythmic movement of qi from the lung.

FUNCTIONS OF THE LUNG

Responsible for respiration

The term 'respiration' should be considered in its broadest sense. Besides the act of breathing, the lung is also responsible for the infusion of qi

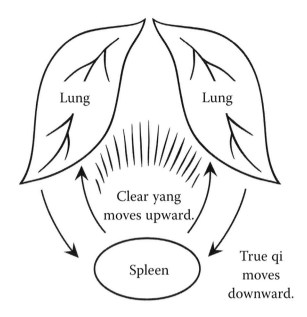

Fig. 5.7

Upward and downward movement is fundamental to *tài yīn* qi transformation.

throughout the body. Many texts describe the lung as 'ruling the hundred vessels' (主百脉 *zhǔ bǎi mài*). Lung function is therefore thought to be everywhere in the body—wherever vessels can be found. Either at the cellular level or within the lung organ itself, *tài yīn* lung function is associated with the separation of clear and turbid qi from the external environment. Inhalation brings the true qi of the environment into the body while exhalation sends turbid qi out. At the cellular level, there is a similar transfer of clear and turbid qi (oxygen and carbon dioxide) through the extra-cellular fluids. This is an important part of the *tài yīn* function of maintaining the nutritive quality of fluids within the body. While the spleen provides nutrition through the nutritive aspect of the blood, the lung is the ultimate source of qi in the fluids. Thus both nutritive and true qi travel in the fluids on their way to the cells of the body (Fig. 5.8).

Besides being balanced by the upward movement of spleen qi transformation, the lung has an upward-downward movement of its own. Specifically, the lung's upward and outward diffusing and dispersing action (宣發 *xuān fā*) also balances the clarifying and descending action described above. The diffusing action of the lung sends qi and fluids up and out to the skin. The descending action facilitates inhalation, balances the middle

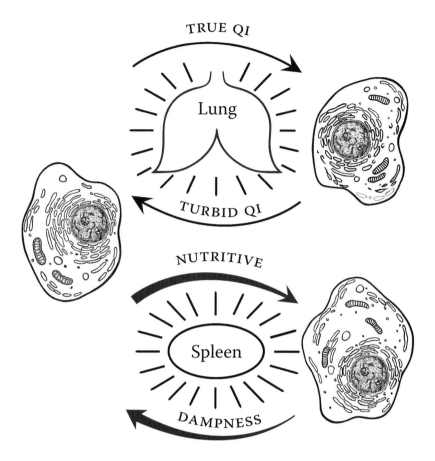

Fig. 5.8
The transformations of the spleen and lung within the interstitial fluids

burner (spleen), and facilitates movement in its paired large intestine organ. Problems with respiration involve dysfunction in or imbalance between these upward and downward movements. The treatment principles for herbs or acupuncture will vary depending on how the qi dynamic (氣機 *qì jī*) is compromised. In general, the treatment principles for lung pathology fall into one of four categories: diffusion (宣 *xuān*), descending (降 *jiàng*), moistening (潤 *rùn*), and contraction (收 *shōu*). One or more of these approaches may be required in cases of compromised respiratory function, and are particularly relevant when developing herbal strategies (Fig. 5.9).

Responsible for the skin and body hair

The second lung function is related to the first in that the nourishment

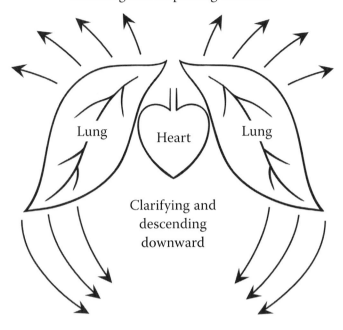

Diffusing and dispersing outward

Lung   Heart   Lung

Clarifying and
descending
downward

Fig. 5.9
The respiration of the lung has both an outward-diffusing and a
downward-clarifying action. Either action may be compromised in illness.
The rhythmic balance of the two movements guides the beating of the heart.

of the skin and body hair depends on proper outward diffusion. As stated above, the lung is responsible for the respiration of qi throughout the body. This also includes the breathing of the skin. The health of the lung is therefore reflected in the quality of a person's skin. Textbooks often state that skin elasticity is a reflection of the 'ampleness' (充 *chōng*) of the lung. When lung qi is ample, it has the ability to fill and diffuse upward and outward. A deficiency of lung qi is therefore often associated with a dry, dull skin tone.

Acts as prime minister

As previously noted, the lung is prime minister to the heart. It assists the heart in administering and regulating the physiology of the body. The heart is responsible for the flow of blood through the body and the lung for initiating the movement of qi. Together, they work in the upper burner to regulate the metabolic pace of the other organs. The prime minister provides the rhythm that helps set the pace. Once again, one can see the importance of rhythm in *tài yīn*. The pace of the breath guides the beating of the heart.

Holds the corporeal soul (魄 pò)

The corporeal soul is reflected in the physical strength of the body. It is also a sense projected by a person that 'whatever is undertaken can be completed'. The confidence that a person inspires in others can therefore be affected by the state of that person's corporeal soul. A relatively yin-natured mind, the corporeal soul radiates upward and outward to the surface with the qi of the lung. It is not directly observable, but is a strength that can be sensed by others.

 Q: *It is sometimes hard to understand why a particular psychic aspect is associated with a certain organ. Why, for example, is the lung associated with the corporeal soul?*

DR. WANG: The key to understanding why an organ is associated with a particular psychic aspect lies in considerations of organ function. In other words, the activities of a particular organ influence and are influenced by the emotional/psychological states represented by the associated psychic aspect. In addition, the psychic aspect is rooted to each organ because of the nature of that organ's physiology. In the case of the lung, the associated psychic aspect is the corporeal soul.

This is a fairly complex idea. Let's turn for a moment to the classics to shed a bit of light. There is a particular passage in the *Inner Classic* that describes the relationship of essence and spirit to the corporeal and ethereal souls: "That which follows the spirit in its comings and goings is called the ethereal soul. That which matches the essence as it goes in and out is called the corporeal soul."[6] First, this passage emphasizes a particular relationship between the essence (kidney) and the corporeal soul (lung) on one hand, and the spirit (heart) and the ethereal soul (liver) on the other. This concept was explained further by Zhang Jie-Bin (張介賓) in the Ming dynasty work, the *Classified Classic* (類經 *Lèi jīng*, 1624 A.D.). As I understand it, the idea is that both essence and the corporeal soul are relatively yin while spirit and the ethereal soul are relatively yang. Now, within those two categories, one might make further distinctions, namely, that essence is yin within yin while the corporeal soul is yang within yin. Conversely, the spirit is yang within yang and the ethereal soul is yin within yang (Table 5.4).

This brings me to my original statement about the importance of considering organ function when trying to grasp what is meant by each of the five psychic aspects. I just mentioned that essence is

	Mind		Organ	Relationship
Yang	Yang within yang	Spirit	Heart	Yang-natured ethereal soul is attracted to the deep yin-blood of the liver.
	Yin within yang	Ethereal soul	Liver	Like the beating of the heart, the spirit moves the ethereal soul (the spirit within the blood).
Yin	Yang within yin	Corporeal soul	Lung	The active qi of the lung attracts the yin-natured corporeal soul.
	Yin within yin	Essence	Kidney	The moving corporeal soul then stimulates essence. Qi stimulates prenatal.

Table 5.4

Relationships of psychic aspects in *Divine Pivot*, Chapter 8

relatively yin to the yang of the spirit. At the same time, the corporeal soul is an essentially yin-natured soul while the ethereal soul is yang-natured. Sorting these four psychic aspects in this manner helps one to grasp why each is associated with a particular organ. Being yin-natured, the corporeal soul is drawn to the active qi of the lung, and in fact depends on the rhythm of lung qi in order to move about the body.[7]

Remember that the corporeal soul 'matches the essence as it goes in and out', and also that essence is the most yin-natured substance in the body. Essence, in fact, is pure yin and requires movement in order to actualize. The movement of essence is facilitated by the corporeal soul. Of course, this is actually woven into the physiological relationship of the kidney and the lung organs as well. Prenatal essence requires qi that arises from the lung in order to actualize. One might think of this as the classical Chinese version of the concept that genetic potential requires stimulus from the external environment in order to take form. A seed needs sunshine in order to sprout. This is the relationship of essence to the corporeal soul, and thus of the kidney to the lung.

Now, what have the classics told us here that might be useful in the clinic? In everyday Chinese, if someone is said to have 'corporeal soul

[83]

strength' (魄力 *pò lì*), this means that they have the ability to endure and stick with a task. Why is this quality associated with the lung in particular? It is because the relationship of lung qi to kidney essence means that strong lung function provides the qi that allows kidney essence to manifest as a strong body—one that is able to endure physical challenge. A person with a strong body must have strong lungs. The lungs are not the root of a strong body; that is provided by kidney essence. However, without the qi of the lung, the essence cannot effectively take root to become material strength. Therefore, the corporeal soul can be seen in the clinic in the strength of a person's body, and particularly in that person's ability to stick with physically challenging work over a long period of time. This is called 'corporeal soul strength.'

An interesting thought that occurred to me about this concept is that singing basically arises from the lung—another reference to rhythm in *tài yīn*. The essence from our ancestors is drawn to the lung, which gives rise to song. One might then think of singing as another manifestation of essence brought about by the qi of the lung.

In the clinic, the practitioner must try to determine the quality and influence of the psychic aspects in each patient. This is not an easy task. Experience with patients is the key to developing this ability and involves perceiving the patient's subconscious, a difficult skill to put into words. The subconscious nature of the five psychic aspects is alluded to in the very structure of the written characters. As previously noted, 'corporeal soul strength' is a sensed quality that an observer can't always put their finger on. The Chinese character for corporeal soul, *pò* (魄), has two components. On the left is the classifier meaning 'white' (白), and on the right is a classifier meaning 'ghost' (鬼). A ghost is something that can't be seen or felt most of the time. It changes form and cannot be completely understood. Similarly, a patient's corporeal soul is difficult to ascertain but is reflected in this quality that is called 'corporeal soul strength.'

Because little is written about them elsewhere, we will focus on the five psychic aspects in this book, and less on the seven emotions. However, we do need to say a few words about how the emotions interact with the psychic aspects. Among the seven emotions, the lung is associated with the emotion of sorrow (悲 *bēi*). The Chinese character for sorrow also conveys a meaning of pessimism, as its structure combines the character for a negative with that of the heart/mind. When the lung is in a healthy state, the corporeal soul is usually also healthy and a person will maintain the optimistic outlook that helps prevent a susceptibility to pessimism or sorrow. This optimism often depends on the physical strength of the body, that is, a strong corporeal soul.

Conversely, when sorrow affects the qi transformation of the lung, it also affects the ability of the corporeal soul to manifest as a strong physical body. The *Inner Classic* (*Basic Questions*, Chapter 39) discusses the effects of sorrow on *tài yīn* physiology:

> Sorrow causes the collaterals of the heart to become agitated and disturbs the lobes of the lungs. The upper burner does not have open movement and the nutritive-protective is not disseminated. There is heat in the middle.

This is a description of a 'backing up' in the *tài yīn* system. Earlier (see Table 5.3a) it was noted that sorrow is said to 'dispel qi'. By dispelling qi in the upper burner, the upward-downward movement of the lung and spleen is compromised, and with the lack of movement, heat is created in the spleen. One can see how a vicious circle thus begins wherein grief compromises postnatal qi production and leads to weaker 'corporeal soul strength'.

A person with a congenital deficiency of corporeal soul strength might also have a tendency to become sad. The health of the psychic aspect can thus also be reflected in a tendency to experience an excess of a particular emotion. Also, a tendency to experience sorrow that is inappropriate to its cause may be a clue to lung organ dysfunction. Of course, serious life events that give rise to grief can damage even the healthiest lungs. The relationship among sorrow, the corporeal soul, and lung function is thus multifaceted. Weak lungs or a lack of corporeal soul strength may leave one susceptible to sorrow, but excessive sorrow can also damage the strongest lungs.

The most important thing to remember about the lung is that it governs the qi of the entire body. For this reason, palpable channel changes will be found along the lung channel in a wide variety of pathodynamics. This means that *tài yīn* channel points can be used in the treatment of many types of dysfunction in qi transformation. Use of *tài yīn* is thus by no means limited to issues with the spleen and lung. This concept is sometimes under-appreciated by practicing acupuncturists.

Clinical pearls of wisdom about lung pathology

Some urinary problems are associated with the lung. If the urine is dark in color, it may reflect an inability of the lung to properly diffuse upward, thus causing heat to be trapped inside. In addition, problems with urinary control during the daytime may be due to an inability of the lung to bring qi upward. Treatment of daytime urinary problems thus often involves *tài yīn* point pairs. (See the narrative following this chapter which discusses the use of the source points LU-9 and SP-3).

Q: *What about the great collateral of the spleen (脾大絡 pí dà luò)? What does that refer to?*

DR. WANG: The great collateral of the spleen has long been a subject of debate in Chinese medicine. When I first began practicing, I really didn't know what it meant. It was always said to treat 'pain throughout the body' (一身之痛 *yī shēn zhī tòng*) or 'softness and weakness' (鬆軟無力 *sōng ruǎn wú lì*), and most doctors leave it at that. I originally tried to use the spleen associated point SP-21 *(dà bāo)* for arthritic conditions, as this certainly seemed to be a type of pain throughout the body, but I didn't get very good results. At one point I had a patient, an older woman, who was extremely thin. She complained of severe pain in her ribs and upper body. At the time, because of the location of her pain, I thought of SP-21 *(dà bāo)*. The point was very effective. Afterwards, I began to think that the reason this particular area has a network vessel of its own is to supply the intercostal muscles. This musculature never really gets to rest, as breathing never stops. When these muscles become weak and the fatty tissue in the area becomes thin, pain often results. So far, my understanding and experience with the great collateral of the spleen stops there. I do, however, suspect that the point can also be beneficial for other types of breathing and qi movement problems. After all, the *tài yīn* system involves nourishment of muscles and it involves the lung. This needs further confirmation in the clinic.

Q: *We see a lot of patients outside of China who tend to have a combination of spleen qi deficiency patterns with stomach heat symptoms. For example, the patient might be fatigued, overweight, and have a puffy tongue or other symptoms of dampness, but also an extremely strong appetite and maybe strong-smelling breath. What do you think about this presentation?*

DR. WANG: The very first thing that comes to mind are the various Drain the Epigastrium (瀉心 *xiè xīn*) formulas, especially Pinellia Decoction to Drain the Epigastrium *(bàn xià xiè xīn tang)*. A formula like this can strengthen the spleen while clearing stomach heat. The general treatment principle, as far as the channels are concerned, is to strengthen *tài yīn* while clearing *yáng míng*. One might use the spleen source point SP-3 *(tài bái)* in conjunction with CV-12 *(zhōng wǎn)* and ST-44 *(nèi tíng)*. If dampness and heat are more pronounced, SP-4 *(gōng sūn)*, the collateral point, and ST-45 *(lì duì)* might be even better. The collateral point can help reestablish the qi transformation of the spleen-stomach while ST-45, the well point, can clear excess heat from the *tài yīn/yáng míng* channels.

Q: *It seems that in many complex cases, you prefer to use tài yīn channel treatment approaches. Why is this approach so frequently chosen?*

DR. WANG: In general, many of the conditions of modern society are due to changes in qi transformation, as opposed to structural/organic problems. These are the types of problems that modern medicine often has difficulty treating, but are ones that respond especially well to Chinese medicine. This is not to say that qi transformation problems are not serious. Immune system disorders and metabolic dysfunction often fall in this category. When regulating qi, it is often appropriate to choose *tài yīn*. Moreover, difficult cases are like untying a knot: Sometimes you must clear the air by regulating the qi dynamic first so that you can expose the core of the knot. For this reason, it may appear that I am choosing *tài yīn* fairly often, but actually I use *tài yīn* to regulate, and then proceed to other channels in later stages of treatment as the root condition becomes more evident.

Case Studies

Certain types of skin disorders are appropriate for treatment with the *tài yīn* channel. In these cases, there is often a loss of the normal nourishing/cleaning functions of the surrounding tissues. This is in contrast to skin disorders caused primarily by heat and/or deficiency of the blood. Given the appropriate diagnosis, *tài yīn* skin problems are often treated with the point pair LU-5 *(chǐ zé)* and SP-9 *(yīn líng quán)*. This pair regulates *tài yīn* qi transformation to reestablish healthy fluid metabolism, which in turn helps to nourish the skin.

The pair LU-5 *(chǐ zé)* and SP-9 *(yīn líng quán)* is often used in treating other conditions as well. Because of its regulating nature, this pair is useful for many patterns associated with dampness or qi counterflow. The ability of the pair to regulate derives from the combination of two uniting (sea) points, which are said to 'reverse counterflow'. In general, counterflow is a qi-level functional disharmony, thus the treatment principle involves the regulation of qi. A functional disharmony is one that involves the metabolism of the organs, as opposed to a condition involving observable physical changes in the organs or channels, which more often involves stagnation of phlegm or blood.

Besides skin disorders, this point combination is useful in the treatment of patterns that include cough, asthma, or edema due to *tài yīn* counterflow. The first three cases below illustrate a few of the applications for regulating *tài yīn* qi transformation.

■ Case No. 1

44-year-old female

Chief complaint   Allergic dermatitis

History of present illness   The patient presented with dry, red, slightly raised papules. Lesions were focused around the wrists, dorsal surface of the hand, ankles, and dorsal surface of the foot (generally *yáng míng* areas). The lesions were scaly and itchy, but without a tendency to bleed or become purulent. The condition was chronic, having first appeared 7–8 years previously. It usually appeared in the fall, continued through the winter, and cleared in the spring. Intensity of outbreaks seemed to be worsening in recent years. Use of detergents, soap, or warm water tended to irritate the condition, even to the point where she had found it necessary to drastically limit hand washing and bathing. There was some worsening of itchiness and redness before the onset of menstruation. Menses were irregular (varying late/early) and began with a scanty flow for 2–3 days. The patient's appetite and sleep were normal, while her bowel movements were generally dry, sometimes occurring once every 2–3 days. She also suffered from recurring nosebleeds.

A doctor at a local hospital diagnosed the condition as allergic dermatitis and treated with a mid-potency topical corticosteroid. Although steroid treatment provided temporary relief, the condition returned when treatment was discontinued. Another doctor prescribed the herbal formula Rambling Powder *(xiāo yáo sǎn)*, which had no effect on the skin problem, but did seem to improve the frequency of bowel movements.

Channel palpation revealed soreness and palpable changes along the lung channel at LU-6 *(kǒng zuì)*, on the spleen channel at SP-6 *(sān yīn jiāo)* and SP-9 *(yīn líng quán)*, and on the liver channel at LR-3 *(tài chōng)*. There were also some palpable changes on the heart channel at HT-3 *(shào hǎi)* and HT-6 *(yīn xī)*, and on the stomach channel at ST-40 *(fēng lóng)*. Nodules on the *tài yīn* channel have a tendency to be fairly deep and are generally harder than those found on the heart, liver, and stomach channels.

The tongue body was puffy/enlarged and slightly purplish, with a crack in the center toward the back. The tongue coating was sticky/slippery and white. The pulse was slippery.

Diagnosis   *Tài yīn* disharmony; dysfunction of fluid circulation

In this case the condition worsens in the fall and exhibits dryness, both associated with lung *tài yīn*. The patient's dermatitis was generally located on the *yáng míng* surfaces of the arms and legs. Here, a disharmony of the yin channel was manifesting along its paired yang channel: a *tài yīn* condition appearing on the *yáng míng* channel. For these types of conditions, it is often appropriate to use yin channel points to treat a yang channel condition. Traditionally, this approach is called 'choosing yin to treat a yang disease' (陽病取陰 *yáng bìng qǔ yīn*). Nevertheless, the chronic nature of this condition and the pattern of menstrual irregularities indicate the presence of blood dryness as a secondary aspect.

Treatment   Treatment focused on regulating *tài yīn* function. As the patient had never received acupuncture before, only four points were used in the first treatment: LU-5 and SP-9 bilaterally. One-inch needles were used with a very gentle radiating sensation on all four points. Subsequent treatments used the original four points, and added LI-5 *(yáng xī)* and ST-41 *(jiě xī)*—patches of redness and itchiness were just distal to both of these fire and river (經 *jīng*) points. (See the section on the five transport points, beginning on page 441, for more discussion of the river points.)

Results   The patient reported a reduction in itching immediately following the first treatment. The next week, the patient reported that the condition had continued to improve. She received treatments once weekly for eight weeks. Lesions began to clear first on the lower limbs, where the redness and scaling also declined. Healing and reduction of the affected areas on the upper limbs followed. The area around LI-4 *(hé gǔ)* was the last to heal, two months after treatment began. At that point, the condition had completely cleared from the *yáng míng* surfaces of the arms and legs, with one final area on the dorsal surface of the hand remaining (now on the triple burner *shào yáng*).

Addendum   As treatment progressed, the patient reported that she had experienced frequent nosebleeds for some time. Palpation revealed tenderness at LU-3 *(tiān fǔ)*. There is often a reaction on the *tài yīn* channel at this point when there are abnormalities in nasal vasculature. Bilateral needling of LU-3 was added to subsequent treatments, and the frequency of nosebleeds decreased.

Analysis   As previously noted, this is a case where a condition involving the yang channel is treated by regulating function of the paired yin channel. Strengthening yin nourishes yang. *Tài yīn* qi transformation was thus regulated using the four uniting points on the arm and leg aspects of *tài yīn*. This is different from a simple case of deficiency of the yin channel where other, more tonifying points (such as source points) might have been chosen. Here there was little indication of deficiency in the *tài yīn* system and thus regulation of function was more appropriate. The *yáng míng* channel, on the other hand, showed obvious signs of dryness. Besides the clear pattern of skin changes along the *yáng míng* pathway, there was also a tendency to dry bowel movements and the general dry nature of her dermatitis, all of which pointed to *yáng míng* as the location of the condition. As yin channels and organs provide nourishment, it is often necessary to utilize the approach of treating yin channels in cases of yang channel or organ deficiency.

A secondary aspect of the original diagnosis included dryness in the blood. This is also due to the underlying *tài yīn* dysfunction. Given the dysfunction in *tài yīn* fluid metabolism, it is not surprising that there are patterns in the menstrual cycle (scanty and irregular menses) that also indicate dryness due to lack of healthy blood production. Fundamentally, it is difficult to separate the nourishing role of *tài yīn* fluids in the skin from the concept that full, healthy blood nourishes the skin. While the *yáng míng* channel is said to be full of qi and blood, it is ultimately dependent on its paired *tài yīn* channel to sustain this fullness via the nutritive aspect of blood. Considerations of underlying physiology thus serve to highlight the importance of choosing yin to treat yang.

In Chapter 14 of this book we provide a detailed discussion of how to choose appropriate channels for treatment. The fact that the channel chosen here was not the channel that showed the clearest signs of disease reflects a fundamental principle of traditional acupuncture, namely, that the qi transformation of the entire channel system must be considered when choosing a channel for treatment. In addition, only after a channel has been chosen can one proceed to consider specific points.

The thought process that led to the selection of these specific points in this patient should be considered. As previously noted, both LU-5 and SP-9 are uniting points used to treat counterflow of qi by reestablishing proper movement in the channel. In particular, the ascending/descending function of the lung was compromised in this patient, a kind of counterflow of qi. The counterflow affected the *tài yīn* system and led to improper nourishment of the paired *yáng míng* channel.

In many modern acupuncture treatments for dermatology, points are chosen based on function much the same as herbs are chosen in a formula. Points such as LI-11 *(qū chí)*, LI-4 *(hé gǔ)*, GB-31 *(fēng shì)*, SP-6 *(sān yīn jiāo)*, or BL-18 *(gān shū)* are generally used to clear wind and benefit the blood in cases of allergic dermatitis. The approach described above focuses more on regulation of channel and organ function than on clearing and removal of wind and/or heat from the blood. While the use of herbs in a situation such as this would be quite effective for clearing, removing, and/ or tonifying, acupuncture is best suited for regulation with a goal of helping the body restore normal qi (正氣 *zhèng qì*) on its own. Often, problems with right qi are not due to deficiency, but are rooted in a lack of regulated movement of qi and blood in the body. In these cases, acupuncture is often more effective than qi-regulating herbal approaches.

■ CASE NO. 2

47-year-old female

Chief complaint Constipation for 5 years

History of present illness Upon presentation the patient's bowels were moving only once every four to six days and would not move without suppositories. Constipation had been a problem for the last five years, but the condition had worsened considerably during the last six months. The day of the first visit was the fifth day since her previous bowel movement. She complained of chronic abdominal distention and a poor appetite. Her hands and feet were cold.

The patient's tongue was pale with a thick, white coating and the pulse was wiry.

Channel palpation showed changes on the *tài yīn* and *yáng míng* channels. There was tenderness and a soft, fairly shallow nodule just below LU-5 and a similar tender spot around LI-10 *(shǒu sān lǐ)*. There was also pain with pressure above and to the right of the umbilicus. Further palpation of the abdomen revealed an egg-like mass to the right of the umbilicus, a likely fecal accumulation.

Diagnosis *Tài yīn* qi transformation counterflow leading to over-assimilation of fluids

Treatment LU-5, SP-9, ST-25 *(tiān shū)*, ST-40 *(fēng lóng)*

Stimulation A draining technique was applied at LU-5 until a radiating sensation down to the thumb was achieved. The same technique was used at SP-9, with radiation down to the foot. Sensation was immediately felt in the abdomen. A draining technique was also used at ST-25 and ST-40. One-and-a-half-inch needles were used on all points.

Results The patient felt movement in the abdomen following treatment. The following day she was able to move her bowels without a suppository. Treatments continued every other day for a week. At the end of that time, the patient was able to move her bowels every other day and her appetite began to recover, while her hands and feet warmed up. Course of treatment was eight visits over a two-month period. At the end of that time, the patient was able to move her bowels on her own (without suppositories or acupuncture) every one to two days with a concurrent reduction in other symptoms.

Analysis Note that the organ diagnosis of spleen deficiency is relatively clear given her low appetite and abdominal distention. The relatively chronic nature of the condition is also a hint to the involvement of the yin channel. One might be tempted to use only the *yáng míng* or possibly *shào yáng* triple burner channels in treating a patient like this. However, organ diagnosis, refined by considering palpated changes, indicates that both the *tài yīn* and *yáng míng* channels were involved. There are cases, of course, where constipation is more of a pure *yáng míng* excess type.

In general, even in many chronic cases, it is best to regulate first and tonify later. It might have been possible to get decent results here using more tonifying points, but the constipation indicated the presence of stagnation. It is often best not to tonify in cases of stagnation. If the condition had improved but did not resolve completely, then it would have been advisable to consider tonification in later stages of treatment. Finally, regulating with uniting points does have a slightly draining effect because they promote movement. The technique in this case also affected the outcome, as a draining technique was used on the pair LU-5 and SP-9.

■ CASE NO. 3

28-year-old female

Chief complaint Leukorrhea

History of present illness Upon presentation, the patient complained of excessive, foul-smelling leukorrhea of a yellowish color. The condition began three weeks previously. She also complained of constipation and a dry throat.

Her tongue was puffy and her pulse was deep. Channel palpation revealed a swollen tenderness around SP-6 *(sān yīn jiāo)* and general tenderness all along the *tài yīn* channel (both spleen and lung aspects). There was also tightness below the skin at CV-12 *(zhōng wǎn)* and hardness of the musculature around ST-40.

Diagnosis *Tài yīn* qi deficiency combined with *yáng míng* excess. Because of the inability to properly maintain fluid metabolism, fluids were unable to effectively nourish the body (dry throat and bowels) and thus accumulated as dampness that drained downward as leukorrhea. *Yáng míng* excess is reflected in the relatively recent onset of the constipation and the palpable tightening of the muscles around ST-40. *Yáng míng* deficiency, on the other hand, would more likely manifest as soft or weak muscles along the *yáng míng* pathway below the knees.

Treatment LU-5, SP-9, CV-3 *(zhōng jí)*, and SP-4 *(gōng sūn)* in the first treatment. Later treatments saw the substitution of CV-12 and ST-40 for CV-3 and SP-4.

Stimulation Even technique on all points except ST-40, which was drained in later treatments.

Results The patient reported slight reduction in leukorrhea following the first treatment, after which the point prescription was modified as indicated above. After the second treatment, leukorrhea had improved further, while constipation continued. The addition of ST-25 and two more weeks of treatment regulated the bowel movements as well.

Analysis Note the addition in this case of the collateral points of the *tài yīn* and *yáng míng* channels (SP-4 and ST-40). Both collateral points were not used at the same time: the spleen collateral point was used in the first treatment, and the stomach collateral point was substituted in later treatments. In this case, there was both a deficiency of qi transformation combined with excess in the paired yang channel. Treatment involved regulating the yin channel first, followed by draining of the yang channel (ST-40 was drained) in subsequent treatments. Collateral points were used to open up the circulation of qi between the paired yin and yang channels, in this case facilitating *tài yīn/ yáng míng* fluid metabolism.

■ Case No. 4

32-year-old female

Chief complaint   Bleeding between periods (spotting: 漏 *lòu*)

History of present illness   Upon presentation the patient reported 20 consecutive days of light spotting. The color of the blood was pale and the volume light. She had been extremely busy with work in recent months and also complained of fatigue that was exacerbated by a generally weak constitution. Her back was also achy and sore. She was sensitive to cold and had cold hands and feet.

Her tongue was pale with a slightly thinner coating than normal. Her pulse was deep and thin. Channel palpation revealed small, string-like nodules in the area around LU-8 *(jīng qú)* and in the area on the knee above SP-9 and below SP-10 *(xuè hǎi)*.

Diagnosis   *Tài yīn* qi deficiency

Treatment   LU-9, SP-3 *(tài bái)*, BL-64 *(jīng gǔ)* (source point of the bladder)

Stimulation   Tonifying technique was used on all three points.

Results   The patient reported that spotting had slowed greatly on the evening of her treatment. She received another treatment two days later, after which spotting stopped completely. The patient was later given herbs, a variation of Eight-Treasure Decoction *(bā zhēn tāng)*, to support her constitution

Analysis   This case should be compared to the previous two in which accumulation of qi or dampness was the primary diagnosis. In this case, the diagnosis was qi deficiency and therefore called for the use of three source points. These points are used to draw source qi from the triple burner into the channel with which they are associated, a concept that will be discussed further in Chapter 17. Here, channel palpation was crucial for differentiating between *tài yīn* and *shào yīn*, as the symptom pattern could have indicated either spleen or kidney qi deficiency. There was little palpable change in the area between KI-3 *(tài xī)* and KI-6 *(zhào hǎi)*. Nevertheless, the presence of low back pain indicated that the menstrual irregularity also likely involved cold stasis in the bladder channel, which called for tonification of bladder channel qi.

Note also that the area between SP-9 and SP-10 on the knee often shows changes in the presence of *tài yīn*-type gynecological conditions (Table 5.5).

Point Pair	Case	Effects on Qi Transformation in each Case
LU-5 *(chǐ zé)* and SP-9 *(yīn líng quán)*	1	Regulates *tài yīn* to facilitate provision of fluids to the skin (even technique)
LU-5 *(chǐ zé)* and SP-9 *(yīn líng quán)*	2	Regulates/drains to strongly reestablish *tài yīn / yáng míng* dryness-dampness relationship (draining technique)
ST-25 *(tiān shū)* and ST-40 *(fēng lóng)*	2	Collateral/local point combination reestablishes fluid circulation in large intestine organ
LU-5 *(chǐ zé)* and SP-9 *(yīn líng quán)*; SP-4 *(gōng sūn)* and CV-3 *(zhōng jí)*; ST-40 *(fēng lóng)* and CV-12 *(zhōng wǎn)*	3	LU-5 and SP-9 pair regulates to support SP-4 and CV-3 pair and ST-40 and CV-12 pair (even technique on all points except ST-40, which was drained)
LU-9 *(tài yuān)* and SP-3 *(tài bái)*	4	Source points used in a case where deficiency is primary (tonifying technique)

Table 5.5

Analysis of point pairs from case studies

. . . .

■ Narrative

THE URGE TO MOVE

Transportation *of* nourishment is the function of *tài yīn*, while transportation *to* nourishment was always the function of Dr. Wang's small, boxy car. The morning clinic shift would generally end around noon and we would consider options for lunch. The streets around the clinic itself, situated in one of Beijing's busiest shopping districts, were full of restaurants, but Dr. Wang always preferred to drive to less redeveloped sections of the city. He was never in a hurry as we negotiated the chaotic traffic that has begun to afflict a city most recently redesigned for bicycles, buses, and the occasional official in a large black sedan.

The small two-door that Dr. Wang drives moved through the traffic at a pace which seemed to frustrate some of the taxi drivers and young professionals in black Audi sedans. He remained only marginally aware of their protestations as he described with enthusiasm one place or another that we drove past: "That small alley over there is where I lived with my mother and father right after I was born. I still remember that old milling stone that you can see in there." Or, as we moved along at a relatively quick pace on the ring highway that surrounds the central part of the city: "This highway is built on top of what used to be Beijing's city wall. Originally, there was also a moat next to the wall where my friends and I would swim and try to catch fish." He would often point to huge glass-sheathed skyscrapers and remember a school or a market that was once in the same place. Sometimes we would get lost or turned around as he negotiated roads so newly altered that even last year's city map couldn't explain the way out.

Eventually we would find one of his favorite restaurants, or we might settle for a favorite style of cooking when one of his preferred establishments had been torn down to make way for a new Kodak store or even an entire shopping mall. In the northern part of the country, most Chinese consider a meal to be incomplete without noodles, while those in the south maintain a similar attitude about rice. As Beijing is solidly part of north China, we would most often eat noodles. This isn't as monotonous as it may seem given that the styles of noodle preparation available in Beijing are many. We would have noodles in soup, noodles in a variety of sauces, fried noodles, or noodles baked in clay pots. There would always be side dishes as well, and these could also vary considerably. A visitor in a large Chinese city like Beijing is often staggered by the variety of Chinese food after experiencing the more limited menus and regional options that overseas restaurants provide.

On a cloudy day toward the end of summer, Dr. Wang and I were eating in one of the old Beijing restaurants that had survived the recent onslaught of urban 'renewal.' It had originally opened one-hundred-fifty years ago as a restaurant specializing in clay-pot cooked dishes and continues to turn out stews and broiled meat today. The walls were covered with detailed paintings of people in Qing dynasty clothing preparing and cooking dishes much like the ones before us on the table. I set down my chopsticks on the edge of the bowl and looked around for the restroom. As in any other language, asking for the location of a restroom during a meal generally requires a careful choice of words to maintain tact. "Where is the hand-washing room?" I asked. This term can be used to mean bathroom in Chinese and is certainly more polite than the usual word meaning toilet, but it can sometimes lead to confusion in a restaurant as there may be a separate area just for washing hands when there is no toilet available. Dr. Wang looked around the room and then asked, "Do you want to wash your hands after the clinic shift?" I replied that I was looking for a more full-service facility and he laughed while pointing me upstairs. When I returned, he chuckled at the recollection of a story from the clinic...

DR. WANG: I remember a patient I had in the mid-1980s. She was a woman who had given birth to her first child over a year before and had since been afflicted with urinary incontinence. In fact, by the time I saw her, she had to visit the restroom almost twenty times a day. She had been to see a host of doctors, both Western-trained and some trained in Chinese medicine. Nothing had helped. As a clinician, one is often surprised at how difficult a seemingly simple condition can be to treat, and also how profoundly they can affect a patient's life.

Take this case for example. The woman was in her late twenties and worked at a government-owned factory back before many of them were privatized in the late 1990s. Government factories like this one provided good jobs in the sense that there was no way one could be fired. However, they were tedious, especially if you got one of the boring jobs that hardly required any work at all. Before her pregnancy, this patient had one of the better jobs in the factory as she worked along the most active assembly line with all of her friends. They would all keep very busy but had a good time talking as the day passed.

After she returned to work following her pregnancy, however, she found that she had to use the bathroom much more often than before. Her job involved calibrating one of the large machines on the assembly line and thus, whenever she left for the bathroom, the whole line would have to stop for a few minutes.

This hadn't been a problem in the past when the whole line would stop every few hours for a break and everyone could go to the restroom. Now, however, she found that she had to stop every half hour to forty-five minutes. Sometimes she had to go even more often than this.

Her boss took note of the change in productivity in her work cadre and reassigned her to a less demanding position in packaging across the room. Yet even the packaging section had a certain rhythm to its work that was interrupted every time she had to duck out to the bathroom. So she was transferred again, this time to the small office next to the production line where she was charged with answering the factory phone. If someone from another part of the factory called to speak with one of the supervisors, she was to go out onto the factory floor to find them. But even *this* job proved difficult for her, as she would often make detours to the bathroom after answering a call before she could notify the recipient, or she might miss calls altogether due to the frequent absences from her post. Eventually, the factory manager placed her in front of the bathroom door where she was charged with distributing toilet paper, a job familiar to those of us who lived in that era when we had to ration even the most basic of daily supplies. But she hated the job, since now she only saw her friends when they took breaks. This was her condition when she came to see me, and she was quite unhappy.

I began by reviewing the course of her previous treatment. As is often the case in postpartum urinary incontinence, the woman had been diagnosed with a displaced urethra. Because the position of the urethra had shifted, she had become less able to control her urine and thus avoided urinating in her pants by making frequent trips to the bathroom. There was no indication of urinary tract infection or neurological problems that might have been the cause. In most cases, this problem is temporary and resolves within a few months. But hers hadn't resolved, and she had sought treatment from a variety of doctors. The Western-trained doctor had given her medications that, while helping a bit, caused her to have dry mouth and blurred vision. She stopped taking those and then went to see a Chinese medicine practitioner who diagnosed kidney deficiency, because the symptoms began after pregnancy and were accompanied by some low back pain as well. After months of using herbs, she felt less urgency but still had to make frequent trips to the bathroom.

She had then visited an acupuncture clinic where the doctors used fairly strong needling techniques around her abdomen on the *rèn* (conception) vessel, which sent strong radiating sensations to her bladder. They had also used strong moxa treatments in the lower abdomen and on KI-3 *(tài xī)* to strengthen the kidney qi and yang. She even had some scars on her abdomen from the use of direct moxa. Despite the strength of these treatments and the relatively large number of needles that were used, she had failed to respond to acupuncture and moxa. Now, over a year after giving birth, she was sitting before us in the clinic. I asked questions but wasn't able to come up with a definitive diagnosis with that method. Apart from the incontinence, she was basically healthy.

It was during the channel palpation stage of her intake that some headway was made. Palpation revealed a small string-like line of nodules along the lung *tài yīn* channel in the area of LU-7 *(liè quē),* but a relatively normal state of affairs along her *shào yīn* channel (heart and kidney). The spleen channel was tender, especially in the area between SP-3 *(tài bái)* and SP-4 *(gōng sūn).* There was also an area of tenderness around SP-9 *(yīn líng quán).* Although her previous treatments had focused on strengthening the grasping and securing functions of kidney qi, it seemed to me to be a case of *tài yīn* qi deficiency which was failing to transform fluids. Another way of describing this diagnosis would be to say that *tài yīn* qi deficiency had led to a loss of regulation and circulation of the waterways (脾胃失調通水道 *pí wèi shī tiáo tōng shuǐ dào).* We chose the pair of source points LU-9 *(tài yuān)* and SP-3 *(tài bái).* I used a gentle tonifying technique and focused on obtaining a light radiating sensation down to the thumb on LU-9 and a distended radiating sensation at SP-3.

The next day the woman came into the clinic beaming. She had only gone to the bathroom eight times the previous day—improvement, believe it or not. I continued treating her with these four distal points for six treatments, twice weekly for three weeks. There were some days where the urinary frequency would increase, then other days that were quite good. Overall, however, the general trend was toward less frequent urination. After six treatments over a period of a month, she had basically returned to normal. It was a great relief for her to return to the factory line and to her friends at work.

A patient like this provides a few interesting insights. The first is the obvious lesson that urinary problems can be quite effectively treated with the *tài yīn* channel. However, in this case we didn't use spleen points on the abdomen, or even a point like SP-9 *(yīn líng quán),* which is traditionally indicated for urinary difficulty. Instead, a clear diagnosis of *tài yīn* qi deficiency failing to transform fluids led us to the source points of the channel.

Only with a clear understanding of the qi dynamic in the *tài yīn* system could we arrive at this treatment principle. If we had gone down the road of thinking only of the functions of individual points, we might have repeated the treatment strategy of other doctors who focused on the kidney and bladder channels and on the lower abdomen. Effective acupuncture involves the use of traditional concepts of organ physiology. It should also be noted that the treatment here involved relatively few needles and gentle stimulation. She had already endured months of strong stimulation, to no avail, and it seemed to me that this probably weakened her channel system. Sometimes a seemingly simpler and gentler treatment will actually be quite profound in its effect. However, there are times when I use more needles, and each patient must be taken in the context of the evolution of their own condition.

By this point we had long finished our noodles and sat thoughtfully for a moment, watching the customers in the restaurant. A few minutes later Dr. Wang dropped me off at a nearby subway stop. As the old squeaking subway cars moved quickly under the busy streets of Beijing, I thought about the small factories above me.

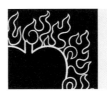

少陰

THE *Shào Yīn* (LESSER YIN) SYSTEM

The General Nature and Function of *Shào Yīn*

THE *shào yīn* (lesser yin) channel regulates the physiology of fire (火 *huǒ*). It is the conduit and regulator of extreme heat from the external environment, and the source of fire and blood movement in the internal environment. The channel weaves together the functions of the heart and kidney and is at the center of the yin aspect of the body. It is the pivot between the opening at *tài yīn* and the deep closing inward of the *jué yīn* level. The pivot of *shào yīn* is moved by the beating of the heart and movement in the gate of vitality (命門 *mìng mén*) between the kidneys. Within the three yin systems, movement at *tài yīn* is broadest, as nourishment spreads outward to meet the three yang channels; movement at *shào yīn* is characterized by the refined regulation of prenatal qi and the movement of blood; at the *jué yīn* level, yang movement decreases as the channel system moves toward a brief stillness before return.

The *shào yīn* channel is used clinically to drain fire and clear the heart (泄火清心 *xiè huǒ qīng xīn*) while also dredging and opening the yin collateral vessels (疏通陰絡 *shū tōng yīn luò*). The nature of the channel is thus to invigorate blood and transform stasis of blood and heat. While the channel clears pathogenic fire, the *shào yīn* organs are the source of metabolic fire.

The role played by *shào yīn* as the pivot of the three yin channels and its association with fire are interrelated: the presence of fire assures proper movement at the pivot. Specifically, *shào yīn* fire includes the gate of vitality (命門 *mìng mén*) of the kidney and the sovereign fire of the heart (君火 *jūn huǒ*). The fire of *shào yīn* regulates the *tài yīn* dispersal of fluids and nourishment outward and facilitates the storage and assignment of blood (sending blood to where it is needed) in the interior at the *jué yīn* level. It seems counterintuitive that a yang-natured entity like fire might arise from a yin channel system. The key to understanding this apparent contradiction lies in the concept of kidney essence (精 *jīng*). Inherited by a person from their ancestors, kidney essence is a fundamental yin substance that gives rise to the fire at the gate of vitality, discussed below (Fig. 6.1).

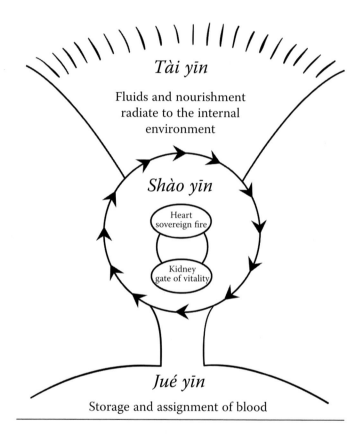

Fig. 6.1
The *shào yīn* level is the pivot. Its fires regulate movement among the yin levels.

The *shào yīn* organs are also responsible for maintaining the body's warmth. This is different from the spleen *tài yīn* function of warming the yin organs. *Tài yīn* warming is provided by nourishment while *shào yīn* warming is provided by the movement of blood and the physiological fundamentals of the gate of vitality and the sovereign fire.

Q: *If shào yīn is intimately related to the sovereign fire and the fire at the gate of vitality, then why is the primary clinical application of the shào yīn channel to clear heat, stasis, and fire? Why isn't it used instead to provide warmth in cases of deficiency?*

DR. WANG: The answer to this question provides insight into the unique nature of *shào yīn*. Each of the six channels has its own nature and unique roles in physiology. At the *shào yīn* level, there is a sort of functional balance between the organs and the channel, in contrast to the synergy seen at the *tài yīn* level. The most difficult concept in *shào yīn* revolves around the meaning of 'fire'. While the *shào yīn* channel and heart and kidney organs are all part of *shào yīn*, the nature of fire is a bit different in each organ, and in the channel itself. As I mentioned before, the channel is often a conductor and regulator of fire, while the organs themselves are sources of physiological fire.

For a moment, try to separate channel and organ in your mind. This is done to underline the fact that the channel is often subject to fire-type disorders while the organs generate warmth. Organ dysfunction can readily lead to fire that can become trapped in the channel system; thus the specific use of the *shào yīn* channel in the clinic. The concept of fire stasis in the channels is particularly applicable to the concept of heat stasis in the yin collaterals, which we'll talk about in a bit. At this point, a helpful image is that of the pivot and movement. When the movement of the pivot (organs) is compromised or over-active, it may give rise to heat and fire in the channels.

This could manifest as heat or fire from either excess or deficiency. However—and this is important—if the ultimate cause is related to *shào yīn*, then there is deficiency at the root. In other words, while channel symptoms may often look like excess, the underlying organ dysfunction in *shào yīn* is deficiency. It is important to understand the implications of what I'm saying here. In the first case, the *shào yīn* channel itself is the location of heat or fire and thus the two primary functions of the *shào yīn* channel are to drain fire and clear the heart while dredging and opening the yin collaterals. But another, decidedly different, clinical use of the *shào yīn* channel is to regulate the qi dynamic of the heart or kidney organs. This is quite distinct from the goal of clearing the heart or opening the yin collaterals. This second, qi-dynamic regulating application of the *shào yīn* channel is more familiar to students and practitioners of Chinese medicine and includes such common applications as using the heart *shào yīn* channel in cases of heart qi deficiency, or the kidney *shào yīn* channel for kidney yin deficiency.

Basically, just remember that *shào yīn* is a channel where one should be especially aware of the unique relationship between channel and organ functions. Your choice of points or technique will be determined by the effects you are trying to achieve in either the channel or organ. Each of the channels is different and should be understood both individually and as a part of the larger channel system. I know this seems a bit complex; just keep thinking it over and over in your mind and, most importantly, while working in the clinic (Table 6.1).

Shào yīn channel	Invigorates and transforms to clear fire stasis
Shào yīn organs	Source of the body's metabolic fire

Table 6.1
Functions of the *shào yīn* channel and organs

There is another concept that adds depth to the concept of *shào yīn*. This is the function of the pericardium as protector of the heart. Often, fire or heat that one might expect to be trapped in the *shào yīn* becomes trapped instead in the *jué yīn* pericardium channel. Therefore, when diagnosing the location of pathogenic fire or heat, one must always consider the *jué yīn* channel as well. Remember that the *jué yīn* pericardium is also a fire-phase organ: it is associated with ministerial fire (discussed later in the chapter). In fact, in many cases where the diagnosis is one of heat or fire in the heart channel, it is the pericardium channel which is nonetheless chosen for treatment. As many students may already know, during the early history of channel therapy the heart channel was considered inappropriate for needling. Because the heart is the house of the spirit and the emperor of the body, problems associated with heart channel dysfunction were often treated with the nearby pericardium channel.

Even though heart *shào yīn* channel points are often used now, there is nonetheless a real clinical tendency for heat-type problems to manifest as palpable changes on the pericardium *jué yīn* channel. It is helpful to remember that the heart and pericardium organs are physically connected. Clinical experience has shown that, in general, the pericardium channel is associated with problems with the heart muscle and cardiac blood supply while palpable changes along the heart channel are seen more often in cases of conductivity problems in the heart, leading to irregular heart beat. Emotional conditions can manifest in either, but are seen more often in the pericardium. An exception is anxiety, which often reflects with a palpable change between HT-5 *(tōng lǐ)* and HT-7 *(shén mén)*. As usual, one must palpate the channels in order to ascertain their condition (Table 6.2).

Channel	Usually shows palpable change when there are...
Heart *shào yīn*	problems with the qi of the heart (conductivity problems affecting heartbeat and some emotional problems)
Pericardium *jué yīn*	problems with the blood of the heart (problems with the vasculature of the heart organ and some emotional problems)

Table 6.2

Cause of changes in heart and pericardium channels

The Five-Phase Relationship of the Heart and Kidney

Because of the unique relationship of the heart and kidney, a few more things should be said about the nature of the *shào yīn* channel. While *tài yīn* involves a clear synergistic relationship between the lung and spleen organs, *shào yīn* is instead characterized by a dynamic tension. Five-phase theory provides helpful insight. While the lung and spleen have a relationship of mother-child (earth gives birth to metal), there is a mutually controlling relationship between the heart and kidney (water controls fire). In fact, there is also a mother-child relationship between the *jué yīn* liver and pericardium (wood gives birth to fire) thus highlighting once again the unique relationship of the *shào yīn* organs to each other. Within the yang levels there is a similarly unique relationship between the bladder and small intestine, for the same reasons (Fig. 6.2).

This diversion into the five-phase relationships of the yin organ systems has clinical implications, namely, that there are fewer situations where one regulates the *shào yīn* qi dynamic in the same way that one might in the other two yin channel pairs. The heart *shào yīn* and kidney *shào yīn* organs do not always work together in synergy, but instead have a relationship based on a balance of mutual strength. The pivot of the *shào yīn* system is

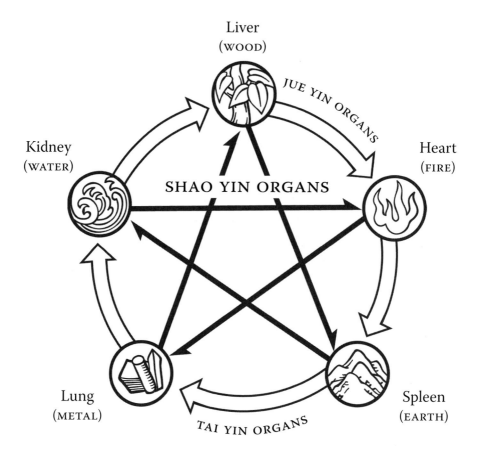

Fig. 6.2
Among the yin organs, the *shào yīn* have a unique five-phase relationship.

turned by two organs balanced like spinning magnets. Of course, in this metaphor, one of the magnets has a water nature and the other a fire nature. The net result of this unique physiology is that the heart and kidney organs have a tendency not to communicate or interact. In the clinic, this pathodynamic (called heart-kidney disharmony) is the cause of a variety of symptoms including insomnia, irritability, excessive dreaming, palpitations, and/or seminal emissions (Fig. 6.3).

Nevertheless, there are situations in the clinic where the combination of points from both the heart and kidney *shào yīn* channels creates a synergy similar to that seen in lung-spleen *tài yīn* treatments, especially in cases where movement is the desired result (see case studies below). The difference is that there are more situations where *shào yīn* is combined with other

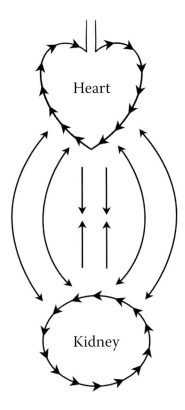

Fig. 6.3
The heart and kidney organs balance each other in mutual strength,
much like a fire-water pair of spinning magnets.

channels in actual clinical practice, especially when deficiency is involved. For example, in cases of heart blood deficiency, heart channel points are often combined with *tài yīn* spleen points, while kidney yin deficiency often involves the use of *jué yīn* liver points or even *tài yīn* spleen and lung points. (Specific treatment strategies will be discussed later.)

What should be remembered at this point is that even the most coherent theories are helpful only insofar as they facilitate real-world applications. In the case of channel and five-phase theory, one must not forget the yin and yang organ relationships when developing treatment strategies. The most difficult part of developing effective treatment strategies is learning how to fine-tune an understanding of the relationship of the channel system to organ *(zàng-fǔ)* theory. This is a slow process, and clinical experience is the best teacher. The goal of this book is to provide a framework from which practitioners can more quickly develop their own understanding.

THE CONCEPT OF HEART-KIDNEY DISHARMONY

Before proceeding, a few more things should be said about the balance of fire and water in the functions of the heart and kidney organs. This grows out of considerations of what is actually meant by the commonly used diagnostic term 'heart-kidney disharmony' (心腎不交 *xīn shèn bù jiāo)*. In order to more fully understand the relationship of these organs, it is helpful to remember that there are multiple layers of relationship that affect *shào yīn* physiology. First, there is the place of the *shào yīn* channel within the channel system as a whole; then there is a relationship inside the *shào yīn* system between the heart and kidney organs to each other; finally, there is a relationship within the kidney itself at the level of the gate of vitality. All of these relationships can affect *shào yīn* physiology and lead to heart-kidney disharmony. It is helpful to begin by looking at the kidney organ alone, then proceed outward to the place of the heart-kidney within the channel system as a whole (Fig. 6.4).

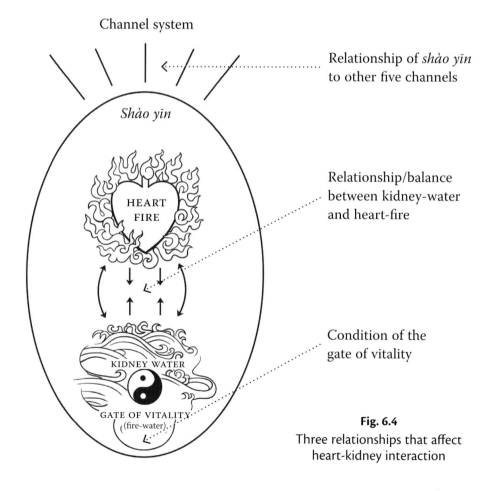

Channel system

Relationship of *shào yīn* to other five channels

Relationship/balance between kidney-water and heart-fire

Condition of the gate of vitality

Fig. 6.4
Three relationships that affect heart-kidney interaction

Beginning with the kidney organ, it was noted earlier that yin essence generates fire in the gate of vitality. Thus the kidney is a fundamentally yin, water-natured organ that paradoxically gives rise to a physiological process that is termed 'fire'. It is helpful to resist the temptation to think exclusively in either/or terms when considering the fire/water nature of the kidney. A more useful image is that of the *tài jí* (太極) or yin-yang symbol. While essence can be thought of as a yin substance, it has within it the seed of the yang-natured fire at the gate of vitality. At the same time, while the fire at the gate of vitality is decidedly yang-natured, it is rooted in essence. By thinking of the *tài jí* symbol, one can begin to understand how classical Chinese physicians conceived of a water-natured organ that nonetheless gives rise to fire. This fire coming from the kidney is the ultimate stimulus of the qi transformation in all the other organs of the body.

Besides the fire-water balance within the kidney, there is another type of fire-water balance occurring simultaneously between the heart and kidney organs. In this second relationship, the kidney is likened to water and the heart to fire. The relationship between the kidney and heart is familiar to students of Chinese medicine as being one of yin essence (kidney) and yang sovereign fire (heart). This is the relationship that characterizes the *shào yīn* system in the broadest sense.

When sovereign fire becomes either excessive or deficient, kidney essence acts to regulate it. Here is the balance which was earlier compared to two spinning magnets. When the water magnet spins too slowly, fire is added to speed it up, and if the fire magnet spins too quickly, water is added to cool and slow it down. When they are in balance, their interaction is smooth and constant, but when they are out of balance, the condition of heart-kidney disharmony often develops. Most often, this disharmony involves a deficiency of kidney yin that leads to heat from deficiency in the heart. A review of the treatment principles and herbal actions within the formula Emperor of Heaven's Special Pill to Tonify the Heart *(tiān wáng bǔ xīn dān)*, for example, gives clear insight into a common treatment approach for this type of *shào yīn* dysfunction (Table 6.3).

Having considered the two aspects of the heart-kidney relationship which occur within *shào yīn*, the third general factor that might lead to heart-kidney disharmony involves the channel system as a whole. In other words, sometimes the healthy balance of heart-kidney function becomes disturbed by a pathodynamic in other organs. When devising a clinical approach to problems with heart and kidney not connecting, it is therefore important to also revisit the multiple channel relationships.

For example, the most common channel-to-channel relationship in-

Herb	Main Function in Formula	Effects on Qi Dynamic
Ziziphi spinosae Semen (suān zǎo rén)	Nourishes heart yin/ calms the spirit	Calm heart fire
Asparagi Radix (tiān mén dōng)	Clears heat from upper burner (nourishes yin of lung and kidney)	
Ophiopogonis Radix (mài mén dōng)	Clears heat from upper burner (nourishes yin of lung and stomach)	
Schisandrae Fructus (wǔ wèi zǐ)	Calms heart (stabilizes kidneys)	
Platycladi Semen (bǎi zǐ rén)	Nourishes heart blood (calms the spirit)	
Salviae miltiorrhizae Radix (dān shēn)	Clears heat and restlessness (moves blood)	Stimulate the process; open circulation between upper and lower
Platycodi Radix (jié gěng)	Opens lung qi; releases the heart	
Ginseng Radix (rén shēn)	Benefits qi	
Poria (fú líng)	Benefits spleen qi	
Polygalae Radix (yuǎn zhì)	Calms the spirit; opens fluids through the triple burner	
Angelicae sinensis Radix (dāng guī)	Nourishes the blood	Build blood to unify
Longan Arillus (lóng yǎn ròu)	Nourishes the blood	
Scrophulariae Radix (xuán shēn)	Nourishes kidney yin	Nourish kidney water
Rehmanniae Radix (shēng dì huáng)	Nourishes kidney yin	

Table 6.3

Analysis of Emperor of Heaven's Special Pill to Tonify the Heart
(tiān wáng bǔ xīn dān)

volves the familiar one of 'interior-exterior' organs. In the case of *shào yīn*, the interior-exterior relationship of the kidney and the bladder is of special significance. As a yang organ at the most exterior of the three yang channels *(tài yáng)*, the bladder provides a direct conduit to the outside through which the kidney can regulate internal fire and heat. The bladder channel removes heat outward by venting (煦發 *xù fā*) over the large surface area of the *tài yáng* pathway on the skin. On the other hand, the bladder can create net warmth in the body by removing fluids through the bladder organ. Damp fluids can lead to cold; thus long, clear, profuse urination is a sign that the body is trying to remove fluids in an effort to create net warmth. This type of urination, in fact, is often a symptom of cold from deficiency in the kidneys.

On the other hand, the herbal formula Guide Out the Red Powder *(dǎo chì sǎn)* is used in situations where heat in the *shào yīn* system (particularly heart fire) is drained through the *tài yáng* bladder organ. In this case, the appropriate pattern would involve urination that is dark and relatively scanty, indicating heat. Promoting and increasing the volume of urine can thus also drain excess fire from the body. These are just a few examples of how the balance between the kidney and heart is facilitated by the internal-external *shào yīn-tài yáng* relationship (Fig. 6.5).

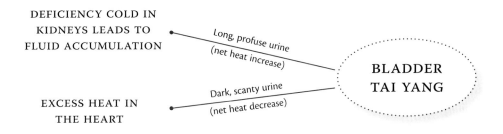

DEFICIENCY COLD IN KIDNEYS LEADS TO FLUID ACCUMULATION

Long, profuse urine (net heat increase)

BLADDER TAI YANG

EXCESS HEAT IN THE HEART

Dark, scanty urine (net heat decrease)

Fig. 6.5
Imbalances in *shào yīn* can also be regulated
via the paired *tài yáng* system.

There are of course other channel-to-channel relationships that affect *shào yīn* physiology. For example, the movement of the *shào yīn* pivot is affected by the quality of blood stored at the *jué yīn* level. Problems with quality of blood (particularly heat in the blood) can affect the relationship of the heart and kidney, a concept discussed in the next chapter.

Finally, the pathway of connection between the heart and kidney involves maintenance of fluid movement within all three burners. Here one can see how *tài yīn* lung and spleen physiology might affect heart-kidney communication. If dampness or phlegm is allowed to collect in the interior, fire and water cannot interact smoothly. Once again, the strategy underlying the combination of herbs in the formula Emperor of Heaven's Special Pill to Tonify the Heart *(tiān wáng bǔ xīn dān)* is illustrative.

To summarize the three levels affecting the heart-kidney relationship:

1. Within the kidney organ there is a fire/water relationship in the generation of fire at the gate of vitality. Ultimately, the result of the interaction of this fire and essence within the kidney is the production of source qi, discussed below.

2. Within *shào yīn*, there is a balance of fire and water between kidney essence and the sovereign fire of the heart.

3. In the channel system as a whole, there is a regulating effect that maintains heart-kidney connection. This is most clearly seen in the interior-exterior organ pairings. In the case of *shào yīn*, the pairing with *tài yáng* provides a venue for heat regulation through contact with the external environment. Nevertheless, the role of the other organs in blood and fluid physiology also plays an important role in healthy *shào yīn* function.

Once again, it is the channel system that provides the communication network for all of these physiological processes. Problems at any of the levels affect *shào yīn* physiology and can lead to the familiar diagnosis of heart-kidney disharmony. Ascertaining the state of water and fire (yin and yang) is of primary importance in making a clear diagnosis in *shào yīn* disharmony. If one can refine that diagnosis further based on a clear idea of location (e.g., within the kidney as opposed to the kidney-bladder) the diagnosis will be more precise. This, in turn, will yield clear treatment principles and more consistent clinical results.

SPECIAL CLINICAL CONSIDERATIONS FOR *SHÀO YĪN*

As noted above, problems in the *shào yīn* channel can be either excessive or deficient, while the root often lies in organ deficiency. Nevertheless, there may be 'hyper-function' (亢進 *kàng jìn*) of the heart organ due to kidney deficiency. This is one of the most familiar causes of heart fire seen in the clinic. It is still rooted in (kidney) organ deficiency, although it presents clinically as excess. The pattern might involve dryness in the body, mental disturbances such as irritability and restlessness, or heart organ disorder such as palpitations and arrhythmias. Pure deficiency of both *shào yīn* organs, on the other hand, involves weakness of the sovereign fire in the heart and/or kidney gate of vitality. This might eventually involve symptoms similar to congestive heart failure where the fluids fail to move, leading to swelling, cold limbs, and fluid in the lungs or kidney-related types of low libido or edema.

It is interesting to note that edema caused by kidney dysfunction generally manifests in the face (upper burner) while that associated with the heart is found in the lower extremities (lower burner). This is a point agreed upon by both modern allopathic and Chinese medicine, but is explained in different ways. In the case of kidney (qi) deficiency, the qi from the lower burner can't reach the face, while in the case of heart (yang) deficiency, the yang is unable to descend to the lower extremities. Again, these conditions are not associated with the channel per se, but involve dysfunction of the organs themselves. This careful differentiation of channel versus organ symptoms may seem trivial, but it does help guide treatment by aiding in the selection of acupuncture points and herbs.

To summarize, the *shào yīn* channel is both a part of and more than the individual *shào yīn* organs. Specifically, the *shào yīn* channel is both a clearer of heat (from the organs and exterior) and an important part of the functional balance of the *shào yīn* organs. It is the channel which drains fire, clears the heart, and dredges and opens the yin collaterals. The *shào yīn* organs, on the other hand, are associated with warming the body. Together, channel and organs regulate the complex physiology of fire.

Finally, having described in theory how the *shào yīn* channel can be associated with excess heat symptoms, a few of the most common pathomechanisms involving heat trapped in the *shào yīn* channel should be noted. These include patterns where there are:

- Heat pathogens blocked internally (熱邪內閉 *rè xié nèi bì*)
  These are generally heart-type symptoms associated with anxiety and agitated movement.

- Sores or fire toxins (瘡瘍火毒 *chuāng yáng huǒ dú*)
  Some types of shingles and boils are included in this category.

- Stagnation in the collateral vessels of the heart or brain
  (心腦絡瘀 *xīn nǎo luò yū*)
  Microcirculation issues in the heart or brain. This broadly applies to stroke, cognition, and developmental issues.

The Heart

> The heart holds the office of emperor and is the issuer of spirit clarity.
>
> *(心者．君主之官也．神明出焉。 Xīn zhě, jūn zhǔ zhī guān yě, shén míng chū yān.)*
>
> —*Basic Questions*, Chapter 8

This is the opening passage in *Basic Questions*, Chapter 8. In the space of just ten characters, the stage is set for all the other organs that follow. The heart is placed clearly above all others with "spirit clarity" as its guiding principle. The term *shén míng* (神明) is translated quite literally here as "spirit clarity." In this case, a literal translation seems appropriate, as any attempt to render more common English phrases would suggest a meaning that is not present in the original. It is especially important to avoid that pitfall with this term.

The term 'spirit' in conjunction with Chinese medicine brings to bear certain cultural preconceptions outside of China. Therefore, a clear understanding of this word should first begin with an explanation of what the writers of the *Inner Classic* might have meant. Simply put, spirit is the intelligence of existence itself, while 'spirit clarity' is a manifestation of that intelligence. Any time that the term spirit (神 *shén*) is used in Chinese, it is in connection with something that cannot normally be seen or felt. In reference to the heart in Chinese medicine, spirit clarity involves an unseen intelligence that allows a being to recognize and interact with its environment. The word 'recognize' does not necessarily refer to something at the conscious level, but instead represents the innate ability of an organism to perceive and respond to its environment. In the case of human beings, there are three levels of recognition:

1. Recognition of the external environment: the six qi
2. Recognition of the internal environment: the movement of the qi dynamic
3. Recognition of the social environment: interactions with people/animals

Because of its role as the 'recognizer', the heart is said to be preeminent among the twelve organs and the source of the intelligence of life (spirit).

The heart is located above the diaphragm and below the lungs at the level of the 5th thoracic vertebra (GV-11 *[shén dào]*). Ancient anatomists may have also noted the attachment of many of the small ligaments that hold the heart in place to the area around the 7th thoracic vertebra. In any case, palpable changes along the spine between the 5th and 7th thoracic vertebrae often coincide with heart dysfunction. Traditionally, the heart was described as looking like a peach or a lotus with openings at the top.

The heart is the pivot for the movement of blood in the body, between the internal storage of blood in the pericardium and liver at the *jué yīn* level and the infusion of external qi and nourishment into (and beyond) the blood at the *tài yīn* level in the lung and spleen. The heart moves blood around the body after it has been infused with qi from the environment and nutrition from food and grains. As we noted in the last chapter, external true qi (真氣 *zhēn qì*) enters the body through the lungs while food and grains are transformed by the spleen. Together, the *tài yīn* organs create the essence of blood (nutritive and protective) which is then moved by the heart.

FUNCTIONS OF THE HEART

Commands the blood vessels [1]

This refers to the heart function of moving blood through the vessels of the body. Difficulty sometimes surrounds this concept due to various interpretations of the character 主 (*zhǔ*) in the phrase "The heart commands the blood vessels" (心主血脈 *xīn zhǔ xuè mài*). Based on the variability of interpretation of this character, it is sometimes said that blood is "created" in the heart.[2] But it is more accurate to say that blood *comes from* the heart, meaning that blood moves about due to the beating of the heart organ.

A discussion of the blood vessels should also include the concept, mentioned earlier, of the yin collaterals. Considered the smallest vessels in the yin channels, the yin collaterals may be likened to the microcirculation of blood. As previously noted, the *shào yīn* channel is used clinically both to drain heat from the body and to dredge stagnation from the yin collaterals. In some cases, the generation of heat in the body can be due to stasis in the yin collaterals. Here the underlying deficiency involves an inability of the heart to properly move blood at this level of circulation. Stasis of blood leads to heat, which finally can cause boils (瘡癤 *chuāng jiē*) and pustulating sores (皰瘡 *pào chuāng*). Longer-term stagnation in the yin collaterals can lead to mental disorders, memory problems, speech difficulties, or even stroke. In general, heat and stasis in the yin collaterals is harder to clear than heat in the yang collaterals. The yin collaterals are most effectively dredged using the *shào yīn* channel, while yang collateral heat is cleared by treating the affected yang channel. Yin collateral stagnation is generally stagnation of blood, while the yang collaterals tend to have stagnation of qi, which might also lead to heat. In both yin and yang collateral stasis, however, the important underlying concept is microcirculation.

Q: *We have discussed the statement in the Inner Classic that the heart "commands the blood vessels." What are the relationships of the other yin organs to blood?*

DR. WANG: Generally speaking, the relationship of each yin organ to blood can be summarized in single characters. The liver stores (藏 *cáng*), the heart moves (行 *xíng*), and the spleen controls (统 *tǒng*) blood (Table 6.4). Let's take each one separately.

Organ	Term	Meaning
Spleen	统 *tǒng*	CONTROLS—The Spleen gathers the blood and keeps it within the vessels at the capillary level.
Heart	行 *xíng*	MOVES—The Heart moves blood like a pump and also moves consciousness.
Liver	藏 *cáng*	STORES—Blood is held deep for rejuvenation and also assigned to where it needs to go.

Table 6.4
Yin organs and the blood

The term associated with the liver blood function is 'storage'. In classical texts, the word *cáng* is used to describe substances held within the yin organs. It suggests putting the blood away somewhere deep and safe. We'll discuss this more in connection with *jué yīn*, but let me say for now that there are two basic subcategories of the liver blood-storing function:

1. The holding of blood at the deepest yin level for storage and rejuvenation.

2. The careful assignment and distribution of blood to where it is needed in the body.

The term associated with the heart blood function is 'movement'.[3] There are also two aspects of the heart blood-moving function. The first relates to the body and the second to the spirit:

1. The heart moves the blood throughout the body by pumping. This is similar to the modern physiological understanding of heart function.

2. The heart moves consciousness. This can be loosely thought of as the need for the spirit to have an adequate supply of blood in order to function.

Finally, the spleen is said to 'control' blood. This involves the process of keeping blood in bounds. There is also the idea of 'gathering up' that brings to mind my metaphor of spleen function at the capillary level. The spleen functions to bring the blood back into the vessels after it interacts with the internal environment.

Stores the spirit

As noted above, in the most general sense, the term spirit refers to the intelligence of existence. This is an intelligence that is in all living things. In plants, for example, it is seen in their ability to respond to changes in the seasons and, on a daily basis, to turn toward the sun (heliotropism). In human beings, this concept also includes the capacity for understanding or comprehending and involves an innate ability to make associative leaps from one concept to another. Thus the more common English definition of intelligence also falls within the idea of spirit.

Previously, it was noted that the spirit was more yang-natured and the essence more yin-natured. Essence is the ultimate material basis of the body, while spirit is the ineffable presence of the supernatural in the human body. While intent, associated with the spleen, involves the logical 'digesting' of information, only spirit can make leaps of inspiration. The quality of spirit in each individual has a broad effect on the five psychic aspects. Without clear recognition by the spirit, the other psychic aspects may become confused. Once again, the position of the heart as emperor is relevant.

Another common image is that of the heart as a pool of water. When the surface of the heart is calm, it can clearly reflect perceptions from the outside world. When the surface is stirred by the wind-like movement of the seven emotions, then the reflection becomes muddled and a person has difficulty perceiving the real nature of a situation. The nature and health of the spirit has a direct effect on the ability of a person to keep the 'heart mirror' polished and calm (Fig. 6.6).

Opens to the tongue

The relationship of the heart to the tongue is of particular importance in the context of speech and communication. Problems moving the tongue and expressing ideas are most likely due to heart dysfunction. The relationship of the heart to the tongue is related to its ability to house the spirit. One aspect of the spirit described above was its ability to clearly 'recognize' the

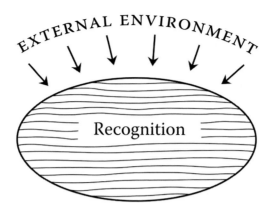

The heart mirror recognizes the true nature of the
external environment when calm and undisturbed.

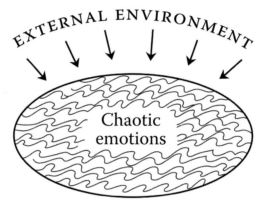

When clouded by the winds of the seven emotions,
reality may become obscured.

Fig. 6.6
Heart mirror

world at large. This is both similar to and greater than the idea of consciousness. A person is conscious if they are awake, but may not necessarily be
able to clearly recognize. In the case of a stroke, for example, a patient may
appear completely conscious but often seems unable to recognize the world
around them in the same way. This is a case in which the qi transformation
of the *shào yīn* channel has been affected. In these types of stroke patients,
the ability to speak is often compromised. More specifically, the patient may
have relatively normal tongue movement, but be unable to properly vocalize
ideas because of changes in the brain itself. In this type of case, where the
'spirit' is disturbed, one should again consider the concept of microcircula-

tion and the yin collaterals.

The kidney, spleen, and *yīn qiāo mài* (yin heel vessel) are also related to tongue function. (Appendix 2 provides a more detailed examination of tongue conditions in Chinese medicine.)

CLINICAL PEARLS OF WISDOM ABOUT HEART PATHOLOGY

- Classical texts often say that itchy sores are related to the heart. Sores, especially those in the upper part of the body and face, are associated with heat toxins in the heart channel. This may include some types of acne or mouth sores. Palpate the *shào yīn* channel for confirmation.

- The area on the back associated with the heart, between the 5th and 7th thoracic vertebrae, is often involved in problems with cognition (神志 *shén zhì*). It is therefore used in treating many types of developmental problems in children, including physical difficulties/muscle coordination and problems with cognition and speech. This area may also have tenderness (as will the parallel bladder channel points) where there are emotional problems. Furthermore, the area is important in the treatment of dementia, Alzheimer's, and other cognition and emotional disorders in the elderly that are related to brain function. The heart channel in general is often important in these types of conditions. For this reason, the point pair HT-5 (*tōng lǐ*) and KI-6 (*zhào hǎi*) is often added to treatments designed to affect the brain.

- Insomnia and a tendency toward fear or being easily startled often involve heart *shào yīn*. This is more often a yin/blood deficiency type.

- Pain in the genitals is sometimes due to excessive accumulation of heat in the *shào yīn* channel due to an underlying deficiency of kidney yang. As noted earlier, this is a case which presents as excess that is actually rooted in deficiency—a lack of yang qi to drive circulation.

- Urinary incontinence may often involve heart *shào yīn*. Note the use of HT-7 (*shén mén*) with KI-3 (*tài xī*) in bed-wetting and problems controlling urine, especially at night.

The Kidney

The kidney holds the office of forceful accomplishment
and is the issuer of wondrous talent.

*(腎者．作強之官．伎巧出焉。Shèn zhě, zuò qiáng zhī guān,
jì qiǎo chū yān.)*

—*Basic Questions,* Chapter 8

Despite suggesting something more mystical, this phrase from the *Inner Classic* is firmly rooted in reality. Of course, this is apropos the concept of the kidney as a repository of essence, that most important of material substances. A more literal translation than "office of forceful accomplishment" might be "an organ of doing and striving"; this is a reference to the importance of the kidney as the material root of the body. It is the root strength from which one rises to the challenge of urgent need. Moreover, the physical strength that develops in the presence of healthy kidney essence also gives rise to the body's "wondrous talent" for reproduction. The term "forceful accomplishment" refers to the association of the kidney with the will (志 *zhì*). The will is the ability of a person to steadily do and strive in the world, with the eventual goal of reproduction. This is the realm of the kidney.

The kidney is said to collect at the level of the 2nd lumbar vertebra, roughly level with the umbilicus.

FUNCTIONS OF THE KIDNEY

Stores essence

Essence is the yin-natured root of the gate of vitality, the driving force behind all life processes. It is the most fundamental physical manifestation of a human being's inheritance from their ancestors. The interaction of essence with the qi derived from fluids, food, and air is the basis for the physiological activities that make up daily life. Essence provides the guidance that creates human form from the fruits of the earth. Furthermore, essence is the fundamental spark that begins the qi dynamic of all the other organs. The urge to take the first breath of life comes from essence stored in the kidneys. Essence moves with the corporeal soul found in the lung. The lung is the commander of qi in the body while the essence is the spark that begins the qi dynamic. Essence is yin to the yang of spirit, and thus the strength of the physical body (yin-material) ultimately depends on essence. The stages of growth and development are manifestations of essence, and the decrepitude of old age reflects the outward signs of its decline.

In Chapter 5, the relationship of the spirit to the ethereal soul was noted. Specifically, the 'comings and goings' of the spirit are said to be with the ethereal soul, which is housed in the liver. The relationship of spirit to essence (heart-kidney) is different from the relationship of spirit to the ethereal soul (heart-liver). Essence balances and roots spirit in the body by bringing the insights of 'intelligence' into reality. It is the balance of fire and water. By contrast, the ethereal soul, associated with the liver and blood, provides a different kind of root for the spirit in the body. Essence is a prenatal rooting while the ethereal soul (via liver blood) provides a rooting based on an abundance of postnatal qi. The ethereal soul, in turn, is moved by spirit as the beating heart moves the blood. (The nature of the ethereal soul will be discussed in Chapter 7 on *jué yīn* physiology.)

Governs the bones

The kidney is responsible for the growth and development of bones, especially during childhood. This is actually part of its function in governing the stages of development. The growth of bones in childhood is regarded as the most visible manifestation of the fullness of essence.

Stores the will

The character usually translated as 'will' (志 *zhì*) also means steadfastness (堅定 *jiān dìng*). A person's ability to persist, to put their mind to something and follow through with plans, is linked to the kidney. The concept of will in Chinese medicine is also inexorably linked to the concept of essence. Simply put, the will depends on essence. The ability to remain steadfast depends on the quality and metabolism of essence. Activities that 'waste essence' will also eventually begin to compromise a person's will.

Consider again the relationship of the heart and kidney in the context of the five psychic aspects. The psychic aspect associated with the heart is spirit and that of the kidney is essence/will. Spirit has been described as the "intelligence of existence" and manifests as the ability to recognize and extend one's vision to the outside environment (intuitive leaps 悟志 *wù zhì*). It is the spirit that perceives. By contrast to the relatively yang-natured spirit, essence roots the physical body. The balancing act maintained by essence and spirit is yet another aspect of *shào yīn* physiology. The inquisitive, curious, and agile mind that we in the West call intelligence must be supported by the physical strength of the human body. This is the crux of the relationship between spirit and essence (Fig. 6.7).

The Chinese word for 'will' might also be translated as 'intention'. In order for the ideas generated by intelligence to take on form in the world, they

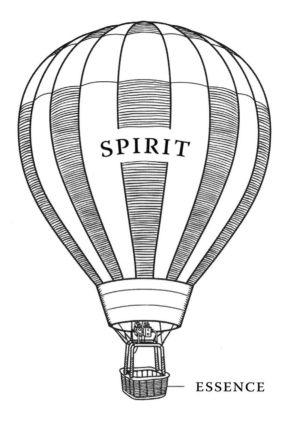

SPIRIT

ESSENCE

Fig. 6.7
Essence roots the spirit so that leaps of intuition can be held and realized.

must be held in place and brought to fruition through sustained will. This is 'keeping one's eye on the ball'. When the heart and kidney are not 'communicating', a person may have an abundance of interesting and insightful ideas, but they are not held or brought into reality. One therefore might also say that essence and will are two sides of the same coin. Without the tenacity that arises from proper manifestation of prenatal essence, it is impossible to maintain intention. At the same time, without the yang-natured stimulus provided by the intelligence of spirit, the life potential represented by essence does not take on its best form. In other words, it is important to keep the reflective pool of the heart calm and clear so that will/intention can focus on real and attainable goals. Ultimately, the will to live and take on the challenges of life arises from the physical body (essence). Without this material foundation, the drive to live and press forward eventually fades. A person who has a strong will to live in the midst of severe disease still maintains an adequate supply of what ancient physiologists called 'essence'.

Opens to the ears

Many take the association of the kidney with the ears to mean that all hearing problems are related to the kidneys. In fact, this is not categorically true. When considering the kidney, think of the small bones of the middle ear. If problems arise with the health or flexibility of movement in these bones, the kidney is more likely to be involved. The process of aging often leads to problems of this type. Problems involving the flexibility or nourishment of the eardrum also tend to be kidney related. However, for ringing in the ears or other types of gradual deafness due to problems with the auditory nerve, the kidney may not be involved at all. Ringing very often involves injury to the qi dynamic of the liver-gallbladder, most often due to heat. Alternatively, problems with clarity of hearing can be due to an accumulation of dampness in the inner ear, which requires spleen-type treatment approaches. However, as the case study below will show, dampness-type inner ear problems can also be due to a lack of kidney qi transformation. A modern perspective on the treatment of ear conditions is also provided in Appendix 2.

CLINICAL PEARLS OF WISDOM ABOUT KIDNEY PATHOLOGY

- The statement in the *Inner Classic* that the kidney holds the "office of forceful accomplishment" suggests an association of this organ with bursts of adrenaline in stressful situations. The ability to rise and perform in highly stressful situations is associated with the kidney. Similarly, excessive stress will eventually damage the kidney.

- Many types of allergic and autoimmune disorders are related to the kidney. This might be thought of as hyperactivity of the "forceful accomplishment" aspect of kidney's nature. In other words, the kidney is responding with force in an untimely way. These cases require strengthening of the kidney yin. For example, in the case of seasonal allergies, the point pair LU-5 *(chǐ zé)* and KI-7 *(fù liū)* is helpful in harmonizing the lungs and benefiting the yin aspect of the kidney. Similarly, herbal formulas designed to benefit kidney yin can be used for chronic allergies, sinusitis, or allergic asthma.

- Problems with the endocrine system are often related to the kidney qi dynamic. Hormone imbalance or hyper- or hypoactivity of endocrine glands are often treated with acupuncture and herbs that regulate the kidney.

Q: *What is the difference between the fluid metabolism functions of the kidney and spleen?*

DR. WANG: In order to answer this question, we should first differentiate between the *tài yīn* function of 'commanding' (主 *zhǔ*) the body's fluids and the kidney's 'control' (統 *tǒng*) of water metabolism. An easy way to understand the difference is to consider the image of a tree. A tree absorbs and metabolizes fluids through its roots but depends on the warmth and nourishment of the earth (literally, the 'qi of the ground' 地氣 *dì qì*) to stimulate the process. In this case the tree can be likened to the spleen and the earth below to the gate of vitality of the kidney. When one hears that the kidneys 'control' water, remember that the function is fundamentally related to the gate of vitality. The gate of vitality rises up, like the qi of the earth, to warm and stimulate *tài yīn*. It thus 'controls' water by providing the prenatal source for the rate of fluid metabolism. The warmth from the gate of vitality radiates from the kidneys to provide the driving force in not only the *tài yīn* system, but in the body as a whole. The warm, generative power of the gate of vitality is known as source qi when it moves through the channel system. At *tài yīn*, source qi stimulates the process of fluid metabolism, thus allowing the spleen to effectively 'command' the transformation of fluids and dampness (Fig. 6.8).

A common fluid metabolism disorder such as edema might be caused by dysfunction of either *tài yīn* or *shào yīn*. *Shào yīn* type edema would necessarily involve a deficiency of yang in the kidney or heart, while *tài yīn* edema is generally a case of spleen qi deficiency, although it may involve excessive accumulation of dampness as well. *Shào yīn* edema is more often pitting edema, while *tài yīn* edema more often accumulates in the abdomen and waist.

Q: *I know we haven't talked about shào yáng yet, but I'm wondering how you differentiate these two 'pivots' in the channel system?*

DR. WANG: Well, the most obvious answer is that *shào yáng* pivots the three yang channels while *shào yīn* pivots the three yin channels. In both cases, the idea of regulation is extremely important. As you've probably noticed by now, I emphasize the importance of *shào yīn* as a place of movement. The heart beats to move the blood while the prenatal stimulus of the kidneys drives metabolism. I must admit that I am informed by the concept of hormones, as understood by

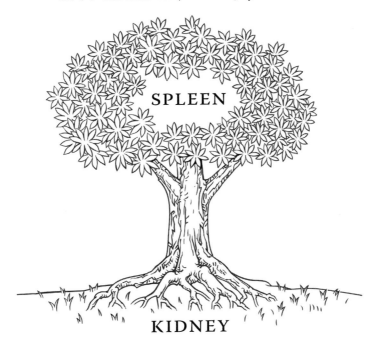

Fig. 6.8
Like a tree to the earth, the spleen depends on the kidney
for warmth and nourishment to initiate its transformations.

modern medicine, when I think of the kidney. The understanding of the adrenal hormones, for example, certainly plays a role in what has been traditionally called kidney qi and yang. Of course in this case, as in almost all others, there is not a direct equivalence between the Chinese and modern physiological concepts, just a striking and helpful similarity.

The differentiation of *shào yáng* and *shào yīn* might also be approached from a completely different angle. Consider the two formulas Minor Bupleurum Decoction *(xiǎo chái hú tāng)* and Frigid Extremities Powder *(sì nì sǎn)*. In the most basic sense, Minor Bupleurum Decoction regulates the yang pivot while Frigid Extremities Powder regulates the yin pivot. In Minor Bupleurum Decoction, the movement created by first warming and transforming the stomach with Pinelliae Rhizoma *(bàn xià)*, Zingiberis Rhizoma recens *(shēng jiāng)*, Ginseng Radix *(rén shēn)*, Jujubae Fructus *(dà zǎo)*, and Glycyrrhizae Radix *(gān cǎo)* is then lifted upward and outward by Scutellariae Radix *(huáng qín)* and Bupleuri Radix *(chái hú)*. The overall movement of Minor Bupleurum Decoction is thus in the yang organs and channels. On the other hand, Frigid Extremities Powder, with the inclusion of Paeoniae Radix alba *(bái sháo)*, has a different focus. That formula also regulates with Bupleuri Radix *(chái hú)*, but the regulation tends more to affect the yin organs. Specifically, Paeoniae Radix alba homes deeply to the blood of *jué yīn*, thus bringing the focus of the formula down into yin levels.

Sure, both formulas are moving and thus yang in nature, but their influences differ: they affect different pivots. Once this basic principle is kept in mind, the realm of modification for the formulas is quite large. When thinking about the difference between the *shào yáng* and *shào yīn* pivots, these two formulas provide an interesting way of thinking.[4]

The Various Fires of the Human Body

I'm a bit confused about the term 'fire' in Chinese medicine. The opinions vary in different texts and in different historical periods. What is your interpretation of the nature of the various 'fires' in the body?

DR. WANG: Any discussion of fire or warmth in Chinese physiology should begin with a look at *shào yīn* function, but will certainly include concepts associated with other channels as well. The warming function of *shào yīn* can be summarized in two basic concepts: the gate of vitality in the kidney and sovereign fire in the heart. The gate of vitality should be considered first, followed by a discussion of a few other concepts related to fire and metabolic stimulus, as understood by Chinese medicine.

GATE OF VITALITY

Fundamentally, kidney function has both a fire and a water aspect. The water aspect is the essence or 'primal yin' (元陰 *yuán yīn*), while the fire aspect is the gate of vitality or 'primal yang' (元陽 *yuán yáng)*. The two together are necessary in order for the gate of vitality to enliven the body. Many classical texts use the metaphor of a pot of boiling water to describe the gate of vitality. When the fire at the gate of vitality and the water-essence are balanced in kidney function, the pot is boiling strongly, but not excessively. Excessive use of the fire at the gate of vitality can boil away the water-essence and lead to signs of heat from yin deficiency. A lack of fire at the gate of vitality, on the other hand, slows down the boiling and reduces the amount of stimulus that can be sent outward to nourish and facilitate the qi dynamic in the body. This will manifest in generalized yang deficiency. One could also say that the gate of vitality is the fire aspect of prenatal qi (that which comes to a person from their ancestors). The water aspect of prenatal qi would of course be essence. The two are inseparable.

It is also interesting to note parallels between the Chinese medicine concept of the gate of vitality and the endocrine system in Western medicine. Ideas about growth, development, libido, and metabolism tend to follow similar lines in both frames of reference. Specifically, the systemic influence of hormones might be likened to gate of vitality theory in Chinese medicine. Also, modern research is showing that many herbal formulas that are said to 'strengthen the gate of vitality' and 'benefit kidney yang' affect the complex interactions of the endocrine system. This idea is exciting and is only just beginning to be understood in the context of modern science (Fig. 6.9).

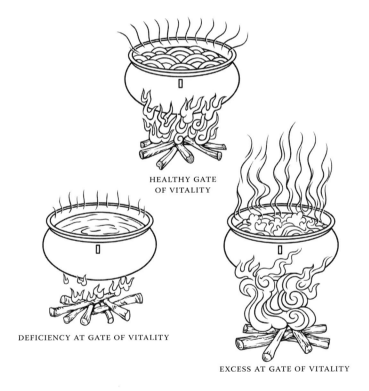

HEALTHY GATE
OF VITALITY

DEFICIENCY AT GATE OF VITALITY

EXCESS AT GATE OF VITALITY

Fig. 6.9
Within the gate of vitality, there is a balance between fire at the gate of vitality and essence (water). Excess and deficiency affect systemic metabolism.

Turning now to the other 'fires' of the body, it is helpful to carefully differentiate between commonly used terms and related concepts. These include ministerial fire (相火 *xiàng huǒ*), sovereign fire (君火 *jūn huǒ*), chest yang (胸陽 *xiōng yáng*), and gathering qi (宗氣 *zōng qì*).

MINISTERIAL FIRE

The term 'ministerial fire' is most commonly seen in three cases:

1. As a synonym for the gate of vitality.

2. In five-phase discussions when trying to categorize the somewhat incongruent 'sixth yin organ'—the pericardium—and its paired yang organ, the triple burner. Some texts describe the pericardium and triple burner as also being fire organs; generally speaking, this is true. To be more specific, however, one should remember that the heart and small intestine are considered to be fire-phase organs, while the pericardium and triple burner are categorized as ministerial fire-phase organs.

3. In discussions of pathology, particularly pathology associated with the liver-gallbladder.

These three uses of the same term are not mutually exclusive. Ultimately, ministerial fire is derived from the *shào yīn* system and arises from the gate of vitality. The interchangeability of the terms 'gate of vitality' and 'ministerial fire' in many texts is representative of the fact that the term changes depending on where in the body this particular fire is located. When in (or between) the kidneys, the term gate of vitality is appropriate. On the other hand, once outside the lower burner, there is some variation and occasional confusion about terminology.

As mentioned above, the pericardium and triple burner are categorized in five-phase theory as ministerial fire-phase organs. Thus the two organs are defined as having a distinctly different nature than the fire-phase organs (heart and small intestine). In addition, the nature of ministerial fire is slightly different in each of the two ministerial fire organs.

The pericardium ministerial fire represents the overflow of heart sovereign fire. A metaphor may be helpful to envision how the pericardium gets its ministerial fire. The heart can be likened to a cooking pot on a flame. The heat in the pot is the sovereign fire of the heart, pumping blood around the body. The excess heat radiating off the sides of the pot, or flowing up from the flames past the pot, may be likened to ministerial fire reaching the pericardium. This metaphor also helps one to imagine how the pericardium protects the heart by absorbing and removing excess heat. Therefore, although ministerial fire in the pericardium ultimately arises from the sovereign fire of heart *shào yīn*, it takes on a different name and nature when entering *jué yīn*. In the case of the pericardium, the ministerial fire is considered to be part of the normal functioning of the organ. When the heart beats, heat is created that is naturally absorbed by the pericardium (Fig. 6.10).

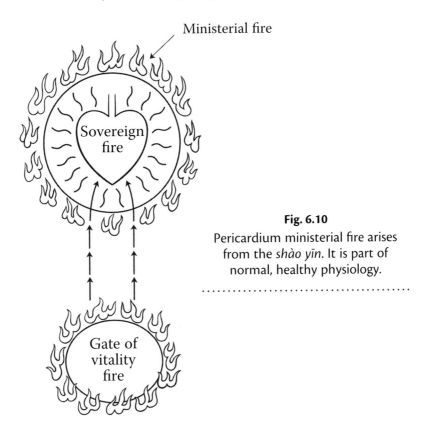

Fig. 6.10
Pericardium ministerial fire arises from the *shào yīn*. It is part of normal, healthy physiology.

To review what has already become a fairly complex concept, in the kidneys there is the gate of vitality, which is related to the ministerial fire of the pericardium via the heart. Earlier in this chapter the sovereign fire of the heart and its relationship to the kidneys was described (see Fig. 6.1).

In the triple burner (a yang organ) the ministerial fire takes on yet another nature. Traveling through the ditches of all three burners, arising from the gate of vitality at *shào yīn*, ministerial fire in the triple burner is crucial to source qi. Specifically, ministerial fire is the motive force underlying source qi. Source qi ultimately arises from the kidneys and can be thought of as the pervasive influence of inheritance (prenatal) in the body. Like the gate of vitality, source qi has a polarity: its yang aspect derives from ministerial fire and its yin aspect from essence. Source qi, perhaps likened to the guiding force of genetics in modern physiology, provides the ultimate stimulus for life activity. Thus the source qi, while not created in the triple burner, travels through it to permeate all aspects of life in the body. In the pathways of the triple burner, the source qi intermingles with the nutritive aspect of blood from food and drink and the qi of the external world drawn from the breath. This is the fundamental interplay of prenatal and postnatal qi in the fluids of the body, a concept that will be discussed in Chapter 9 on *shào yáng*. At this point, it is important to note the use of the term ministerial fire in relation to the triple burner and to understand that this fire also ultimately arises from the gate of vitality at *shào yīn* (Fig. 6.11).

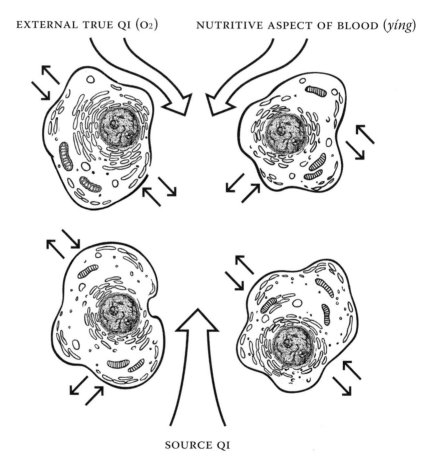

EXTERNAL TRUE QI (O_2)   NUTRITIVE ASPECT OF BLOOD (*yíng*)

SOURCE QI

Fig. 6.11

In the fluids of the triple burner, external true qi (真氣 *zhēn qì*)
and the nutritive aspect of blood (營 *yíng*) interact with source qi.
The source qi is driven by the motive force of ministerial fire.
This is the cellular level interplay of prenatal and postnatal.

Thus ministerial fire, associated with the pericardium and triple burner, can be understood as a type of fire that arises from *shào yīn* and is part of the normal, healthy metabolism of those organs.

The final reference to ministerial fire is its association with the development of disease and involves the interior-exterior paired organs of both the triple burner and the pericardium. In the case of pathogenesis, ministerial fire 'leaves' the pericardium and triple burner and can damage the qi in their paired liver and gallbladder organs. Here the term ministerial fire involves fire gone astray. In this case either the liver, gallbladder, or both is affected by a fire-type pathodynamic. In the case of the liver, the pathodynamic is often a dual deficiency of kidney and liver yin, leading to liver yang rising. Liver yang rising is thus sometimes termed 'ascendant hyperactivity of ministerial fire'. Healthy ministerial fire has left the *shào yīn* and is affecting the liver. In the case of the gallbladder, hyperactive ministerial fire has more of an excess nature and leads to constrained heat patterns, sometimes called 'internal blazing of ministerial fire' (相火內熾 *xiàng huǒ nèi chì*).

In the massive, fifty-two volume *Grand Materia Medica* (本草綱目 *Běn cǎo gāng mù*), compiled by Li Shi-Zhen (李時珍) over a thirty year period in the 16th century, there is description of a pattern of ministerial fire disorder associated with the liver-gallbladder. This is found in a discussion of the herb Saigae tataricae Cornu *(líng yáng jiǎo)*:

> [When the] ministerial fire lies in the liver and gallbladder, anger is created in the qi level, illness develops, producing irritability and fullness with qi counterflow, hiccuping obstruction, chills and fever resulting from injury by [external] cold and deep-lying fever, then Saigae tataricae Cornu *(líng yáng jiǎo)* can be used to direct downward.[5]

In this case, the herb is being used to direct ministerial fire downward and back into the kidney.

Finally, some texts describe the ministerial fire as being "held" in the liver/gallbladder, and there is a tradition of using the term in conjunction with the yang energy of the gallbladder that helps to move the *jué yīn* liver; this will be discussed further in Chapter 9 on the *shào yáng*. Nevertheless, many physiological models describe ministerial fire as moving in the pericardium and triple burner; it is only associated with the liver/gallbladder in cases of pathogenesis.

As is often the case with other concepts, given the long history of Chinese medicine, a survey of historical texts will uncover conflicting ideas about the location and nature of ministerial fire. What is most important to remember about ministerial fire is that:

• It arises from the gate of vitality.

- It is associated with the warmth drawn to the pericardium from the heart.

- It inspires the movement of source qi in the triple burner.

- It is associated with patterns of disharmony in the liver and gallbladder.

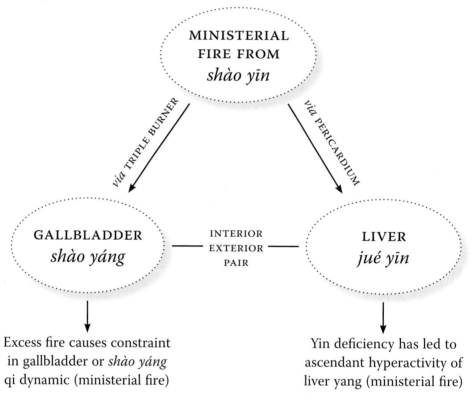

Fig. 6.12
When associated with pathology, ministerial fire has left the *shào yīn* and ministerial fire organs.

SOVEREIGN FIRE

The sovereign fire is associated with the heart and is exemplified in the actual movement of the heart organ. This movement sends warm blood throughout the body and is directly dependent on the stimulus from the gate of vitality. This is the crux of the heart-kidney relationship at the fire level. The fire at the gate of vitality, balanced by the water-essence of the kidney, provides constant and regulated impetus to the warming movement of the heart. Therefore, while sovereign fire is considered to be a 'fire' in its own right, it ultimately depends on the gate of vitality for stimulus.

Sovereign fire is a simpler concept than ministerial fire, but is nonetheless crucial. There is a fire in the heart that stimulates its beating. If this fire wanes, the movement of blood is slowed and an array of associated symptoms may arise. The sovereign fire might also become excessive due to heat from deficiency rising up from the kidney. In this case, the normal warming of sovereign fire has the potential to become heat which damages the body. The first line of defense is the pericardium, which absorbs the fire of the heart in the creation of ministerial fire. Again, this ministerial fire is ultimately coming from the kidney, but is moving through the heart as it stimulates the sovereign fire.

CHEST YANG

Related to the concept of fire in the body is the term 'chest yang'. It is not actually a fire, but instead describes the warmth of yang which fills the upper burner. It is the result of the combination of ministerial fire from the pericardium with postnatal qi from the lungs and spleen. Chest yang has no material form (in contrast to gathering qi) and is often a fairly generic term for warmth in the upper part of the body.

GATHERING QI

This term is also translated as 'ancestral qi', and, like chest yang, is not a fire but is related because of its dependence on fire in the upper burner for its creation. It is the broadest of the three fire concepts associated with the upper burner (the other two being sovereign fire and chest yang). Gathering qi involves the combination of chest yang with lung and heart yin. Thus constituted, gathering qi is another way of describing the physiological functions of the upper burner. This is what is often termed the ascending and descending (升降 *shēng jiàng)* function of the lung and the warming movement of blood in the chest. An important feature of gathering qi is the incorporation of yin nourishment in its definition. Gathering qi, while sharing some aspects of fire, is actually the final expression of a classical conception of a complex physiological process. In the case of gathering qi, yang warmth has now taken yin form (Fig. 6.13).

Case Studies

An illustrative point combination to demonstrate the *shào yīn* channel function of 'dredging the yin collaterals' is HT-5 *(tōng lǐ)* and KI-6 *(zhào*

[133]

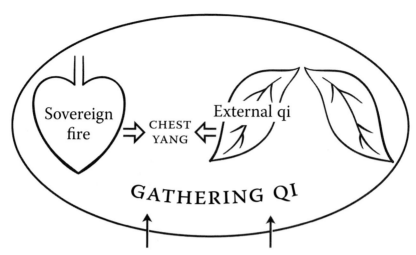

Includes yin aspect of the lungs and heart,
arising from the spleen and kidney

Fig. 6.13
Gathering qi

hǎi). This combination is often used to address problems with microcirculation in the brain and/or heart leading to cognition or speech difficulties. Clinically, this might also include treating problems with brain development. These two points are also especially effective for stroke associated with speech problems or esophageal dysphagia (choking easily). In the case of stroke, treatment should begin as soon as possible because the benefits from acupuncture are less after six months. 'Problems with speech' can also refer to dementia, the early stages of Alzheimer's, or even vocalization problems in children. In these cases, the points can be beneficial at any time.

HT-5 *(tōng lǐ)* is the collateral (絡 *luò*) point of the heart channel and helps to open collateral circulation not only in the heart and brain, but, because the heart is the prime mover of blood, it also dredges the collaterals throughout the body. KI-6 *(zhào hǎi)* is the command point of the *yīn qiāo mài* (yin heel vessel). This vessel affects the function of the involuntary (smooth) muscle tissue and also internal muscles such as the tongue or heart (see the discussion of *yīn qiāo* in Chapter 11). KI-6 *(zhào hǎi)* also helps reestablish circulation in the collaterals around the throat and tongue, which explains its use for loss of voice as well.

[134]

■ CASE NO. 1

4-year-old male

Chief complaint Developmental difficulties following a fever of unknown origin during infancy.

History of present illness At six months of age, the child developed a very high fever (42°C) which lasted for approximately four days. During the febrile episode, he experienced seizures and profuse sweating. After the fever abated, he was left with brain damage that manifests primarily as difficulty with speech and coordination of the lower limbs. The child also has diplopia (double vision), likely due to damaged cranial nerves or brain tissue. This is alleviated by wearing a patch over one eye. Treatment before the initial visit involved the use of low-dose steroids for two months following the episode in conjunction with herbal formulas to clear toxic heat. Previous acupuncture treatment by other doctors included local points for speech difficulties such as CV-23 *(lián quán)* and GV-15 *(yǎ mén)*, and *yáng míng* channel points such as ST-36 *(zú sān lǐ)* and LI-10 *(shǒu sān lǐ)*, to strengthen postnatal qi. Earlier acupuncture treatments seemed to have helped some, but the parents were dissatisfied with the rate of change and thus decided to consult Dr. Wang.

Upon arrival at the clinic, the child had received no acupuncture or herbs for six months. On the first visit, he was unable to vocalize with any significant volume. He was able to speak basic words and small sentences, but with a weak voice and unclear articulation. Motor difficulties included an inability to balance when sitting and an inability to stand or walk. Despite the various neuromuscular difficulties, the child maintained significant cognitive ability and an awareness of surrounding people and places. He was extremely irritable, crying often, and sometimes refusing to eat. Bowel movements tended to be normal to slightly dry. The child would go to sleep fairly easily, but would often wake with violent crying episodes.

Palpation of channels revealed tightness of the muscles and fascia in the yin aspect of the arms. There was a noticeable tightness in the muscles and a lack of skin elasticity along the pericardium *jué yīn* and heart *shào yīn* channels. The areas below T_5 and T_6 also had tightness that was comparatively greater than around other vertebrae in that part of the spine. The 'qi pass' area on the second joint of the child's index finger showed red, full vessels, while the tongue was also slightly red.

Diagnosis Five retardations (五遲 *wǔ chí*)

The term 'five retardations' is from classical Chinese pediatrics and describes a condition characterized by slower rates of development for standing, walking, hair growth, tooth growth, and speech. Not all children given this diagnosis will necessarily have all five symptoms. The five retardations may be caused by either a congenital (essence) deficiency or by postnatal external pathogens. In this patient, the cause was postnatal. This case involved heat trapped in the *shào yīn* system affecting the yin collaterals. Here, the term 'yin collaterals' refers specifically to the collaterals (microcirculation) of the brain.

Treatment   Treatment of this patient continued for over a year. In the initial stages, the child was treated 2–3 times each week. Frequency declined over time but never went below twice monthly. During the course of treatment, channel and point selection varied, but followed certain themes, as described below. In all cases, 1-inch needles were inserted to a shallow depth, stimulated, and removed quickly.

Clearing of yin collaterals

In the initial stages, treatment focused on clearing heat from the yin collaterals. The lead point pair during this stage was HT-5 *(tōng lǐ)* and KI-6 *(zhào hǎi)*. There was also heat trapped in the pericardium, evidenced by the findings in channel palpation and the frequent crying episodes. Excessive crying in children is a sign of heat, most often associated with stasis in the *jué yīn* pericardium. Consequently, the point pair PC-7 *(dà líng)* and LR-2 *(xíng jiān)* was used at the same time to clear and transform *jué yīn* (see discussion of point pairs in Chapter 20).

Opening the *dū* (governing) vessel

Problems with motor skills in children usually also include a lack of open circulation in the *dū* vessel. In this case, palpation revealed tightness in the *dū* vessel area associated with the heart (T_4–T_6). After the initial clearing of heat toxins (approximately three months), the focus of treatment shifted to warming and opening the *dū* vessel. Stimulation of the entire *dū* vessel on the back is especially helpful in these cases. Specifically, GV-14 *(dà zhuī)*, GV-12 *(shēn zhù)*, GV-9 *(zhì yáng)*, GV-8 *(jīn suō)*, GV-6 *(jǐ zhōng)*, GV-4 *(mìng mén)*, and the command point pair SI-3 *(hòu xī)* and BL-62 *(shēn mài)* were used.

Strengthening postnatal qi

Throughout the course of treatment, but especially after heat had been cleared from the yin collaterals, there was also a focus on strengthening the child's ability to absorb nourishment and support the nutritive aspect of blood. This included the use of *yáng míng* channel points like ST-36 *(zú sān lǐ)* and ST-40 *(fēng lóng)* in conjunction with the *tài yīn* points SP-3 *(tài bái)* and LU-9 *(tài yuān)* to facilitate the interrelated qi dynamic of *tài yīn* and *yáng míng*. Note that ST-40 *(fēng lóng)* is the stomach *yáng míng* collateral point and that SP-3 *(tài bái)* and LU-9 *(tài yuān)* are both *tài yīn* source points. As many textbooks point out, source-collateral point combinations serve to bring nourishment from a yin channel to its paired yang channel.

Balancing the *shào yáng* pivot

In later stages, the *shào yáng* channel was used in conjunction with treatments to strengthen postnatal qi. The *shào yáng* channel is especially helpful for treating problems with balance and walking. *Shào yáng* points included GB-30 *(huán tiào)*, GB-34 *(yáng líng quán)*, and GB-39 *(xuán zhōng)*, the influential point for marrow.

Results Initial changes in the symptom pattern involved the gradual reduction of heat in the *jué yīn* pericardium. Specifically, there was a reduction in the frequency of violent crying episodes and an improvement in the ability to sleep through the night. The pair PC-7 and LR-2 was discontinued after these symptoms abated. After continued treatment (six months) to clear the yin collaterals using the pair HT-5 and KI-6 as lead points, the child began to exhibit improvement in communication skills, followed by improvements in balance. The following stages (six months to one-year) involved alternation and sometimes combination of the yin collateral clearing treatment with *dū* vessel treatment. Gradually, the yin collateral pair was used less often as treatment focused more on improving postnatal qi and *shào yáng* circulation, as described above.

After one year, the child was able to vocalize at significantly greater volume, with clearer articulation. Problems with balance improved significantly, allowing for the development of motor skills in his legs and, eventually, the ability to walk unaided. There was still a tendency to fall more often than other children of the same age, and his problems with vision remained. Of significance to the parents was a dramatic improvement in the child's mood. Whenever he came to the clinic during the final six months of treatment, he would smile and laugh with other patients and would only barely cry during treatments. At this point, due to increased participation in school, the frequency of visits was slowly reduced to once weekly, then bimonthly, and finally was discontinued with plans for another course of treatment after one to two years.

Analysis   When treating children with developmental problems, the general goal is to reestablish proper circulation of qi and blood in the channel system in order to facilitate normal development. While strengthening treatments are used, this case emphasizes the importance of clearing excess (heat and blood stasis) as a preliminary goal. Remember that the diagnosis was 'five retardations' due to heat trapped in the yin collaterals. Of course, the heat in this case is a lingering result of the initial high fever. After first clearing heat from the yin collaterals, the focus of treatment shifted to opening the *dū* vessel and finally to the regulation of postnatal qi production and *shào yáng* balance. During the course of treatment, the evolution from one stage of treatment to the next was not always clearly defined but involved a gradual shift. The points used during each phase of treatment varied accordingly. For example, while clearing heat from the yin collaterals was the goal of treatment in the early stages, points to regulate the *dū* were eventually included before heat was totally cleared. Similarly, in later stages, while the goal was to strengthen production of postnatal qi, *dū* points were still used (Fig. 6.14).

This is a difficult type of case that involves a great deal of patience on

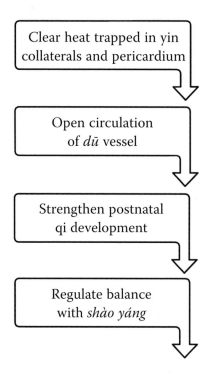

Fig. 6.14

General evolution of treatment for Case No. 1

the part of both the practitioner and the parents. Changes are gradual and must be gauged against the severity of initial presentation. Of course, in cases involving significant brain impairment, like this one, complete recovery is extremely unlikely. Nonetheless, by improving the child's mood and by facilitating normal development, the parents were very pleased with the results.

In general, acupuncture can be useful in helping children along the path of development when there is any type of slowness in development. The child's own body often facilitates the process. It is assumed that this particular child will require repeated courses of treatment. In such cases of long-term treatment, it is often helpful to stop treatment for periods of up to (but not more than) a year so that the doctor and parents can evaluate effectiveness while also reducing economic strain.

Now, compare the application of *shào yīn* treatment in this case with the following one.

■ CASE NO. 2

70-year-old female

Chief complaint   Hearing loss (with tinnitus)

History of present illness   The condition began four months prior to the first visit, with low-pitched ringing in both ears. The patient had experienced periodic bouts of tinnitus and numbness on the right side of her face below the cheek and mouth since a cervical surgery six years before. In this recent bout, both the tinnitus and numbness became constant, gradually leading to severe hearing loss in the right ear and slight loss of hearing in the left ear.

The patient was thin but appeared to be generally healthy. She had a slight deviation of the mouth toward the left (away from the area of numbness). Her pulse was thin and slightly wiry, and her tongue was red with reduced coating. Channel palpation revealed a line of thin, tender nodules along the heart *shào yīn* channel near the wrist. There was also a puffy, tender area on the kidney *shào yīn* channel around KI-4 *(dà zhōng)*. On the face, the *shào yáng* channel behind the ear did not show nodules or tenderness (less likely *shào yáng* involvement) while small, hard nodules could be felt to the right of CV-24 *(chéng jiāng)*.

Diagnosis   *Shào yīn* qi deficiency failing to send the clear yang upward

Treatment   The lead points in this case were HT-5 and KI-4. Both *shào yīn* collateral points, this pair has a more specific effect on the collaterals of the *shào yīn* channel, as opposed to the yin collaterals of the brain and heart in the pair HT-5 and KI-6. KI-7 *(fù liū)*, the mother point on the *shào yīn* channel in the five-phase system, was used as well to benefit kidney yin in order to facilitate the generation of clear yang. A 1-inch needle was also inserted at a very shallow depth into the nodule at CV-24.

There were a total of three treatments over a two-week period, with the second and third treatments involving the addition of CV-6 *(qì hǎi)* to facilitate the clear yang and ST-7 *(xià guān)* to improve qi circulation on the face.

Stimulation   One-inch needles were used at all points, with a radiating sensation at HT-5 and a distending sensation from KI-4. An especially gentle technique was used at the point next to CV-24, likened to dropping a stone into a pond. A very light twirling technique was used with the intent of creating a gentle radiating sensation throughout the right side of the face (Fig. 6.15).

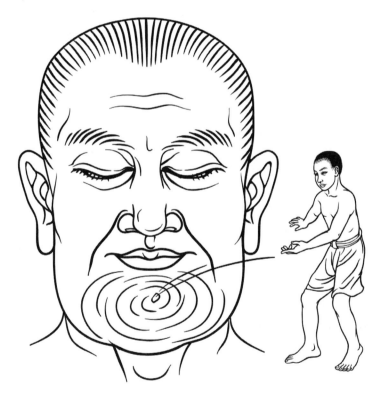

Fig. 6.15
Stimulation of a nodule found next to CV-24 *(chéng jiāng)*
was likened to "dropping a stone in a pond", i.e.,
gentle-twirling with a faint radiating sensation.

In the final two treatments, a 1.5-inch needle at CV-6 was combined with a heat lamp to warm the kidney yang. A 1-inch needle was also used at ST-7 with the same gentle twirling technique described above.

Results   The patient reported immediate improvement in the ringing of the ears and, when she came for the second treatment four days later, reported that the ringing continued to diminish. The addition of CV-6 in the second treatment seemed to broaden the scope of improvement, as she reported that her hearing had dramatically improved and that the ear ringing was only barely noticeable when she came for the third treatment. The deviation remained to some degree on her face, while the numbness was less.

Analysis   This is an interesting case both for the relative simplicity of the treatment and the quickness of the patient's recovery. The case highlights the importance of careful channel palpation in facilitating proper point selection, as KI-4 is not always the first point that comes to mind in cases of hearing loss. As a collateral point, however, it is appropriate to benefit microcirculation (collaterals) in the ears. Also, it is often the case that a sudden symptom presentation like this might lead to a diagnosis of *shào yáng* involvement. Of course, as the pathway of source qi in the body, the *shào yáng* channel may have been helpful in this case, but recovery time would likely have been longer. Considerations of *shào yīn* qi dynamic led to the inclusion of CV-6 to benefit the ascending of clear yang.

Checking on the face itself for small changes and nodules along the channel pathways is also a very important aspect of all treatments involving the head. The small lymph nodes of the face and neck often show small changes in chronic conditions and should be palpated very slowly and carefully.

It is also significant in this case that the general yin collateral point pair HT-5 and KI-6 was passed over in favor of the very specific *shào yīn* collateral point pair HT-5 and KI-4. In this case, because the condition seemed clearly to be associated with *shào yīn* in particular and not with microcirculation in general, it was deemed less appropriate to use the *yīn qiāo* command point (KI-6). As mentioned above, the *yīn qiāo* command point, when combined with HT-5, has a specific effect on collateral circulation in the heart, brain, and speech areas.

■ CASE NO. 3

41-year-old female

Chief complaint   Dementia

History of present illness   This patient had a history of high blood pressure. During the previous year she had also begun to develop signs of disorientation and dementia along with increased irritability. Recently, her family had even found her standing in the bathroom for hours in the morning in a state of disorientation. Pharmaceutical and herbal medications had stabilized her blood pressure, but the cognitive symptoms remained months later. Channel palpation revealed noticeable change along the *shào yīn* heart channel.

Diagnosis   Heat in the yin collaterals

Treatment   The pair HT-5 and KI-6 were needled bilaterally with 1-inch needles. These were the only points used.

Stimulation   Slight draining technique twice weekly for three weeks.

Results   The cognitive symptoms resolved fairly quickly over the period of a few weeks. The patient continued to use medication to stabilize her blood pressure.

Analysis   This short case highlights the importance of clearing heat and stasis from the yin collaterals in the early stages of what was likely a series of minor strokes. If the patient is treated fairly quickly, the prognosis is much better.

■ Narrative

THE SPIRIT OF CHINESE MEDICINE

The concept of spirit was discussed in the previous chapter. In our discussions about the functions of the *shào yīn* system, I would often try to steer the conversation toward the subject of how Dr. Wang's understanding of the five psychic aspects and the interplay of the seven emotions applied in the clinic. The discussion would inevitably be very interesting, not only because these are concepts about which Dr. Wang has thought a great deal, but also because of what it revealed about my own preconceptions. Specifically, we both came to realize that there were some fairly profound differences in what we meant by the term 'spirit' (神 *shén*) and 'spiritual' (心靈的 *xīn líng de*).

Many students who come to China in the early 21st century are looking for the 'spiritual side' of the medicine and are disappointed to find huge, underfunded hospitals full of poor people with non-existential complaints. A two-week tour of a major big city hospital or even a four-year course in undergraduate TCM training in China leaves gaping holes of expectation. So many have had these types of experience that we often hear complaints about how the communists have vacuumed the 'spirit' right out of the *Inner Classic* in their efforts to create a traditional medical edifice worthy of respect from their Western scientific colleagues.

What happened to Chinese medicine? Where is the qi of the medicine today? Did it ever "have qi" as we understand that statement outside of China? In fact, the very concept of qi seems to always be the goal on the ever-receding horizon, that unattainable philosopher's stone within the mind's eye of Chinese medicine. What is a clear, concise, and (especially to the mind of the 21st century) 'provable' definition of qi? Is it possible that we have built up a romanticized idea that existed neither in modern China nor in the mists of history? These are the questions that many students are asking as the field enters a new stage of maturity, where texts are not accepted without question, and the claims that we make as healers are coming under increasing scrutiny. Of course, my conversations with Dr. Wang didn't answer all of these questions, as these are subjects that could fill books or stretch over an entire career.

Just finding a way to convey these questions as a non-Chinese student in China is a challenge. First of all, what exactly is the question? What do we mean as students when we say that we are interested in the 'spiritual side' of Chinese medicine? Are we talking about *qì gōng*, about applications for psychology, about mystical Daoism, or the Chinese understanding of the somatization of disease? Often, students don't even know specifically what it is they want to learn. Instead, there is simply a sense that there must be more going on beneath the surface, given the tantalizing hints in basic textbooks about spirit, souls, and destiny.

The problem of framing the question is compounded by the fact that one of the greatest gulfs that exists between the Chinese TCM establishment and non-Chinese students of Chinese medicine is caused by subtle stereotypes. These have led to different expectations about the basic goals and motivations of each side. For example, many Chinese practitioners who have had less experience with foreigners believe that non-Chinese have a lack of interest in what are often termed "superstitions." This belief is compounded by a widely-held conviction in China on the part of many TCM professionals and the Chinese public at large that Chinese medicine is a web of mystery upon mystery that the occidental mind will never be able to fully penetrate. Now, contrast these perceptions with the expectations of practitioners who arrive in China to study and are often seekers of esoteric knowledge. They are often met by teachers and Chinese friends who are under the impression that they could not possibly have any interest in the "mysterious" sides of Chinese medicine. In any case, most Chinese believe that any such knowledge is beyond the comprehension of a non-Chinese mind. This is not a setting for good communication.

One cool fall day, Dr. Wang and I came back to the clinic after lunch to talk over a backlog of questions that I had gathered while trying to understand qi transformation in the *shào yīn* system. We had been going over and over the concepts of essence and gate of vitality and I had asked variations on the same questions from a variety of angles. We were both a bit frustrated, I think, by the inability of the other to understand what was being said. This was one of those situations where it wasn't so much that we were misunderstanding each other's words, but that we couldn't quite get to the heart of what the other person meant. It was a clear case of a cultural gap.

I had been confused and frustrated by a few concepts that had actually seemed fairly straightforward to me a few years back. Basically, I kept asking questions along the lines of what is the relationship of the essence to the fire at the gate of vitality? And exactly how do the heart and kidney regulate each other's qi dynamic? Of course, I had in my mind the explanations of many teachers, textbooks, fellow students, and Dr. Wang himself to this same question. It just didn't seem to be enough that, simply put, "the water-natured kidney acts to balance the fire-natured heart in a raising and lowering pivot that provides movement." Thinking back on the conversation, I think that I wanted an answer that spoke of 'ancestors' and 'spirit'. Because of those expectations, I wanted to hear something like "The yin essence of the ancestors is enlivened by the yang presence of the spirit." Even more confounding, though, was the fact that sometimes Dr. Wang would in fact make 'spiritual' statements about the relationships of the organs to the five psychic aspects.

After about an hour of conversation that ranged from the etymology of the Chinese character we translate as 'essence' (精 *jīng*) to the various uses of the term 'spirit' in modern Chinese, we put the question aside. The results of that conversation, and many others like it, are drawn out as carefully as possible in the previous chapter.

Finally, we both sat back for a moment, and I put the question to him in a different way.

QUESTION: Dr. Wang, you've taught in foreign countries and run into students of all types who are interested in Chinese medicine. You must know what I mean when I describe the tendency of students to want to hear more about the 'spiritual side' of Chinese medicine. We often hear people say that the communists removed everything that had soul and left a shell that tries to satisfy a Western scientific approach. Students always wake up if the teacher makes any mention of the seven emotions or ghost points or Daoist acupuncture styles. What do you make of all of this? Is it accurate to say these things? Is it worthwhile to pursue these aspects of classical Chinese medicine?

DR. WANG: I know what you mean by asking this question. In the 1970s, during the early stages of the recent interest in Chinese medicine, there were more than a few instances where foreign students came to me wanting to study such things as stem and branch point selection (子午流註 *zǐ wǔ liú zhù*), five periods and six qi (五運六氣 *wǔ yùn liù qì*), and the Daoist spiritual turtle tradition (靈龜八法 *líng guī bā fǎ*). We studied some of these acupuncture styles as part of our training back in the 1950s and I was initially very interested as well. It's a misconception, in my opinion, to say that the Communist Party conducted an active campaign to "remove superstitions" from Chinese medicine in the early stages of developing the system that we now call TCM (中醫 *zhōng yī*). It might be true to say that, in the realm of religion or other aspects of daily life, government policy later (especially during the Cultural Revolution) did serve to eliminate what were termed "feudal relics of thought." With regard to Chinese medicine, however, the official policy at first was to collect under one roof all of the traditions that could possibly be found and then to research which ones had merit.

You should remember that this codification was going on during the decade before the especially disruptive Cultural Revolution. In the 1950s, we studied with teachers who taught detailed methods for determining the 'open' point in stem and branch theory, and others who discussed the possibilities for using the five periods and six qi to predict in advance the onset of illness and to guide herbal treatment. These ideas were very prevalent in the early decades at the Beijing University of TCM. In fact, there are still official textbooks today on some of these subjects.

I spent some time in the clinic with the doctors who taught these theories, however, and found that often they wouldn't really be applying the approach on real patients. For example, if they were treating a patient using the stem and branch approach, they might use the open points but would always add a few others that addressed the patient's chief complaint. Whether or not this is part of that style of acupuncture, the most important thing to me is that there didn't seem to be a difference in clinical results when they used the open points versus simply using more common acupuncture approaches. Also, I tried using the stem and branch approach myself for awhile in the clinic in the 1970s and was never impressed with the results. These approaches may still have some validity; I just don't see it in my own work.

In my opinion, the same is true for many of these styles that don't emphasize symptom differentiation and physiological considerations as the primary determinants of treatment strategy. Yes, they have survived for centuries in China, often as a means by which doctors created a mystique around themselves while enhancing their reputation for depth of study and breadth of perception. Of course, as we know, there is a certain benefit to treatment outcomes when a patient believes strongly in the skills of the doctor. In the end, however, the reason there has been less emphasis on these traditions in recent decades is not because of any concerted effort on the part of the TCM authorities. Instead, it is a reflection of the fact that they have proven to be less effective for treating actual patients. I think these ideas are important as a reflection of Chinese culture and the history of Chinese medicine, but they shouldn't become the object of much effort by students who are searching for clinical efficacy.

Nevertheless, there are aspects of Chinese medical theory that, in my mind, represent under-researched areas of development for the future. I think that the concepts of the seven emotions and the five psychic aspects, for instance, actually represent a very subtle understanding of psychology as practiced here in China for centuries. At first glance, they may seem very simplistic, but by keeping these general guidelines in mind, the practitioner can gain some very helpful insights into pathology.

For example, do you remember that patient who came in here this morning with chronic cough, chest pains, and dizziness who was absolutely terrified of getting SARS [severe acute respiratory syndrome] after the outbreak here a few months ago? She has undergone a battery of Western medical diagnostic tests without any definitive conclusion. Channel palpation and organ diagnosis also showed no real indication of a serious disorder, but she is nevertheless obviously coughing and has pain in her chest. This is a type of patient that can best be addressed in Chinese medicine by using what you might term the 'spiritual' ideas from our tradition. This woman's condition remains one that involves the seven emotions, specifically the *shào yīn* kidney, as her overriding emotional state is one of fear. The condition is not so advanced that it has actually affected a psychic aspect, to the point where a modern psychologist might diagnose 'psychosis'.

Thinking along these lines can produce clinical results. The specific lessons that classical Chinese medicine provides about psychology are ones that do merit further research. Other ideas that you or others might call 'spiritual' (and that I personally believe to have merit) include the eight extraordinary vessels and the multitude of techniques to improve qi circulation through breath and movement, among others.

I continue to believe that, by and large, those who wrote the ancient texts that have survived the test of time were not kidding us. Problems with utilizing all of the information that those texts provide are largely due to our inability to really understand what they are talking about. Sometimes, modern readers misinterpret classical texts and end up going down pathways that are interesting in an academic sense, but of little clinical value. This problem, of course, is heightened by difficulties with proper translation and I therefore hope that the information in other languages can be as good as possible. To be honest, by the way, I have no idea what term you are using in English for this idea of 'spiritual'. Even in Chinese, the term means different things to different people. Remember that, to me, the character *shén* (神) refers to the intelligence of existence. It is an innate intelligence that, when the heart is healthy, any person or animal might have. This intelligence is also present in the world at large. I know that the definition is broad, but so is its meaning. People in China today even speak of the sounds of thunder or earthquakes as somehow representing the mysterious intelligence of *shén*.

Whatever you might call them, there are certainly concepts in classical texts that have been underemphasized in our schools that at least deserve further study. In many cases, the main reason this hasn't happened is that resources and priorities have been elsewhere. Resources have been primarily focused on addressing the pressing issues of more commonly seen diseases.

Now, there is another trend in schools of Chinese medicine since the 1950s that may also have contributed to the impression that many foreign students have after coming to China to study. This is the trend toward an emphasis on Western medicine at the expense of Chinese medicine. When I studied at the Beijing University of TCM, around twenty percent of our coursework involved Western science and treatment. Of course, we spent time learning modern anatomy and physiology and basic principles of Western medical treatment, but, when it came down to preparing for clinical practice, it was about learning Chinese medicine. In fact, some of the best teachers those days talked very little about Western medicine. Anyone will tell you now that up to sixty percent of the coursework and clinical work these days involves Western medicine. Because of this shift in emphasis, many TCM doctors are more comfortable talking about diseases within the framework of Western medicine and are less inclined to discuss some of the classical physiological concepts that inevitably interest foreign students.

Another trend that began in the 1950s was a more Western-style differentiation of disease into strict types (分性 *fēn xìng*).

Although this approach still separated disease into classical categories, it created a kind of artificial structure with very clear lines that were previously not there. For example, most modern TCM practitioners in the West, and even in China, think very strictly in categories like 'spleen qi deficiency' and 'heart blood deficiency' as ways of describing dysfunction in the qi dynamic. While this is not necessarily a direct infusion of Western medicine into our tradition, it does represent a fundamental change in the way we see things. It takes away some of the flexibility inherent in a system of interrelated channels. This is a hard thing for me to explain clearly.

QUESTION: Well, is there a better way that you can think of to understand pathomechanism in Chinese medicine?

DR. WANG: That's just the thing. If you are going to teach students in a large university setting, there really isn't a better option. It isn't hopeless, however. The thing to remember is that the differentiation of disease taught in the TCM schools is just a starting point, a structure that you must eventually outgrow. So maybe the 'spirit' is found when you outgrow that initial structure!

厥陰

The *Jué Yīn* (Terminal Yin) System

The General Nature and Function of *Jué Yīn*

Jué yīn RESTS at "the inside of the inside" of the channel system. Composed of the pericardium and liver, the *jué yīn* level is one of retreat, storage, and rejuvenation. Of the six external qi, *jué yīn* is associated with wind. The movement and chaos of wind is anathema to the restfulness of *jué yīn*. Thus healthy qi transformation by the liver and pericardium help create an environment in which the destructive power of wind cannot arise. To be specific, both the disease-bearing winds of the external environment and the moving diseases of internal wind are calmed by the fullness of *jué yīn* blood. As nourishment defines the nature of *tài yīn* and regulation the nature of *shào yīn*, the *jué yīn* level is specifically associated with the blood. The pericardium, a broader concept in Chinese medicine than in other medical systems, protects the heart with yin blood. The liver holds blood in reserve and distributes according to need by dredging and draining (疏瀉 *shū xiè*) the pathways of qi.

Many classical texts assert that "blood is the mother of qi, and qi is the commander of blood" (血為氣之母, 氣為血之帥 *xuè wéi qì zhī mǔ, qì wéi xuè zhī shuài*). *Jué yīn* plays an important role in the qi-blood relationship. The pathways of qi are maintained by the liver, and qi depends on the fullness of *jué yīn* blood for nourishment. When the body sleeps, blood returns to *jué yīn*, where it settles and clarifies. Within *jué yīn*, the blood is stored and clarified by the liver while the qi of emotional excess is held, calmed, and released by the pericardium. Among the six yin channels, *jué yīn* closes inward (闔 *hé*).

In the Chinese names for each of the six levels, one is struck by the fact that both the innermost yin and yang levels seem to have unique nomenclature. The first two levels in both the yin and yang aspects have the same characters in the first position. The most outward level of yang is called *tài* (太) *yáng* and is mirrored by the most outward level of yin at *tài yīn*. In both cases, *tài* means largest or greatest. This suggests expansiveness, which is reflected in the descriptive term *kāi* (開) used to describe the open, outward-directed movement of the *tài* levels. Similarly, the second yin and yang levels are termed *shào* (少) *yáng* and *shào yīn*; in both cases, *shào* means lesser, as in less than that which came before. Channel theory asserts that both *shào* levels are pivots (樞 *shū).* (This *shū*, by the way, is not the same character as that used to refer to the back *shū* 腧 points, which conveys a meaning of transport or conveyance through muscle.) Finally, both the yin and yang levels reach their innermost at the *yáng míng* and *jué yīn* respectively. The *yáng míng* (陽明) characters will be discussed later, but their unique status should be noted[1] (Table 7.1).

		Defining Character	General Meaning
Open 開 *kāi*	*tài yáng* (太陽)	太 *tài*	Highest, greatest, excessive, extreme
	tài yīn (太陰)		
Pivot 樞 *shū*	*shào yáng* (少陽)	少 *shào*	Lesser, young
	shào yīn (少陰)		
Close 闔 *hé*	*yáng míng* (阳明)	明 *míng*	Bright, clear
	jué yīn (厥陰)	厥 *jué*	Reverting, retreat

Table 7.1

The defining character of the six levels

The medical meaning of the Chinese word *jué* (厥) has been difficult to understand for both modern Chinese and Western students. In modern colloquial Chinese, the character most often means to faint or collapse. This reflects another traditional medical use of the same character, originally found in *Essentials from the Golden Cabinet,* where it refers to a reversal of qi flow that leads to the specific condition of loss of consciousness. The term usually translated as rebellion or counterflow (逆 *nì*) also refers to a reversal of qi flow, but in a situation where qi transformation is compromised but there is no loss of consciousness; stomach qi or liver qi ascending are examples. *Jué* can also be used to describe a situation where the yang, instead of flowing to the extremities, is retreating inward; this is referred to as 'inversion cold' or 'reversal cold' of the extremities.

Elsewhere the term *jué yīn* is translated as 'terminal yin', reflecting its position at the end or apex of yin. Wiseman translates *jué* as 'reversal' and thus *jué yīn* as 'reverting yin'. This is because the term *jué* is said to imply that, as yin reaches its apex, it reverts to yang. To the image of reverting, it is helpful to add the idea of retreat and all that this term might imply. In other words, *jué* does describe a reversion toward yang, but also something more: a retreat away from the exterior toward rest and rejuvenation. This apparent contradiction highlights the dual nature of *jué yīn*: it is a closing inward, but within itself holds the seed for a reversion toward yang.

The character for *jué* (厥) has an interesting construction. The outside of this character comes from the obsolete character 厂 (*hàn)*, a partial enclosure that means cliff, as on the side of a mountain. The inside of the character is a variant of the commonly used *quē* (缺), which usually means lacking, but can also mean vacant or an opening. The character 厥 (*jué*) therefore suggests an opening or vacancy on the side of a mountain. It is a place of absolute stillness and retreat from which one begins the process of 'reverting' back to yang. Recall the Daoist influence on Chinese medicine, and it is not difficult to imagine the adepts of a thousand years past retreating to their caves in the mountains. This is a helpful image for *jué yīn* but is at odds, in some respects, with a commonly held belief by many modern practitioners who think of *jué yīn* as a moving cauldron of emotions. Of course, for many modern patients, the cave of retreat may in fact be filled with just such chaos! In such cases, yin and blood will not have a place for restoration (Fig. 7.1).

厂	Partial enclosure; an opening in the side of a mountain; a cliff
欮	Variation of 缺 *quē;* lacking; absent

Fig. 7.1
The defining character (厥 *jué*) in the term *jué yīn* is composed of two classifiers, which bring to mind an empty cave in the side of a mountain.

Returning now to the *jué yīn* channel, its functions are to foster yin (育 陰 *yù yīn*), nourish blood (養血 *yǎng xuè*), and regulate the distribution of blood to the other channels (調血 *tiáo xuè*). Many modern texts also assign to the *jué yīn* organs and/or channels the function of 'spirit calming'. While not strictly a function of the liver and pericardium, there is nonetheless an important relationship between the concepts of blood and spirit in Chinese medicine. The blood must ultimately nourish the spirit, which is stored in the heart. The specific relationship of the liver to spirit is exemplified by the ethereal soul-spirit relationship, discussed below.

The concept of wind and its relationship to blood is important for understanding both the physiology and pathology of *jué yīn*. The *Inner Classic* associates wind with the season of spring. This is likely due to the strong spring winds experienced along the Yellow River (around modern Shanxi), the locale from which the *Inner Classic* emerged. However, as Chinese medicine evolved over the centuries, so too did the physiological concept of wind. Later physicians associated sudden changes in the weather at any time of year with wind, as they did sudden changes in the body's inner landscape. Chapter 42 of *Basic Questions*, entitled "Discussion of Wind," says that wind "has a tendency to move and frequently change" (善行而數變 *shàn xíng ér shuò biàn*). Patients who suddenly become ill or whose illness changes quickly are therefore said to be afflicted with a wind-type pathogen. Diagnosis in these cases should include palpation of the *jué yīn* channels.

Symptoms associated with wind include twitching and muscle spasms, skin rashes which come and go, and nearly any other condition that involves a sudden onset or tendency to change. When properly functioning, the *jué yīn* channel facilitates the body's infusion of the gentle winds of springtime while preventing injury from the strong and potentially destructive winds of autumn. The operative concept here is that when healthy blood fills the vessels, it can prevent the invasion of pathogenic wind. Wind fills the vessels in the absence—or 'insufficiency'—of blood.[2] This could be blood insufficiency in general, or a problem with proper assignment of blood by the liver to the area that is afflicted. Both causes can arise from a dysfunction of *jué yīn*, and will be discussed below.

The two terms most often associated with the *jué yīn* function of preventing damage from wind are dredging (疏 *shū*) and extinguishing (熄 *xī*). Dredging is associated with the thrusting of external wind pathogens out of the body, while extinguishing relates to calming internal wind. Different *jué yīn* functions are associated with the two treatment approaches. In the case of dredging external wind, the liver *jué yīn* function of dredging and moving qi is particularly helpful, as movement lifts wind upward and outward to the yang levels of the body where it can be released from the surface. Extinguishing internal wind, on the other hand, depends more on the provision of blood from both the pericardium and liver so that the reckless movement of internal wind can be calmed by the fullness of blood. Different treatment principles will require different acupuncture points and herbs. Nevertheless, even in the case of dredging external wind, the blood provides a vital role. If *jué yīn* blood is deficient, then dredging (especially with herbs) may actually generate wind rather than releasing it outward.

Pericardium

"The center of the chest [i.e., pericardium] holds the office of governmental envoy; happiness issues from it."

(膻中者．臣使之官．喜樂出焉。Tán zhōng zhě, chén shǐ zhī guān, xǐ lè chū yān.)

—*Basic Questions*, Chapter 8

The pericardium is the envoy of the heart. The Chinese term for envoy is *chén shǐ* (臣使), which can also be translated as official or secretary. In China this term usually refers to government officials who have weathered the fire of the imperial civil service exam system. Considering the functions of the pericardium, the term envoy is most appropriate. Like modern envoys, the function of the pericardium is to facilitate communication. But unlike modern envoys, the pericardium must also act as a defender, guarding the palace from attack, and protecting the emperor from treachery. The pericardium is thus charged with both cushioning the effects of assaults from the outside and disseminating the commands and moods inside from the heart.

It is important to differentiate the functions of the pericardium from those of the lung in its relationship to the heart. The *Inner Classic* describes the lung as being, "like a prime minister, the issuer of management and regulation," while the pericardium is likened to an envoy. An envoy is entirely dependent on its monarch for instructions and guidance; its functions are interwoven with those of the heart. By contrast, the prime minister has distinct functions of his own, as delegated by the emperor. Moreover, the functions of the lung are quite different from those of the heart: the lung commands the qi while the heart moves the blood. In the case of the pericardium, its sole purpose is to serve as envoy/protector of the heart; the functions of the heart and pericardium are thus more difficult to separate (Fig. 7.2).

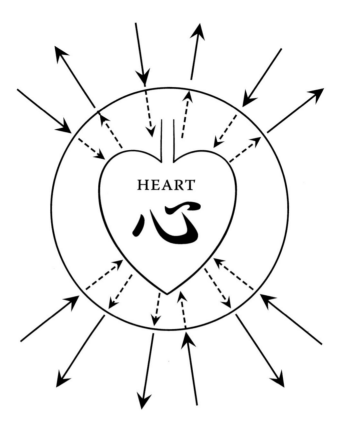

Fig. 7.2
The pericardium, woven to the heart, protects from exterior excess
while facilitating outward communication.

. . . .

The *Inner Classic* also says that happiness issues from the pericardium.
Like an envoy to the emperor, the pericardium keeps the lines of communication open to and from the heart. If pericardium function is compromised,
the ability of heart qi to disseminate is effectively blocked. Proper pericardium function keeps the heart open, while dysfunction can lead to constriction and emotional disorders. Therefore, while the influence of the seven
emotions can be felt by the heart, it is the pericardium that helps maintain
the peace. Stagnation of qi and blood in the pericardium may consequently
affect the ability of the heart to properly integrate the emotions.

The pericardium is situated below the heart and above the diaphragm. It
connects to the heart on the inside and to the lungs on the outside. Usually
called 'the sixth yin organ', the pericardium is also sometimes viewed as a
sub-category of the heart.

FUNCTIONS OF THE PERICARDIUM

Protects the heart

Because of the unique status of the pericardium as the 'sixth yin organ', its functions are discussed less than the other organs in early classical sources. Descriptions are more frequent in later centuries, particularly in discussions of heat-type disease in the late Ming and Qing dynasties. Texts such as the *Discussion of Warm-Heat Pathogen [Disorders]* (溫熱論 *Wēn rè lùn*) by Ye Tian-Shi (葉天士) and the *Systematic Differentiation of Warm Pathogen Diseases* (溫病條辯 *Wēn bìng tiǎo biàn*) by Wu Ju-Tong (吳鞠通) emphasize the importance of the pericardium as a protector from and recipient of external heat. Like a bodyguard, the pericardium is said to integrate pathogens that might otherwise damage the heart. In the estimation of these texts, if the pericardium has a deficiency of blood, then the heart is more likely to be damaged.

It is important to once again emphasize that, in addition to protecting the heart from external pathogens, the pericardium integrates excess coming outward from the heart. For example, where there has been an excess of physical activity, the pericardium provides blood and nourishment while absorbing and releasing generated heat. Similarly, emotional excess in the heart is absorbed and released via the pericardium.

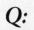

Q: *In my mind, I still can't separate the pericardium from the heart. What exactly is meant by the pericardium? Is this the same thing as the lining around the heart referred to in modern anatomical textbooks?*

DR. WANG: In my experience, what we refer to in Chinese medicine as the pericardium includes both the lining and important aspects of the heart organ itself. Remember that *jué yīn* is more yin and therefore more materially substantial than *shào yīn*. *Jué yīn* is deep in the blood vessels and thus the pericardium might be thought of as being equivalent to the blood engorging the heart muscle. *Jué yīn* is the reservoir of blood that surrounds the heart to support movement in the pivot of *shào yīn* (Fig. 7.3).

This idea is supported by clinical experience. For example, in cases of angina where there is a blockage in coronary blood circulation, the *jué yīn* pericardium channel will often have palpable changes along the arm below the elbow. In this type of case, *jué yīn* points like PC-4 (*xī mén*)—the cleft (*xī*) point—are appropriate for treatment. What

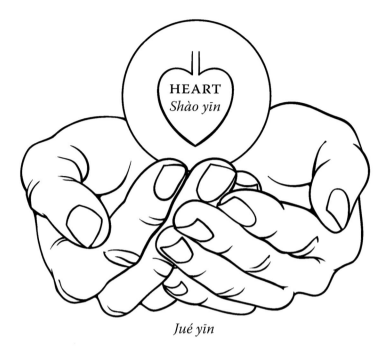

Jué yīn

Fig. 7.3
Blood from *jué yīn* protects and holds the heart.

is called the heart, on the other hand, to me is associated with the movement and function of the heart organ. For example, cases of irregular heartbeat, where there are problems with the conduction system in the heart, are more often associated with palpable changes on the *shào yīn* heart channel, especially in the area between HT-5 *(tōng lǐ)* and HT-7 *(shén mén)*. In general, you shouldn't get too caught up in thinking about the pericardium organ as being physically outside of and surrounding the heart organ. Instead, think about *jué yīn* and the deep abundance of yin-blood that arises from there. By reflecting on the functional relationship of *jué yīn* blood to *shào yīn* movement, you will proceed further in your understanding of patients in the clinic.

Also, as I've pointed out before, descriptions of the heart and pericardium often overlap in classical texts. We always say that there are five yin organs and six yang organs while ignoring the obvious fact that, when you count the pericardium, there are actually six yin organs. If you consider the most ancient information that we still have (much has been lost), one might actually conclude that the so-called five yin organs actually include the pericardium and *not* the heart.

This is because the ancient texts considered the pericardium as a 'stand in' for the heart as its envoy. In any case, there is a clinical tendency for both the pericardium and heart channels to show palpable change in the presence of heart disease. More important is the ability of both channels to be helpful *in the treatment* of heart disease. The key is to know which pathodynamic is more likely to be associated with each channel, and then verify with palpation.

Clinical pearls of wisdom about pericardium pathology

• *Discussion of Warm-Heat Pathogen [Disorders]* describes the pathodynamic whereby externally-contracted heat disease progresses from the external *tài yáng* level to the lung *tài yīn* and, from there, to the pericardium, where it becomes 'trapped' in the chest. Symptoms of this pattern include high fever that doesn't abate and breathing difficulty with tightness in the chest. Externally-contracted disorders may therefore quickly affect the pericardium.

• Because of the association of the pericardium with the blood and muscle of the heart, arteriosclerosis often manifests as palpable changes on the pericardium channel. These changes are most commonly found around (and can be treated with) the cleft point, PC-4 *(xī mén)*.

Liver

> "The liver holds the office of general and is the issuer of strategies and planning."
>
> (肝者. 將軍之官. 謀慮出焉。 *Gān zhě, jiāng jūn zhī guān, mó lǜ chū yān.*)
>
> —*Basic Questions*, Chapter 8

The comparison of the liver to a general is likely to be familiar to students of Chinese medicine. The passage cited above is the first known use of this metaphor. The liver is also often described as being prepared to "storm the fortifications in pursuit of bandits" (攻堅伐賊 *gōng jiān fá zéi*). It can be quick and resolute in developing strategies for both protection and attack.

At first, the image of a general seems to be at odds with the idea of *jué yīn* as a place of quiet refuge. Remember, however, that a general commands the chaos of war from the relative calm of a strategic headquarters. Resting at the level of *jué yīn*, the liver stores great reserves of yin blood. When healthy, the liver is like a general with all his supplies at the ready, both peaceful and alert.

The liver has the ability to react quickly to changes in the diverse environments of the internal landscape. Despite coming from a place of deep stillness, the liver is charged with mobilizing the body's defenses. While protective qi has a similar function on the surface of the body, the liver moves in the deep interior, making strategies and clearing the pathways of qi.

The liver organ collects around the 9th thoracic vertebra. Classical anatomy places it in front of both the right aspect of the large intestine and the right kidney, at the same level as the stomach.

FUNCTIONS OF THE LIVER

Dredges, drains, and regulates (疏瀉調節 shū xiè tiáo jié)

The word translated as dredging (疏 shū) is associated with the dredging of ditches and describes the role of the liver in maintaining the flow of qi, especially among the internal organs. The dredging function also facilitates the draining of accumulated qi. Referring again to the metaphor of the general, an effective strategist keeps all options open and keeps the supply lines open and moving. While possessing the resolution to "storm the fortifications," the liver also dredges the pathways to maintain communication when more aggressive methods are not needed.

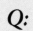 **Q:** *When hearing this, I'm reminded of some of the uses of tài yīn in regulating qi. You mentioned that the lung is the "commander of the entire body's qi" and thus has a regulating effect. What is the difference in the clinic between tài yīn versus jué yīn in cases of qi counterflow?*

DR. WANG: *Tài yīn* is the ultimate source of qi regulation, as the lung is the commander of the entire body's qi. The liver, on the other hand, is charged with dredging and draining and thus loosens and opens the pathways of qi when they're blocked. But it doesn't regulate qi in the same broad way that one sees at *tài yīn*. This, by the way, is the reason why I begin treatment of so many patients with the pair of uniting *(hé)* points LU-5 *(chǐ zé)* and SP-9 *(yīn líng quán)*. Uniting points are said to reverse counterflow; that is, when qi is flowing the wrong way, the uniting points are used to get it back in the right direction. In the end, the special effect of the pair LU-5 *(chǐ zé)* and SP-9 *(yīn líng quán)* as a regulator draws on the lung's responsibility for the entire body's qi.

The use of *jué yīn* points may also have some regulating effects on qi transformation when there is counterflow. In cases where the qi is really stuck and heat is beginning to form, one might want to 'dredge and drain' *jué yīn*. Again, the liver opens up the passageways. In this case, *jué yīn* treatment might be considered a form of 'regulating' in that it regulates by opening and facilitating the flow. This is different than the lung *tài yīn* function of regulating the rhythms of qi for the entire body.

Now, to make things even more complicated, if there are chronic *jué yīn* problems where a lack of proper dredging and draining has led to heat, I wouldn't choose the *jué yīn* channel for treatment. Instead, this is a situation where one would use the paired yang channel to drain yin channel excess. I would consider using the point pair TB-5 *(wài guān)* and GB-41 *(zú lín qì)* when heat is present, or TB-6 *(zhī gōu)* and GB-34 *(yáng líng quán)* where there is significant qi stasis. The affected channel is still *jué yīn*, but the channel chosen for treatment is *shào yáng*. (The selection of channels for treatment will be discussed in Chapter 14.)

To summarize, *tài yīn* regulates when the qi is going the wrong way, while *jué yīn* dredges and drains when the qi is stuck and not moving (Table 7.2).

	Effect on Qi Transformation	Illustrative Point Pair
Tài yīn	Regulates / re-establishes proper movement in qi counterflow	LU-5 *(chǐ zé)* and SP-9 *(yīn líng quán)*; *hé*-sea points regulate counterflow
Jué yīn	Dredges and opens the pathways of qi	TB-5 *(wài guān)* and GB-41 *(zú lín qì)*; when heat is present
		TB-6 *(zhī gōu)* and GB-34 *(yáng líng quán)*; qi stasis dominates

Table 7.2
Tài yīn, jué yīn, and qi transformation

Stores blood and nourishes the sinews (藏血養筋 *cáng xuè yǎng jīn*)

The liver function of storing blood includes the determination of where blood should go. In this case, the concept that yin 'reverts' is illustrative.

Namely, after circulating to the *jué yīn* level to settle and clarify, blood reverts outward to where it is needed. Consequently, metabolic functions which involve the regulation of blood flow to particular organs or to the sinews and muscles involve liver function in Chinese medicine. Specifically, there are three aspects to the relationship of the liver to blood:

1. The storage of blood.
2. The assignment of blood to particular organs.
3. The impetus for movement of blood.

Should *jué yīn* qi transformation be compromised, problems could arise with any of these three aspects. In the first, storage, the problem could involve not holding back the blood from flowing out into the vessels; this would include certain types of menorrhagia (see the related question below). Storage of blood also involves the maintenance of blood quality, what might be termed 'cleaning' the blood. Problems with cleaning the blood while it is stored could cause such symptoms as insomnia, irritability, or even dermatological issues should the ability to remove heat from the blood be compromised.

The second type of liver blood condition involves problems with the assignment of blood to areas of the body. Symptoms include muscle twitching or spasms due to an inadequate blood supply in a particular area.

The third type of liver blood disorder involves problems with the function of providing impetus for blood movement. This function is closely related to that of dredging the pathways of qi. If the smooth flow of qi is compromised, there will be concurrent problems with blood flow. A typical symptom pattern might involve congealing and astringing of blood with such symptoms as metrorrhagia (irregular onset of period). Thus, while the beating of the heart moves the blood, there is also an important role played by the liver in blood circulation. Namely, by facilitating the smooth movement of qi, one also helps the circulation of blood.

Treatment goals will differ slightly in each of these cases. For problems with storage and cleaning, the liver yin might be nourished. For problems with the assignment of blood, the liver qi dynamic should be regulated. And for problems with the movement of blood, dredging and draining is required (Table 7.3).

As always, careful differentiation of the cause and location of disease (病因 *bìng yīn*) is a necessary precondition for determining the appropriate treatment strategy. A clear understanding of qi transformation is a prerequisite for accurately determining the cause of a disease.

	Common Symptoms of Dysfunction	Treatment Strategy
Storage and cleaning (藏 *cáng*)	Storage: certain types of menorrhagia Cleaning: insomnia, irritability, skin problems	Nourish liver yin and blood
Assignment (分配 *fēn pèi*)	Twitching, organ dysfunction, tendon nourishment	Regulate *jué yīn* qi transformation
Impetus for movement (流動 *liú dòng*)	Irregular menstruation (metrorrhagia)	Dredge and drain

Table 7.3
Liver and the blood

. . . .

Stores the ethereal soul (魂 *hún*)

The ethereal soul involves a psychic aspect that manifests as courage. This is not foolhardiness or aggression, but the courage to pursue plans first seen clearly by the spirit, held in the heart. Yin-yang theory is helpful for understanding how this type of courage relates to liver function. It was noted earlier that the *Inner Classic* describes the liver as the organ from which strategy and planning issue. When developing and planning strategies for the pursuit of one's goals, it is important to maintain the delicate balance between courage and rashness. In normal physiology, the liver must be able to make swift, fearless decisions about the distribution of blood or removal of toxins, while also maintaining a degree of caution. There is a need to balance strategies for action with a careful assessment of the dangers at hand. When the assessment has been made, courage is then in order. The ethereal soul facilitates the ability of a person to wait and observe situations, relationships, or emotional conditions until the time is ripe for action, when courage is needed.

Insight into the use of medicinals such as Paeoniae Radix alba *(bái sháo)* and unprocessed Haematitum *(dài zhě shí)*, which are said to preserve (斂 *liǎn*) the liver, might be gained by considering the ethereal soul. When a patient shows a tendency to act rashly with excessive courage or foolhardiness, then preservation is an appropriate treatment strategy. Specifically, the goal is to preserve liver blood, which in turn houses the ethereal soul.

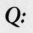

This brings to mind our discussion of the corporeal soul and its relationship to lung function. Do you have any useful insights from the Inner Classic regarding the ethereal soul and liver function?

DR. WANG: First, recall from our earlier discussion of the *Divine Pivot* that essence and the corporeal soul are said to 'enter and exit' together, while the 'comings and goings' of the spirit are with the ethereal soul (see Chapter 5). Thus, on one hand, essence (kidney) and the corporeal soul (lung) are paired, and on the other hand, spirit (heart) and the ethereal soul (liver) are paired. We also noted that the spirit-ethereal soul pair is relatively yang in nature while the essence-corporeal soul pair is yin. Furthermore, within the two yang-natured psychic aspects, the spirit is thought of as being yang within yang while the ethereal soul is yin within yang. Thus we see that these aspects have relative yin-yang relationships (Table 7.4).

		Mind	Organ	Relationship
Yang	Yang within yang	Spirit	Heart	Yang-natured ethereal soul is attracted to the deep yin-blood of the liver.
	Yin within yang	Ethereal soul	Liver	Like the beating of the heart, the spirit moves the ethereal soul (the spirit within the blood).
Yin	Yang within yin	Corporeal soul	Lung	The active qi of the lung attracts the yin-natured corporeal soul.
	Yin within yin	Essence	Kidney	The moving corporeal then stimulates essence. Qi stimulates prenatal.

Table 7.4

Relationships of psychic aspects in *Divine Pivot*, Chapter 8

Ultimately, the answer to your current question involves the relationship of the heart (spirit) to the liver (ethereal soul) and includes the concept of blood metabolism. In the most basic sense, the reservoir of *jué yīn* blood requires movement from the heart. At the same time, the heart depends on the quality of blood settled and clarified by the liver. There is a similar relationship between the ethereal soul and the spirit. Specifically, the ethereal soul is moved by the spirit, while the spirit is rooted in the body by the ethereal soul.

Also recall that when we talked about the relationship of the heart and kidney, we also said that essence helps to 'root the spirit' in the body. Essence is a prenatal rooting, which is more fixed, almost a personality-type rooting. The blood, on the other hand, is postnatal in nature and thus the ability of blood to root the spirit might be compromised by problems with the quality of blood. Both essence and blood are of course yin-natured, but relatively speaking, essence might be said to be "more yin."

In Chapter 6 on the *shào yīn* we also talked about the nature of spirit as it relates to the heart. Spirit was described as the 'intelligence of life' and was associated with the ability to clearly perceive and recognize the world around us. Thus the spirit involves the ability of a person to clearly achieve communion not only with other human beings, but even more importantly, with the qi transformation of the larger environment. The spirit, located in the heart, is 'awareness' and 'consciousness' in the largest sense (see Fig. 6.7 in the previous chapter).

Although there is a similar yang-natured movement of the ethereal soul, it is more firmly rooted because of its association with the deep yin of the liver. As was said before, the ethereal soul is associated with an observable trait that manifests as a certain kind of courage. This is courage that knows restraint. The ability to restrain and balance the courage of the ethereal soul comes from the health and quality of liver blood. A yang-natured entity, the ethereal soul is balanced by the deep yin of liver *jué yīn*.

Now, how do the spirit and ethereal soul interact? Let's first reconsider the natures of these two psychic aspects. The spirit is relatively yang-natured and, when healthy, perceives the outside world with clarity. The ethereal soul is thought of as being even more yang-natured and is associated with the trait of courage. The courage of the ethereal soul must be guided by the clear perception of the spirit. Without a clear spirit, courage may become misguided. Rashness may ensue, and the blood will become deficient in an effort to keep the ethereal soul rooted.

The *Divine Pivot* describes the ethereal soul as "coming and going" (往來 *wǎng lái*) with the spirit. It is the spirit that leads the ethereal soul, just as the beating of the heart leads the movement of blood. It is the leadership of an emperor to his general. Clear insight is crucial. When considering these more philosophical aspects of classical physiology, the key to understanding is a return to the basic concepts of qi transformation in the organs. With a clear understanding of how the organs relate to each other, one can begin to develop a picture of these relatively difficult concepts associated with the five psychic aspects.

This brings us to the manifestations of the ethereal soul in the clinic. A patient who can maintain control of their courage in stressful situations where rash action is unwarranted has a strong ethereal soul. On the other hand, a tendency toward rashness or sudden anger indicates a problem with the ethereal soul (or with perception by the spirit). Once a person gives way to uncontrolled anger, this is no longer a healthy manifestation of the psychic aspect. I have seen many patients in my life who repeatedly give in to anger and cause serious physical damage to their bodies. I truly believe that chronic, uncontrolled anger can lead to serious illness. By the way, this doesn't mean 'control' in the sense that we bottle up our anger when things happen to us. Instead, it means finding appropriate ways to view the situation (the function of the heart-spirit) and direct our actions (courage) accordingly.

One final thought. Remember that in our discussion of the corporeal soul and the lung we highlighted the fact that the essentially yin-natured corporeal soul is attracted to the movement of qi in the lung. Similarly, the yang-natured ethereal soul is attracted to the calm restfulness of the blood in the liver. Furthermore, as just noted, the corporeal soul and essence are thought to 'exit and enter' (出入 *chū rù*) together and are considered to be the more yin-natured pair. While the ethereal soul-spirit pair is yang-natured and is involved in the recognition and interaction with the outside world, the corporeal soul-essence pair is associated more with the physical body. Essence is the most fundamental material substance in the body, and the corporeal soul manifests in the strength of the body as a whole (Fig. 7.4).

Opens to the eyes

Not all eye problems are associated with the liver, but there are two significant aspects of the liver that relate to the eyes. Both are actually concerned with the relationship of the liver to the sinews.

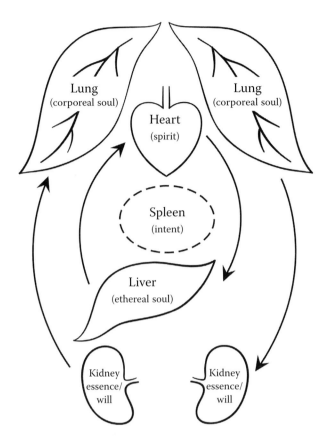

Fig. 7.4
Among the five minds, the essence (kidney) and corporeal soul (lung)
are said to 'exit and enter' together. The spirit (heart) is said to 'come
and go' with the ethereal soul (liver). Intent, housed in the spleen,
maintains a position in the center.

• Movement of the musculature of the eyes

The minute muscles of the eyes are among the 'sinews' that are nourished by the liver. Problems with the ability of the eyes to move together in
a coordinated manner would also be included in this category.

• Dilation and contraction of the pupils

Again, this is an aspect of sinew function. The inability of the eyes to
properly respond to changes in light may involve the liver. However, more
chronic problems with the pupils can be related to the kidney.

• Problems with the optic nerve

This is less a function of the relationship of the liver to the sinews than it is the liver function of assigning blood through normal dredging and draining. Just as the sinews are unable to function properly without adequate nourishment, so too is the optic nerve.

The treatment of liver-type eye problems should therefore always consider the liver's ability to nourish through proper distribution of blood. Treatment principles should involve nourishing and protecting the liver yin and blood or dredging the liver so that the proper distribution of blood is maintained.

By contrast, cases involving redness and/or increased inter-ocular pressure tend to involve the paired gallbladder organ. In these types of cases, benefiting the liver is less likely to help, and the treatment principle should instead focus on draining *shào yáng*.

Finally, a problem with relatively severe swelling and crustiness around the eyes is a damp condition and more likely involves deficiency of the spleen combined with heat (Table 7.5). (See Appendix 2 for a more extensive discussion of the treatment of eye problems.)

Organ	Common Associated Symptoms	Treatment Principle
Liver	Problems with movement of the eyes or optic nerve	Dredge and drain or regulate *jué yīn*
Gallbladder	Redness or increased inter-ocular pressure	Clear *shào yáng* excess
Spleen	Swelling or discharge from the eyes	Regulate *tài yīn* to clear damp and heat

Table 7.5

Simplified overview of organ involvement in eye conditions

CLINICAL PEARLS OF WISDOM ABOUT LIVER PATHOLOGY

- There are cases where one might diagnose an invasion of external wind into the yin collaterals. Here, an external pathogen has moved to the interior and led to chronic moving conditions that often combine with heat. For these patients, a helpful combination is PC-7 *(dà líng)* and LR-2 *(xíng jiān)*. This point pair has the effect of extinguishing wind by strongly clearing and dredging the pathways of qi (see further discussion in Chapter 20).

Additionally, this point pair is used to disperse in cases where qi stagnation in the liver coincides with blood stagnation in the pericardium. This pattern is often seen during menopause and usually also involves heat. Both uses for the pair draw from its ability to strongly clear the *jué yīn* channel (of qi stasis, wind, and heat) by dredging qi. It is helpful to take note of the interesting fact that the yin collaterals can become blocked by wind pathogens to cause chronic, moving conditions. This is in contrast to the concept of blood stasis in the yin collaterals that leads to problems with cognition/development that are associated with the *shào yīn* channel.

• Deficiency in *jué yīn* can lead to congealing and binding (凝澀 *níng sè*) due to lack of dredging, which may cause irregular bowel movements and urinary difficulty. In particular, while constipation is usually associated with the spleen or large intestine, *jué yīn* should also be considered when other signs and symptoms point in that direction.

Q: *How do you differentiate the tài yīn spleen function of 'holding blood' from the jué yīn blood functions?*

DR. WANG: My experience is that problems associated with bleeding from larger vessels are generally of a *jué yīn* type while bleeding problems associated with reuptake at the capillary/lymphatic level are more spleen type. Bleeding problems associated with heavy, severe blood flow are generally liver type. Slow, gradual leakage of blood, or problems with reabsorption, are associated with spleen dysfunction.

A clear example of this concept can be seen in the diagnosis and treatment of irregular uterine bleeding. This term has been known in Chinese medicine as 崩漏 *bēng lòu*. It includes two separate diagnoses. The first, profuse uterine bleeding (崩 *bēng*), is heavy bleeding and is associated with the liver. The second, leaking (漏 *lòu*), is characterized by smaller amounts of blood that may come at irregular times throughout the month and is associated with the spleen. The first type is often treated with LR-1 *(dà dūn)* and LR-3 *(tài chōng)* while the second calls for SP-1 *(yǐn bái)* and SP-3 *(tài bái)*. Generally, the liver type will be an excess condition and thus needling is appropriate for the liver points. In fact, if the condition also involves heat, LR-1 *(dà dūn)* can be bled for better results. The spleen type, on the other hand, is usually more of a deficient presentation and moxa is thus more appropriate on the spleen points. In both cases, the well/source point combination both stimulates qi transformation in the channel and sedates a bit to secure bleeding.

Q: *I'm still a bit confused by shào yīn and jué yīn. How can the liver-pericardium be deeper than the heart-kidney? Somehow in my mind there is a conflict with this and the fact that we have always been taught that the "kidney is the root."*

DR. WANG: There are basically three perspectives from which this question might be addressed. The first involves returning to the concept of the six levels, the second considers five-phase relationships, and a third is drawn from an analysis of the functions of the organs associated with *shào yīn* and *jué yīn*.

When considering the six levels of the channel system, *jué yīn* is traditionally thought to be 'deeper' than *shào yīn*. The general physiological principle, as discussed earlier, is that *shào yīn* is a 'pivot' while *jué yīn* 'closes' to the inside. The pivot is a place of movement and activity while the closing of *jué yīn* involves holding large reserves of yin-blood. At *jué yīn*, yin comes to its interchange point (交接 *jiāo jiē*) before returning to yang. From the vantage point of the six levels then, *jué yīn* is deeper in that it has relatively more yin substance (blood).

The second perspective from which to view *shào yīn* and *jué yīn* is five-phase theory. This is part of where the idea that the kidney is the 'root' of the liver comes from. In five-phase models, water (kidney) gives birth to wood (liver). The key to understanding exactly what is meant by this, however, involves the more nuanced model provided by an understanding of organ physiology.

This brings us to the third perspective. When considering organ functions, one notes that the kidney relationship as the 'mother' of the liver involves its role as the source of prenatal stimulus. The stimulus provided by the gate of vitality initiates a cascade of physiology, via the spleen-stomach and lungs, which eventually gives rise to blood (among many other things). From this angle, the kidney is most certainly the 'root'. When the kidney, due to a deficiency of yin, is out of balance, fire may flare up through the liver leading to the familiar pattern of fire from deficiency of the liver-kidney yin. There is often liver blood deficiency in this pattern as well.

Among the *jué yīn* organs, the liver stores blood to nourish the body while the pericardium stores blood for the nourishment of the heart. In each case, the primary concept is one of storage of significant amounts of yin (blood). *Shào yīn*, on the other hand, is not the repository of such great amounts of solid yin substance. While *jué yīn* can be thought of as the repository for large amounts of the postnatal yin derived from food and drink, *shào yīn* is the repository of prenatal yin essence. Both are important; one is at a deeper level than the other and represents a larger volume of yin substance (*jué yīn*), while the other adds the vital stimulus of prenatal fire along the way (*shào yīn*). There is then a relative depth of *jué yīn* in relation to *shào yīn*, but not necessarily a relative importance. The body obviously requires both to function.

Besides the vital catalyst provided by *shào yīn*, the *jué yīn* level is also stimulated by its paired organs at the *shào yáng* level. In the clinic, considerations of liver-pericardium physiology must include an appreciation of the yang moving function provided by the *shào yáng* gallbladder and triple burner. In order for yin to begin its transformation to yang at *jué yīn*, there must also be stimulus from the paired *shào yáng* organs. Without the strong yang stimulus of *shào yáng*, *jué yīn* would not move from the depths. These concepts should be kept in mind when devising both herbal and acupuncture treatment strategies (Fig. 7.5).

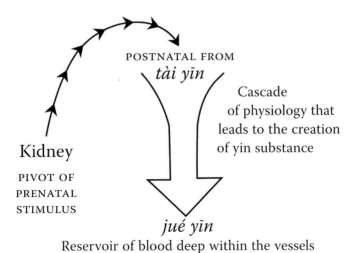

Fig. 7.5

The kidney is the root of prenatal stimulus while the depth of *jué yīn* is a postnatal reservoir, storing blood and assigning flow.

■ Case Study

13-year-old male

Chief complaint Attention deficit hyperactivity disorder (ADHD)

History and current condition At the age of six, the patient began to complain of neck tightness and pain. Massage by the parents was usually helpful for relieving symptoms, but they continued to recur. By the age of nine, the child was often noticeably irritable and restless and continued to frequently complain of neck discomfort. During the past two years, in addition to the other symptoms, the child had also begun to have trouble concentrating in school and often talked in class inappropriately. His grades in school had declined and his teachers had expressed some concern. Nevertheless, in general the child was relatively normal and physically active, with the exception of a recent trend toward angry outbursts. He had no problems in relationships with other children his own age and, in fact, often felt remorse over his inability to behave.

On presentation, the boy appeared to be a bit thin and slightly small for his age. Despite his parents' descriptions of hyperactivity, he was actually quite subdued in the clinic. His mother described him as a very picky eater, refusing to eat any vegetables at all and generally eating very little. His bowel movements and urination were normal. He had trouble sleeping due to the neck discomfort and often had active dreams. The boy did not like heat and became lethargic on hot, muggy days. In fact, he often wore short-sleeve shirts in weather where others wore coats. His pulse was slippery and his tongue was reddish with a slight crack in the tip.

Channel palpation revealed a thickening of the fascia along the *jué yīn* pericardium channel in the medial forearm. The heart *shào yīn* channel showed tenderness around the elbow while the liver *jué yīn* channel was tender throughout, especially around LR-3 *(tài chōng)*, where small nodules could be palpated. There was also a small nodule with tenderness on the spleen channel at SP-4 *(gōng sūn)*. Observation of the spine revealed a clear enlargement of C_7 and tenderness between T_5 and T_6, in the vicinity of GV-10 *(líng tái)* and GV-11 *(shén dào)* (Table 7.6).

Diagnosis *Jué yīn* channel stasis. This is a case of liver qi constraint and stasis of pericardium blood.

Where a patient is suffering from what modern biomedicine terms ADHD, there is a tendency of the symptom-pattern in Chinese medicine to move rapidly and change frequently. Thus the name might be thought of as describing both the symptoms of the patient and the nature of the condition (see discussion in Appendix 5).

	Organ	Palpated Findings	Possible Significance
Tài yīn	Lung		
	Spleen	Nodule at SP-4 (collateral point)	Phlegm accumulation in collaterals ('slow' spleen)
Shào yīn	Heart	HT-3 area tender	Heart qi transformation affected; lack of regulation (*hé*-sea point affected)
	Kidney		
Jué yīn	Pericardium	Thicker fascia on medial forearm	Blood stasis in the pericardium leading to heat that affects heart
	Liver	Tender throughout low leg (especially LR-3)	Qi stasis in *jué yīn* with lack of dredging and draining
Dū vessel	C$_7$ enlarged; tender between T$_5$ and T$_6$ (GV-10 & GV-11)		Congenital cervical irregularity; accumulation of blood, heat, and phlegm in upper burner

Table 7.6
Summary of palpation for case

· ·

Treatment   Treatment lasted for nine months and included both acupuncture and herbs.

Acupuncture treatment

Initial treatments focused on clearing and transforming stasis and heat from the *jué yīn* channel and collaterals. Treatment was once a week using the primary point pair PC-7 *(dà líng)* and LR-2 *(xíng jiān)*. (See Chapter 20 for a discussion of this pair.)

Many prenatal (congenital) conditions with children involve the kidney channel and *dū* (governing) vessel. Therefore, on visits where heat symptoms were less pronounced, treatment shifted to include SI-3 *(hòu xī)*, which is the command point of the *dū* vessel, GV-19 *(hòu dǐng)*, and KI-7 *(fù liū)* to support the yin.

The symptoms on the neck involved the upper back along the *tài yáng* channel. Most treatments therefore also included BL-10 *(tiān zhù)*, an 'a-shi' point in the area around BL-10 which showed palpable tightness, and BL-64 *(jīng gǔ)*, the source point of the bladder channel. BL-10 is often used in connection with developmental problems and has a stimulatory effect on the governing vessel and brain.

A fourth general treatment principle was a response to the tendency in children with ADHD to have pathomechanisms involving phlegm. During the second three months of treatment, the child came every 2–3 weeks. ST-40 *(fēng lóng)* and ST-36 *(zú sān lǐ)* were included to support *tài yīn / yáng míng* qi transformation (dampness and dryness) and aid in the elimination of phlegm. A variation of Warm the Gallbladder Decoction *(wēn dǎn tāng)* was also used during this phase (see below).

Maintenance in the later stages of treatment involved cupping along the bladder channel and short doses of a *dū* vessel invigorating formula (see below). In this final phase of treatment, the child came only once every 3–5 weeks.

Herbal treatment

Herbal therapy was introduced in the third month of treatment. At that time, the parents expressed interest in reducing frequency of visits and asked about the possibility of using herbal therapy as an adjunct. Based on a diagnosis of wind and damp phlegm, and in consideration of the extremely hot and humid weather in Beijing at the time, a modification of Warm the Gallbladder Decoction *(wēn dǎn tāng)* was prescribed:

Testudinis Plastrum *(guī bǎn)*–15g; cooked first for 10 minutes

Haliotidis Concha *(shí jué míng)*–20g; cooked first for 10 minutes

Arisaema cum Bile *(dǎn nán xīng)*–6g

Pinelliae Rhizoma *(bàn xià)*–10g

Poria *(fú líng)*–10g

Citri reticulatae Pericarpium *(chén pí)*–6g

Fossilia Dentis Mastodi *(lóng chǐ)*–20g

Ziziphi spinosae Semen *(suān zǎo rén)*–12g

Paeoniae Radix rubra *(chì sháo)*–10g

Nelumbinis Semen *(lián zǐ)*–10g

Carthami Flos *(hóng huā)*–6g

Angelicae sinensis Radix *(dāng guī)*–6g

Menthae haplocalycis Herba *(bò hé)*–3g; added in last five minutes of cooking

Uncariae Ramulus cum Uncis *(gōu téng)*–10g; added in last five minutes

Results Within the first few weeks, there was a marked improvement in the ability of the child to sit still in class. His irritability at home also showed clear improvement. By the second month of treatment, his sleep had improved and he reported a decrease in the intensity of his dreams. During the second stage of treatment—month three to six—his symptoms presented more often as a tendency toward spleen qi deficiency and food stagnation. At this time, the herbal formula listed above was added. For a few weeks during this period, M-UE-9 *(sì fèng)* on the tips of the fingers were bled to stimulate a 'slow spleen' (慢脾 *màn pí*).

The final stage of treatment proved to be the most difficult. By the sixth month, the boy was much more able to sit still in class and his sleep and performance at school had improved to the satisfaction of his parents. However, he reported that the pain in his neck and upper back continued to trouble him. Cupping produced improvement for up to a week at a time, but the pain continued to return. At that point, the addition of the *dū* vessel invigorating formula (discussed above) helped to relax his shoulders and neck.

After eight months of treatment, all of the child's symptoms had improved significantly, but had not disappeared completely. The pain/discomfort in his neck and upper back proved to be quite tenacious. This is likely due to the quite obvious enlargement (hyperostosis) or malposition of the C_7 vertebra. He therefore continued to come for regular treatments once every three weeks and was encouraged to maintain regular visits to a local hospital for orthopedic observation.

Analysis While generally successful, this case highlights an important aspect of the clinical experience: that of patients whose conditions fail to completely resolve. While experience has shown that ADD/ADHD responds quite well to Chinese medicine, there are occasionally difficult issues which are not fully resolved. In this case, most of the child's symptoms—sleep problems, irritability, difficulty concentrating—did resolve, but he continued to have upper back and neck pain.

■ Narrative

RESTING AT THE INSIDE

Because the *jué yīn* system represents the inside of the body and the innermost aspect of our exploration of the six levels, it seems appropriate at this point to explore some of the innermost workings of Dr. Wang's mind. With the necessary disclaimer about the inherent inability of one person to understand another's mind, I must say that I tried as hard as I could. One of the subtleties of apprenticeship that is most difficult to convey in words is the sense of interconnectedness that eventually develops between teacher and apprentice. Interconnectedness, in this case, means a sense of how a person goes about doing things not directly related to seeing patients and healing sickness that will nevertheless reflect a particular outlook that shapes one's clinical approach.

Specifically, I tried to pay attention to how Dr. Wang understands the process of learning. What were the processes that he went through during and after his formal training? The favorable conditions that existed at the Beijing College of Traditional Chinese Medicine during the 1950s have already been mentioned. This period was obviously quite important for Dr. Wang in his formative stage. Despite the best efforts of all of us working both in China and in other countries, I believe it may still be awhile before a meeting of so much clinical experience with classical Chinese medicine, such as existed at that time and place, will again occur under one roof.

In any case, upon graduation, where did Dr. Wang start? Did he also have that moment of panic when the first patients entered the door expecting him to heal their ailments? I was often most surprised in this regard when he commented on the relative importance of teachers in helping him develop clinical approaches. While he often spoke with reverence about certain practitioners with whom he had worked, or teachers who had been important in shaping his thought, he emphatically stated many times that the best teachers of all had been his patients. More than once he told me that neither the greatness of your teachers nor the mysteries and secrets that one or another practitioner passes along will make you successful over the long run at clinical work. Rather, it is an attentiveness to the results of your treatments and a willingness to return over and again to critically evaluate the experience of others and the concepts of the classics that will improve clinical efficacy.

Dr. Wang and his wife would often invite me and my wife to their apartment for dinner. On one of these occasions, I asked him about the concept of book learning versus on the job training. We had just finished a feast of dumplings, crispy radish, steamed fish, and beer. Here's what he said.

> **DR. WANG:** Those first years in the clinic in the early 1960s were the hardest of all for me. As you might expect, I started out with a host of points and herbal formulas in my head and memorized lists of all the conditions that they might treat. I would treat patients based on classical 'point songs' or from notes I had taken in my classes. The results in those days were often decent, but not always what I had hoped for. I had hoped that 90 percent of the patients who came through the clinic door would show improvement. I found instead that clear improvement happened only maybe 30 percent of the time in those early days. Another 35 percent might get slightly better, while as many as 35 percent of the patients wouldn't improve at all, and might even get worse. I poured all of my attention into that last, unimproved 35 percent. There are two things I might recommend based on the approach I finally worked out in those days:
>
> ▶ *Keep a clinic notebook*
>
> At the end of each day, sit down for a few minutes and write a quick summary of the especially difficult cases and what you're thinking about treatment. This serves as a reference to track the patient's progress (or lack thereof). Also, write down your successes or discoveries. When something works well or you think that you have come up with an effective new approach, write that down as well. I know that it seems quite basic, but I would often write down all of the symptoms of the really difficult patients in the book and try to figure out all of the possible changes in qi dynamic that might have caused that symptom. By figuring out the likely cause of the major symptoms in these patients, I was often able to come up with a more accurate diagnosis.
>
> I was very rigorous about doing this for over ten years. I can't believe it now, but in the chaos of the Cultural Revolution, I threw all of my notebooks away. In those days it was unfortunately quite

common for Red Guards to suddenly appear, rifle through your belongings, then find things you had written and use them against you during 'reeducation' campaigns. I was fortunate to have had few problems during that period, but I did get caught up a bit in the prevailing paranoia of the time. In any case, the great benefit of a clinical notebook comes from the process of writing and thinking through difficult issues. I learned a lot this way.

▶ *Return over and again to the clinical experience of others*

After searching through many different texts and speaking with my teachers about their favorite books, I settled on three favorite works and developed a study method based on those. The works were:

Gathering of the Blossoms of Acupuncture (針灸聚英 *Zhēn jiǔ jù yīng*). Published in 1529 during the Ming dynasty by Gao Wu (高武), this text is basically a collection of ideas and approaches from various schools of the time.

Compilation of Channel Examination and Point Inspection (循經考穴編 *Xún jīng kǎo xuè biān*). Published around 1575 during the Ming dynasty by an unknown author, this text is an illustrated analysis of channel pathways with discussion of points used for particular conditions.

Classic of Nourishing Life with Acupuncture and Moxibustion (針灸資生經 *Zhēn jiǔ zī shēng jīng*). Published in 1220 during the Jin dynasty by Wang Zhi-Zhong (王執中), this text is generally believed to be more of a collection of the author's personal experience. With forty-six accompanying illustrations, the text discusses acupuncture approaches according to the chief complaint. It also discusses point location and channel theory.

My strategy for using these books was as follows. In those days I would first determine an organ-based categorization of the disease type using mainly differential diagnosis. Then I would see which points the *Classic of Nourishing Life with Acupuncture and Moxibustion* would recommend for treatment. I would next go to the sections on those individual points in both of the first two books and compare and contrast how the two books understood the functions of each point. The other two texts didn't break disease down into organ syndromes, so getting into the author's mind involved making some intuitive leaps. For example, in order to determine the function of the point, you had to look at the other diseases that each book listed as being appropriate (Fig. 7.6).

This process gave me considerable insight into how great scholars and clinicians from other eras understood the effects of the points on the qi dynamic. You see, I would get this multi-layered picture that began with the disease that I had a question about, and some points that might be helpful, followed by the opinions of two other doctors about what other conditions might be treated with the same points. Based on all of this, I could then

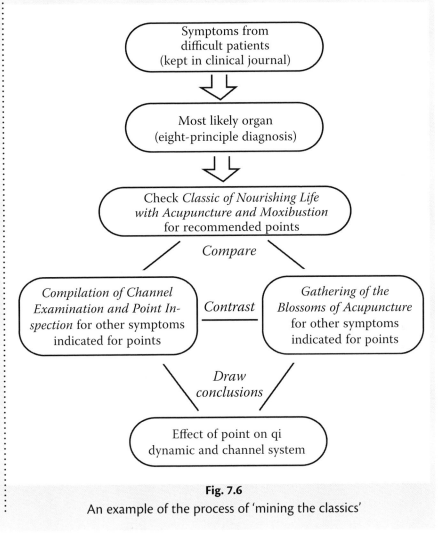

Fig. 7.6

An example of the process of 'mining the classics'

make a fairly good educated guess about how those doctors understood the effects of each point on the qi dynamic. The exciting thing for me was that much of the time, not only were they in agreement, but I found that the easiest way to reconcile it all was by considering channel theory. This process was actually the beginning of much of my understanding about the qi dynamic and channel theory. It therefore wouldn't be inaccurate to say that, although I certainly had some wonderful teachers for fundamental theory, my greatest lessons came from my patients. Every time a person came with another difficult condition, I was sent back to the books. I really felt like I got to know the authors of those old books during those days!

At this point, we were finishing the last of a huge plate of dumplings that Dr. Wang's wife had made for us. He had gotten up a few times during the conversation to go into his study to retrieve the books he spoke about. His study is dominated by a huge floor-to-ceiling bookshelf that fills an entire long wall of the room. Dr. Wang estimated that seventy percent of the books on that wall relate to Chinese medicine. The other thirty percent cover a range of subjects from Western philosophy to travel handbooks, and a huge contingent of works about Chinese history. In front of the books on many shelves are pictures of Dr. Wang in foreign countries posing next to famous sites with students of every color and age. There is a treatment table in his home office for friends and relatives, and a large desk with a powerful halogen reading light. Next to the desk is a large window that looks north to a small stand of trees. The room is very clean and comfortable and has recently been furnished with new, classically-styled furniture. Dr. Wang and his wife had lived in the same building near her work unit for twenty-five years, but just recently moved to this new, modern apartment on the outskirts of the city near the Summer Palace. Like so much of Beijing in the 21st century, Dr. Wang has raised his standard of living considerably in recent years.

After dinner and a meandering discussion about other books on his shelves, the four of us moved to the living room for tea, and the conversation turned, as is so often the case in China, to the subject of food and how to find the best of China's ten thousand flavors. But that is the subject for another entire lifetime!

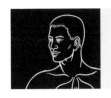

太陽

THE *Tài Yáng* (GREATER YANG) SYSTEM

THE NEXT THREE chapters will discuss the qi dynamic in the three yang levels. Although less emphasis is placed on yang organ function in most texts, the channel system at these levels is no less important. In general, the yang levels are more dynamic and expansive than the yin channels. The surface area covered by the pathways of the bladder, stomach, and gallbladder channels alone is greater than all of the other channels combined. Because of their size, and the need for constant movement, the yang channels and their related sinew vessels are especially prone to pain disorders associated with circulation along their pathways.

The organs associated with the yang channels are said to be "replete but not filled up" (實 而 不 滿 *shí ér bù mǎn)*. In other words, as yang organs, they are hollow pathways that must be kept moving at all times. Accumulation leads to dysfunction.

While the yang organs play the important role of transporting the material products of the yin organ qi dynamic, they also provide functional balance. The concept of functional balance is important to an understanding of how the yin and yang channels interact in physiology. Simply put, the tendency of the yin organs toward restful accumulation is balanced by the active stimulus of their yang organ pairs. This occurs at each level in the body (Fig. 8.1).

In addition, the concept of a metabolic system comprised of balanced poles will be important to the process of choosing channels for treatment (see Chapter 14). Before proceeding with our discussion of the specific yang levels, it will be helpful to first consider a question that often comes up in the context of yin-yang channel pairs.

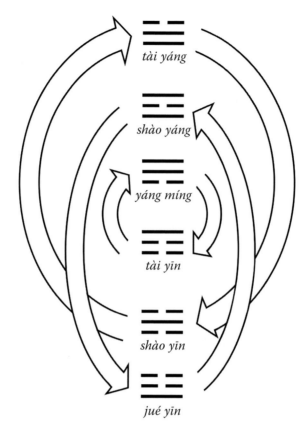

Fig. 8.1

The channel system at a glance. Movement from the yang levels activates the creation of yin substance. Nourishment from the yin levels supports yang activity.

Q: *Some of the yin-yang organ pairings are easy to understand, but others are more difficult. For example, the liver-gallbladder, kidney-bladder, and spleen-stomach pairs make sense, even in a modern medical context. However, it is difficult to discern why the lung and heart organs are paired with the large and small intestines?*

DR. WANG: This is a question that often comes up with students. In fact, it is basically the same question asked in Chapter 35 of the *Classic of Difficulties*. There the question is posed, "How can organs that are so far away from each other physically and functionally be considered to be paired?" We'll review the answer provided by the *Classic of*

Difficulties in a moment. An important way to understand these pairings is to appreciate the fact that their connection is more therapeutic than physical. As I've said many times, theories in Chinese medicine are only valid insofar as they help to deepen one's understanding of what happens in the clinic.

The most useful aspects of these pairings have been historically drawn, first and foremost, from observations in the clinic about how they correlate to treatment. In other words, when there seemed to be a verifiable connection to the treatment of one channel or organ with that of another, early theorists began to delve into how these relationships might be understood. When the explanations led to effective clinical approaches, they were recorded and refined by generations of physicians in a process that has been going on now for well over a thousand years. While the theoretical framework that this process created is quite different from that of modern medicine, the clinical results are repeatable and measurable.

To answer your question, let's first develop an answer based on classical theory, as described in the answer to the question posed above, and follow that up with a look at some common applications in the clinic. The classical answer begins by noting that the heart and lung are located in the pure, refined environment of the upper burner, while their paired yang organs are deep in the trenches of the lower burner. As you may recall from our discussion about the qi dynamic of the yin organs, the lung and heart are involved in the movement of qi and blood respectively. The movement of heart blood carries the nutritive (營 *yíng*) aspect, while qi incorporated by the lung is responsible for the liveliness of the protective (衛 *wèi*) aspect. For a pair of yin organs, these functions are relatively yang, as they involve the upward and outward movement of nutrition and the body's defenses.

Turning to the large and small intestines, one should note that here we have two yang organs in a very yin area of the body charged with transporting large amounts of yin-turbidity. This pair of yang organs has a relatively yin existence. Both intestines are transporting the most turbid aspects of the body's metabolism, the unneeded dregs from digested food. This is in direct contrast to the pure, refined essences from the digestive process moved around the body by the activities of the heart and lung. With this in mind, one can begin to see how, in the body as a whole, the functions of these paired organs have a balancing effect. The tendency of the yin heart and lungs to yang movement is balanced by the relatively yin nature of their paired yang organs (Fig. 8.2).

Chapter 35 of the *Classic of Difficulties* describes the physiological rationale underlying the interior-exterior pairing of the heart-small intestine and the lung-large intestine.

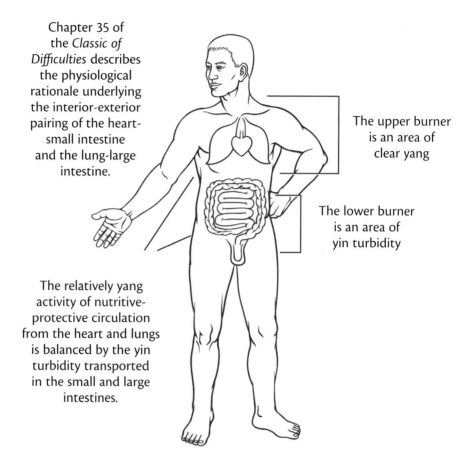

The upper burner is an area of clear yang

The lower burner is an area of yin turbidity

The relatively yang activity of nutritive-protective circulation from the heart and lungs is balanced by the yin turbidity transported in the small and large intestines.

Fig. 8.2
Yin-yang balance between upper and lower burners

A few common clinical treatment strategies are best understood in this light. For example, points on the large intestine channel such as LI-11 (*qū chí*) and LI-4 (*hé gǔ*) can be used to treat exterior conditions often associated with the lung. How does this happen functionally? Accumulated yin-turbidity is moved by stimulating the abundant qi and blood in the *yáng míng* large intestine channel. This facilitates the upward diffusion of yang qi from the lung, and is similar to the idea of lightening the load of a hot air balloon. The formula Ephedra, Apricot Kernel, Gypsum, and Licorice Decoction (*má xìng shí gān tāng*) is often explained in this way. In a similar vein, many students are familiar with the use of herbal formulas like Guide Out the Red Powder (*dǎo chì sǎn*) to clear heat in the heart through the *tài yáng* small intestine / bladder. An understanding of the specific type of balance provided by these paired organs helps explain why, for example, we learn that heat in the heart is cleared through the small intestine, but we don't hear of clearing spleen heat through the stomach.

The separation of these four organs from each other in distance and function actually becomes the root of their strength and a necessary counterbalance to their own relatively extreme natures. While other yin-yang organ pairings are based more on a similarity in function and location, these four are paired because of their dissimilarity: balance is achieved through contrast. In any case, the theories are certainly borne out in the clinic. That's always the final consideration.

Finally, when you consider the pairing of the 'sixth yin organ'—the pericardium—with the triple burner, it is important to remember the particular relationship that these organs have with the ministerial fire (see discussion in Chapter 6). The similarity of these organs is rooted in the concept of fire. (More on this later.)

The General Nature and Function of *Tài Yáng*

The *tài yáng* level is broad and expansive, rising to the surface of the channel system like the vapors off the top of a bamboo dumpling steamer. Connected internally with the heat of *shào yīn*, the *tài yáng* level nourishes and discharges through the skin and hair with warm moisture radiating from the qi dynamic of the yin organs. Now that the discussion has turned to the three yang channels, the reader should note that movement now supersedes yin substance. Movement is particularly important to *tài yáng* as it is classically described as opening outward (開 *kāi)*. Note that the same term, *kāi*, is also used to describe the outward opening of the *tài yīn* level. While *tài yīn* is the 'external aspect of yin' in the body, *tài yáng* is the external aspect of yang, opening out to the world at large.[1] The character 太 (*tài*) looks very similar to the Chinese character 大 (*dà*), meaning big, but it also includes a small stroke of emphasis on the left leg. *Tài* is therefore bigger than big; significantly, it is the first character in the term *tài jí* (太極), often translated as the 'supreme ultimate', which is best known as the yin-yang symbol (Fig. 8.3).

Tài yáng, the ultimate yang, is thus large in both its functional scope and surface area on the body. As the most external of the six channels, *tài yáng* is the first line of defense against external invasion. Defense is achieved by warming and discharging the exterior (煦發表 *xù fā biǎo)*. This function of *tài yáng* explains the channel's responsibility for protecting the body from cold (寒 *hán)*.

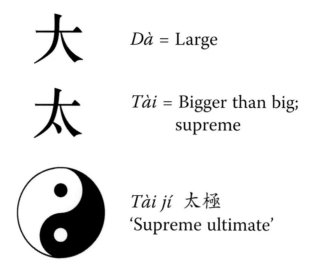

Dà = Large

Tài = Bigger than big; supreme

Tài jí 太極
'Supreme ultimate'

Fig. 8.3
Yin-yang symbol

Another short diversion into terminology is warranted here. It was just noted that the *tài yáng* level 'warms and discharges' the surface of the body. The character translated here as warms is 煦 (*xù*), which actually has a broader meaning. It is most commonly used in colloquial Chinese in the term *xù rì* (煦日), meaning a warm, comfortable day. Therefore, when modern Chinese doctors use this term to describe the function of *tài yáng*, there is an implied meaning of comfort as well. The *tài yáng* channel might thus be said to provide 'warm comfort' and to 'discharge'. This explains the association of the *tài yáng* syndrome in the *Discussion of Cold Damage* with pain and discomfort in the body. In this type of syndrome, there is blockage at *tài yáng* that has compromised the normal warming and discharging, which causes discomfort.

Other symptoms associated with the *tài yáng* syndrome in *Discussion of Cold Damage* can also be more clearly understood by considering the qi dynamic of the *tài yáng* channel and its relationship to cold. In the case of external invasion, the channel raises yang to disperse cold from the exterior by warming the skin through the interstices (腠理 *còu lǐ*). The interstices are understood to be the area below the skin and above the muscles. Functionally, they are an important part of the barrier between the body and the environment.

The body's ability to control its temperature also involves the interstices. This is similar to the modern understanding of dilation and constriction of skin capillaries in response to environmental change. When cold invades from the external environment, the *tài yáng* channel reacts. The ability of *tài yáng* to 'open and close' the interstices is crucial to this reaction. 'Opening' means to effectively send protective qi to the area, while 'closing' implies the constriction of the interstices to prevent cold from invading (Fig. 8.4).

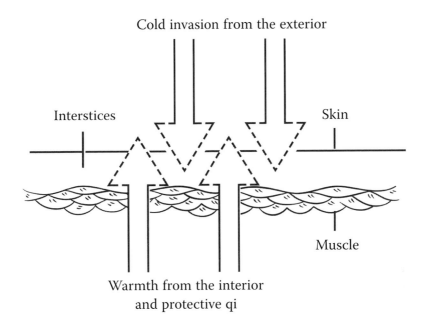

Cold invasion from the exterior

Interstices

Skin

Muscle

Warmth from the interior
and protective qi

Fig. 8.4
The normal opening and closing of the interstices allows heat to radiate outward with protective qi, while also closing to prevent invasion from external cold.

Once cold has invaded the body, the goal of the *tài yáng* qi dynamic is no longer to close the interstices but to reestablish proper opening; thus the use of the term 'blockage' (閉 *bì*) in discussions of the *tài yáng* syndrome. When the *tài yáng* level is blocked by cold, the patient may feel chills. Another symptom mentioned in the *Discussion of Cold Damage* is headache. Because the interstices are blocked and yang is unable to discharge outward, the yang qi rises upward to the head, causing pain. Blockage of yang also explains why the *tài yáng* syndrome might involve a fever or sense of warmth.

A chronic inability of *tài yáng* to protect the body from external cold is traditionally treated with moxa at CV-6 (*qì hǎi*). Similarly, if a patient has systemic yang deficiency, moxa at BL-10 (*tiān zhù*), BL-11 (*dà zhù*), GV-

14 (*dà zhuī*), and ST-36 (*zú sān lǐ*) can strengthen the *tài yáng* function of warming and moving the yang qi to the surface. Incidentally, in administering this treatment, ST-36 (*zú sān lǐ*) should be the final point treated in order to direct the yang downward from the head. Traditionally, moxa has been applied to these points as a general tonic around the time of the winter and summer solstices (December 21st and June 21st).

It should be emphasized that the *tài yáng* channel is primarily associated with the protection of the body from external cold. Heat may sometimes become trapped in the interstices, leading to signs of heat without sweating and pain in the body, but this is less common than cold. Rather, external heat (a yang entity) is more likely to affect the lung *tài yīn* and pericardium *jué yīn* in its early stages, or possibly the spleen *tài yīn* where there is also dampness. The tendency of external heat to directly affect the more internal yin levels underlines the fact that the six-level channel model does not always represent a fixed progression from *tài yáng* to *shào yáng* to *yáng míng* and so forth, like so many steps on a ladder. Instead, each of the six levels is responsible for integrating one or another of the six environmental qi (see Chapter 2).

As noted earlier, the surface area covered by the *tài yáng* channel is greater than that of any other channel. The two separate pathways of the *tài yáng* bladder channel on the dorsal surface of the trunk reinforce this idea. Because of the wide net of yang qi cast by the flow of the *tài yáng* channel, it interacts with all of the other internal organs. This is evidenced by the varied uses of the back transporting points (腧穴 *shū xué*) along the spine. In fact, because of its association with the surface, the *tài yáng* system plays a part in connecting all the organs to the external environment.

It has been mentioned before that the *tài yáng* interior-exterior pairing with *shào yīn* serves as a means by which warmth and moisture from the qi dynamic of the yin organs is transported outward. There is also a corresponding relationship of the functions of the *tài yáng* and *shào yīn* organs. Besides clearing the urine produced by the kidney, the bladder is also dependent on the fire from the gate of vitality to initiate its wide dispersion of warmth and fluids to the surface. Without this primary warmth from *shào yīn*, the *tài yáng* level would be overwhelmed by yin fluids. In fact, the interplay of *shào yīn* and *tài yáng* (as represented by the kidney and bladder) describes one mechanism by which edema can be understood. This will be discussed further in the bladder section below.

In another interior-exterior relationship, the small intestine was observed by the ancient Chinese to be associated with the absorption of nutrients, thus helping the heart in its traditional function of moving the blood (行血 *xíng xuè*). Specifically, food that has already been initially transformed by the spleen-stomach passes through the small intestine, which then further removes vital substances (the 'clear') which are transferred back to the spleen, absorbed into the blood as nutritive qi, and eventually sent to the heart. Small intestine function might therefore be said to be an important part of the 'transformation to red' (化赤 *huà chì*),[2] that is, the building of blood.

Excess in the *tài yáng* channel is associated with urinary disorders or problems with sweating. This includes too much or too little sweat or urine due to problems with either the interstices or the bladder organ. In fact, it is helpful to think of urination and sweating as two aspects of the same fluid substance. If there is excessive sweating, then urination will be less, and vice versa. One important difference, obviously, is that other waste substances are eliminated through the urine, so it is especially important to keep this passage open. There is a common saying in China that people urinate more in the winter and less in the summer. In light of *tài yáng* function, this might be explained by considering the rather obvious fact that we tend to sweat less in the cold of winter, thus leading to increased urination during those months of the year.

Deficiency of the *tài yáng* channel is associated with sensitivity to cold or cold extremities and also with urinary problems, usually difficulty in controlling urination.

An interesting aside to *tài yáng* function involves the classical explanation for the 'shake' that often occurs at the end of urinating. First remember that, in the process of eliminating excess fluids from the bladder organ, there is a net loss of heat from the body. The 'shake' at the end of urinating is understood as the *tài yáng* channel's effort to reestablish yang qi on the surface in response to this rather sudden expulsion of heat.

Small Intestine

> "The small intestine holds the office of receptacle of plenty; the transformation of substances issue from it."
>
> (小腸者．受盛之官．化物出焉。 *Xiǎo cháng zhě, shòu chéng zhī guān, huà wù chū yān.*)
>
> —*Basic Questions*, Chapter 8

Another reading of the characters translated here as "receptacle of plenty" (受盛 *shòu chéng*) might be "holder of plenty," which would bring to mind the image of a bowl to a Chinese reader. While the large intestine is compared to a pathway, the small intestine is viewed as a brief stopping place for assimilation and modification. Thus the compilers of the *Inner*

Classic not only noted the presence of large and small 'intestines', but also recognized significant functional differences between them. In the small intestine, remnants of food essence passed along from the stomach undergo modification. The stomach is likened to an official charged with the collection of grains, and the small intestine to a lower functionary charged with classification (分類 *fēn lèi*).

In an image similar to that presented by modern physiology, the small intestine in Chinese medicine is charged with taking in food fermented by the stomach and then further separating out (classifying) constituent materials to be used by the rest of the body. The process of 'separation' in the small intestine is preceded by the transformation of lighter qi from food and fluids in the spleen. Consequently, when one thinks of the small intestine as 'separating the clear from the turbid' (分別清濁 *fēn bié qīng zhuó*), it should be in the context of a process already begun in the stomach and spleen (Fig. 8.5).

The 'turbid' separated out by the small intestine is not all passed along as waste, however. This is an important and sometimes overlooked aspect of small intestine function. While many textbooks describe this function rather simplistically as removing clear fluids from waste, classical physiologists likely had a more subtle idea of the 'clear and turbid' in mind. For example, some aspects of the heavier turbid materials are important for the production of thick fluids (液 *yè*) in the body, especially those associated with glandular secretions. There are, in fact, some interesting associations that can be made regarding the functions of both *tài yáng* organs and the modern physiological understanding of glands. These parallels will be further explored below.

FUNCTIONS OF THE SMALL INTESTINE

As noted, the function of the small intestine is to 'separate the clear from the turbid'. There are four primary aspects of this separation and classification function:

Transforms red to maintain blood (化赤維血 huà chì wéi xuè)

This function is a reference to the interior-exterior connection of the small intestine to the heart, which 'moves the blood'. Some of the substances separated out by the small intestine go directly to the blood through the heart, particularly those that 'become red'.

Provides essential substance (精微之物 jīng wēi zhī wù) to the spleen

The small intestine participates in a process that begins with the spleen-stomach. One might compare the actions of the stomach to that of a warehouse manager who takes raw materials from disparate sources and then cleans and separates them. Next, the spleen removes most of the essential substances from food, which is then received and held by the small intestine. The activity of separating the clear from the turbid in the small intestine involves a process of further classifying and separating. The resulting 'clear' essential substances are transported back to the spleen where they are processed into the nutritive aspect. As noted above, some turbid substances are used in the production of thick fluids, while most are transported downward to the large intestine (Fig. 8.5).

Removes excess water

The removal of excess water involves the passage of turbid fluids down to the large intestine for eventual discharge from the body. One might also consider the relationship within *tài yáng* to the bladder as another means by which the small intestine affects water removal.

Removes waste

After all of the above has occurred, the small intestine sends the remaining waste turbidity out of the body through the large intestine.

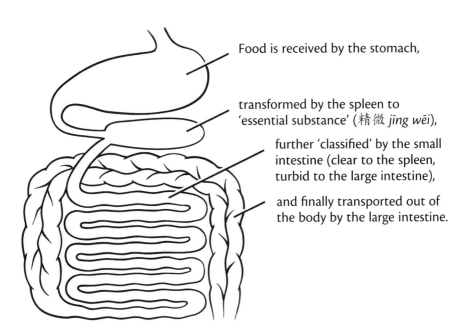

Food is received by the stomach,

transformed by the spleen to 'essential substance' (精微 *jīng wēi*),

further 'classified' by the small intestine (clear to the spleen, turbid to the large intestine),

and finally transported out of the body by the large intestine.

Fig. 8.5
The general functions of the digestive organs in classical physiology

CLINICAL PEARLS OF WISDOM
ABOUT SMALL INTESTINE PATHOLOGY

- Cervical disorders are most often associated with the small intestine channel. This is especially true of problems with the ligaments or small joints of the neck, but less true in osteosis (formation of bony tissue). The early stages of displacement of cervical vertebrae are often treated along the small intestine channel. With this type of condition, there are often very small nodules that can be palpated in the area between SI-3 (*hòu xī*) and SI-6 (*yǎng lǎo*).

- Problems in the shoulder joint (especially ligaments) often involve the small intestine channel.

- Sometimes back pain affecting the bladder *tài yáng* channel will manifest instead on the small intestine channel. In such cases, the manifestation will often be contralateral, that is, right side back pain will manifest on the left small intestine channel, in the area around SI-3 (*hòu xī*) in particular.

- Eye, ear, and throat problems often involve the small intestine channel.

- Heart conditions may cause palpable changes along the small intestine channel.

- Ligament problems in the elbow are often treated via the small intestine channel.

- Excess in the collaterals of the small intestine channel is associated with elbow joint problems and pain. Consider using the collateral point of the channel, SI-7 *(zhī zhèng)*.

 Q: *Although this discussion presents a fairly clear understanding of the classical conception of the small intestine, there seems to be a gap between this understanding and its clinical application that is unique to this organ. Why is that?*

DR. WANG: Points on the small intestine channel are used fairly rarely, except in the treatment of pain along the pathway of the channel itself. This might indicate a lack of thorough understanding of the qi dynamic of the small intestine. Also, you shouldn't forget that the yang channels are generally less directly associated with the functions of the yang organs with which they are associated than is the case with the yin channels and their associated organs. This is particularly true of the large and small intestines. Nevertheless, there are a few concepts that have occurred to me which might be worth exploring in the clinic.

For example, symptoms associated with the small intestine channel include swelling and pain in the throat and lower jaw. This is an area full of important glands. When considering the responsibility of the small intestine organ for "separating the clear from the turbid," one might think about the glands and their turbid secretions.[3] It therefore seems possible to me that our understanding of not just the glands in the neck and jaw, such as the thyroid or saliva glands, but also those throughout the GI tract, might benefit from remembering that the small intestine is an organ of 'classifying'. For example, the enzymes present in saliva are understood by modern physiologists to initiate the first steps in the chemical breakdown of food; this is a type of sorting or classification. Other glands in the digestive tract that continue this process might also be said to be separating the clear from the turbid. Even the lymphatic vessels which surround the GI tract might be included, as they too are engaged in separating the clear from the turbid. These are ideas that have occurred to me only recently, and I have yet to verify them in the clinic.

On a similar note, consider CV-4 (*guān yuán*). This is a point that I sometimes use for treating anemia. It is the alarm (幕 *mù*) point of the small intestine. There may be other uses for small intestine points in treating blood conditions, and I encourage you to explore this possibility for yourself in the clinic.

Bladder

> "The bladder holds the office of regional rectifier; yin and yang fluids are stored in it and can be excreted when qi is transformed."
>
> (膀胱者．州都之官．津液藏焉．氣化則能出矣。*Páng guāng zhě, zhōu dū zhī guān, jīn yè cáng yān, qì huà zé néng chū yǐ.*)
>
> —*Basic Questions*, Chapter 8

The bladder is the last of the twelve organs discussed in Chapter 8 of *Basic Questions*. Maybe this is because the organ is situated lowest in the body, in front of and below the kidneys. As administrator of the waterways, the bladder holds the fluids of the body in reserve. The use of "yin and yang fluids" here is a very broad, inclusive term that encompasses both the thin and thick fluids (津液 *jīn yè*) everywhere in the body. Every type of liquid in the body is somewhere along the spectrum of viscosity between the thicker yin fluids (like mucus) to the thinner yang fluids (like tears). The bladder, which maintains the fluid volume, determines how much fluid is stored in the body and how much is to be released.

However, especially in the case of the bladder, it is important to remember that the concept of 'organ' is much broader in classical Chinese medicine than in modern anatomy. When considering the bladder, not only the fluids inside the organ itself, but also the fluid reserves held throughout the body are affected by its qi transformation.

The passage from Chapter 8 of *Basic Questions* cited above also includes an interesting additional piece of information. It says that the fluids stored by the bladder "can be excreted when qi is transformed." Because the *tài yáng* channel covers a very large surface area, it is particularly dependent on strong qi transformation to move the fluids and warmth outward. Here, without specifically saying so, the *Inner Classic* is likely referring to the presence of the gate of vitality in close physical proximity to the bladder and to the importance of that fundamental fire to the qi transformation of this organ. Thus the bladder, warmed by the presence of the fire at the gate of vitality in the kidney, radiates clear fluids and warmth upward and outward to the outermost *tài yáng* level.

FUNCTIONS OF THE BLADDER

Stores fluids (藏津液 *cáng jīn yè*)

The function of the bladder is not limited to the storage and passage of urine. A broader meaning is implied which includes the *tài yáng* function of sending the beneficial fluids upward and outward. Thus the bladder in Chinese medicine is concerned not just with the waste fluids, but also with the quality of the healthy fluids. Once again, one should keep in mind the interior-exterior connection of *tài yáng* to *shào yīn*, and the importance of the fire at the gate of vitality to the ability of the bladder to effectively move the fluids that come under its administration. Through the interior-exterior connection to the warm yang of the kidney, the bladder is able to warm and discharge fluids to the surface.

Secretes and differentiates the clear and the turbid
(泌別清濁 *mì bié qīng zhuó*)

This concept contains the idea of filtering the fluids of the body to maintain net volume. This should be distinguished from the function of the paired small intestine that is also said to "separate the clear from the turbid." The small intestine receives food from the spleen-stomach and further sorts/classifies to remove more essential nutrition, which is then returned to the spleen. The residual turbidity (not including those 'turbid' materials used to make thick fluids) moves down to the large intestine. The concept of the bladder, on the other hand, is thought of in a larger, more systemic sense as reflected by the size of the channel on the body surface.

The 'clear' in this case are clear fluids that radiate outward to become the warm, fluid movement at the surface of the body. The fluids of the blood and the warm, fluid movement at the *tài yáng* level are in constant interplay. Both the nutritive aspect (in the blood) and the protective aspect (surrounding the blood vessels) travel up and out to the *tài yáng* level where they circulate in the interstices. Turbid fluids separated by the bladder are eventually expelled from the body in the form of urine. Note that both the small intestine and the bladder separate 'clearness'. The clearness of both eventually interacts with the nutritive aspect of blood. There is constant interchange (Fig. 8.6).

When considering the interplay of fluids and blood, remember that both *tài yīn* and *tài yáng* are considered to 'open outwards' (開 *kāi*) among the three yin and yang levels, respectively. As noted above, both *tài yīn* and *tài yáng* have a relationship to the nutritive-protective aspects. *Tài yīn* is charged with generating the nutritive-protective aspects through the transformation of food (spleen) and external qi (lung). *Tài yīn* then opens to the interior by providing the nutritive-protective aspects in the blood. *Tài yáng*, on the other hand, has the more yang-natured function of providing movement and separation, while simultaneously radiating to the very border of the body's interface with the external world. *Tài yáng* is thus said to open to the exterior. Remember as well that it is the function of spleen *tài yīn* to maintain the quality (nutritive action) of the fluids at the capillary level. Additionally, recall that it is the spleen which 'transforms dampness', while the bladder is charged with maintaining net fluid volume. Both the spleen and bladder also depend on the warming stimulus from the gate of vitality in the kidney. Consequently, when treating dampness, it is important to consider the interactions of the spleen, bladder, and kidney in fluid metabolism.

The *Discussion of Cold Damage* formula Cinnamon Twig Decoction (*guì zhī tāng*) helps to bring the theoretical into the realm of the clinical. Used as a treatment for cold from deficiency in the exterior, the formula contains both *tài yīn* and *tài yáng* elements. The pair Cinnamomi Ramulus (*guì zhī*) and Paeoniae Radix alba *(bái sháo)* is said to regulate the nutritive-protective aspects through a combination of outward spicy dispersion by Cinnamomi Ramulus (*guì zhī*) and cool, sour astringency on the part of Paeoniae

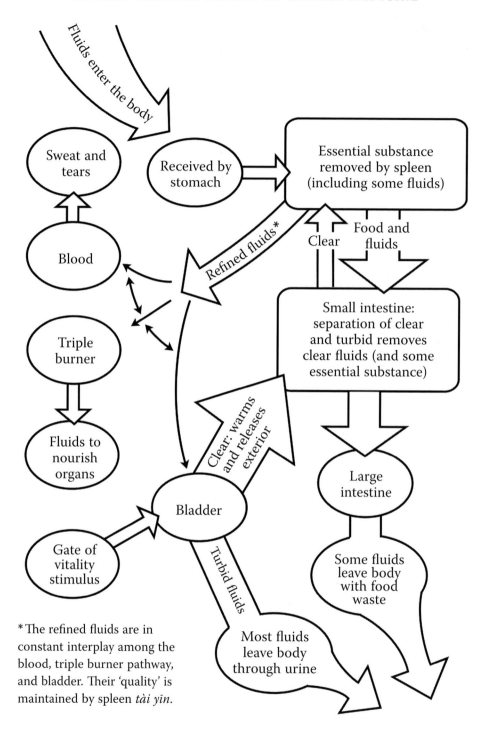

Fig. 8.6
The pathways of the fluids

Radix alba *(bái sháo)*. Thus these herbs are said to affect the surface of the body—at the *tài yáng* level in the interstices. By contrast, the other three herbs in the formula, Zingiberis Rhizoma recens *(shēng jiāng)*, Jujubae Fructus *(dà zǎo)*, and Glycyrrhizae Radix *(gān cǎo)*, enliven the *tài yīn* by stimulating and nourishing the spleen-stomach. Together, the formula 'opens' both the outermost yin level and the outermost yang level in an effort to harmonize both the generation *(tài yīn)* and the outward distribution *(tài yáng)* of the nutritive-protective aspects so that they can more effectively remove an externally-contracted pathogen from the body. Like so many formulas from the early imperial era, those of the *Discussion of Cold Damage* can often be more clearly understood when considering the qi dynamic and channel theory as understood by physicians of that time (Table 8.1).

Incidentally, one should take note of the fact that the qi transformation of both organs in the *tài yáng* level involve a separation of clear and turbid that facilitates both the production (small intestine) and movement (bladder) of the nutritive-protective aspects. As previously noted, each channel system includes not just the two organs, but also the channels themselves with their unique set of functions.

Another commonly-used formula from the *Discussion of Cold Damage* reflects another aspect of *tài yáng* function. In contrast to Cinnamon Twig Decoction, which clearly reaches the surface area of the *tài yáng* channel, the formula Five-Ingredient Powder with Poria *(wǔ líng sǎn)* has more of an effect on the function of the *tài yáng* bladder organ. This formula is used for a variety of damp conditions ranging from exterior invasion of the damp pathogen to the accumulation of internal dampness. As in Cinnamon Twig Decoction, Cinnamomi Ramulus *(guì zhī)* plays a pivotal role in promoting

Herb	Effects on Qi Dynamic
Cinnamomi Ramulus *(guì zhī)*	Stimulates the bladder qi transformation while stabilizing the nutritive in the interstices
Paeoniae Radix alba *(bái sháo)*	
Zingiberis Rhizoma recens *(shēng jiāng)*	Enlivens *tài yīn* production of the nutritive-protective aspects; radiates upward and outward
Jujubae Fructus *(dà zǎo)*	
Glycyrrhizae Radix *(gān cǎo)*	

Table 8.1

Cinnamon Twig Decoction *(guì zhī tāng)* and the qi dynamic

qi transformation. The use of Poria *(fú líng)* and Atractylodis macrocepha-lae Rhizoma *(bái zhú)* stimulates the spleen. However, in this formula, the *tài yīn* function of damp transformation is encouraged. The other two herbs in the formula, Polyporus *(zhū líng)* and Alismatis Rhizoma *(zé xiè),* have a more direct effect on the bladder organ function of fluid removal.

To summarize, the bladder plays an important role in fluid maintenance. Specifically, fluids throughout the body are differentiated into clear and turbid by the bladder. The clear fluids are reintegrated by the spleen at the microcirculation level to become the fluids within the blood. Turbidity is released from the body through the urine. The classical understanding of the bladder is thus fairly complex and represents a systemic process of both transformation and distribution. While some part of distribution involves the removal of waste fluids from the body as urine, there is also an impor-tant contribution to the fluid aspects of the blood.

Finally, bladder qi transformation is also associated with gland physiol-ogy in the lower abdomen. The discussion of fire at the gate of vitality in Chapter 6 on the *shào yīn* outlined some parallels between the classically-defined role of the gate of vitality in Chinese medicine and the biological understanding of hormones (the endocrine system). The discussion above of small intestine function also introduced a possible association of that channel with exocrine gland secretions in the digestive tract. Similarly, the modern understanding of exocrine glands in the lower abdomen finds par-allels in some classical concepts regarding the bladder. A review of bladder organ pathomechanisms reveals, for example, disease patterns similar to what Western medicine defines as dysfunction of the prostate gland, semi-nal vesicles, or bulbourethral glands in men.

Thus both *shào yīn* and *tài yáng* disease patterns present some interest-ing parallels to pathology in the Western medicine-defined endocrine and exocrine systems. But as always with comparisons of this type, there are limitations. While providing an interesting foundation for discussion, they should not be considered clinical equivalents. Both modern medicine and Chinese medicine are unique systems for analyzing the human body. Any similarities between them are ultimately due to the fact that they are both analyzing the same subject.

The important thing to keep in mind about the bladder is that there is a broad qi dynamic at play in the *tài yáng* system. Because of the broad scope of the channel pathway and the location of the organ in the lower burner with the gate of vitality, it is a particularly important yang organ. Although less closely related to the fire at the gate of vitality than the kidney, the blad-der is the pathway through which primary fire transforms and distributes the fluids of the body.

■ Case Study

The relationship of the bladder qi dynamic to the kidney gate of vitality was discussed above. While this idea has a sort of elegant theoretical balance, it is sometimes difficult to appreciate how the idea might be used in the clinic. Specifically, how might one integrate the idea of bladder qi transformation with the more commonly described pattern of kidney qi/yang deficiency? The following case study provides a helpful start.

69-year-old male

Chief complaint Urinary incontinence

History of present illness The patient had been suffering from chronic urinary incontinence for two years due to benign prostatic hyperplasia. Symptoms included frequent, short urination throughout the day with occasional incontinence. At night, incontinence was more pronounced and included frequent bed-wetting. The patient also complained of a lack of sweating in the lower body. During normal exertion in warm weather, he was able to sweat around his chest, but found that there was no sweating from his low back or legs. Consequently, his ankles and legs were dry. His hands often felt warm, while his feet felt cold throughout the day.

The patient was very thin and seemed prematurely bent over for his age. His voice was quiet and his energy level was fairly low. The pulse was racing and slightly floating, while the tongue was swollen and normal in color, with a white sticky coating.

Palpation Channel palpation revealed tenderness mainly along the *tài yīn*, *shào yīn*, and *tài yáng* channels. There was also softness in the muscles along the *yáng míng* stomach channel. The muscles in the area around LU-6 (*kǒng zuì*) were thick and particularly tender, while nodules could be palpated at KI-5 (*shuǐ quán*), LR-3 (*tài chōng*), and BL-62 (*shēn mài*).

Diagnosis *Tài yáng* qi transformation deficiency: heat above, cold below. Due to lack of proper discharging of *tài yáng* there is a blockage in the interstices above, characterized by heat, and obstruction of the bladder organ below leading to difficult urination, incontinence, and cold lower limbs.

Treatment The course of treatment was four months. Treatment goals evolved during the course of treatment and can be generally divided into the following stages:

Regulation

The first three treatments were once weekly for three weeks, with the general goal of regulating qi throughout the body. In the first treatment, the LU-5 (*chǐ zé*) and SP-9 (*yīn líng quán*) point pair was combined with KI-7 (*fù liū*). During the second treatment, some eye swelling was also noted, so LI-6 (*piān lì*), the collateral point of the large intestine channel, was added to the original point prescription to drain *tài yīn* excess through *yáng míng*. CV-3 (*zhōng jí*), the alarm point of the bladder, was added in the third treatment. LI-6 was not used later due to quick improvement in the eye swelling.

Tonification

While aspects of regulation were often a part of subsequent treatments, the focus of later treatments shifted to tonification of the kidney and bladder qi. Over the course of three months, point prescriptions were used in the following order:

• 'The Three *Tài*': For two weeks, LU-9 (*tài yuān*), SP-3 (*tài bái*), and KI-3 (*tài xī*), all source points on their respective channels, were used. To these points, CV-3 and BL-64 (*jīng gǔ*), the source point of the bladder channel, were often added. One-inch needles were used at all four source points, with a twirling technique to cause distending sensation. A 1.5-inch needle was used at CV-3, with deep insertion (1.2 inches) and stimulus radiating downward, followed by lifting the needle to a depth of 0.5 inches after which it was retained for 25 minutes.

• *Shào yīn* focus: For the next six weeks, once weekly treatments shifted to the *shào yīn* channel and most often included HT-7 (*shén mén*), KI-3, KI-6 (*zhào hǎi*), and/or KI-7 (*fù liū*) combined with CV-6 (*qì hǎi*) and either BL-64 (*jīng gǔ*) or moxa at BL-67 (*zhì yīn*), the mother metal point on a water channel. One-inch needles were used at HT-7, KI-3, KI-6, and BL-64, and 1.5-inch needles were used at KI-7 and CV-6. Like CV-3 above, needling at CV-6 involved an initial insertion to a depth of 1.2 inches to facilitate a radiating sensation, followed by retraction to a depth of 0.5 inches and retention for 25 minutes.

Back treatments

During the fourth month of treatment, the rate of improvement seemed to slow and treatment thus shifted to points on the *dū* vessel and bladder channels on the back. In general, back-transport (*shū*) points and *dū* vessel points are considered more warming and moving, and slightly less tonifying, than source points. Points at this stage included variations of the following: GV-4 (*mìng mén*), BL-26 (*guān yuán shū*), BL-28 (*páng guāng shū*), the transport point of the bladder, and the sacral foramina points BL-31 ~ BL-34 (*bā liào*). Needles of 1.5 inches in length were used at all of these points. GB-30 (*huán tiào*) was also needled in some treatments, with a medial insertion angle, for the goal of getting radiation toward the genitals; a 4-inch needle was used for this purpose.

Results The patient reported a reduction in the frequency of urination during the day after the second visit. After the first month of treatment, daytime urination was occasionally frequent, but did not involve incontinence. Urination at night responded more slowly but did show constant improvement. By the second month of treatment, the patient was no longer wetting the bed and had to wake up less frequently at night to urinate. By the fourth month of treatment, he was waking 1–2 times a night, and sometimes not at all. Interestingly, he found that his ability to sweat in the lower half of his body slowly improved over the course of treatment. First, he noticed that his back would sweat on exertion, and later that he began sweating lower and lower on his legs. He eventually noticed that the dryness at his ankles and feet had also improved. Two months into the treatment, the patient's daughter called to report that the whole family had noticed a marked increase in his appetite and that he had gained approximately 5 kilograms in weight.

Analysis Despite the relatively clear nature of the diagnosis in this case, there are a few symptoms that require further consideration. Most notably, there seems to be a slight contradiction in the presence of a racing, floating pulse. One might consider the floating pulse to be an indicator of blockage in the *tài yáng* level. A racing pulse, however, would seem to also indicate heat. Although the patient reported a feeling of warmth in the palms, and palpation revealed warm skin, his tongue and symptom pattern were generally one of deficiency and cold. Throughout the course of treatment, despite improvement in all symptoms (including the cold feet), he continued to have a pulse rate of between 80–90 beats per minute. Incidentally, blood testing had ruled out thyroid disorder or any other metabolic irregularity. In the end, the racing pulse was thought to be an indication of heat from deficiency rising from the kidney, reflected in the warm sensations in the palms. Because of this suspicion that some degree of yin deficiency was present, KI-7 was used in many treatments. While KI-3 is generally considered to be useful in supplementing kidney qi, KI-7 is more often used in the presence of yin deficiency. In some treatments, both points were used together (Table 8.2).

Throughout the course of treatment, a variety of point pairs were used including LU-5 and SP-9, LU-9 and SP-3, CV-6 and KI-7, and CV-6 and KI-3. Further discussion of the functions of these pairs can be found in Chapter 20. In addition to these, one might add the source point pair HT-7 and KI-3, which was used here to strengthen *shào yīn* fire.

It is interesting to note the relationship between the *tài yīn* and *tài yáng*

Phase	Treatment Goal	Main Points Used	Symptom Change
One	Regulate fluid metabolism	LU-5 *(chǐ zé)* and SP-9 *(yīn líng quán)* CV-3 *(zhōng jí)* and BL-64 *(jīng gǔ)* LI-6 *(piān lì)*	Improvement in frequency of daytime urination
Two	Tonify	LU-9 *(tài yuān)*, SP-3 *(tài bái)*, and KI-3 *(tài xī)*; CV-3 *(zhōng jí)* and BL-64 *(jīng gǔ)*; HT-7 *(shén mén)* and KI-3 *(tài xī)*	Improvement in frequency of nighttime urination
Three	Warm and move	GV-4 *(mìng mén)*, BL-26 *(guān yuán shū)*, BL-28 *(páng guāng shū)*, BL-31~BL-34 *(bā liáo)*, GB-30 *(huán tiào)*	Gradual normalization of sweating, improvement of skin moisture, weight gain

Table 8.2
Summary of treatment plan

systems that this case highlights. Consider the discussion of Cinnamon Twig Decoction *(guì zhī tāng)* above. There, the importance of both channels to the nutritive-protective aspects was described. Because both channels are said to 'open' outward, a case such as this one involving *tài yáng* also requires transformation of dampness by *tài yīn*. Note that the initial treatments here included regulation of the *tài yīn* qi dynamic with the uniting point pair LU-5 and SP-9, and that subsequent treatments involved the use of both the spleen and lung source points. This is a reflection of the importance of 'opening' both the *tài yīn* and *tài yáng* in cases of nutritive-protective disharmony. The disharmony in this patient manifested clearly as a problem with sweating and moisture in certain areas of his body.

Fundamentally, this is a case of a yang channel deficiency pattern affecting its paired yin channel. The primary symptoms are generally associated with bladder deficiency, but are also rooted in the paired *shào yīn*. As stated in the passage from the *Inner Classic* at the beginning of this section, bladder function ultimately depends on stimulus from "qi transformation" (the gate of vitality). Chapter 14 will further explore the principle applied in this case that, where there is yang channel deficiency, it is often desirable to supplement the paired yin channel.

The clinical reality in this case also dictated that the practitioner constantly reevaluate progress. While the general principle in the second step of treatment was to tonify, three different tonification strategies were utilized. These strategies do not represent a magic formula for the treatment of bladder qi transformation deficiency, but instead reflect the need for continued reappraisal and modification of channel approaches, based on the rate of improvement as described by the patient and observed by the doctor. In other cases, a different approach might have been used depending on the evolution of the symptoms and changes in the palpated condition along the channel pathways.

■ Narrative

A Story about the Back *Shū* Points

The following story was related after asking Dr. Wang about a treatment for shortness of breath that had utilized the back associated (腧 *shū*) points lateral to the spine.

DR. WANG: In the early 1970s a couple came into our clinic with their son. I remember this case so clearly because it provided unexpected insight into the use of the back associated points. Like most practitioners, I used the points along the bladder channel on the back quite often to treat problems with the internal organs. Then, as now, I used the 'inner line' of back *shū* points closer to the spine when there were physical or structural problems with the internal organs. This is in contrast to problems with what Chinese medicine calls the qi dynamic, which are often best treated by using the five transport (輸 *shū* or 'phase') points on the extremities as lead points. A kidney infection, for example, might call for the use of BL-23 *(shèn shū)*, while kidney qi deficiency is better treated with KI-3 *(tài xī)*.

In any case, this 12-year-old boy was brought to our clinic with the unusual chief complaint of sleepwalking. By the time his parents brought him to me, the boy was moving around the house every few nights. The problem had begun a few months before and, at first, his parents didn't even know that he was sleepwalking. The boy would awake a few hours after going to sleep and go to the kitchen to prepare a snack. He would boil an egg with some noodles and sit quietly in the kitchen eating before going back to sleep. His parents believed that he had not eaten enough at dinner and was simply rambling around the kitchen looking for a midnight snack. It didn't occur to them that he might actually be asleep while doing these things.

It was only after the boy had done this two or three more times that the parents addressed the issue at dinner. The mother encouraged the boy to eat more this time so that he wouldn't have to get up in the middle of the night and wake every one else up with his clanging in the kitchen. "What are you talking about?" asked the boy. "I haven't been getting up at night." The father, believing that the boy was intentionally lying to them, upbraided his son and told him rather sternly that he would not stand any more of his deception or nighttime snacking. The boy, confused, agreed to try to be better, and the matter was seemingly resolved.

However, two nights later, the boy again awoke in the middle of the night and began frying rice in the kitchen. The father, annoyed at being awakened by the sound of spatula on steel, snapped his son on the top of his head and said, "What in the heck are you doing making such a racket here in the middle of the night? Get back to bed!" The boy seemed startled to find himself in this argument with his father and immediately returned to his bed to sleep. The next morning, the father again asked his son with some irritation how he could wake the whole family with his after-hour stir-frying. "Dad, I didn't get up! Why do you keep accusing me when I'm telling the truth?" Impressed with the sincerity of his son's denial, the father began to suspect that something was amiss. He watched his son's face a week later when he awoke to eat soup and realized that he wasn't completely conscious.

The parents first took the boy to their local hospital where he was seen by a neurologist. The doctor diagnosed the boy as a "sleepwalker" and prescribed a mild sedative to be taken before bedtime. Unfortunately, the medication was not helpful and the child continued to wake up and head for the kitchen a few times each week. At this point, the parents brought the child to the Xuan Wu Hospital of Chinese Medicine, where I was working.

Now, in my training, very little had been said about the use of Chinese medicine for sleepwalking. I did remember a discussion of classical texts concerning the concept of the five psychic aspects (五志 *wǔ zhì*). The ethereal (魂 *hún*) and corporeal (魄 *pò*) souls are often said to be involved in sleep disorders. In fact, students are often familiar with the diagnosis of "ethereal soul failing to be stored by the liver" in cases where there are problems with sleep. This case really brought that idea from the textbooks to life for me. With this in mind, I palpated along the lateral urinary bladder line on the back and, in fact, found that the "corporeal soul door" point BL-42 *(pò hù)* and "ethereal soul gate" point BL-47 *(hún mén)* were both very tender. It had always made theoretical sense to me that these points might be helpful for sleep problems, but here was a real-life example of a situation where the points were not only indicated, but also showed palpable change. I treated both points bilaterally. After three treatments, his parents reported that his sleepwalking had abated.

The doctors in our ward thought the case interesting and a few other children with similar complaints came to the clinic. Most were able to get over their sleepwalking issues fairly easily by using these points. I remember another one of these children as well, because this little boy complained not of sleepwalking, but of crying out at night in his sleep. The interesting thing was that he didn't cry out with a voice that sounded like his daytime voice, but instead made sounds almost identical to the braying of a donkey! His parents, city dwellers, were perplexed as to how a boy growing up in Beijing could suddenly develop an aptitude for imitating the sounds of a donkey in his sleep. He responded surprisingly well to treatment with the five psychic aspects points on the back. In his case, I also added the source point of the lung, LU-9 (*tài yuān*), because the braying was likened to sobbing sounds by his parents—a type of sound associated with the lung—and the very act of making braying sounds was likely very stressful on the lung.

Over the years, I occasionally have had cases that make me think of disharmony in the psychic aspects and I then check the condition of the back points associated with each aspect. Furthermore, over the years I have broadened my understanding of the five psychic aspects to include this concept of a kind of prenatal, innate personality or subconscious that I describe. In cases where one suspects that problems stem from these aspects of innate personality, the appropriate points should be checked for changes. It seems that these points are particularly applicable for children, as the problem might be looked at as a kind of developmental issue involving the maturation of the psychic aspects. One might also find severe tenderness along the lateral bladder line representing generalized stasis in these cases.

It is my belief that there is much more to be relearned by modern practitioners about the application of Chinese medicine to psychology. There is a tendency sometimes by modern practitioners to view concepts such as the five psychic aspects as "superstitions." While the concepts have, in some instances, been given various religious meanings by the Daoists and Buddhists, I think that there is still more to these ancient ideas than meets the eye. Problems with applying these ideas in the modern clinic may very well stem from problems understanding exactly what ancient physicians meant when they diagnosed a patient as having disharmony in the psychic aspects. In other words, we still haven't gotten a very precise understanding of which cases apply to which "aspect." This problem, in turn, leads to a loose grasp of the points said to treat each of the five aspects. Because the concepts have still not been fully understood in the modern era, diagnostic precision suffers.

It has been my experience that the key to consistent use of any concept in Chinese medicine depends on a clear understanding in the doctor's mind of the diagnosis. The clearer the diagnosis, the more precise the treatment. In the case of acupuncture, different points have different natures. They are kind of like people in that respect. Some people are adept at doing a wide variety of things: jacks-of-all-trades. Other people have only very specific skills. Commonly-used acupuncture points like ST-36 *(zú sān lǐ)*, SP-6 *(sān yīn jiāo)*, CV-12 *(zhōng wǎn)*, and GB-34 *(yáng líng quán)* are points of very broad application. On the other hand, other points that are rarely used have very precise applications for particular illnesses.

In the case of these rarely used points, the key is to get to know them. One must know their specific strengths and not attempt to apply them too broadly. This, to me, is one of the most subtle and difficult aspects of acupuncture to teach. Experience and careful study is the only way to get to know the very precise personalities of some of the points. The lateral line of transport points on the bladder channel represents just such a dilemma. These are points that are rarely used (except in cases of local pain) and are thus more difficult to get to know.

Psychic Aspect	Back Transport Point	Point Name in English
Ethereal soul (魂 *hún*)—liver	BL-47 (魂門 *hún mén*)	Gate of the ethereal soul
Spirit (神 *shén*)—heart	BL-44 (神堂 *shén táng*)	Hall of the spirit
Intention (意 *yì*)—spleen	BL-49 (意舍 *yì shè*)	Abode of intent
Corporeal soul (魄 *pò*)—lung	BL-42 (魄戶 *pò hù*)	Door of the corporeal soul
Essence (精 *jīng*)/ Will (志 *zhì*)—kidney	BL-52 (志室 *zhì shì*)	Residence of the will

Table 8.3
The five psychic aspects and their associated back transport points

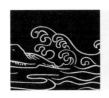

CHAPTER 9

少陽

THE *Shào Yáng* (LESSER YANG) SYSTEM

The General Nature and Function of *Shào Yáng*

Shào yáng is the pivot (樞 *shū*) between the opening of *tài yáng* at the surface and the closing of *yáng míng* inward toward yin. The yang pivot weaves together the triple burner and gallbladder organs. Classical sources, most famously the *Discussion of Cold Damage*, describe *shào yáng* as being "between the interior and the exterior." Thus, while the skin and external surfaces of the body are associated with *tài yáng* and the pathways of digestion are within the scope of *yáng míng*, all the other yang areas of the body are encompassed by *shào yáng*. This is largely due to the vast scope of the *shào yáng* triple burner 'organ', a unique and important concept that will be developed at length in this chapter. Like the yin pivot *shào yīn*, the *shào yáng* channel is associated with movement and regulation—now in the areas outside of the internal organs. Also like the *shào yīn* pivot, the channel regulates in normal physiology and is used clinically to drain in cases of excess accumulation. Specifically, the channel is used clinically to "clear and drain [heat] while dispersing clumped [qi]" (清瀉疏結 *qīng xiè shū jié*). Ultimately, *shào yáng* pathology revolves around the concept that, when regulation is compromised, heat and qi become clumped in the interior.

One of the metaphors used in the *Inner Classic* to describe the nature of *shào yáng*—"balanced in the center and spotless" (中正潔淨 *zhōng zhèng jié jìng*)—is often associated with Confucian ideas about governance. This is an allusion to two basic Confucian principles: a balanced 'middle road' between extremes in governance, and the maintenance of 'spotless principles' free from corruption. These principles reflect the physiological role played by *shào yáng*. Charged with making decisions about the distribution of source qi (in the case of the triple burner) and absorption in digestion (in the gallbladder), the *shào yáng* must remain free of corruption. 'Corruption' here refers to stasis of any kind that might prevent movement through this far-reaching pivot between the interior and exterior of the body. As yang organs, the primary functions of the triple burner and gallbladder involve the maintenance of movement through passageways.

The concept of movement through a physiological pivot may be summarized in the single word 'regulation' (調理 *tiáo lǐ*). In particular, the pivot of *shào yáng* regulates the flow of qi and fluids in the passageways surrounding the internal organs. The concept of an internal pivot was discussed earlier with regard to *shào yīn*, where it was said to regulate the metabolic fires of the yin organs (see Chapter 6). By contrast, *shào yáng* regulates the various 'climates' surrounding not only the internal organs, but all the other structures of the body as well. It is important to remember that *shào yáng* regulation occurs in the middle of the three yang levels. In the case of the triple burner, it warms and moistens the internal organs while facilitating the transport of fluids, first separated at *yáng míng* (with the help of *tài yīn*), outward to the *tài yáng* level for distribution as sweat above and urine below. At the same time, the *shào yáng* gallbladder acts as a pivot for the regulation of digestion among the other yang organs (Fig. 9.1).

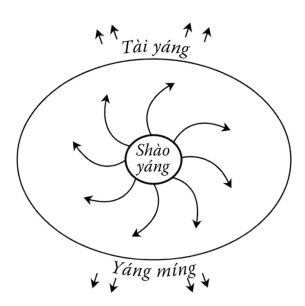

Fig. 9.1
Shào yáng is the pivot of regulatory movement
between *tài yáng* and *yáng míng*.

At this point it would be helpful to recall the metaphor of the dumpling steamer discussed in Chapter 2. In this metaphor, the steamer's ability to regulate the movement of steam is likened to that of *shào yáng*. Like the pressure beneath the lid of the steamer, *shào yáng* acts to allow heat radiating from the more internal *yáng míng* level to move upward and outward to *tài yáng*. The interstices at the *tài yáng* level may be likened to the bamboo latticework of the lid itself. On the other hand, if *yáng míng* heat is insufficient, *shào yáng* prevents heat from being lost by slowing the outward radiation. *Shào yáng* is thus likened to the ability of the steamer to hold in or release steam. Again, the operative word is *regulation*.

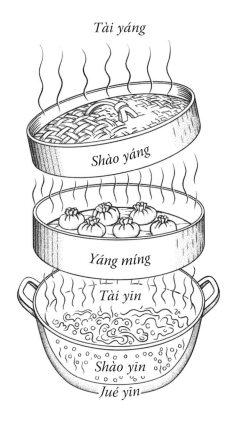

Shào yáng is paired with *jué yīn*, providing fire and movement to enliven the stillness of the deepest yin. The liver and pericardium, reservoirs of blood, are stimulated by their paired yang organs. The presence of the yang gallbladder assists the liver by facilitating decisions about the distribution of blood to the organs. The pairing of the triple burner and pericardium is quite interesting. Both organs have been the subject of much debate over the centuries, turning largely on the so-called 'formless' nature of both organs. Despite the fact that the pericardium is associated with the tissue surrounding the heart muscle, the functions of that organ are quite different from those described by modern physiology. There is an even greater gulf between modern science and Chinese medicine in the case of the triple burner, discussed below.

Shào yáng is also associated with the 'sinew-bones' (筋骨 *jīn gǔ*).[1] This concept should be carefully distinguished from both the liver function of nourishing the sinews and the kidney's role in bone development. The liver nourishes the sinews through the medium of blood while the kidney facilitates the development of bones through the essence and marrow. By contrast, *shào yáng* is associated with movement in the joints (a pivot). Thus, while the liver nourishes the sinews and the kidney facilitates bone development, *shào yáng* is responsible for movement in the spaces between the sinews and bones. It is important to distinguish nourishment, a yin function, from movement, a yang function. If either the sinews or bones lack nourishment, treatment should be directed at benefiting the liver or kidney. On the other hand, if there are problems with moving the joints due to poor fluid circulation, look to *shào yáng* (Fig. 9.2).

The movement of fluids by *shào yáng* is the vehicle by which nourishment is brought to the sinew-bones and metabolic waste is taken away. One might therefore think of the synovial membranes and fluids when interpreting a passage from the classics that asserts, for example, that "the water pathways issue from the triple burner."[2]

Among the six external qi, *shào yáng* is associated with summerheat (暑 *shǔ*). This is a slow-moving, external pathogen characterized by both dampness and heat. Healthy movement through the *shào yáng* pivot is needed to

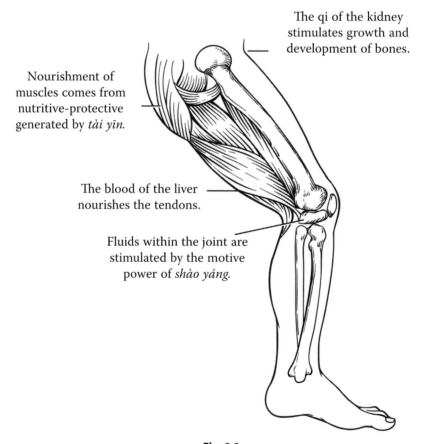

The qi of the kidney stimulates growth and development of bones.

Nourishment of muscles comes from nutritive-protective generated by *tài yīn*.

The blood of the liver nourishes the tendons.

Fluids within the joint are stimulated by the motive power of *shào yáng*.

Fig. 9.2
The movement of muscles and joints depends on the coordinated functions of multiple organs and channels.

deal properly with this external pathogen. For this reason, sluggishness in *shào yáng* circulation, or cold in the gallbladder, can be a predisposing factor for susceptibility to this external pathogen. Internally, *shào yáng* conditions are often associated with the flaring of ministerial fire. Remember that this is not the sovereign fire of the heart, but the fire rising from the gate of vitality. When not properly rooted by yin, ministerial fire can flare upward to affect *shào yáng* (see Chapter 6).

It is important to understand the relationship of the healthy ministerial fire associated with kidney *shào yīn* and the pathological ministerial fire associated with *shào yáng*, discussed in Chapter 6. To review, ministerial fire comes from the gate of vitality, associated with the kidney. It enlivens the beating of the heart (its paired *shào yīn* organ) while also traveling through *shào yáng*. Normal movement of the *shào yáng* organs requires this primary fire. Another metaphor might be helpful. *Shào yīn* ministerial fire may be likened to the heat radiating from a cup of tea while *shào yáng* ministerial fire is more like a flame. In normal physiology, the flame stays within the bounds required to stimulate the *shào yáng* organs. But if it flares up due to kidney yin deficiency (not 'rooting' fire) or gallbladder stagnation, the flame becomes the 'ascending counterflow of ministerial fire' (相火上逆 *xiàng huǒ shàng nì*) (Fig. 9.3).

Symptoms of this pattern, most often associated with the liver and gallbladder, include headache, dizziness, red face, dry mouth, and a stuffy sensation in the chest. Since the fire is often due to lack of movement through the *shào yáng* pivot, symptoms such as constipation may also present.

The pathogenesis of ministerial fire may also include deficiency. For example, a deficiency of *shào yáng* fire may reduce the dredging and draining by the liver. When this function is compromised, it affects the ability of the body to clear waste. In a circle of pathology, the resulting stasis can lead to heat and the associated flaring of ministerial fire.

In fact, the interaction of *shào yáng* deficiency and *jué yīn* excess is often under-appreciated. Symptoms such as urinary and bowel difficulties combined with dryness of the mouth, eyes, and nasal passages may be indications of this relatively common pattern. The individual may also be less responsive to the external environment and present with symptoms similar to those seen in patients who take certain antidepressants: a lack of strong emotional highs or lows. Or to turn this around, these antidepressants might be understood to have a sedating effect on the dredging and draining functions of the liver. From the perspective of Chinese medicine, this might explain why stopping the medications can cause the original symptoms—strong highs and lows—to return or even worsen. This pattern can

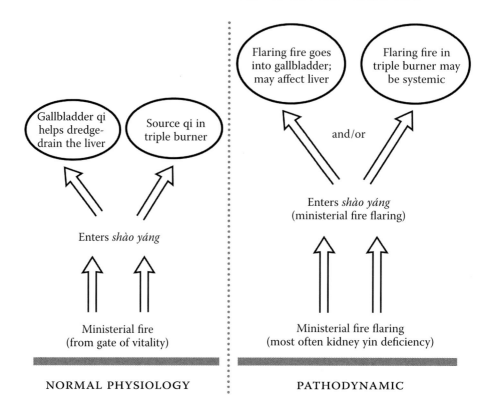

Fig. 9.3

The relationship between the pivotal fires of *shào yīn* and *shào yáng*

be understood as a type of stagnation that has not been properly cleared. Although often associated with *jué yīn*, the fire of *shào yáng* may be needed to activate healthy liver dredging in these types of cases. One might warm the gallbladder with Warm the Gallbladder Decoction *(wēn dǎn tāng)*, modified, of course, to include herbs to help dredge the liver.[3] If severe, the treatment principle would also necessarily involve a focus on improving the flow of ministerial fire *(shào yīn)* upon which the *shào yáng* organs depend.

It should now be clear that internal symptoms associated with *shào yáng* are rooted in a lack of movement. Movement is most often compromised due to stagnation or a deficiency of ministerial fire. All excess-type *shào yáng* disorders can be reduced to this fundamental cause—a lack of movement leading to compromised regulation and thus the generation of heat. This is why the most common use of the channel in the clinic is to 'clear and drain [heat] while dispersing clumped [qi]'. While a significant deficiency of *shào yáng* fire (just described) would be an obvious exception, most clinical applications of *shào yáng* focus on clearing and moving. Even when deficiency is part of the picture, tonification must be accompanied by maintenance of movement in the channels and organs. A helpful image might be that of the moats and ditches that surround ancient Chinese city walls. If, over time, there is a lack of movement, leaves, sticks, and waste build up. In the body, such build-up in the ditches of *shào yáng* leads to heat, and treatment almost always involves reestablishing movement.

The principle of movement is key to the effectiveness of other herbal approaches to *shào yáng* conditions as well. The formula Minor Bupleurum Decoction *(xiǎo chái hú tāng)*, for example, clears heat by reestablishing movement in the pathways of *shào yáng*. Consequently, the formula has a wide variety of clinical applications that go beyond its common use in treating external conditions trapped between the exterior and the interior. In herbal therapy, when thinking of *shào yáng*, the key is to consider the movement and regulation of fluids as a means of clearing heat. Again, however, when it is more a case of pure deficiency, the idea of generating ministerial fire from *shào yīn* must also be taken into account.

In acupuncture, modern clinical texts present a fairly limited use of the *shào yáng* channels in treating internal disorders. Nevertheless, as many practitioners know, texts on musculoskeletal conditions often include a wider variety of gallbladder and triple burner channel treatments. The frequency of *shào yáng* treatments for musculoskeletal disorders underlines the association of the channels with the spaces between the joints, bones, and organs. These same areas, of course, may be associated with more internal disorders involving inflammation as well. Consequently, *shào yáng* should also be considered in cases of goiter, lymphatic conditions, cysts, and boils—all instances of fire and toxicity 'between the interior and the exterior'.

Two pairs of points illustrate the concepts underlying the use of *shào yáng* in the clinic. The first, TB-6 *(zhī gōu)* and GB-34 *(yáng líng quán)*, is used to dredge constraint and clumping (疏鬱結 *shū yù jié*) from the *shào yáng*. This pair can be used in the treatment of diverse patterns ranging from constipation to pain, whenever constrained qi is the cause. It may be likened to 'shaking the channel out' so as to promote movement. The second pair, TB-5 *(wài guān)* and GB-41 *(zú lín qì)*, is used to clear when heat in *shào yáng* is more primary. Conditions such as tinnitus, conjunctivitis, dizziness, or high blood pressure due to rising heat can be treated with this second pair. If a patient presents with *both* heat and stagnation, a helpful approach is to use the second pair until the heat symptoms recede, then follow up with the first pair to facilitate movement.

Triple Burner

"The Triple Burner holds the office of irrigation design; the water pathways issue from it."

(三焦者．決瀆之官．水道出焉。 *Sān jiāo zhě, jué dú zhī guān, shuǐ dào chū yān*.)

—*Basic Questions*, Chapter 8

The concept of the triple burner is one of the most debated topics in historical Chinese medical literature. Records of that debate begin with the above-cited passage from the *Inner Classic*. Some scholar-physicians over the centuries focused on determining which (if any) anatomical structures comprise this unusual 'organ', while others focused on defining its physiological functions.

As reflected in the passage above, the *Inner Classic* succinctly describes the triple burner as an organ of irrigation and waterway management. Thus the earliest extant text on the subject describes the triple burner as the maintainer of the fluid passageways.

Approximately three-hundred years later, the *Classic of Difficulties* tried to clarify the meaning of the triple burner. Chapter 31 of that text begins by asking:

> How is the triple burner supplied and what does it generate? Where does it begin and end? At which places [in the body] might one treat the triple burner? Is it even possible to know these things? [4]

Even from a great distance in time and culture, it can be seen that the concept of the triple burner, and questions about its form and functions, confounded physicians as far back as the Han dynasty. The answers to the questions raised in this passage begin with the statement that the triple burner is the "passageway for water and grains," thus linking the organ to the transport of postnatal essence. The text goes on to say that the triple burner is the "beginning and end of the pathways of qi," that is, both the creation and the eventual use of qi in normal physiology occurs in the triple burner. In sum, this chapter states that the postnatal essence moves, and qi is transformed, within the passageways of the triple burner.

What does this mean? In many ways, this statement has parallels in modern biochemistry. As understood by ancient physicians, the transport of nutrition and the generation of activity are said to occur within the confines of the triple burner. In modern parlance, when one speaks of "the ultimate destination of postnatal essence and the beginning and end of qi," one might be discussing the cells of the body. It is to the cells that nutrition ultimately goes and it is in the cells that activity begins and ends. The extracellular environment that bathes this process might be likened to the triple burner. While acknowledging the obvious limitations of trying to create equivalents across such a formidable conceptual distance, the comparison between the triple burner qi transformation and the extracellular environment provides relevant insight into classical concepts.

QI TRANSFORMATION WITHIN THE TRIPLE BURNER

The pathways of the triple burner are involved in all qi transformation in the body. All of the myriad transformations of qi, at every moment during the process of metabolism, are occurring within the environments maintained by the triple burner. As just noted, in modern physiological terms, the triple burner might be thought to represent the fluid pathways within which the complex process of cellular metabolism occurs. In other words, references to the triple burner as the location of the "beginning and end of qi" involve concepts similar to the modern understanding of the conveyance and removal of nourishment and waste from the cells.

There are three basic preconditions for proper triple burner qi transformation:

There must be a primary stimulus that initiates transformation. In classical Chinese physiology this stimulus is called source qi, which comes from the gate of vitality and is associated with (or located between) the kidneys. This is the process of fire distribution from *shào yīn* to *shào yáng* shown in Fig. 9.3 above. This primary stimulus is also viewed as being 'prenatal', thus implying its quintessential nature. It may also be likened to the modern understanding of genes as arbiters of the processes of conception, growth, development, and ultimately decay. Chapter 66 of *The Classic of Difficulties* states that "The triple burner is the director of separation for the source qi and is responsible for the movement of the three qi through the five yin and six yang organs."[5] Source qi is thus the spark that stimulates function (功能 *gōng néng*) in every organ of the body.

There must be a location and a proper environment for qi transformation to occur. As noted earlier, because the *Inner Classic* asserts that "water pathways issue from" the triple burner, we imagine this environment to be aqueous and all-pervasive. Like a living river, the organ is both a pathway *and* an environment for the primary stimulus of source qi. Unless this environment is properly maintained by the triple burner, the primary genetic stimulus of the gate of vitality cannot be actualized.

[217]

There must be free and easy movement within that environment. The use of the term 'environment' in describing the triple burner is instructive. The nature of the different environments in the three 'burners' will be discussed below, but in general, as so many Chinese concepts are derived from observations of the natural world, it may be helpful here to analyze the environmental images which are used as metaphors for triple burner qi transformation.

One such image is the movement of water from the oceans and glaciers on the planet surface to the clouds above, when it is stimulated by the warmth of the sun. With evaporation, water travels to the skies above the continents and falls to the ground as rain. Rain nourishes the plants and animals of the continental biosphere as it passes through streams, creeks, and rivers on its way back to its ultimate destination in the seas. Remember too that the fluids passing through rivers and streams contain more than just water. Minerals and other substances that nourish plants and animals are also carried along the earth's waterways. Eventually, after passing through the multitude of interweaving rivers, streams, and lakes, water makes its way back to the sea and the circle begins again.

Of course, this description is an oversimplification. Within each area irrigated by the earth's waterways are many varieties of plants and animals that are themselves nourished not only by water, but also by the minerals and climate of their particular region. There are countless microclimates all over the planet which use the earth's water in different ways and at different rates. Concentrations of plants and trees, which thrive in areas of rich soil, themselves become sources of fluids which evaporate from the surfaces of their leaves. Thus the giant circuit of fluids from the oceans through the rivers and back to the oceans contains within it many smaller circuits that are dependent on their varied geography (Fig. 9.4).

Just as the environment of the planet teems with complexity, so too does the human body. Within the seemingly simple concepts of triple burner and channel theory in Chinese medicine, there is an appreciation of the complexity of the human ecosystem. It is a disservice to assume that generations of physicians in China were unable to grasp this fundamental concept. As previously noted, ancient scientists were able to look beyond what they could see by utilizing the tool of metaphor. Often, by observing and reflecting upon the complexity of their natural environments, scientists in ancient China (and other premodern cultures) were able to make astute inferences about the nature of the world within themselves. The often underappreciated complexity inherent in the concept of triple burner qi transformation as maintaining 'environments' represents one of the great achievements of classical Chinese medicine.

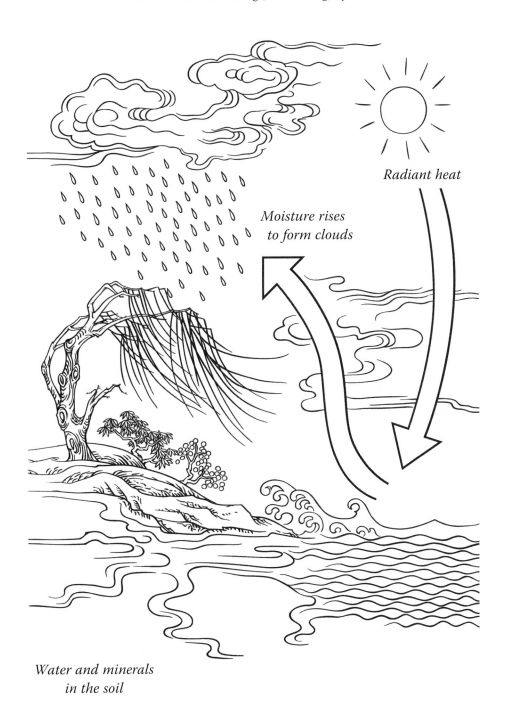

Radiant heat

*Moisture rises
to form clouds*

*Water and minerals
in the soil*

Fig. 9.4
Like the climates and microclimates of the natural environment,
the triple burner regulates through the medium of water.

THE SHAPE OF THE TRIPLE BURNER

Returning to the *Classic of Difficulties*, Chapter 31 goes on to carefully describe the location of each of the three burners. What is important to note at this point is that, according to the authors, both the functions and location of the triple burner can in fact be defined. The *physical form* of the organ, however, is not described. While there is a 'location' for each of the three burners, Chapter 38 says that the organ "has a name but no form" (有名而無形 *yǒu míng ér wú xíng*). This would suggest that the triple burner is a kind of overarching concept for metabolism which occurs in three separate sections of the chest and abdomen. It is not a physical organ that might be taken out of the body and observed on a laboratory table.

This statement, that the triple burner "has a name but no form," is the crux of much debate over the centuries. Classical authors struggled with the concept of an organ with a name, location, and function but "no form." Some authors felt that the triple burner was only an anatomical dividing line between three sections of the body, while others insisted that its lack of form meant that it was an all-pervasive influence in the internal environment of the body, a kind of Daoist formlessness. Some felt that the triple burner had no form of its own, but took on the form defined by other internal organs. In this conception, the triple burner is like a piece of clothing (or an exterior casing) that has no form until worn. Once it was put on (as it were), the triple burner would take the form of the organs folded within it. This idea provides a means by which the ancient concept might be understood in a modern light (Fig. 9.5).

Some sources also use the term 'corridor' to describe the form of the triple burner. The character translated here as corridor (隙 *xì*) can also mean a crack or fissure. If, as above, one views the shape of the triple burner like a piece of clothing that takes its form from the organs held within, this might also include the fissures, or spaces, within that clothing. In fact, as a hollow yang organ, the triple burner is more about the spaces within the clothing than the clothing itself. In any case, this 'clothing' exists not only around the organs in the chest and abdomen, but also around the muscles, nerves, and vessels in the peripheral limbs.

This is a newer and broader understanding of the triple burner. No longer limited to just the three sections of the chest and abdomen described in many modern texts, the triple burner may be associated with the fluid-filled spaces of the body. In the most general sense, these are the spaces inside the mesenteric linings and connective tissues described by modern physiology, all effused with interstitial fluid. Perhaps the description found in some modern texts of the triple burner as the "corridor of the five yin and six yang

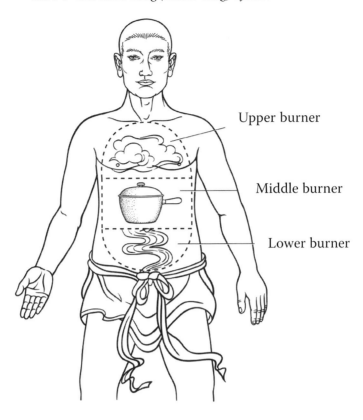

Fig. 9.5
Classical view of the triple burner

organs" (五臟六腑之所隙 *wǔ zàng liù fǔ zhī suǒ xì*) is a reference to the important role played by those spaces in physiology. This concept is linked to the role of fluids in the triple burner as the location of qi transformation.

Before going on, it is important to point out the relationship between blood and the fluids in the triple burner. Although the concept of the triple burner does not include the blood, the fluids of the triple burner are just as important in both classical physiology and pathology. This is because all of the fluids within the linings of the triple burner ultimately come from and return to the blood. Modern physiology provides a picture that mirrors this concept in descriptions of blood circulation at the capillary level. Physiology textbooks describe how the division into smaller and smaller vessels ends in the space where the tiniest capillaries enter the interstitial fluid. At that point, plasma from the arterial capillaries leaves the vessels to become interstitial fluid that circulates around the cells and is later reabsorbed into the circulatory system by the venous capillaries (Fig. 9.6).

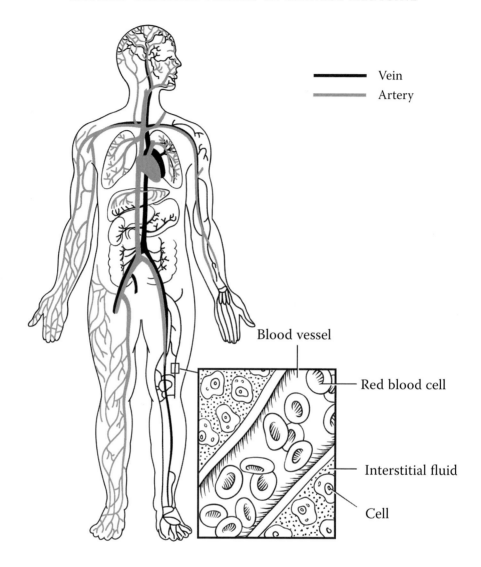

Fig. 9.6
The modern understanding of capillary circulation provides
some interesting insight into the triple burner as a classical model for
understanding interstitial fluid flow within connective tissue (fascial) pathways.

It is at this level that nutrition generated by the breakdown of food leaves the blood system and travels through the interstitial fluid to the cells. As described in Chapter 5 on *tài yīn*, the nutrition in the interstitial fluids is supported by the spleen and enters the fluids through the blood in the form of the nutritive (營 *yíng*) aspect. The transfer of waste from the cells into the venous capillary system involves a similar interstitial leap. Incidentally, the waste includes not only the by-products of cellular metabolism, but also dead cells, unwanted bacteria, and viruses. All of these substances pass through the interstitial fluids on their way back into the circulatory system. Note that, in this context, the concept of 'circulatory system' also includes the lymphatic system. To be precise, the modern understanding of fluid circulation also takes note of the role of lymphatic circulation in helping to bring fluids back into the blood after filtration. In any case, the triple burner involves interstitial spaces that are also beyond the level of the lymphatic capillaries. The quality and movement of the interstitial fluids vary in different parts of the body, and change over time. These aspects of interstitial fluid circulation can be likened to what classical physicians termed the 'corridors' of the triple burner.[6]

A picture is thus drawn of an organ that is pervasive in the fissures of the body, but has no distinct form of its own. Furthermore, one can see how the triple burner comes to be involved in one way or another with the vast majority of physiology and pathology.

Another classical concept that relates to the form of the triple burner is that of the 'membrane source' (膜原 *mó yuán*). Classical anatomy texts seem to associate this membrane with the mesenteric lining that attaches the internal organs to one another and to the abdominal cavity.[7] Thus the membrane source is a classically-defined structure that might also fall within the definition of the triple burner organ. This spongy lining is also suffused with interstitial fluid and includes both the raw materials and by-products of cellular metabolism.

In any case, wherever they are found, the nutrients, ions, and hormones moving within the interstitial fluids may be likened to the "water and grains" and "beginning and end of qi" that are said to be within the purview of the triple burner. At this point, the mind of ancient China might make tentative contact with the anatomy labs of the 21st century. But common ground, of course, does not mean equivalency, and the concept of the triple burner represents a unique understanding of these spaces, with a special emphasis on the importance of the fluids found within. Like its paired yin organ, the pericardium, the triple burner is a tissue lining whose significance is broader than anything found in modern anatomy. Most importantly, classical physiology posits that the lining surrounding the organs is the pathway of source qi—the diffuse presence of inheritance (prenatal) in the body. This concept is quite foreign to modern physiology. Therefore, in order for the modern practitioner to fully understand the triple burner, it is important to have a clear idea of what is meant by the term 'source qi'.

THE ROLE OF SOURCE QI IN THE TRIPLE BURNER

Chapter 38 of the *Classic of Difficulties* describes the triple burner as "the disseminator of source qi and determiner of all other qi" (原氣之別 焉，主持諸氣 *yuán qì zhī bié yān, zhǔ chí zhū qì*). In other words, source qi, traveling in the triple burner, is distributed throughout the body where it sparks the development of all other types of qi. The clinical application of source points is based on this passage, and on the related Chapter 66 of the *Classic of Difficulties* as well (see Chapter 17 of our text). The Chinese character 原 *(yuán)*, from which the English term 'source' is derived, literally means original, primary, or unprocessed. In classical physiology, source qi arises from the primary movement of the gate of vitality.

Earlier we introduced the idea that source qi has some tentative parallels with the concept of genetics and hormones in modern physiology. While these parallels help the modern mind get through the door, so to speak, they are still quite different from the original meaning of source qi. In Chinese medicine, the qi transformation of all organs ultimately depends on the stimulus from source qi. It is the first breath of life. All other types of qi in the body are infused with it. To restate another concept developed earlier, both ministerial fire and source qi arise from the gate of vitality, but each has different functions in the body. Ministerial fire is the warming and moving aspect of the gate of vitality, while source qi can be likened to the fundamental spark of life. In the fluids of the triple burner, source qi intermingles with the nutritive aspect of blood from food and drink and the qi of the external world drawn from the breath. This is the biochemistry of ancient China (Fig. 9.7).

Traveling in the triple burner, described above as corridors filled with interstitial fluid, source qi exerts its broad influence on metabolism. In fact, it is possible to conceive of a unique system in the body comprised of the interplay of the gate of vitality, source qi, and the triple burner. Fundamentally, it is a system that provides the spark of life at the cellular level. In classical physiology, source qi is not only the primary spark of qi transformation but also determines the length of a person's life. Chinese medicine links the quality of the kidneys and the gate of vitality to longevity. Source qi is the medium through which longevity is attained. As a person ages, the quality of source qi arising from the gate of vitality begins to decline and the tissues of the body and marrow of the bones are no longer properly nourished. Hollowing of the marrow weakens the bones and slows the workings of the brain.

Treatment strategies to slow the aging process don't focus on 'strengthening the brain' or 'brightening the skin' but on maintaining an even flow of

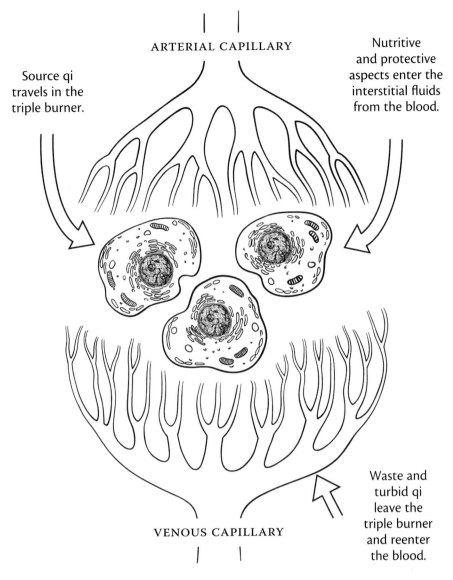

ARTERIAL CAPILLARY

Source qi travels in the triple burner.

Nutritive and protective aspects enter the interstitial fluids from the blood.

Waste and turbid qi leave the triple burner and reenter the blood.

VENOUS CAPILLARY

Fig. 9.7
Detail of a view of the triple burner at the cellular level

source qi by benefiting the kidney and keeping the passageways of circulation open. (The treatment of chronic or serious illness with gate of vitality herbal tonics follows a similar line of thought.) Because source qi follows the pathways of the triple burner, the ability of the other organs to receive this vital stimulus depends on the health and smooth flow of this multilevel organ.

THE THREE BURNERS

Up to this point, our discussion has focused on clarifying the definition of the triple burner and broadening its location to include not just the three 'burners' described in basic textbooks, but also the fluid-filled spaces that surround the cells of the body. Now we must return to another basic Chinese medicine concept, the tripartite nature of the organ within the thoracic and abdominal cavities. No discussion of the triple burner would be complete without addressing this concept. However, before doing so, let's again consider the basic terminology.

The term 'triple burner' is a translation of the Chinese characters 三焦 (sān jiāo). It has also been rendered as 'san jiao' or 'triple energizer'. While in most cases the translation of a term into English will provide greater clarity, in the case of the triple burner, translation requires careful consideration of the unique meaning of the original Chinese. The first character, 三, represents the number three and thus needs no further elaboration. The second character, 焦, most often means burnt, worried, or agitated. Thus the most straightforward English rendering of the term is, in fact, triple burner. In its classical sense, the word burner is helpful only insofar as it provides an image of a warm place of transformation.

But there is more to the meaning of 三焦. Modern students, often confused by the lack of clear definition when first encountering the term, tend to emphasize the concept of 'burner' at the expense of 'three'. But it is important to remember that the triple burner is a three-in-one organ encompassing three distinct sections of the body. All three sections might be described as 'burners' only if that term is understood to mean an environmental system. In other words, each of the three sections should be thought of as unique micro-climates within the body's internal topography, with its own specific requirements for temperature, pH, and relative pressure.

Upper burner   The uppermost of the three burners is said to "take in but not send out" (主納而不出 zhū nà ér bù chū).[8] The upper burner takes in food and external qi through the mouth and directs them downward. It encompasses the esophagus, lungs, and heart and can be treated at CV-17 (tán zhōng). The *Divine Pivot* likens the environment of the upper burner to mist (霧 wù).[9] It is a light environment with lower relative pressure around the lungs. It is empty (虛 xū) and clean so as to provide space and nourishment for the inhalation and exhalation of the lungs and the beating of the heart.

Middle burner   The *Inner Classic* likens the middle burner to a compost or pickling pot (漚 òu). This is the warm cauldron of the spleen and stomach where the reception and transformation of food and water occur. The middle burner is said to "receive and decompose food and water" (腐受水谷 *fǔ shòu shuǐ gǔ*). The direction associated with the middle burner is not so much upward or downward, but more like moving around the pivot of the umbilicus. Its activity is transformative, and is thus roughly analogous to the stomach and small intestine in modern physiology. (In Chinese medicine the functions of the stomach and small intestine tend to overlap.) The middle burner is treated at ST-25 *(tiān shū)*.

Lower burner The lower burner is likened to a ditch (瀆 *dú*). It is said to facilitate the draining and removal of waste from above. This lowest of the burners can be found below the umbilicus, extending to the lower aspect of the bladder. It is said to both "take in and send out" (主納而出 *zhū nà ér chū*). Its pathways include the large intestine, small intestine, and bladder. The goal of metabolism in the lower burner is to make the final separation of the clear and turbid from food and fluids. The lower burner is treated at CV-7 *(yīn jiāo)*.

Putting it all together

The next question that naturally comes to mind is, How can one reconcile the concept of three separate burners in the chest and abdomen with the earlier notion of the triple burner as the small spaces in the body? The answer to this question can be found in a common thread that runs between the two models: the regulation and integration (調和 *tiáo hé*) of internal environments. In the chest and abdomen, there are three different internal environments for the major organs that are maintained fairly precisely by the three burners. By contrast, the presence of the triple burner in the extremities is more diverse, as it surrounds the peripheral muscles, nerves, and vessels. The body's matrix of connective tissue unifies the entire system, and it is within this matrix that one can find the interstitial fluid pathways, the "beginning and end of the pathways of qi" that occur in cellular metabolism. Thus the concept of the triple burner as three parts of the chest and abdomen, on one hand, and as spaces in the peripheral limbs, on the other, finds common ground in the fact that both are describing pathways that maintain the internal environment.

To summarize, there are two perspectives from which to view the triple burner:

1. *The 'cavity' (腔體 qiāng tǐ) concept of the triple burner as three parts of the chest and abdomen.*

This is the most common understanding and, historically, may also involve equating the triple burner with the digestive process in general.

2. The spaces surrounding the tissues of both the internal organs and the peripheral limbs.

This concept also includes areas near the surface of the body, beneath the skin, and "between the external and the internal." Interestingly, when one contrasts the muscle tissue surrounding the organs with that found in the limbs a difference emerges: the muscles in the peripheral limbs are larger and thus the spaces around them are also much larger. By contrast, the muscles of the body trunk are smaller, often smooth muscles that have less peripheral space. This leads to the rather counterintuitive assertion that stimulating points in the larger inter-muscle spaces on the arms and legs can have a greater effect on triple burner qi transformation than points on the body trunk. This may be one reason why the points on the distal limbs are so powerful in the clinic. (The relative effects of points on the limbs versus the trunk will be further explored in Chapters 16 and 17.)

Recall again that the *shào yáng* level is the pivot of the three yang levels, with the *tài yáng* above and the *yáng míng* below. The function of the pivot of the yang levels is to regulate movement. The triple burner regulates the movement of "fluids and grains" among the environments within its purview. It also integrates the three burners of the thoracic and abdominal cavities by "opening the ditches" and maintaining smooth interchange and communication among its three micro-climates.

Because of its internal pairing with the pericardium, the triple burner is sometimes associated with helping to regulate movement between the heart and kidneys. The pivots of *shào yīn* and *shào yáng* are in fact interwoven by the physiology of the pericardium and triple burner. In the clinic, formulas to treat problems with heart-kidney interaction often include herbs to stimulate triple burner circulation. For example, the formula Emperor of Heaven's Special Pill to Tonify the Heart *(tiān wáng bǔ xīn dān)* contains three herbs that help regulate fluids and stimulate movement in the triple burner. Polygalae Radix *(yuǎn zhì)* calms the spirit by transforming phlegm and opening the passageways of source qi. Poria *(fú líng)* percolates dampness in the middle and lower burner to create fluid movement below, while Platycodi Radix *(jié gěng)* facilitates the upward/downward movement of *tài yīn*. Together, these three herbs keep the pathways of the triple burner open so that the more tonifying herbs in the formula have an avenue through which to connect the kidney below to the heart above.

Regulation and integration also come to mind when considering the place of the triple burner among the other five yang organs. Like those organs, the triple burner is a hollow organ charged with transporting substances through or out of the body. It was previously noted how the triple burner is sometimes thought of as a regulator and integrator of movement along the pathway of the GI tract. In this context, the functions of the triple burner are associated with peristaltic movement: the wave of physiological activity from esophagus to colon. This provides another application for the triple burner in the clinic. In the abdomen, one might consider the triple burner to be 'digestion' in the most general sense. This is because the organ holds within itself the stomach, large intestine, small intestine, and gallbladder.

Points along the triple burner channel are in fact helpful clinically for general digestive regulation. If a patient has problems throughout the GI tract, and it is difficult to determine which organ is primarily affected, then the triple burner may be the place to start. It might be thought of as the 'central command' since the triple burner oversees movement in the small spaces surrounding the organs throughout the system. This is especially true in the case of digestive yang deficiency, usually associated with the spleen and kidney. Deficiency of this type is due to a lack of stimulation from source qi in the digestive system. In this case, the source point of the channel, TB-4 *(yáng chí)*, can be treated with moxa.

Thus a fairly complex picture of the triple burner system is painted. One must hold in mind the more common understanding of the triple burner as three separate regions of the chest and abdomen while at the same time broadening it to include the 'spaces' throughout the entire body and the fluids within. All of this, of course, is enlivened by the presence of source qi, which stimulates the entire triple burner. Taken together, this is a dynamic system which can be used to broaden both acupuncture and herbal approaches in the clinic.

With this background in mind, we can now summarize the basic functions of the triple burner.

THE FUNCTIONS OF THE TRIPLE BURNER

The triple burner is a pathway for source qi
(原氣之道路 *yuán qì zhī dào lù*).

Source qi arises from the interplay of essence and kidney fire at the gate of vitality; it is distributed throughout the body by the triple burner. The ability of the triple burner to maintain free and easy movement determines the rate of flow for both source qi and fluids to the various parts of the body.

The actual flow of source qi into the channels, however, is determined by a more complex physiological process described by the growth of channel qi in transport point theory. This will be discussed at some length in Chapter 16.

The triple burner manages the various types of qi (主持諸氣 *zhǔ chí zhū qì*).

The management of qi by the triple burner essentially involves the transmission of information. 'Management' (主 *zhǔ*) here should be understood as the passing along of messages that lead to modifications in the qi transformation of the yin and yang organs. This includes information about normal physiology as well as pathology. This concept may be difficult to grasp at first, but the idea is that the fluids and substances that fill the spaces of the triple burner have 'information' that moves from one part of the body to the other through the triple burner.

An example from modern physiology might be helpful. Hormones and enzymes pass through and interact with—that is, transmit information to—the areas through which interstitial fluids circulate; these are areas we have tentatively associated with the triple burner. Information about the presence of disease is similarly relayed: When there is dysfunction in an organ, this information is carried through the medium of the triple burner and causes reactions throughout the body in an effort to reestablish balance.

For example, in the fairly common clinical presentation of heart qi deficiency leading to symptoms of shortness of breath, agitation, and insomnia, information about this imbalance travels through the triple burner. The other organs respond to these changes in the 'weather' of the internal environment in different ways: The liver qi may dredge and drain to increase circulation to the heart, or the kidney may provide water to balance the deficiency of heart fire. The medium through which this information travels is the triple burner. This occurs in both the so-called 'peripheral' triple burner and in the three parts of the 'chest and abdominal' triple burner. It should be clear by now that these two different aspects of the triple burner are actually part of the same thing. By maintaining the free flow of communication, the triple burner 'manages', in a very broad sense, the types of qi transformation that occur throughout the body.

If the passageways of the triple burner are unable to accommodate the flow of information, there may be a sudden occurrence of disease. To extend the example above, a sudden heart attack may be due to the chronic failure of other organs to balance heart function due to faulty internal communication. Should that be the case, while the root of the condition may still lie in a deficiency of heart qi, the process of recovery must also address *shào yáng* function. Again, the role of certain herbs in the formula Emperor of Heaven's Special Pill to Tonify the Heart *(tiān wáng bǔ xīn dān)* may be instructive (see above).

The triple burner is a place where yin and yang meet and transform (陰陽交會 *yīn yáng jiāo huì*).

As noted above, the spaces within the triple burner are sites of transformation. This is the same idea referred to in Chapter 31 of the *Classic of Difficulties* where it says that the triple burner is the "beginning and end of the pathways of qi." In both instances, this refers to the function of the triple burner as a passageway for the postnatal qi of "water and grains." Remember that the fluids of the triple burner circulate *outside* the blood vessels and may be thought of as comprising the extra-cellular environment. In order to understand what is meant by the phrase "yin and yang meet and transform," it is helpful to focus on that level. As noted earlier, it is here that nutrition leaves the blood vessels and enters the realm of the triple burner spaces where it is taken into the cells and metabolized. In the process, waste is created. In the classical view this might be described as a transformation from yin (nutrition) to yang (energy/potential) and then back to yin (waste). This process occurs continuously in every moment of life.

Thus, while the first function of the triple burner is to serve as a passageway for the dissemination of prenatal qi, this function relates to the distribution of postnatal qi. In other words, the triple burner carries both the spark of source qi that begins the transformations in the body as well as the fuel—the "water and grains"—that sustains that spark throughout the body (Table 9.1).

• Pathway of source qi (prenatal)
• Pathway of information about physiology & pathology
• Meeting place for the transformation of water and grains

Table 9.1
Triple burner: basic functions

The tendency of modern practitioners to focus on the triple burner as a representation for the three sections of the chest and abdomen has led to some misunderstandings about channel theory. Specifically, it is only through the concept of a pervasive triple burner that one can fully appreciate the idea that the channels and collaterals are everywhere in the human body. In other words, ultimately, all of the channels of the acupuncture system fall within the various environments represented as the pathways of the triple burner (see Chapter 17).

The three functions of the triple burner outlined here all involve large, systemic activities, which highlights the broad domain of the organ. Simply put, anywhere in the body where there are open spaces filled with interstitial fluid falls within the scope of the triple burner. The circulation of fluids within this connective tissue matrix is underemphasized, not only in modern Western medicine, but also in modern Chinese medicine. These fluids, circulating through the local capillaries, have a systemic function that is not well understood. One might speculate that the circulation of these interstitial fluids presents patterns that correspond to what classical physicians called 'channel theory', and that the effects of acupuncture can be explained in this light.

CLINICAL PEARLS OF WISDOM
ABOUT TRIPLE BURNER PATHOLOGY

- The fact that the greater omentum (a part of the peritoneal lining that surrounds the organs) actually drapes over the lower abdomen and often has large deposits of fatty tissue provides insight into why the *shào yáng* channel is important in the treatment of obesity. When palpating obese patients, pay attention to the quality of the triple burner channel. There is often a bumpiness all along the channel that frequently corresponds to a lack of free circulation in the organ. If accompanied by heat, the channel may also be tender (and the tongue body likely red).

- This same sensation of bumpiness along the triple burner channel is also often found in patients who are not obese, but have a type of systemic inflammation or autoimmune condition. In these cases, one might think along the lines of ministerial fire pathology.

Gallbladder

"The gallbladder holds the office of rectifier and is the issuer of decisions."

(膽者.中正之官.決斷出焉。 *Dǎn zhě, zhōng zhèng zhī guān, jué duàn chū yān.*)

—*Basic Questions*, Chapter 8

The *Inner Classic* metaphor for the gallbladder is particularly Confucian. It is difficult to convey in a single word the meaning of the term translated here as "rectifier" (中正 *zhōng zhèng*). A modern *Inner Classic* commentary describes the term as meaning impartial and unbiased (不偏不倚 *bú piān bú yǐ*).[10] It conveys both incorruptibility and a clear sense of judgment. The term is used in other contexts to denote the unwavering moral sense of a gentleman, and in classical times was actually used as a title for an official charged with ranking and classifying men in their jurisdiction for higher office. Similarly, the gallbladder is charged with 'choosing' what should and should not be taken in during the process of digestion. In order to do so, the movement of the *shào yáng* pivot must be smooth and free of corruption. 'Corruption' of *shào yáng*, most often in the form of dampness and heat, creates lethargy and dissipation. This is similar to the nature of summer-heat, also associated with *shào yáng*.

The stringent moral qualities associated with the gallbladder in the *Inner Classic* are a reflection of its physiological function. Unique among the six *fu* organs, substances emerging from the gallbladder are regarded as clean by classical physiologists. Recall that the gallbladder is not only a yang organ, but also one of the 'extraordinary organs' (奇恆之腑 *qí héng zhī fǔ*). The other five yang organs are conduits through which substances pass and less clean substances are excreted. By contrast, the bile produced by the gallbladder is a clear (清 *qīng*) substance. As a result, the gallbladder is also often described as the "yang organ of clear essence" (清精之腑 *qīng jīng zhī fǔ*).

At the beginning of this chapter, the *shào yáng* pivot was described as "balanced in the center and spotless." This is a middle road between excess and deficiency. In the case of *shào yáng* gallbladder function, this means avoiding taking too much or too little from the food passing through the digestive system. This idea has some interesting similarities to the role of bile in modern physiology.

The gallbladder must also be balanced and morally upright so as to help the liver make clear decisions about strategy. Besides the obvious anatomical reasons for the pairing of the liver with the gallbladder, classical physiology attaches importance to the clarity of the bile as a determinant of proper dredging and draining by the liver. If gallbladder function is impaired, the liver will be less effective.

Treatments designed to drain the gallbladder or facilitate gallbladder qi might be thought of as helping to reestablish the upright position of the organ in cases of excess. For gallbladder qi deficiency (often manifesting as 'cold' in the gallbladder), the formula Warm the Gallbladder Decoction *(wēn dǎn tāng)* is used. Again, the original, warmer version of the formula, with 12g of Zingiberis Rhizoma recens *(shēng jiāng),* is more appropriate.

In classical anatomy, the gallbladder is located "behind the leaf of the liver" and is in the middle burner with the spleen and stomach. The gall-bladder is also said to be "between the liver and the stomach," a pivotal po-sition between the yin of the liver and the yang of the stomach/intestine. It assists those organs with decisions about keeping that which is wanted and expelling that which is not.

FUNCTIONS OF THE GALLBLADDER

Maker of decisions

As noted above, the gallbladder is described as a decision maker. In the body, its ability to decide depends—like the triple burner—on healthy movement.

The functions of the gallbladder are more clearly understood by consid-ering the organ's internal-external relationship with the liver, and the role of these two organs in digestion. The liver function of dredging and drain-ing has a kind of symbiotic relationship with the movement of *shào yáng.* Many cases of liver qi stasis are actually related to a kind of yang deficiency. In these more deficient cases, there is often a corresponding gallbladder qi deficiency (with the possible involvement of cold). The net result is com-promise of the decision-making function of the gallbladder in the digestive system. In other words, because of deficiency in the liver-gallbladder, there is inefficient digestion. This may involve either over-absorption of foods, leading to ever-increasing weight gain, or under-absorption of foods, lead-ing to a more systemic postnatal qi deficiency.

Thus in the clinic, compromised gallbladder function often involves di-gestive complaints that are sometimes confused with spleen patterns; this is especially true where the liver is also involved, leading one to suspect liver-spleen disharmony. Careful differential diagnosis and pulse/channel palpation is therefore important.

On the other hand, the long-term compromise of gallbladder function can eventually lead to stagnation that gives rise to heat. When severe, this may develop into the common condition of gallbladder heat, which often includes bilateral headaches, redness in the eyes, dizziness, tinnitus, dry throat with a bitter taste, and possibly alternating sensations of heat and cold *(shào yáng* symptoms).

Q: *What's the connection between the functions of the gallbladder and those of the triple burner? Why are they paired?*

DR. WANG: Once again, the most important concept is 'regulation' (調理 *tiáo lǐ*). As noted with reference to the gallbladder, the *shào yáng* level, as a pivot, is associated with regulation and with decisions about distribution. The triple burner is charged with regulating the various environments that surround the organs. The gallbladder, on the other hand, regulates by deciding what should be absorbed during the digestive process. In both cases, as yang organs, they are actually the conduits through which these decisions are made and are therefore involved in that process.

Q: *It seems that you are saying that the regular channels are all moving within the triple burner. Is that true?*

DR. WANG: What I'm saying is that the triple burner function of managing the various types of qi means that the organ is providing the environment in which the regular channels are moving. I'm not saying that all the channels are the triple burner. That would be a mistake. I'm trying instead to clearly define the physical location of the triple burner organ and to describe how that organ is involved in what we call the acupuncture channels.

In the body, there are spaces that are called the triple burner. The regular channels utilize these spaces in rather defined ways to convey particular information about what Chinese medicine calls the 'yin and yang organs'. When one inserts a needle into a point, one is affecting a channel. The channel has a pathway that includes both qi and blood. The information following insertion of the needle may travel through the spaces of the triple burner but there is still more to the 'channel' than these spaces. There are blood, sinews, muscles, and even bony areas that are also associated with each channel.

Think of the triple burner concept as analogous to various neighborhoods in the body. The channels are the things happening within the neighborhood. There are people going about their daily business, cars and bicycles coming through, and buildings along the roads. The triple burner represents the pathways and roads—but not the activities happening within the neighborhood. The ability of source qi and postnatal qi to move through the neighborhood depends on the quality of the roads. The maintenance of quality involves this careful regulation of environments that I've been talking about.

[235]

The key here is to remember that the triple burner concept represents the spaces that are themselves the fluid pathways along the course of the 'channel'. Information is conveyed across these spaces through the medium of interstitial fluid. This is the main point. Through many, many years of careful observation, practitioners of acupuncture have begun to discern particular groupings of these spaces that are associated with what we call 'organs' in the classical sense. This is a complex idea that we will return to again later.

Q: *I understand that the triple burner can be thought of as an overall regulator of digestion, but I still have some difficulty understanding when one might use the triple burner for treatment versus the stomach, large intestine, or even spleen. How do you decide?*

DR. WANG: As I said before, the triple burner is a very broad concept with regard to the digestive system and is thought of as having a general regulating effect. Remember that the triple burner is thought to maintain the environment around the internal organs due to its presence in the fissures or small spaces of the chest and abdomen. Therefore, the triple burner is more often chosen to treat broad systemic problems. For example, Crohn's disease is a systemic condition potentially affecting any part of the GI tract. Often, there are also fevers and a sense of warmth, more clues suggesting the involvement of *shào yáng* ministerial fire. Constipation is another issue that might be caused by a lack of coordinated movement along the GI tract. One should remember, however, that constipation could have many other causes as well, especially dryness in the large intestine.

The triple burner is used when there is a need to regulate among more than one digestive organ. But sometimes using the triple burner to treat digestive issues isn't appropriate, and it is best to use other channels. For example, when one sees clear patterns of stomach heat or spleen qi deficiency, better results will be obtained by focusing on the primary organ. I like to think of the triple burner as a kind of inter-departmental regulator for digestion. If one uses the back office to treat a problem best handled by subordinates, confusion sometimes arises or commands become diffuse and imprecise.

By the way, this concept of regulation as a form of treatment is especially important in Chinese medicine. Doctors sometimes spend a great deal of time tonifying in cases of deficiency or draining excess when a much more effective approach would be to regulate. Regulation is a treatment principle that is all too often overlooked. The triple burner, an organ at the pivot of *shào yáng*, is particularly effective at harmonizing communication between multiple organs and channels. We will discuss later how the extraordinary vessels play a similar function. Broadly speaking, the triple burner has four movements through which it regulates. It can raise (fluids), direct downward (waste and fluids), move (qi), and facilitate (water circulation).

Q: *I'm a bit confused by the relationship of the triple burner to the fluids of the internal environment. It seems that earlier, when we were talking about the spleen and its relationship to fluids, you mentioned that the 'cellular bath' of interstitial fluid can be thought of as an aspect of tài yīn function. What's the difference here?*

DR. WANG: Yes, we did say before that the spleen maintains the health of the interstitial bath surrounding the cells. This is helpful, but as usual, is an oversimplification. In fact, the fluids in the spaces or 'fissures' (隙 *xì*) between the organs are affected by both spleen and triple burner function. The spleen is responsible for the yin function of supplying the nourishing aspect of fluids while the triple burner is charged with the yang function of moving the fluids and nourishment, along with source qi, around the internal environment. The spleen provides material substance, while the triple burner provides the movement of qi. As a yang organ, the triple burner is a passageway and does not create. Think about boats on a large river carrying many different material things; this is like the spleen. The pathway, the movement of the river water which carries these material things along, is like the triple burner.

In fact, this discussion provides a great example of the interaction of yin and yang within the body. It is really difficult to completely separate the two. Strictly speaking, the fluids in the triple burner are affected by the physiology of all the organs and channels—not just the spleen. They are an end result of physiology and, as we've said before, they come from the blood. Therefore, while the spleen and triple burner may be of special importance to the fluids, they are really only part of the picture.

The whole triple burner concept is really a kind of metaphor, and is difficult to understand by thinking exclusively within the concepts of modern (or even classical) anatomy and physiology. We have linked the classical concept of the triple burner to the connective tissues and interstitial fluids but we both know that classical physicians didn't understand these concepts in the same way that they are understood in modern biology. Like many of the metaphors I use, the goal is to get one's mind into a process of thinking that will eventually lead to more accurate diagnoses in the clinic. Of course, the process of understanding and teaching the complexities of the human body requires the use of words and theories, which can never completely convey the reality. As soon as you start talking about it, you're a step away. It's like discussions with friends about the beauty of music: One might be able to give others clues for listening, but you can never quite describe the emotions stirred by hearing a favorite piece using words alone. Among the organs of the body, the triple burner is especially so.

Nevertheless, many diseases associated with the *shào yáng* level can be thought of in light of the functions of the triple burner that I have outlined. Of course, the most common is the '*shào yáng* disease' of the *Discussion of Cold Damage* wherein a pathogen is trapped between the exterior (skin) and interior (organs). This brings to mind the connective tissue, doesn't it? In this type of condition, the classical approach is to move the pivot to release outward by increasing triple burner circulation. How exactly do you increase triple burner circulation? It is helpful to think across centuries of scholarship on the subject.

For example, the *Systematic Differentiation of Warm Pathogen Diseases* describes a type of disease affecting the membrane source that we described earlier as a lining in the chest or abdomen. As I said before, this is likely a reference to the triple burner. Disease in the membrane source is classically treated with the formula Reach the Membrane Source Decoction (*dá yuán yǐn*), which relies on warm, aromatic, and moving lead herbs like Tsaoko Fructus (*cǎo guǒ*), Magnoliae officinalis Cortex (*hòu pò*), and Arecae Semen (*bīng láng*) to activate circulation in the triple burner. You can take this concept and apply it more broadly. In fact, my experience would seem to indicate that many diseases associated with the Western medical concept of collagen—including rheumatoid arthritis, lupus, scleroderma, and Sjogren's syndrome—respond well to treatments designed to facilitate circulation in the triple burner.

Q: *Now I'm a bit unsure how to differentiate the function you just described of the triple burner from our earlier discussion of the bladder. It seems to me that both are 'pathways' of fluids in the body on a large scale.*

DR. WANG: There is a difference here. The best way to differentiate between the bladder and the fluid circulation functions of the triple burner is with the image of irrigation. In classical Chinese farming villages, irrigation was maintained by a complex system of ditches interspersed with gates to regulate the flow. If a particular field was in need of water, gates could be raised and the flow diverted. Now, in the larger sense, the entire system was often dependent on an original water source, often a large river. Each village would divert water into its own system from the river. In the body, the bladder may be likened to the river while the triple burner is more like the irrigation systems. While the bladder function involves fluids in the most broad and general sense, it is within the pathways of the triple burner that fluids in the spaces surrounding the internal organs and appendages are regulated. Also, you shouldn't forget that, while the bladder depends on the gate of vitality as a source of initial warming to activate its qi transformation, the triple burner is considered to be a pathway for source qi. While both have a relationship to the gate of vitality, once again, the triple burner is more specific. The bladder distributes diffused warmth to the surface while the triple burner carries the very specific source qi that eventually joins in channel flow.

Q: *This information brings to mind the concept of channel palpation for diagnosis. In the clinic, you are palpating changes along the course of the channels to clarify or modify your diagnosis. What about a condition like the one described earlier? If a patient has an underlying deficiency of heart qi but the body is not regulating due to problems with conduction of information by the triple burner, will you find palpable changes on the triple burner channel as well as the heart channel?*

DR. WANG: This is a good question and involves a few concepts that we haven't covered yet. It is quite true that, in the clinic, I am palpating the channels for nodules, softness, tension, or other changes in an attempt to determine the proper diagnosis. We will discuss this process at great length later. However, you must remember that all of the separations between muscles as well as the spaces these separations create are within the triple burner. In other words, while there is something we call the 'heart channel', the spaces which comprise it are still within the scope of the triple burner. This is a hard concept to grasp (Fig. 9.8).

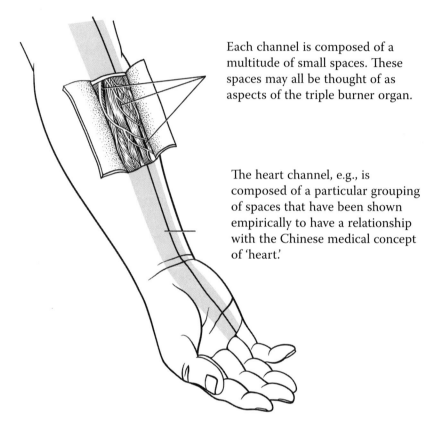

Each channel is composed of a multitude of small spaces. These spaces may all be thought of as aspects of the triple burner organ.

The heart channel, e.g., is composed of a particular grouping of spaces that have been shown empirically to have a relationship with the Chinese medical concept of 'heart.'

Fig. 9.8
Relationship between the triple burner and the channels

In fact, this touches on one of the great unanswered questions at the root of Chinese channel theory, namely, why is it that a particular area on the arm is associated with what Chinese medicine calls the 'heart' while another area nearby is associated with what we call the 'lung'? To be frank with you, I don't know the answer to this most basic of questions. However, I do know that treating these areas has a clear and measurable effect on my patients, and furthermore, that palpating these areas gives me dependable insight into the course and nature of their disease. I think the most likely explanation is that the understanding of channels in Chinese medicine is the result of thousands of years of empirical trial and error. By observing and keeping very thorough records about how stimulus at a particular point affected physiology and disease, classical Chinese scientists were able to develop channel theory. It is staggering to imagine the complexity of the project. It is still going on, you know—every time we treat a patient in the clinic.

In any case, while the spaces between the muscles themselves might be associated with the triple burner, the area along the heart channel still relates to heart function. So, to answer your question, when you are palpating the channels and feel changes along the heart channel, you are feeling a part of the triple burner that is associated with the heart. Therefore, in my experience, when there is a problem with the triple burner function of facilitating the flow of information about an organ condition, it will still manifest as palpable changes along the channel associated with the organ that is primarily affected—in this case, the heart. We will talk a lot more about channel palpation later.

There is one more thing that I should say, though. This also brings us to the question of what, exactly, is going on in an acupuncture treatment. When we insert a needle at a point and you see (or feel) that visible twitch or movement in the patient, this coincides with an opening in the separations along the course of that channel. As the spaces open up, there is a better circulation of fluids along that particular channel. Information about whatever condition exists in the body is therefore more easily conveyed, and the other organs then step in to reestablish balance. This may very well be how acupuncture works. Particular points along each channel have different effects on the flow of information. This is why point selection and location are so important.

Now, as to exactly why different acupuncture points have these different effects, classical Chinese medicine does offer models for explanation. Transport (five-shu [五輸 *wǔ shū*]) point theory is the most common way of explaining the varied functions of the points below the elbows and knees, for example. I personally believe that there is a lot more research to be done to adequately explain why different points have different effects. This will be the work of the next generation. I have found that there is much to be learned by studying the classical models, however. For one thing, if you can really understand this concept of the triple burner that I'm trying to describe, you will have a much deeper understanding of the functions of the transport points. I'm not just saying all of this, by the way, out of some sort of ideological conviction. These statements come from careful observation of patients in the clinic. As I've said many times, actual clinical results should be the ultimate judge of quality for any theory. (For a related discussion, see Chapter 15.)

■ Case Studies

CASE NO. 1

60-year-old male

Chief complaint Headache

History of present illness Two days before, the patient had a cold with headache and sore throat. In the last 24 hours, severe distending pain had developed, especially on the right, radiating from the side of the head toward the ears. Upon presentation, the patient had a low-grade fever, sensitivity to wind, sweating, sore throat, and laryngitis. He also had a cough with white phlegm. The intensity of pain was evident, as he was holding his head and was very irritable. His tongue was red with a white coating, and his pulse was floating-rapid.

Channel palpation revealed changes along the *shào yáng* and *tài yīn* channels. In particular, there was a line of thin, bamboo-like nodules along the gallbladder channel in the area between GB-41 (*zú lín qì*) and GB-43 (*xiá xī*) and puffy tenderness around SP-9 (*yīn líng quán*).

Diagnosis Headache due to upward counterflow from wind-heat (風熱上逆 *fēng rè shàng nì*).

Point Prescription TB-5 *(wài guān)*, GB-41, and LU-5 *(chǐ zé)* bilaterally. Ten drops of blood were also let at LI-1 *(shāng yáng)* on the right side, due to increased distention on that side.

Stimulation Draining technique was used at all points with a 1.5-inch needle. LI-1 was bled using a small lancet.

Results There was immediate relief 30 minutes later. The headache did not return.

Analysis This is a very straightforward case of an exterior pathogen trapped 'between the internal and external levels'. On the *shào yáng* channel, the point pair TB-5 and GB-41 is commonly used to clear *shào yáng* when heat is primary. The presence of sore throat and laryngitis affected the *tài yīn* collateral of the throat. LU-5, the uniting point of the channel, was used to regulate, while LI-1 was an effective way to clear yin channel excess by way of its paired yang channel.

■ CASE NO. 2

51-year-old female

Chief complaint   Dizziness

History of present illness   Upon presentation, the patient complained of ongoing dizziness and a frontal headache for three days. Symptoms began after being severely fatigued. Her blood pressure was 150/100 mm/Hg; it had been higher, but was controlled with medication. Despite relatively normal blood pressure recently, she was still experiencing dizziness. Her eyes were itchy/dry and she was irritable and restless. Her face was a bit red while her tongue was pale with some cracks and a thick white coating. Her pulse was deep and thin. Channel palpation showed a generalized pattern of small nodules all along the liver and gallbladder channels.

Diagnosis   Upward counterflow of liver fire (肝火上逆 *gān huǒ shàng nì*)

Point Prescription   TB-5, GB-41, ST-40 *(fēng lóng)*, GV-21 *(qián dǐng)*

Stimulation   One-and-a-half-inch needles were used. Draining technique was utilized at all points except GV-21, which was tonified. Needles were retained for 30 minutes.

Results   When she came for the second treatment two days later, the patient reported a clear reduction in the dizziness. The same points were used again for a total of four more treatments, after which the dizziness had completely subsided. Treatment then changed to focus on high blood pressure, utilizing LI-4 *(hé gǔ)*, LR-3 *(tài chōng)*, and KI-3 *(tài xī)*. Following 10 biweekly treatments, her blood pressure had also stabilized and the pharmaceutical dosages were reduced.

Analysis   This case underlines once again a clinically useful approach: When there is heat or excess in a particular yin channel, it is often helpful to drain its paired yang channel. This is because of the different functional natures of yin and yang channels. Especially when there is an accumulation of heat in the yang channel, or in its paired yin channel, clearing the yang channel is often appropriate. This approach, mentioned repeatedly in classical texts, is described in the following adage: "When there is yin disease, choose yang, and when there is yang disease, choose yin." In this case, "yin disease" means an illness which arises primarily from the yin organ, but one should still choose yang for treatment.

■ Narrative

THE STORY OF THE WITCH

In the last chapter we discussed the function of *shào yáng* as the pivot of the yang levels in classical Chinese physiology. But there is another pivot that should be kept in a physician's mind, one that is often underemphasized in both modern schools of Chinese medicine and in Western clinical medicine. This is the pivotal role that a patient's emotional state plays in the evolution of disease.

Dr. Wang would often say that the emotional component accounted for 20 to 80 percent of most chronic disease. Emotional/psychological symptoms might themselves be the root cause of the disorder, or, as is often the case, the disorder might be greatly exacerbated by the emotional aspects of physical suffering and disability. An understanding of the emotional state of the patient is therefore often crucial for determining whether or not a condition will continue to deteriorate. While this may seem obvious, applying it in the clinic requires subtlety. Once, when discussing this aspect of patient relationships, Dr. Wang's eyes lit up as he remembered a story from the Great Proletarian Cultural Revolution.

The Cultural Revolution is still very much alive in the mind of any Chinese person who lived through it. Officially spanning the decade of 1966–1976, many Chinese today continue to carry the scars of the chaos that engulfed China when Chairman Mao tried to force Chinese society to make one violent jump out of its feudal past. It has been surprising in recent years to observe the frankness with which both the average Chinese and their government speak of the "mistakes" of Chairman Mao. Dr. Wang would occasionally mention the abuses that some of his teachers suffered at the hands of the marauding Red Guards, who virtually ruled the streets of Beijing during the most tumultuous years of 1967–1969. He even mentioned once that the spirit of one of his teachers, Dr. Qin Bo-Wei (秦伯未), was broken by the assaults he received during those years, and that he died in 1970 largely as a result.[11] However, Dr. Wang was fortunate enough to have completed his training some years before the Cultural Revolution began, while still being young enough during the chaos that followed to avoid the abuses endured by many of his superiors.

Like many doctors at the time, Dr. Wang was sent to the countryside to help develop rural health care while also being given the opportunity to "learn from the peasants." In fact, Dr. Wang did learn a great deal during his year in the small village of Mi Yun (Hebei Province). He would travel through the area each day with a small bag containing basic medicines such as aspirin, antibiotics, and simple surgical tools, along with ample acupuncture supplies and some herbal medicines. Walking the hills with a large stick to ward off the aggressive dogs kept by local farmers, Dr. Wang would set up a small clinic for the day with the help of a nurse who was sent as his assistant…

DR. WANG: "I was the only doctor in the area so people came to me for everything. Mostly, it was for colds, infections, injuries, and complicated births. Nevertheless, I was able to see diseases during that time that simply wouldn't occur in a modern city like Beijing. An interesting example involved the emotional aspect of healing that we were just speaking of. The patient in question happened to be the wife of the village supervisor. She was around 30 years old and was quite beautiful. This woman had been trained by her mother as a shamanistic healer. In those days, small villages throughout China had healers of this sort. They would claim to be representatives of local spirits. Some villages might have a fox spirit, a hawk spirit, or a panther spirit. She was a self-avowed oracle of a snake spirit.

People from all over the surrounding area would come to her for help with illness or problems with other members of the community. I went to watch her at work a few times. She would sit inside her farmhouse with incense and a candle, slowly entering a trance. Suddenly, when we all had begun to think that she had fallen asleep, she would take in a huge breath, with violent hissing sounds. Using a voice very unlike that which I had heard her use before, she would ask the assembled villagers what they had come for. Men and women would then come forward, nervously, to describe whatever problem or ailment they had, sometimes responding to questions from the woman.

She would often mention how certain things that they had done had offended the snake spirit and that their troubles could be traced to this transgression. Remedies would be suggested that frequently involved small gifts for the snake spirit. I remember that the woman was often given the best fruit or little trinkets by other villagers. Most interestingly, the people who came to see her often reported that their conditions improved, or that their problems showed signs of letting up. I figured that people were getting some benefit from her, so I kept my thoughts about her work to myself.

Normally, that would have been that. I would have continued my work in the community, and she would have continued hers. However, political movements from the national government began to filter down to our level. At that time [1967], the Cultural Revolution was just getting started. My trip to the country was but an interesting side trip for me, and I little suspected all of the other 'campaigns' that were to follow. For some time the government had been striving to weaken the hold that shamanistic healers like this woman had on the minds of the rural population, but to no avail. People felt that she was helping them and thus refused to stop seeing her. However, in 1967, other forces began to come into play. Communist leaders began to pressure their subordinates to eliminate superstition with the vehemence that came to characterize that decade. There was less of the gentle persuasion of the past and more of the implied loss of position (or worse) for those petty officials who didn't show results. The village of Mi Yun was not exempt.

As I mentioned before, the woman who carried out the shamanistic healing also happened to be the wife of the village supervisor. As the local representative of the national government, it was he who was charged with rooting out superstition in the local community. You can see his difficulty: He was being asked to eliminate his own wife's activities. Compounding his natural reluctance was the fact that he also believed to some degree in his wife's powers and was genuinely afraid of her. Nevertheless, he began to apply whatever pressures he could and thus slowly curtailed her treatments. Yet the progress of his success was paralleled by a corresponding deterioration in his wife's health. His pressure to stop her work was met with a refusal on her part to eat, drink, or leave the house.

After about a week of this, the village supervisor asked me to come to his home one night saying, 'Old Wang, you have to help me out here. My wife now refuses to eat or drink and I'm afraid she may starve herself to death. On the other hand, if I give in we'll both be ruined by my bosses in Beijing!' I have never been too involved in politics and don't enjoy the grueling courting of favors that this often requires. Thank goodness that I have generally found that, if I work hard to help patients, I can then avoid the complexities of my country's bureaucracy! In this case, however, I did have to act, as she was obviously not well, and her husband had been kind to me and helpful to my work in the village.

I didn't know where to start. At that point, I was still relatively inexperienced, especially with psychological cases such as this. It did seem similar to the types of 'possession' that Sun Si-Miao (孫思邈 581–682 A.D.) had mentioned regarding his 'ghost points,' so I began by using a few of those.[12] Treatment was difficult though, as the room was fairly dark and the woman was screaming out to me, 'I'm not afraid of you, Wang! Your treatments will not work!' and similar protestations. I could see after a few minutes that she was right. It seemed that the harder I pushed to get her out of her state, the more determined she became that she would not. This had obviously been going on for some time and she was determined that she wouldn't give in.

I finished the three needles that I was inserting at the time then walked across the room to where her husband was nervously waiting. 'Well, what do you think, Wang? Is this going to work?' I paused for a moment and an idea suddenly occurred to me. I told the supervisor that I did in fact think that there was a treatment that might be helpful. Suggesting that the current treatment might prove to be enough if we waited a few minutes, I began to tell him (within earshot of his wife) that there were two other points that I might use. However (I went on to say), these points are on her face and the technique I use will likely cause some scarring. It is the best treatment for this type of serious condition, though, as it has a direct stimulatory effect on her brain.

In fact, I knew of no such points but had determined that the woman who was, as I mentioned, very beautiful, would want no part of a treatment that would leave her beauty marred even slightly. The husband thought for a moment then said that if I thought it might help, then I must proceed. She wasn't eating and he didn't know what else to do. I said that I would try the treatment but that we should first wait five minutes to see if the points I had already used might be sufficient. A few minutes later, the woman inhaled forcefully and deeply and let out a loud moaning cry. She was quiet for awhile before asking for a bowl of rice porridge. Within days she had sufficiently recovered and her husband was able to keep his job.

There are a few things that can be said about the importance of a patient's emotional condition in regard to this case. As I have said before, many illnesses are interwoven with threads of psychology. In traditional Chinese villages, the role of shamanistic healers like this woman has been to help alleviate just this aspect of disease. By helping patients to believe that they will get better, and that there is a discernible cause for their illness, she was able to help alleviate that aspect of chronic disease that involves the emotions. By untying the knot of psychology that is very often linked to physical suffering, she was able to do a great service in her community. I personally do not believe, however, that there was a snake spirit that spoke through her. But some people do believe this.

This case was also important for me in that it brought home the vital role that we play as doctors in assisting with all aspects of our patient's healing process. However, personal experience with patients has shown that the use of acupuncture can be effective whether or not the patient 'believes' that it will help them. My work with children and skeptical patients has been enough to verify this for me. Nevertheless, as doctors of all traditions will agree, there are patients who respond more quickly when an aspect of their psychological suffering is somehow alleviated. In fact, Ye Tian-Shi (葉天士 1667–1746 A.D.), a famous doctor whose ideas were later collected in a text written later by Wu Ju-Tong called *Systematic Differentiation of Warm Pathogen Diseases*, often utilized techniques like the one I used with the witch when treating emotional conditions. For these types of patients, emotions are actually the pivot."

At that point, Director Zhang, owner of the Ping Xin Tang, came into the room escorting a group of officials. Days in the clinic would often be punctuated by these rounds of introductions and the flurried exchange of business cards. Despite the decades that have passed since the end of the Cultural Revolution, the cultivation of relationships with the Communist Party continues to be a vital part of keeping a business afloat in modern China. After all, the Ping Xin Tang, unlike the clinics of the 1960s, is a business. Dr. Wang would make jokes and shake hands before turning once again, with a more serious expression, to face the next patient.

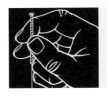

CHAPTER 10

陽明

THE *Yáng Míng* (YANG BRIGHTNESS) SYSTEM

The General Nature and Function of *Yáng Míng*

A T *yáng míng*, the external aspect of the body closes inward toward yin. The channel weaves together the digestive functions of the stomach and large intestine organs and is often described as the "interior of the exterior" aspect of the body. While the organs of the digestive tract are considered to be external because of their connection to food entering from the mouth and leaving through the anus, they also represent the point at which external food and drink meet the internal transformation of the yin organs. Among the yang organs, the pivot at *shào yáng* regulates the digestive process as a whole, while *yáng míng* is particularly associated with movement and fluid balance along the internal pathways of digestion.

Another statement often seen in both modern and classical texts is that *yáng míng* is "full of qi and blood." This level is the warm core within yang and the relatively solid place from which yang begins to grow outward to its eventual dispersal to the external environment at *tài yáng*. Because *yáng míng* is the innermost of the external levels, it also relates closely to the external aspect of yin at *tài yīn*. The fullness of qi and blood at *yáng míng* is dependent on the transformation of water and grains facilitated by one of its paired organs—the spleen.

The chapters on *shào yīn* and *shào yáng* discussed the role of the prenatal fires that rise from the gate of vitality to provide the primary metabolic stimulus in the body. Here at the *yáng míng* level, that stimulus comes to fruition in the generation of abundant radiant warmth as postnatal essence is derived from raw food. Specifically, the stomach begins the process of generating postnatal essence by 'fermenting' recently eaten food and fluids. The process of fermentation involves adding warmth and appropriate moisture so that the spleen can initiate its transformations. At the other end of the digestive tract, the large intestine uses warmth to remove fluids from digestion and then passes unneeded waste downward and out of the body. In the clinic, regulation of *yáng míng* affects the rate and efficiency of the body's food and liquid metabolism. Consequently, *yáng míng* points and herbs are often used in the treatment of chronic disease when there is insufficient generation of postnatal qi.

Another way to understand the nature of *yáng míng* is by returning to the metaphor introduced in Chapter 2, where movement in the three yang levels was compared to the steaming of dumplings. Recall that the dumplings themselves were likened to *yáng míng,* the regulation of the steam surrounding the dumplings to *shào yáng,* and the steam emerging from the top of the steamer to *tài yáng* function. In this metaphor, as in the body, the *yáng míng* aspect is "held on the inside" of yang while being warmed by steam from below (the qi dynamic arising from the yin organs). When heat and steam are abundant, the *shào yáng* pivot allows steam to rise upward and outward to the *tài yáng* level. Conversely, when heat is insufficient, *shào yáng* acts to hold the steam inside the steamer. The image is one in which 'steam' rises from the solid radiant heat of *yáng míng* to the broad surface of *tài yáng* via the regulated passageways of *shào yáng.*

The concept of heat rising from *yáng míng* should be contrasted with the triple burner function of warming the internal organs. In the previous chapter we described how the triple burner provides passage for prenatal fire, in the form of source qi, to circulate through the body. Source qi is a kind of diffuse and vital presence that 'warms' the organs by stimulating function. On the other hand, the heat one feels radiating from a living body comes from the great postnatal reservoir of *yáng míng* qi and blood. It is a relationship similar to that noted earlier between *jué yīn* and *shào yīn,* where the substantive blood of *jué yīn* is activated by the prenatal stimulus of the *shào yīn* pivot. In this case, the *shào yáng* pivot provides a pathway for conveyance of the prenatal stimulus to the digestive system where it interacts with water and grains from the external environment. The two pivots serve as the source *(shào yīn)* and transport *(shào yáng)* of prenatal qi (Fig. 10.1).

Among the six external qi, *yáng míng* is associated with dryness. This concept was discussed in the chapter on *tài yīn* but warrants revisiting here. Both the ability of the *yáng míng* channel to assimilate external dryness and its tendency to develop internal dryness are related to the concept that *yáng míng* is full of qi and blood. Simply put, when qi and blood are abundant, pathogenic dryness cannot take hold. The first step in building qi and blood

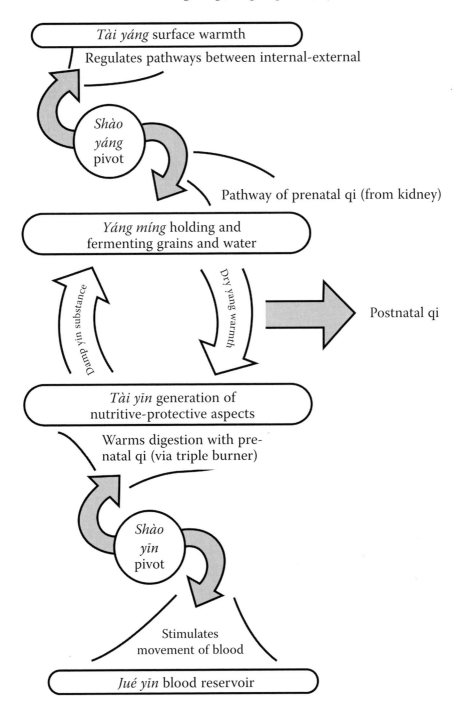

Fig. 10.1

The two pivots serve as the source (*shào yīn*) and transport (*shào yáng*) of prenatal qi, while *yáng míng* begins the process of postnatal qi development.

involves the interaction of *tài yīn* and *yáng míng* in digestion. When dietary factors or problems with the qi dynamic in the spleen-stomach (middle burner) lead to a reduction in food essence, dryness may result. The lack of fluids at the *tài yáng* surface of the body may be due to this lack of food essence, or even to a more basic lack of heat from *yáng míng* in radiating the fluids upward and outward. In the body's internal landscape, *yáng míng* prevents dampness by contributing to the dryness of the internal organs. This important physiological function also draws from the ability of *yáng míng* to hold abundant warmth.

When discussing the digestive system, the concept of 'dryness' is sometimes overlooked. In general, dryness is placed in opposition to dampness. This opposition involves both moisture and temperature. Dryness tends to be warm while dampness tends to be cold. In normal physiology, the internal environment requires dryness in order to transform dampness, but not so much that the organs lack moisture. Too much dryness can begin a chain of pathology reflected in the saying that "dryness is the beginning of heat while heat is the beginning of fire." Dryness, heat, and fire represent a progression along a continuum. In order to prevent dryness from progressing to pathological heat and fire, a balance with dampness is necessary. In much the same way, there is also a continuum of dampness in the body. Fluids accumulating over time will lead to dampness, which can eventually turn to phlegm and then give rise to heat. In the constantly changing dynamic of dryness-dampness, it is the *yáng míng/tài yīn* organs that provide the balance (Fig. 10.2).

Thus the interior-exterior relationship of the *yáng míng* and *tài yīn* channels also involves a balance of fluids. The stomach (*yáng míng*) has a warm-dry nature that "does not like dryness" while the spleen (*tài yīn*), which is the source of fluids in the body, "does not like dampness." The large intestine (*yáng míng*) is responsible for eliminating waste fluids from the digestive process while the lung (*tài yīn*) requires moisture to facilitate the absorption of external qi and also helps to synergize the spleen with its upward/downward movement. The yang organs add dry warmth to facilitate digestion and separation while the yin organs integrate fluids in the process of metabolizing food and external qi.

Imbalance can cause both the stomach and large intestine to become excessively warm and dry, thereby encouraging their tendency toward yin deficiency. Similarly, the inability of the spleen to integrate fluids, or problems with the lung's ability to cause the qi to rise or descend, may lead to the accumulation of dampness. Thus one sees how the yin-yang paired organs act to balance each other's tendencies to excess and deficiency.

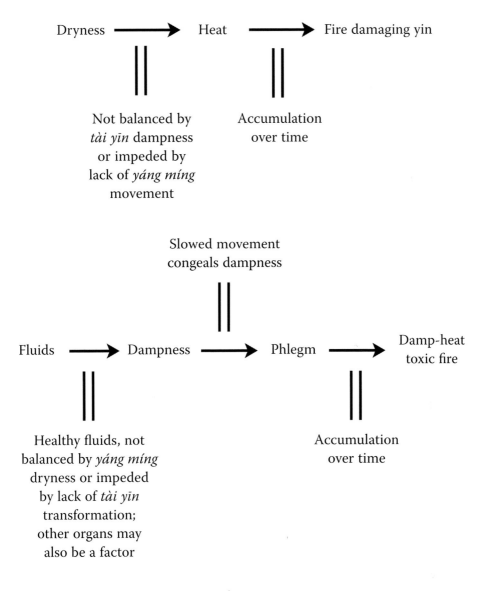

Fig. 10.2
Dryness and fluids can transform into pathogenic fire.

. . . .

The *yáng míng* organs require a constant, even pace and temperature to properly carry out their digestive functions. If movement is too fast, or the dry warmth is insufficient, then the food will not be properly digested and will pass through to the stool. Conversely, if movement is too slow, or the dry warmth is excessive, then constipation and foul odor (food stagnation) will result.

When movement and warmth are unbalanced, one can regulate the *yáng míng* qi dynamic with the uniting (sea) point ST-36 *(zú sān lǐ)*. Incidentally, it is this regulatory effect that allows ST-36 to treat seemingly contradictory conditions, for example, both diarrhea and constipation. In addition, some types of diabetes are also related to dysfunction of the *yáng míng* qi dynamic, a pathodynamic involving stomach fire. This type of diabetes can be understood to arise from excessive heat in the stomach that prevents the body from properly absorbing food. In fact, absorption is a common theme in discussions of *yáng míng* physiology and pathology. The stomach, at the top of the digestive tract, is charged with the initial absorption of raw food, while the large intestine absorbs fluids at the other end. In both cases, a normal pace and temperature are critical to proper function.

Common applications of the point pair ST-36 and LI-10 *(shǒu sān lǐ)* illustrate the use of the *yáng míng* channel to treat problems with absorption. This pair is most appropriate in conditions of *yáng míng* qi deficiency that lead to malabsorption, a condition often similar to the modern medical diagnosis of chronic colitis. As many already know, both of these points are called *sān lǐ* (三里) or "three miles," thus implying an ability to increase strength for "three more miles." This pair is a classic combination for generalized deficiency.

Note, however, that the large intestine uniting point, LI-11 *(qū chí)*, was not combined with the other *yáng míng* uniting point, ST-36. This is because the two uniting points have different natures. ST-36 both moves and strengthens while these two functions diverge on the large intestine channel. In general, LI-11 is most effective in cases where movement and clearing are needed, while LI-10 is better for tonification. Chapter 20 will examine the art of point pairings, but for now, this example underlines how theory can be modified by clinical experience. Unfortunately, point pairs that are elegant in theory are not always the most effective in the clinic, and empirical treatments sometimes confound the strict application of theory.

Another common *yáng míng* point pair is LI-1 *(shāng yáng)* and ST-45 *(lì duì)*. This well (井 *jǐng*) point combination is often used to clear fire-toxin stagnation in the *yáng míng,* manifesting as toothache, hemorrhoids, or sleep disorders involving restlessness or sweating. These points may also be bled in the case of eczema (濕疹 *shī zhěn*) on the face or for teeth grinding at night due to stomach fire flaring upward (Table 10.1). The unique nature of the well points will be further discussed in Chapter 16.

Large Intestine

> "The large intestine holds the office of transport master, issuing change and transformation."

(大腸者．傳道之官．變化出焉。 *Dà cháng zhě, chuán dào zhī guān, biàn huà chū yān.*)

—*Basic Questions*, Chapter 8

In Chapter 8, on the *tài yáng*, reference was made to differences in function between the large and small intestines. Chapter 8 of *Basic Questions* says that the small intestine holds the office of Receptacle of Plenty and that "material transformation" comes from it. Thus it is likened to a receptacle that takes food transformed by the spleen and stomach and then makes further modifications, consisting of more separating and sorting. By contrast, the large intestine is "a transport master" and thus more of a passageway than a receptacle for further refinement. It maintains constant movement and passage of the products of digestion through the organ. While the small intestine too is obviously a passageway, the function of moving the products of digestion through the GI tract is associated more with the large intestine. Paired with the lung and thus benefiting from the rhythmic movement of *tài yīn*, the large intestine commands downward movement in the lower burner.

Yáng míng Points	Effect on Qi Transformation
ST-36 (*zú sān lǐ*)	Uniting point regulates movement and inter-regulation of dryness-dampness
ST-36 (*zú sān lǐ*) and LI-10 (*shǒu sān lǐ*)	Regulates while also tonifying
LI-11 (*qū chí*)	Clears by strongly stimulating movement of qi and blood
LI-1 (*shāng yáng*) and ST-45 (*lì duì*)	Clears excess heat in the channel, especially with bleeding technique

Table 10.1
Yáng míng points and qi transformation

···

FUNCTIONS OF THE LARGE INTESTINE

Transports and transforms waste

Traditional Chinese medicine, like modern physiology, associates the large intestine with the final removal of digestive waste. Because the organ is also involved in the metabolism of dryness, it plays an important role in fluid absorption. Classical physiologists conceived of the large intestine as more than a simple tube for transporting waste from the body. As previously noted, the *Inner Classic* describes the large intestine as an issuer of "change and transformation." The large intestine oversees a process by which digested food undergoes its final transformation. The precise meaning of the term 'transform' (變化 *biàn huà*) is important. The products of metabolism from the spleen-stomach and small intestine reach the large intestine where they are completely transformed from a substance with some remnants of nourishment into waste to be removed from the body. While the *Inner Classic* says that "material modifications" (化物 *huà wù*) issue from the small intestine, it is the large intestine that is charged with complete transformation. In other words, while the small intestine "separates clear from turbid," the large intestine transforms absolutely (Fig. 10.3).

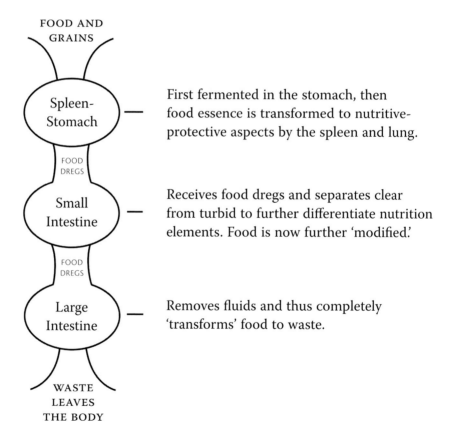

FOOD AND GRAINS

Spleen-Stomach — First fermented in the stomach, then food essence is transformed to nutritive-protective aspects by the spleen and lung.

FOOD DREGS

Small Intestine — Receives food dregs and separates clear from turbid to further differentiate nutrition elements. Food is now further 'modified.'

FOOD DREGS

Large Intestine — Removes fluids and thus completely 'transforms' food to waste.

WASTE LEAVES THE BODY

Fig. 10.3
The large intestine oversees a process by which digested food undergoes its final transformation.

As noted above, rhythm is important to the process of transformation in the large intestine. Keeping in mind the importance to *tài yīn* function of maintaining an even, constant rhythm (see Chapter 5), one can begin to appreciate another aspect of the lung-large intestine pairing. The ability of the large intestine to transform the dregs of food into waste depends on the rhythm provided by the downward-directed aspect of the qi dynamic of the lung (which, in turn, is dependent on the kidney to 'grasp' the qi). As usual, the interaction of the various organs is an important consideration.

Not only is the *tài yīn* lung important to large intestine function, the fluid-regulating aspect of the spleen can also affect the bowels. For example, most students of Chinese medicine are familiar with the association of spleen qi deficiency with loose bowel movements. This is a case where *tài yáng* dysfunction manifests in the *yáng míng*. Less appreciated is the role of the *tài yīn / yáng míng* relationship in the pathogenesis of constipation. Usually regarded as an indication of dryness caused by either dryness in the large intestine organ or a lack of proper fluid circulation in the pathways of the triple burner, constipation can also be rooted in *tài yīn* dysfunction. As noted above, the passage of digested waste through the intestine depends on the proper movement and drying by the *yáng míng* in conjunction with the maintenance of proper fluids and rhythm by *tài yīn*. If the spleen 'over-metabolizes' the fluids, or the lung fails to properly direct the qi downward, the digestive tract may become dry. Think of this as a case where the *tài yīn* qi dynamic requires regulation. In such cases, one would likely find palpable change along the course of both the *yáng míng* and *tài yīn* channels. Regulating treatment with the uniting points LU-5 *(chǐ zé)* and SP-9 *(yīn líng quán)* is often best for these types of patterns.

The reverse is also true. One might regulate the *yáng míng* to benefit the *tài yīn*. The use of the formula Ephedra, Apricot Kernel, Gypsum, and Licorice Decoction *(má xìng shí gān tāng)* was mentioned in Chapter 8 on the *tài yáng* as a common method for treating accumulation of fluids or dampness in the lung by moving and clearing the large intestine.

Removes fluids

While this second function of the large intestine might easily be considered a sub-category of the first, it is important to emphasize the role of the organ in fluid absorption. While the spleen is the source of fluids in the body, the large intestine serves as a final step in fluid metabolism. The failure of the large intestine to remove fluids from digestive waste manifests as 'water diarrhea'. This is diarrhea where undigested food is less obvious and instead has a fairly even consistency. By contrast, diarrhea associated with spleen qi deficiency will contain undigested food.

CLINICAL PEARLS OF WISDOM ABOUT
LARGE INTESTINE PATHOLOGY

- Some types of deafness and/or tinnitus are due to *yáng míng* channel stagnation. This may be an accumulation of stomach heat or a lack of free flow through the large intestine. This type of deafness and tinnitus is often fairly easy to treat and should not be confused with kidney-type patterns. The *yáng míng* condition involves excess in the collaterals of the large intestine channel.

- Deficiency in the collaterals of the large intestine channel can lead to tooth pain that is sensitive to cold. Collateral deficiency may also involve a general sense of coldness in the mouth. Another sensation associated with large intestine collateral deficiency is discomfort or tightness in the chest that does not involve heat. Treatment for any of these conditions should include moxa at the combined source and collateral points, LI-4 (*hé gǔ*) and LI-6 (*piān lì*).[1]

Stomach

"The spleen-stomach holds the office of the granaries and issues the five flavors."

(脾胃者．倉廩之官．五味出焉。 *Pí wèi zhě, cāng lǐn zhī guān, wǔ wèi chū yān.*)

—*Basic Questions,* Chapter 8

As noted in Chapter 5 on the *tài yīn*, only the spleen and stomach are assigned a common metaphor in the *Inner Classic.* One yin and one yang, both organs are placed at the center of the body in both the triple burner and five-phase systems (Fig. 10.4).

In fact, because *yáng míng* meets *tài yīn* at the border between the exterior and interior levels of the body, the functions of the two organs are often blurred in classical physiology. While there are certainly clear distinctions drawn between the yin and yang organs and their respective associations with dryness and dampness, there is a sort of grey area in which both the classics and experience in the clinic acknowledge an overlap. Herbal and acupuncture strategies likewise weave the treatment of stomach disorders into those of spleen disorders and vice versa. Pathogenesis in one organ almost always involves the other.

Chapter 5 on the *tài yīn* pointed out that the description of the spleen-stomach in the *Inner Classic* as holding the "office of the granaries" is an allusion to their role as the primary organs of digestion, and that "issuer of

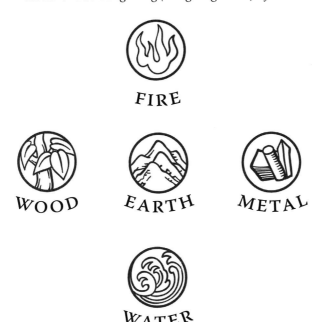

Fig. 10.4

Some five-phase diagrams place earth at the center, the place to which all other elements return. This is also true of diagrams of the 'five' directions—with earth at the center. (In traditional Chinese diagrams, south is placed at the top of the page in deference to the association of that direction with the power of the emperor.)

the five flavors" is a reference to the role of digestion in nutrition. "Flavor" here refers to the relative abundance of the flavors from food and drink that are available for use within the internal landscape.

Stomach pathology often involves heat. Due to the warm-dry nature of *yáng míng*, the large intestine also has this tendency. As noted earlier, over time heat can lead to the commonly-seen yin deficiency patterns of the stomach and large intestine.

FUNCTIONS OF THE STOMACH

Stores and decomposes

All food and fluids that enter the body make their first stop in the stomach. It is here that fermentation (the addition of warmth and maintenance of proper fluid composition) occurs, in advance of the transformation by the spleen of the more refined essence of food and drink into the nutritive aspect of blood. As noted above, practically speaking, the qi dynamic of the spleen and stomach are difficult to separate. Food enters the stomach for fermentation, is transferred to the spleen for refinement into the nutritive aspect, and is then combined with external qi in the lung. The result is nutritive-protective qi, which travels to the rest of the body in (nutritive) and around (protective) the blood (see Fig. 5.5 in Chapter 5).

CLINICAL PEARLS OF WISDOM ABOUT STOMACH PATHOLOGY

- Tooth grinding at night is often due to heat from constraint in the *yáng míng*. The well points LI-1 *(shāng yáng)* and/or ST-45 *(lì duì)* can be bled for treatment.

- Obesity in children is often due to over consumption of damp or even highly nutritious foods that leads to damp-heat in the spleen, eventually affecting the stomach. Consequently, as a preventive measure, children in China are regularly given mild formulas to clear stomach heat.

■ Case Study

50-year-old male

Chief complaint Chronic intestinal inflammation (colitis)

History of present illness During the previous five years the patient had been suffering from chronic, progressive intestinal inflammation. Initial symptoms included diarrhea and fatigue. Symptoms worsened in the last year, with concurrent weight loss. Upon initial presentation, the patient appeared thin and weak.

Channel palpation revealed a lack of muscle tone and tenderness in the area around LI-10 *(shǒu sān lǐ)*. The *tài yīn* channel pathway appeared relatively normal.

Diagnosis *yáng míng* (yang) qi deficiency

Treatment LI-10, ST-36 *(zú sān lǐ)*, and CV-11 *(jiàn lǐ)*—the "three *lǐ*" points (see Chapter 20 for more discussion about this point combination). Treatment continued for 12 weeks.

Stimulation All points were treated with a tonifying technique. Gentle radiation to the hands and feet was achieved at LI-10 and ST-36. CV-11 was needled with a 1.5-inch needle, initially deep, touching the more substantive outer lining of the stomach organ (there was a sense of resistance under the needle), followed by retreat to a depth of 0.5 inches; needles were then retained for 25 minutes. Treatments were twice weekly for the first three weeks, followed by once weekly thereafter.

Results The patient's appetite began to recover by the third treatment. The diarrhea decreased in frequency and volume throughout the first month, with stabilization of bowel movements by the fifth week. The patient showed considerable weight gain by the end of the second month of treatment, and was able to discontinue treatment 12 weeks after initial presentation.

Analysis This rather simple case represents one of the most effective disease categories for acupuncture treatment. Systemic, chronic digestive complaints of this type are some of the most common in Chinese hospitals. However, it is important to impress on the patient that the course of treatment will be 2–6 months and that amelioration of symptoms will be gradual—especially if it is a very chronic condition.

Note: The reader should also take special note of the needle technique used at CV-11 in this case. Following initial insertion, the needle is inserted to a depth of 1.5–1.8 inches in order to stimulate the stomach organ itself. Sensation under the acupuncturist's hand will be of reaching a hard, slightly flexible surface. *Do not needle through this surface.* A very gentle lifting and thrusting technique is then used to facilitate the arrival of the qi sensation. Finally, the needle should retreat to a depth of 0.5 inches and then be retained for 25 minutes. It is especially important to stress that the needle should neither go through the hard surface nor be left at the 1.5-inch depth during retention. The goal is to reach the border of the deep surface so as to strengthen sensation, but not to pierce the organ. This is a more advanced technique that should be approached conservatively in initial treatments. If done correctly, it is extremely safe (Fig. 10.5).

Q: *It is fairly easy to see how the tài yīn spleen and yáng míng stomach and large intestines are involved in digestion. But it has always been harder for me to understand the relationship of the lung to this process. Can you say a bit more about how the lung is related to digestion?*

DR. WANG: One should first think of *tài yīn* as a system of balance between upward and downward movement in the middle and upper burners. The spleen moves clear yang upward while the lung directs qi downward. Together, a synergistic cycle of qi dynamic is created that manifests as the circulation of fluids. The spleen circulates fluids transformed from food and drink to the lung where external qi is

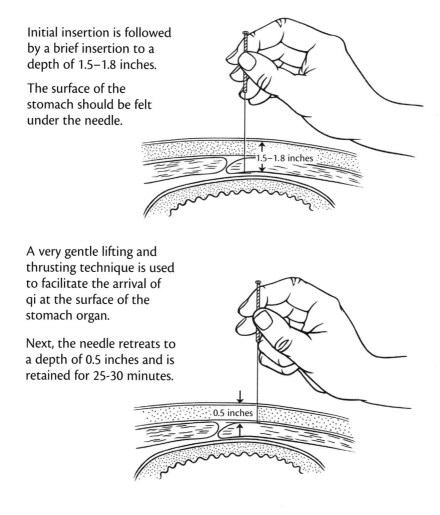

Initial insertion is followed by a brief insertion to a depth of 1.5–1.8 inches.

The surface of the stomach should be felt under the needle.

1.5–1.8 inches

A very gentle lifting and thrusting technique is used to facilitate the arrival of qi at the surface of the stomach organ.

Next, the needle retreats to a depth of 0.5 inches and is retained for 25-30 minutes.

0.5 inches

Fig. 10.5
Needle technique used at CV-11

infused to facilitate transportation. Finally, the qi dynamic of the *tài yáng* bladder effuses fluids outward to the body surface.

Now, the *yáng míng* is always warm and has a tendency toward dryness when not balanced by *tài yīn* dampness. The fluids which move from the most external yin aspect *(tài yīn)* to the most internal yang aspect *(yáng míng)* are vital for proper digestive function. Of course, the *tài yīn* spleen and lung organs have a tendency to accumulate dampness, which is balanced in turn by the drying nature of the stomach and large intestine.

Within this qi dynamic, the lung provides the driving force behind the movement of qi. Again, the lung governs the qi of the entire body. It not only directs qi downward to balance the spleen, but also directs qi upward. Classically, this is called the "raising and descending" of the lung qi. Interestingly, another concept is apropos here: the rhythm of the spleen and its function of "holding intent." This rhythm includes the rhythm of digestion as seen in peristaltic movement. The *yáng míng* depends on the rhythm provided by the *tài yīn* to maintain proper movement. Ultimately, it is a qi rhythm initiated by the even, regular breathing of a normally functioning lung. With this image in mind, one can see right to an aspect of the relationship of the lung and the large intestine. The regular, even movement of the large intestine depends on the regular, even movement of the lung qi (ascending and descending). Descending is particularly important to the large intestine function of eliminating waste, and its impairment may even be a cause of constipation (see related case study in Chapter 5).

■ Narrative

ALLEY LIFE

The people of Beijing are early risers. This became evident immediately after we moved into our apartment in the heart of one of the few remaining sections of Beijing's "*hutong* life." Like the hills of San Francisco, the canals of Venice, or the temples of Bangkok, the *hutongs* (衚衕 *hú tòng*, from the Mongolian *hottog*, meaning 'well') in Beijing provide a unique context for city life. *Hutongs* are maze-like complexes of alleys and small streets. They are both chaotic and intimate, with an almost beehive-like feeling of interrelationship and community.

Living there, one is awakened every morning by the singing calls of street vendors or the brushing sound of the street sweepers who rigorously patrol even the smallest alley every day with their over-sized straw brooms. One also hears the stirring of neighbors who come out of their courtyards and head for the public restrooms, as many homes in the area are still without facilities. While huge, well-lighted supermarkets with shrink-wrapped grapefruit exist in the areas around the new highrises, one still finds vegetable stalls and eggs carefully placed in straw baskets around the tree-lined alleys.

The *hutong* where we lived was originally built in the Yuan dynasty (1300s) but has been modernized in its own way. There are now satellite dishes atop old tile-roofed buildings, and air-conditioners clinging to the sides of ancient brick walls.

Over time, I got to know some of the people who spend entire days without leaving the neighborhood. A man everybody called Old Wang owned one of the small shops in our *hutong*. He sold drinks, snacks, cigarettes and beer. His seat of choice was a small table across from his store, in front of a public toilet. He began each day with strong jars of green tea, then generally switched to beer by 11 A.M. He had a cadre (literally, as we were, after all, in a communist country) of about ten old men who joined him each day for long games of Chinese chess and mahjong. One night, I stopped to have a beer with Old Wang and from that time on he said "hello" to me whenever I passed. He told me once that he wished he could have a day off each week like us lucky foreigners, but that he had to stay there at his post selling beer. "At least I don't have to live like that family there," he said, pointing over his shoulder to the public restroom. "Those guys actually live there! Sure, they have a free place to live for just mopping up a few toilets, but they *really* can't get away from work." He took a sip of beer. "I go home every night at least."

Living in the *hutongs*, whether one likes it or not, everybody notes one's comings and goings. This was the subject on a hot August morning at the clinic. I had mentioned to Dr. Wang that there was a family in my *hutong* who lived in the tile-covered toilet near my bus stop. He laughed and sat back comfortably in his large wooden chair...

DR. WANG: "Life in those small alleys is quite different from what you must have grown up with, and certainly different from the life that my grandchildren experience today. I grew up in a neighborhood not far at all from where you live now. I ran around with my friends in the *hutongs* and went to a middle school behind the old imperial lakes at *Hòu Hǎi*. One of the great things to me about the *hutongs* is their names. Years ago, there was Elephant Nose *hutong*, Little Elephant Nose *hutong*, Itty-Bitty *hutong*, and Well-Handle *hutong*. Those were named for the shapes of the alleys. Some *hutongs* would be named after a famous government minister who lived there, such as Great Hu's *hutong* or Honorable Peng's *hutong*. There was even one called Take a Crap *hutong* that was dirty and full of trash. The names of the places reflect their character, and the people of Beijing love the humor of place names. Back then and, as you have seen, still today, the public restrooms are part of *hutong* life. Your neighbors often know about your most intimate habits. I had a patient in the 1980s that will give you some idea of how health issues are also woven into life in the *hutongs*.

This patient was a 70-year-old woman who came to see me in the spring of 1983. Her chief complaint at that time was diarrhea that had continued for ten months. It began with a stomach flu that started during the hottest weeks of summer. During the week of onset, she had abdominal pain and diarrhea 3–4 times each day. She first went to see a doctor at a small clinic in her *hutong* who gave her antibiotics that proved ineffective. She then went to an herbal pharmacy a few *hutongs* over and bought a prepared extract for summerheat. This was likely some variation of Patchouli/ Agastache Powder to Rectify the Qi *(huò xiāng zhèng qì sǎn)*. This helped a bit with the abdominal pain, so she kept taking the prepared herbs for a week, but the diarrhea continued. By then, the condition had been going on for over two weeks. She decided to get another professional opinion, and this time took a bus to the Beijing Hospital of Chinese Medicine.

The doctor who saw her listened to her case history, asked careful questions, and considered the advanced age of the patient. He gave her another modified summerheat formula, which helped with her diarrhea. After a few weeks, she no longer had abdominal pain or diarrhea during the day, but found that she still had to wake up very early every morning to empty her bowels. At this point, now six weeks after initial onset, a careful eight-parameter diagnosis indicated that her spleen and kidney yang had been damaged (possibly by a combination of antibiotics and over-use of cold herbs). The situation seemed to be what the textbooks call 'daybreak [cock's crow] diarrhea' (五更瀉 *wǔ gēng xiè)*. This pattern is most often treated with variations of the formula Four-Miracle Pill *(sì shén wán)*. For the next six months, she took various modifications of this formula, with added kidney and spleen strengthening herbs, given her age and the chronic nature of the condition. This approach, however, was not very effective.

We should remember here that this woman's travails all played out on the very public stage of her *hutong*. Her neighbors could plainly see her repeated trips to see various doctors, and they asked about her progress (or lack thereof). More importantly, her regular morning trips to the bathroom had become part of other people's daily pattern as well. Because very few of the courtyard homes in the *hutongs* have their own toilets, everyone comes out in the mornings to use the public restrooms. In fact, in most of these restrooms, private stalls don't exist, so her problems were known quite clearly by other women in the neighborhood. When people saw her coming toward the bathroom in the early morning, they would quickly make way for her. It just became part of what happened every day. Of course, for her the situation was not a comfortable one. Around this time, one of her neighbors was coming to see me, and she recommended that this woman give acupuncture a try for her condition.

In those days I was working at the Xuan Wu Hospital of Chinese Medicine. On busy days, I would often see 40 patients each morning and had students and nurses as assistants. One of my students was a doctor and teacher of acupuncture from Guangxi Province who was studying for a year in Beijing. He would often conduct the initial patient intake and channel palpation, then ask my opinion about treatment approaches based on his conclusions. This student was the first to see the woman we've been talking about. After palpating along her channel pathways, he was confused and came to me saying, 'This seems like a tricky case. Her entire symptom presentation is clearly one of spleen-kidney type daybreak diarrhea. She is 70 years old and wakes up at the crack of dawn to go to the bathroom. She can't eat raw or cooling foods either without feeling worse. However, when I palpated her channels, the spleen and kidney channels felt quite normal without any noticeable nodules or soft-weakness, and she doesn't report any tenderness or pain either. On the other hand, the *yáng míng* channel has clear, tender nodules around the areas of LI-10 *(shǒu sān lǐ)* and LI-11 *(qū chí)*. She also has tightness and tenderness around ST-36 *(zú sān lǐ)* and ST-37 *(shàng jù xū)*. The *yáng míng* channel has a fullness that indicates a pattern of excess!'

I verified the student's findings and agreed that the channel palpation in this case clearly differed from the organ diagnosis. The radial pulse, however, was wiry and neither deep nor thin, indicating that she really wasn't severely weak. There was also some tenderness around CV-12 *(zhōng wǎn)*.

I started from the beginning and asked her about the course of her disease. It seems that, despite months of daily diarrhea, she didn't feel very tired. Her face looked fairly bright. The attacks would come very regularly at 6 A.M., which is within the *wèi* (未) two-hour period of the classical Chinese clock and is associated with the large intestine.

The classics mention cases like this where a pulse or channel may say one thing while the eight-parameter pattern seems to indicate another diagnosis. In these cases, one must choose carefully. I believe that if I had been working without the benefit of channel palpation, I would have made the same conclusions as the other doctors and would have proceeded with an acupuncture treatment based on strengthening and warming the spleen and kidney. However, as channel palpation seemed to be showing clear *yáng míng* excess, I chose to move the *yáng míng* by strengthening the channel so as to clear heat. I would likely have used ST-36 no matter what, even if my diagnosis had been one of spleen-kidney deficiency. However, I would probably have also used more kidney and spleen points instead of the pure *yáng míng* treatment strategy that I chose. We used a point prescription that I call the 'three *lǐ*' that includes ST-36, LI-10, and CV-11 *(jiàn lǐ)*. All of these points have the word *lǐ* (里), which means 'mile', in their names and each has the ability to strengthen the *yáng míng* channel to go the extra mile. They are both strengthening and moving. Because this woman was 70 years old, I still wanted to choose an approach that had an element of tonification, but not as strong as that implied by the use of the spleen and kidney yin channels. I use the 'three *lǐ*' prescription very often in the clinic now, but I credit this case with making me aware of its powerful action.

The patient came to see us two days later and reported that she had not awakened early during the previous two mornings and that she had slept much more deeply than before. In fact, on the first morning after the treatment, she was awakened at almost 10 A.M. by her neighbors coming to make sure that she was all right. They hadn't seen her early that morning at the public restroom and had begun to worry. She reported that not only was she okay, but that she in fact felt better than she had in months. She did go to the restroom later that morning, and had diarrhea. However, over the course of seven treatments during a three-week period, the wateriness of the diarrhea continued to decrease until she began to have relatively normal bowel movements.

The fairly rapid recovery that the woman experienced indicates that the condition was in fact more of a *yáng míng* stagnation type of pattern than a kidney-spleen deficiency type. One might have expected a yin organ pattern, given her described symptoms and age, but instead it seems that the condition remained in the yang organs. The yin was not affected, despite the chronic nature.

This woman was greatly impressed with the effectiveness of acupuncture on her condition and became a sort of local walking advertisement. Through her repeated recounting of the long course of her illness, her *hutong* became a source of many new patients for our acupuncture department. Now, more than 25 years later, she's still alive and continues to send her nephews, nieces, grandchildren, and anyone else who complains of illness in her presence to see me."

At that point, another patient came in for treatment and our discussion of how *yáng míng* excess might masquerade as deficiency ended. I never had a chance to meet this woman, but I was reminded of a host of other cases we had seen in the clinic. Dr. Wang would often take not only Western medicine diagnoses, but also the opinions of other Chinese medicine practitioners as reference points only. Even if a new patient came in with what appeared to be a clear diagnosis from another doctor, he would ask about the condition from the beginning. Often, what I might have thought was a clear case of a certain pattern would transform as he asked questions and palpated the channels. Of course, all of us who practice Chinese medicine have found cases where the same patient will have very different diagnoses from two different doctors. Sometimes, both diagnoses can lead to effective treatment strategies. Nevertheless, even if both treatment approaches achieve results, they are not necessarily of equal quality. The above case was but one of many where the clarity of diagnosis led to quicker and seemingly more lasting curative effects. There may be many diagnostic roads to treatment in Chinese medicine, but some are more direct and often more effective.

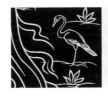

The Extraordinary Vessels
(奇經八脈 *qí jīng bā mài*)

A DISCUSSION OF CLASSICAL physiology would be incomplete without considering the role of the extraordinary vessels. The previous six chapters have explored the functions of the organs and channels. This chapter will first examine some fundamental classical concepts regarding the extraordinary vessels, then describe ways that the vessels are used in the modern clinic.

While the extraordinary vessels are part of the physiological system described in early texts, extraordinary vessel theory and treatment strategies have evolved a great deal over the centuries. The earliest discussion of the eight extraordinary vessels is found in Chapters 27, 28, and 29 of the *Classic of Difficulties* (難經 *Nàn jīng*). Reference to the presence and location of the vessels had been made earlier in the *Inner Classic* (內經 *Nèi jīng*),[1] but full theoretical development and clinical application of extraordinary vessel theory occurred much later. Therefore, before delving into the interesting complexity of extraordinary vessel theory, it is helpful to first draw a few broad brush strokes of the history of this idea that there are 'extraordinary' vessels in the body.

Drawing upon questions and answers outlined in the *Classic of Difficulties* during the Han dynasty (ca. 200 A.D.), generations of doctors developed ways to understand and apply the concept that there are vessels in the body that have a different nature than the twelve 'regular' channels (正經 *zhèng jīng*). As the centuries passed, patterns began to emerge regarding acupuncture points whose influence reached beyond the scope of the channels with which they were associated. Many of these points had already been discussed in references to the extraordinary vessels found in certain chapters of the *Inner Classic* and *Classic of Difficulties*. As the effects of these points were considered, a theoretical system evolved to integrate their implications into traditional physiology. This was a long process that involved literally a thousand years of clinical trial and error combined with careful observation. Eventually, certain points began to be consistently associated with the functions of what are now called the eight extraordinary vessels, a term that was likely introduced in the *Classic of Difficulties*. Many of these points are now referred to in modern acupuncture textbooks as the 'confluent' points (交會 穴 *jiāo huì xué)* of the extraordinary vessels.

Widespread application of extraordinary vessel theory, however, did not occur until the relatively late period of the Yuan dynasty (1271–1368). Heightened interest in the subject at that time was largely due to careful commentaries on the *Classic of Difficulties* and its clinical significance by Hua Bo-Ren (滑伯任) and Dou Han-Qing (竇漢卿). Dou Han-Qing is thought to be the first to promote the 'eight command points' (八會穴 *bā huì xué)*, widely used today, while also codifying his clinical experience with the extraordinary vessels. Development continued during the Ming dynasty (1368–1644) when Li Shi-Zhen (李時珍), the famous author of the *Grand Materia Medica* (本草綱目 *Běn cǎo gāng mù)*, wrote *Examination of the Extraordinary Vessels* (奇經八脈考 *Qí jīng bā mài kǎo)*. Li's text added details to the description of the pathways of the extraordinary vessels beyond the general outlines described in the *Classic of Difficulties*. Later, in the Qing dynasty (1644–1911), Ye Tian-Shi (葉天士) utilized extraordinary vessel points and theory in his analysis of treatment for warm diseases in *Case Records as a Guide to Clinical Practice* (臨證指南醫案 *Lín zhèng zhǐ nán yī àn)*. Ye provided one of the earliest descriptions of chronic illness 'entering' the extraordinary vessels. More recently, the extraordinary vessels have also been associated with midnight-midday point selection (子午流注 *zǐ wǔ liú zhù)* and family lineage styles of acupuncture—topics not discussed in this text.

Throughout the history of the development of extraordinary vessel theory, the questions posed in the *Classic of Difficulties* have been considered as the starting point for discussion. We will begin there as well, before considering some new ways of understanding this important subject. Many of the concepts outlined below owe a great debt to the work of the physicians described above.

We will address the following topics in this chapter:

• What does the *Classic of Difficulties* say about the nature of the eight extraordinary vessels?

• What are some new ways of understanding the eight extraordinary vessels?

- What are the functions of the extraordinary vessels?

- What types of disease patterns in the clinic might lead one to consider extraordinary vessel treatment?

The *Classic of Difficulties* and the Eight Extraordinary Vessels

In Chapter 27 of the *Classic of Difficulties*, the following question is asked:

> "Among the vessels, there are eight extraordinary vessels which are not within the scope of the twelve channels. What does this mean?"

This question is first answered with a list of the eight extraordinary vessels, followed by an affirmation of the statement that they are indeed not within the scope of the twelve channels.

This answer, while providing some clarification, is obviously not enough, so another question is posed:

> It is accepted that there are twenty-seven vessels in the body consisting of the twelve channels and the fifteen collateral vessels. Furthermore, it is said that the qi of the body moves upward and downward throughout the body in these vessels. How can it be that these extraordinary vessels exist outside of the system?[2]

This question is then answered in a way that typifies the *Inner Classic* and the *Classic of Difficulties*. It includes no technical descriptions of the points, their locations on the body, or their physiological functions. Instead, the *Classic of Difficulties* first returns to the use of metaphor to elucidate physiology. In classical (and even some modern) texts, the inner workings of the body are likened to the relationship of human society to the natural world. We saw this earlier in the metaphors used by the *Inner Classic* which compared the organs to officials of the imperial administration. Similarly, Chapter 27 of the *Classic of Difficulties* uses a metaphor of water systems to illuminate the nature of qi and blood circulation in the body:

> The idea came as a result of observations and careful considerations by educated doctors of old about the nature of waterway systems. It was noted that the ditches, streams, and waterworks in a community provide pathways for water raining down from the heavens. However, in some cases, these water pathways are not enough. When there is a flooding of water, the run-off cannot be controlled and the water pathways overflow. Similarly, when the [twenty-seven] vessels are filled, they cannot control the effluence.

Chapters 28 and 29 of this text return to the concept of the extraordinary vessels. Chapter 28 describes the general pathways of the extraordinary vessels (later expanded upon by other physicians), and Chapter 29 describes the specific pathologies associated with each of the eight vessels, discussed below.

From these chapters in the *Classic of Difficulties*, together with other concepts added by later writers, modern textbooks have drawn certain basic principles about the extraordinary vessels (Table 11.1). These can be summarized as follows:

- *The eight extraordinary vessels are something entirely different.*

  This is to say that the very nature of the structures themselves is different from that of the regular channels.

- *They do not flow to the upper limbs.*

  However, indirect connections via the regular channels allow the upper limbs to influence, and be influenced by, the eight extraordinary vessels.

- *They flow only from below to above in the body.*

  Consider possible parallels to lymphatic or interstitial flow patterns—toward the heart.

  The pathway of the *dài* vessel around the waist provides an obvious exception to this principle.

- *They do not have a direct connection to the organs.*

- *They do not have cutaneous regions, channel sinews, or channel divergences (經別 jīng bié).*[3]

- *The basic functions of the extraordinary vessels are to handle overflow of qi and blood from the regular channel system.*

- *They do not fall within the regulatory scope of the channel system.*

Some New Ways of Understanding the Eight Extraordinary Vessels

The use of water systems as a metaphor in the *Classic of Difficulties* is significant in that it points to the physiological realm where the extraordinary vessels are functioning. Elsewhere in this text, the concept of fluids in

Twelve Regular Channels	Eight Extraordinary Vessels
Flow to and from all four limbs to the head (yang channels) and trunk (yin channels)	Flow from the lower limbs to the upper aspects of the body; are not thought to flow directly to the upper limbs*
Weave together and participate in normal organ physiology; this occurs through six distinct two-organ levels/systems	Do not connect directly to the 'twelve organs'**
Each channel participates in developing and communicating the qi transformation of its associated organ (see Chapter 16)	Handle the overflow of qi and blood from the regular channels; act as reservoirs
The twelve channels inter-regulate in a web-like system	The extraordinary vessels are not regulated by the regular channels
The twelve channels have relatively distinct pathways and associated cutaneous, tendon, and divergent pathways	There are no distinct cutaneous, tendon, or divergent pathways;*** they do have intersection and command points

    * The *chōng* vessel has a branch that travels down the leg. The *dài* vessel goes around the waist.

    ** The *dū* vessel wraps around the kidney and passes through the heart.

    *** The *dū* and *rèn* vessels have pathways with points.

Table 11.1

Classical understanding of differences between
regular channels and extraordinary vessels

the body is mentioned in a variety of contexts. The function of the *tài yīn* system is described as maintaining the ability of fluids (and blood) to provide nourishment. The *tài yáng* system, especially the qi transformation of the bladder, is responsible for regulating fluids throughout the body in the most general way—by maintaining net volume of fluids with the assistance of its connection to the kidney *shào yīn* gate of vitality. And our discussion of *shào yáng* develops the idea of the triple burner as a pathway for the movement of fluids (and source qi) through the body. So where, in the classical physiology of fluid circulation, do the extraordinary vessels fit in? This is the crux of the question as to what exactly is meant by the concept 'extraordinary' (Table 11.2).

Regular Channel	Relationship to Fluids
Tài yīn	Maintains ability of fluids to nourish the tissues of the body
Tài yáng	Maintains net volume of fluids with the aid of fire at gate of vitality (from kidney)
Shào yáng	Maintains pathways for fluids in small spaces of the body (in the triple burner)

Table 11.2

Comparison of fluid maintenance functions

First and foremost, it should be said that the eight extraordinary vessels do not actually exist. That is, they do not have definable, fixed pathways that might be palpated in the same manner that one palpates the twelve regular channels. The twelve regular channels and fifteen collateral vessels move in a circuit. Described by some as a kind of circadian (24-hour) cycle, the movement in the regular channels is like the flow of a great river.

Q: *To interrupt here, I'm just wondering how this movement in a circuit relates to midnight-midday point selections (子午流注 zǐ wǔ líu zhù). Do you think that there is "more qi" in one or another of the twelve regular channels at a particular time of day?*

DR. WANG: I personally put less emphasis on midnight-midday point selection. I have seen teachers and colleagues use systems of choosing points based on the theory of circuits and time. In my observations, I notice that they always seem to add other more empirical or channel-based points on top of the point combinations suggested by midnight-midday point selection theory. In other words, it seems to me that the results of their treatment can be explained on the basis of the regular mechanisms of acupuncture, and not necessarily because of the special reactivity of certain points at certain times of day. I believe that one should stick to trying to determine what is going on with a patient by palpating the channels and looking for verifiable changes as a means of diagnosis and as a tool for guiding treatment. However, palpable changes on the channels might change throughout the day and thus influence point choices. I haven't focused on this, however.

It does seem plausible to me that the theories that later gave rise to midnight-midday point selection are reflections of the cultural reality of the time in which they were formulated. Early in the development of Chinese culture, people were very dependent on the rhythms of the sun and the cycles of seasons. Many aspects of their lives, including sleep, diet, and exercise, were therefore also highly dependent on those cycles. By contrast, modern societies are relatively devoid of strict natural rhythm, and thus whatever validity midnight-midday point selection may have is undermined by the very nature of modern life. These are just my personal observations.

As I've said before, the movement in the twelve regular channels isn't like that of a boat, passing through the channels one at a time. Instead, the entire regular channel system is like a river wherein movement is constant and within relatively definable boundaries. Like rivers, however, the boundaries are not hard and fixed, but relatively fluid and changeable. The exact pathways of channel flow change in response to the biography of the person. If there are injuries, illness, or even long-term lifestyle habits, the channels will change accordingly. They may slow, speed up, or alter their paths slightly. There will certainly be a variety of palpable changes along their courses as well. The eight extraordinary vessels are altogether different, however.

The eight vessels represent eight basic physiological principles that are at work in the body outside the scope of the regular channel system. These eight vessels, however, are associated with certain areas of the body—they are just not fixed and defined like the regular channels. To understand this concept, it is helpful to turn for a moment to the original Chinese terminology.

The term *qí jīng bā mài* (奇經八脈), translated here as the eight extraordinary vessels, might be more literally translated as 'extraordinary channels eight vessels'. In other words, there are actually two terms within the concept: 'extraordinary channels' and 'eight vessels'. The extraordinary channels themselves are thought to be innumerable, while the eight vessels are regarded as eight general categories of these channels, which are grouped together to facilitate functional understanding. The eight groupings represent general tendencies within the system of fluid circulation. Remember that this system of fluid regulation is considered to be outside the flow of the regular channels.

A question which then logically comes to mind: What is meant by "outside the flow of the regular channels"? One way to understand this is to think of the eight extraordinary vessels as representing the classical understanding of the slow movement of interstitial fluids, and possibly of cerebrospinal fluid. These fluids are "outside" the flow of the blood, lymphatic vessels, and organs.

By narrowing the definition of the extraordinary vessels to the concept of interstitial fluid movement, one can see how they are both different from the twelve regular channels and how they act as reservoirs without definable pathways. It is also possible to view them in relation to the concept of the triple burner outlined in Chapter 9. The triple burner is the pathway of fluids and source qi, while the extraordinary vessels regulate movement in those pathways in order to integrate. The triple burner is a location while the extraordinary vessels are a broad, regulating function. The interstitial fluids are the medium which is regulated within this location. It is these fluids which commingle with the blood through vessel walls and act as reservoirs of qi constantly interacting with the twelve regular channels.

Once again, a metaphor may be helpful. While the twelve regular channels may be thought of as streams passing between mountain ranges, the extraordinary vessels may be likened to a wetland reservoir lying in the lowlands. In the spring when the streams are full, the wetlands absorb the overflow of water. In times of drought, on the other hand, the wetlands act as a source for filling the streambeds with needed water. Throughout the year, the water in the streams and all of its living organisms constantly interact with the wetland (Fig. 11.1).

Q: *I'm a bit confused about this concept of the eight extraordinary vessels as an environment within which the other channels function. When we discussed the triple burner, you also described an environment within which the organs function. What is the relationship of the triple burner to the eight extraordinary vessels?*

DR. WANG: Yes, both the triple burner and the eight extraordinary vessels are part of the body's internal environment in the broadest sense. The relationship of the triple burner to the extraordinary vessels provides yet another window into what these vessels are. First, let's quickly review a few concepts about the triple burner. As a yang organ, the triple burner is understood to be a hollow pathway. For example, we talked about how the *Inner Classic* describes the triple burner as the "issuer of waterways." Also, as you just mentioned,

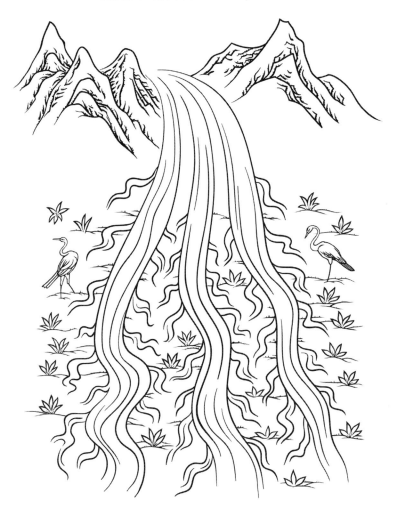

Fig. 11.1
The regular channels are like streams,
while extraordinary vessels are like wetland reservoirs.

when we discussed *shào yáng* we talked about how the triple burner might be thought of as the three-part environment in which the organs function. Finally, the triple burner was described as a pathway throughout the body for movement of fluids and source qi. This pathway is roughly analogous to the spaces inside the connective tissues of the body, filled with interstitial fluid, and surrounding the organs in the thoracic and abdominal cavities. The triple burner is also the pathway of interstitial fluids moving in the spaces around the muscles in the arms and legs. So, we've now developed a model of the triple

[281]

burner that, at least in some ways, brings the organ into the realm of modern anatomical understanding.

There is a degree of overlap between the concept of the extraordinary vessels and that of the triple burner. The triple burner, a yang, hollow organ, is the passageway in the body for fluids and source qi; it is a pathway. On the other hand, the eight vessels can be thought of as the movement of the fluids themselves. The extraordinary vessels represent the more general concept of regulation (調整 *tiáo zhěng*) of the fluids within the triple burner and the integration (聯繫 *lián xì)* that those fluids provide. When I say integration, by the way, I am referring to the fact that the whole body may be said to be linked together through a constantly changing medium of fluids.

This idea was hinted at earlier when we talked about how the *Classic of Difficulties* regards the extraordinary vessels as absorbers of overflow from the twelve regular channels. I think of 'overflow' as a reference to everything *outside* of the blood, lymph, nervous, gastrointestinal, and other organ systems. To me, these other systems are all within what classical Chinese medicine calls the 'regular channels'. So, the overflow may be likened to the modern concept of interstitial fluid. Again, interstitial fluid is not only in the thoracic and abdominal cavities, but can be found surrounding the tissues all over the body. The regulatory function of the extraordinary vessels is therefore at work in the small spaces all over the body, beyond the reach of regular channel circulation. Nevertheless, all of these fluids are still within the pathway of the triple burner organ. The triple burner is the pathway; the quantity and movement of these fluids within the pathways is more related to the extraordinary vessels. In reality, they overlap.

Now, extraordinary vessel function is particularly important at the level of the smallest collaterals. In the collaterals, there is constant uptake and diffusion of fluids. The importance of the collaterals to extraordinary vessel function is highlighted by the fact that four of the eight vessel command points are also collateral points.

Everywhere in the body there is an overarching circulation of fluids. Within what we refer to as the eight extraordinary vessels are eight broad categories of fluid circulation. Classical experience indicates that each of these categories responds to stimulus at one of the eight command points. This is still an exciting and evolving aspect of Chinese physiology. I think that modern research into anatomy and physiology will provide some interesting insights that will help us to refine our understanding and clinical application of the extraordinary vessels.

Remember that our current understanding of the eight extraordinary vessels really didn't begin to develop until the relatively late stage of the Ming and Qing dynasties (1368–1911). The ideas were mentioned in many ancient texts, but there was a long period of time during which the concepts were rarely applied in the clinic. That is, at least according to the texts that are now available, they were discussed, but less often used. My understanding of the extraordinary vessels is based on observation of patients in the clinic combined with repeated readings of classical and more recent texts. Nevertheless, I still have a way to go before I can say that I completely understand this concept. Just think about the broad ideas that I'm outlining here, reflect upon them in the clinic, and see if you can reach an even deeper understanding.

Triple Burner	Eight Extraordinary Vessels
Pathway for fluid movement	Integrate multiple regular channels by influencing the nature of interstitial fluid movement
Maintains pathways by regulating	Integrate using those pathways
Fluids are a medium for the transport of source qi	Fluids are a medium for integrating/connecting regular channels

Table 11.3
Both the triple burner and the extraordinary vessels
are involved in interstitial fluid circulation.

The eight extraordinary vessels thus represent an underemphasized principle of classical physiology. They can be thought of as an important aspect of the environment within which the twenty-seven vessels (twelve regular channels and fifteen collaterals) operate. Just as the natural environment cannot be fully controlled by human beings, the extraordinary vessels are beyond the regulatory control of the regular channel system. Instead, they provide in times of need and receive runoff in times of excess (or pollution). This concept has broad clinical application. When groups of channels are affected by the presence of disease, or when symptom patterns defy all explanation within channel or eight-parameter diagnosis, then it is time to consider the 'extraordinary'.

Functions of the Extraordinary Vessels

At this point the picture should be emerging of the eight extraordinary vessels as general inter-regulators of qi and blood among the twelve regular channels and fifteen collaterals. Their general function is to maintain the connections among the regular channels while also facilitating recovery from disease.

Their function can be described as environmental, but in a different sense than the 'environments' governed by the triple burner. While the triple burner maintains the pathways of fluids and source qi around the organs and periphery of the body, the extraordinary vessels integrate the connections among the channels themselves. The triple burner is associated more with the pathways while the extraordinary vessels comprise an important functional aspect of the fluids within those pathways. For the triple burner, the fluids are a medium through which source qi is transported, but for the extraordinary vessels, the fluids are a medium of connection and integration. While triple burner and extraordinary vessels are different, it is difficult to completely separate them conceptually.

In addition, because of the broad, systemic nature of the extraordinary vessels, clear delineation of specific functions for each of the eight vessels can sometimes be difficult as well. Thus, before considering the functions of the vessels individually, it will be helpful to summarize a few general principles that apply to the vessels as a whole.

The extraordinary vessels integrate the channel system like a series of lakes.

This is the concept introduced earlier that likens the extraordinary vessels to a reservoir into which overflow pours and from which qi and the fluids that make up blood are drawn in times of need. These 'fluids' are not like distilled water, but more like the teeming life that one sees under a microscope when looking at living tissue. Furthermore, when thinking of the extraordinary vessels as reservoirs, it is also important to keep in mind that the reservoirs have an integrating function: they facilitate the constant interaction among groups of regular channels. That is to say, while the twelve regular channels and fifteen collaterals regulate normal physiology, it is the extraordinary vessels that integrate the channels themselves. The effect is like a web of qi dynamic.

Premodern texts therefore liken the extraordinary vessels to a network of small lakes or canals that surround the larger rivers of the regular channels. When pressure builds in the regular channels, qi and blood flow to the eight extraordinary vessels. When pressure is low, these reservoirs fill the deficiency. But just as normal qi (正氣 *zhèng qì*) can flow into the extraordinary vessels, so can pathogenic qi that causes disease. If there is deficiency in the channels, pathogenic qi may flow into the extraordinary vessels like pollution from a slow moving river into streams and lakes. Thus the extraordinary vessels may become involved in chronic disease.

Recall again the metaphor of waterways described at the beginning of this chapter. The concept of the extraordinary vessels, according to the *Classic of Difficulties*, arose from observations about the nature of water systems. Perhaps observers watched the movement of water around Lake Tai in Jiangsu province near the ancient city of Hangzhou. The lake is huge and relatively shallow, with many sandbars and over eighty islands. Water flowing into the lake from the Huai River in ancient times was unpredictable. In some seasons there were floods while in others there was drought. When the water was low, the sandbars in the lake would surface, creating a maze of interwoven streams. In times of flood, the water first filled one area of the lakebed then flowed over the sandbars to fill others until the entire 2,200 square kilometers were once again a large, unbroken lake. The classical understanding of the extraordinary vessels is similar to Lake Tai. Like a lake and its tributary rivers, the system regulates and supplements by its ability to absorb in times of excess and provide in times of deficiency. The most efficient means of flow through any area, however, is always the major river—or regular channel.

The extraordinary vessels act as a supplementary system when the regular channel system cannot function.

When the regular channels are unable to effectively carry out their functions, the extraordinary vessels either temporarily or permanently act as auxiliary channels. For example, in the event of an organ or limb removal, the extraordinary vessels would maintain the functions of the regular channels as much as possible. Or, in the more common situation of blockage in a regular channel pathway, qi sensation might follow instead the alternate 'pathways' of the extraordinary vessels. Indeed, the presentation of unusual pain or needle sensations might be better understood by thinking of the extraordinary vessels.

This tendency of qi and blood to flow into the extraordinary vessels in situations of blockage can be understood by thinking of the concept of electrical resistance. Movement of electrons in a system tends to flow toward the area of least resistance. Flow through the twelve regular channels, when moving normally, can be thought of as having relatively low resistance. When there is stasis of qi and/or blood, however, channel qi flows out of the regular channels and into the extraordinary vessels. This is not to say that qi in the channels is equivalent to the flow of electricity; rather, the metaphor is used to facilitate understanding of how qi moves in the body. There are many types of this diffuse substance that Chinese medicine calls qi. Its meaning is broader than that of electricity, and in the simplest terms, it may be thought of as the smallest possible division of functional potential (功能 *gōng néng*) in the body and its surrounding environment. It exists but has no visible form (無形而存在 *wú xíng ér cún zài*). Thus, while electricity is one type of qi, it is a subcategory of a larger concept (Fig. 11.2).

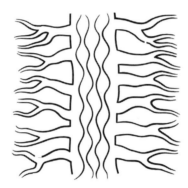

In normal channel flow, qi moves through the regular channels
because they are the path of least resistance.

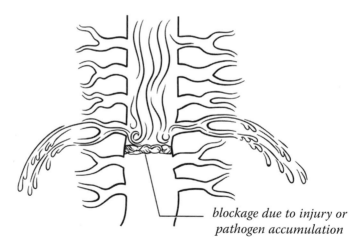

*blockage due to injury or
pathogen accumulation*

When there is blockage in the regular channels,
flow moves into the extraordinary vessels.

Fig. 11.2
Qi flow in the channels

Over time, blockage of qi flow along a regular channel may lead to physiological 'ruts' outside the normal channel pathway. That is to say, if a person has a chronic issue that has led to consistently abnormal flow of qi and blood such that it now affects the extraordinary vessels, then it may be difficult to reestablish normal channel circulation. Simply removing the blockage of qi and/or blood from the regular channel is sometimes not enough. This is another reason why treatment of the extraordinary vessels should be considered during the process of recovery from chronic illness or from conditions that affect groups of channels.

Furthermore, if illness should recur, it is more likely to return to the extraordinary vessels than might otherwise be the case in a patient with no history of that particular condition. This is reflected in the expression "disease traveling familiar roads" (病走熟路 *bīng zǒu shú lù*). In these types of patients, disease can readily return to the extraordinary vessels when the regular channels are blocked.

What is meant when one says that a channel is 'blocked'? Commonly, this means that there is a lack of distention or radiation down the channel pathway during an acupuncture treatment. Or it might be used to describe the condition of a channel pathway that manifests with pain or numbness. The term for blocked is *bù tōng* (不通), which literally means not open, connected, or whole. Fundamentally, a blocked channel has a lack of moving (yang) qi. The cause may be underlying deficiency or excess constraint and/or stasis. In either case, circulation of qi and blood along the channel pathway is compromised, with a consequent lack of nourishment to muscles and nerves.

In the context of classical Chinese physiology, the effects of this lack of nourishment are not only local but also have a systemic effect via the channel system. When circulation at distal points (on the extremities) is compromised, the organs will also be affected. Thus when the qi and blood flow out of the channel system and through the extraordinary vessels, there is a concurrent lack of efficiency. Qi, blood, fluids, and the myriad information that is normally passed along a healthy channel can suffer from this lack of smooth flow or blockage. While the extraordinary vessels act as a supplementary system in cases of compromised qi flow, they are unable to completely mimic the normal functions of the twelve regular channels.

Within the extraordinary vessel system, each of the eight extraordinary vessels has specific functions. While the system as a whole has the regulatory and integrating functions described above, the function of each vessel is best understood by considering the areas of the body traditionally associated with its 'pathway'. This may seem to contradict our earlier assertion that the extraordinary vessels "do not exist." But it means that, unlike the regular channels, the extraordinary vessels do not have strictly defined pathways. Rather, the pathways shown in textbooks might be thought of as 'spheres of influence'.

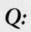

Q: *I'm a bit confused here about how these "vessels that don't exist" can function in the body. If they don't exist, how can they be said to have these spheres of influence?*

DR. WANG: This has been one of the hardest things for me to come to terms with myself. The clearest way to understand this is by thinking of the extraordinary vessels as a means through which the regular channels are interwoven. Each 'vessel', as I've been saying, has a sphere of influence over the interrelationships of particular channels or areas of the body. They serve the function of integration.

For example, the act of swallowing involves the tongue (most clearly associated with the heart and spleen channels), the throat (kidney channel), and the esophagus (stomach channel). The coordination of the various muscle groups involved in swallowing is the function of the extraordinary vessels, specifically, in this case, the *yīn qiāo*. This is what I mean when I say that the vessels themselves "do not exist." Unlike the regular channels, they don't have paths per se, but are instead mechanisms of integration. It would not be incorrect to say that everything outside of the circulation of the twelve regular channels is part of the extraordinary vessel system. What do I mean by this? I'm talking about circulation between blood and lymph vessels at the microscopic level of interstitial fluid circulation. Keep this thought in mind and the concept of channel palpation will make more sense. It will also eventually allow you to get to the next level, as far as choosing pairs of points in the clinic is concerned. The process of understanding is slow and must be based on observing real patients in the clinic.

In the end, the clearest moments of insight will likely come long after reading this information, when some real-life connection is made to an idea discussed here. At this point, however, our discussion will now turn to the functions of each of the eight extraordinary vessels.

The *Rèn* ('conception') vessel

Both the *rèn* ('conception') and *dū* ('governing') vessels are said to come from the same source. In women, the source is the uterus, and in men the area around the testicles or prostate. Others assert that the *rèn* and *dū* vessels arise from the gate of vitality in both men and women. In either case, these vessels that loop around the abdomen and spine are considered to spring from a fundamental prenatal source: the reservoir of essence (yin) and the fire at the gate of vitality (yang).

The *rèn* vessel is the meeting place of yin running up the center of the abdomen and eventually into the throat and eyes. Like a valley between a mountain range, the *rèn* vessel collects yin and blood so that it can ripen. Again, it is not a 'vessel' as such, but represents an anatomical and physiological tendency of the area. Because of the location of the *rèn* vessel, its functions are similar to those of the three yin channels of the leg, which follow parallel paths. Therefore, while the *rèn* vessel is said to link all six of the regular yin channels, it has a particularly close functional relationship to the kidney, liver, and spleen.

The Chinese character for the *rèn* vessel (任) can mean to accept, to take responsibility, to be confided with, or to control. What is it that this vessel is accepting responsibility for? Specifically, it is responsible for the nourishment and development of the fetus. It is noteworthy that substituting the radical for human being on the left side of this character with the radical for woman creates a character meaning to be pregnant (妊 *rèn*). Thus, to most Chinese readers, within the character for the *rèn* vessel there is a harmonic meaning of pregnancy (Fig. 11.3).

The *rèn* and *dū* vessels are unique among the extraordinary vessels. The most obvious difference is that these vessels have their own points. But they also have collateral vessels, while the other six extraordinary vessels do not. Both of these differences illustrate how the *rèn* and *dū* vessels are sort of quasi-extraordinary, in that some of the principles of the regular channels

任	This character in *rèn* vessel also means to accept, take responsibility for, be confided with, or to control
妊	*rèn*—to be with child

Fig. 11.3
Rèn (任) and *rèn* (妊)

still apply. One can needle the *rèn* and *dū* vessels directly instead of working through confluent and/or command points. One might also palpate the *rèn* and *dū* vessels in a diagnostic context—a practice that is often done.

Texts also refer to the *rèn* vessel as a 'sea of blood'—a term sometimes applied to the *chōng* ('penetrating') vessel as well. While the *chōng* vessel irrigates blood to the internal organs, the *rèn* vessel is closely associated with the blood of menstruation and nourishment in the uterus. However, in the clinic, it is sometimes difficult to separate the *rèn* and *chōng* vessels. In fact, points associated with the *chōng* on the abdomen are so close to those of the *rèn* that the two may sometimes be thought of as interweaving and overlapping. In addition, the collateral vessel of the *rèn* vessel mentioned earlier goes inward at CV-15 *(jiū wéi)* toward the heart and stomach, thus also involving the vessel in digestive and circulatory functions.

THE *Dū* ('GOVERNING') VESSEL

As mentioned above, the *rèn* ('conception') and *dū* ('governing') vessels arise from the same source. Before following the familiar path up the spine, the *dū* vessel travels down to the genitals and meets with the *rèn* vessel. The *rèn* and *dū* vessels are thus sometimes said to be two aspects of the same vessel. In fact, in *Examination of the Extraordinary Vessels*, Li Shi-Zhen describes an anterior, deep collateral of the *dū* vessel traveling up the front of the body deep to the *rèn* vessel. The *dū* vessel ends by entering the brain at GV-16 *(fēng fǔ)*. The Chinese character for *dū* (督) means to superintend or govern and the vessel is thought to specifically govern and regulate the yang of the entire body.

The *dū* vessel also has two collaterals traveling along both sides of the spine. In fact, the points 0.5 inches lateral to the *dū* vessel, known as the *Huá Tuō jiá jǐ* 華佗夾脊 points (or M-BW-35) are actually along this collateral vessel. The *dū* vessel also links with all six regular yang channels and is therefore used in cases where there is a lack of movement anywhere in the body (including cases of paralysis).

The following should be kept in mind about the pathway of the *dū* vessel:

- The vessel has an immediate branch forward to the urethra, uterus, and testicles.

- The *dū* vessel directly enters the brain at GV-16.

- M-BW-35 *(Huá Tuō jiá jǐ)* are points that are actually on a collateral of the *dū* vessel.

THE *Yīn/yáng qiāo* ('HEEL') VESSELS

Among the eight extraordinary vessels, both the *qiāo* ('heel') and *wéi* ('linking') vessels consist of yin-yang pairs. The term *qiāo* (蹺) refers to a tightening and loosening of muscles, most commonly in the legs. This is one reason why it is sometimes translated as 'heel' vessel. The *qiāo* vessels are associated with agility and are thought to maintain a balance in the seesaw of yin-yang muscle movement. Like the *rèn* and *dū* vessels, the *yīn-yáng qiāo* vessels connect to each other. While the *rèn* and *dū* vessels meet in the perineum, the *yīn-yáng qiāo* vessels meet in the eyes. This is in contrast to the *yīn-yáng wéi* ('linking') vessels that are not said to meet.

The pathways of the *yīn-yáng qiāo* vessels are often associated with movement in the lower limbs. Some translators thus also use the term 'walker' as a rendering for *qiāo*, although the term actually means to lift up the leg or stand on tiptoe. Nevertheless, the idea that these vessels coordinate walking is helpful. Another common translation, 'springing', is based on this understanding.

In fact, the purpose of these vessels should be broadened further to include the careful coordination of muscle movement anywhere in the body. The movement of muscle groups often involves the channel sinews of more than one channel, and it is the function of the *qiāo* vessels to coordinate these complex muscle movements. The relationship of the two *qiāo* vessels to each other can be understood by considering the fact that, when one muscle tightens, another must loosen to provide free range of movement.

The *yáng qiāo* vessel integrates the three yang channels of the leg as well as the *yáng míng* large intestine channel. The *yīn qiāo* is associated with the *shào yīn, tài yīn,* and *tài yáng* channels of the leg. All of these channels travel to the face as well, and thus the *qiāo* vessels are associated with facial movement. Also, because the *yáng qiāo* vessel is said to enter the outer canthus of the eyes while the *yīn qiāo* vessel enters the inner canthus, both vessels are involved in eye movement and function. In addition, this function includes the opening and closing of the eyes in healthy rhythms of sleep (Table 11.4).

Another important concept should be added to the traditional interpretation of the functions of the *yīn-yáng qiāo* vessels outlined above, namely, that there is an internal muscle aspect of the function of coordinating muscle movement among multiple channel sinews. This relates most specifically to the *yīn qiāo* vessel and involves the movement of muscles in and around the internal organs. In modern physiology, these muscle groups are considered to be involuntary (not controllable by conscious effort) and consist of smooth muscle tissue. Clinical experience indicates that the function

Vessel	Associated Sinew Vessels/Muscle Groups
Yáng qiāo	Gallbladder, bladder, stomach, large intestine, lateral eye
Yīn qiāo	Kidney, spleen, bladder, medial eye

Table 11.4

Yáng and *yīn qiāo* vessels and associated sinew vessels and muscle groups

of these muscles can also be affected by stimulating points associated with the *yīn qiāo* vessel. This concept will be developed below in the course of discussing the clinical applications of the extraordinary vessels.

The most important thing to remember about the *qiāo* vessels is the concept of integration of movement and function among the channel sinews of more than one regular channel. Also, while many modern texts emphasize the association of the *yáng qiāo* vessel with muscle abduction and the *yīn qiāo* vessel with adduction, they do not mention the ability of the *yīn qiāo* to affect muscle movement in the body cavity—especially when multiple channels are involved in problems along the GI tract from throat to intestines.

THE *Yīn-yáng wéi* ('LINKING') VESSELS

The *yáng wéi* ('linking') vessel is associated with the three yang channels of the arm, the three yang channels of the leg, the *dū* ('governing') vessel, and the *yáng qiāo* ('heel') vessel. The *yīn wéi* vessel is associated with the three leg yin channels and the *rèn* ('conception') vessel (Table 11.5).

The Chinese character for *wéi* (維) means to connect, tie-up, integrate, or maintain. In most English books it is translated as 'linking'. It also means to safeguard. While the eight extraordinary vessels in general are regarded as reservoirs and integrators of the overflow from the twelve regular channels, it is the specific function of the *wéi* vessels to integrate the slow irrigation of yin and yang within these areas of overflow. This is an interesting concept that begins in the *Classic of Difficulties*.

Chapter 28 of that text describes the *wéi* vessels as "an integrating network in the body which overflows to fill [when areas] are not circulated and irrigated by the various [regular] channels."[4] These areas, which are not within the orbit of circulation and irrigation of the regular channels, nonetheless require yang stimulation and yin nourishment. The function of the *wéi* vessels is to integrate the distribution of yin and yang at this level, or more specifically, to harmonize the distribution of yin and yang by *multiple* channels into these small areas. The *wéi* vessels do not provide yang stimu-

Vessel	Integrated Channels and Vessels
Yáng wéi	All yang channels, *dū* vessel, *yáng qiāo* vessel
Yīn wéi	Yin channels of the leg (spleen, kidney, liver), *rèn* vessel

Table 11.5

Yīn and *yáng wéi* vessels and associated channels and vessels

lation and yin nourishment themselves; rather, they integrate the distribution of yin and yang by the regular channels.

The ability of the regular channels to provide yang stimulus and yin nourishment to areas of the body outside their reach involves circulation beyond the minute collateral level. Thus both of the *wéi* vessels are influenced via command points, which are also collateral points. The *yáng wéi* command point is TB-5 *(wài guān)*, the collateral point of the triple burner channel. Earlier, the relationship of the triple burner and the extraordinary vessels was described as one of pathway of fluids (triple burner) with categories of function for those fluids (extraordinary vessels). The triple burner is also a pathway of source qi. It is through the minute collaterals of the triple burner that source qi enters the integrating network of yang circulation supported by the *yáng wéi* vessel. In fact, it may be for this very reason that the name of TB-5 is 'outer gate' *(wài guān)*: a gate through which yang is circulated beyond the collaterals.

Similarly, the *yīn wéi* vessel harmonizes the provision of yin nourishment beyond the level of minute collateral circulation. Its command point, PC-6 *(nèi guān)*, also a collateral point, is known as the 'inner gate'. PC-6 is the collateral point of the pericardium, a *jué yīn* organ full of yin-blood. The collaterals of *jué yīn* are a place where abundant yin nourishment enters the deepest inner environment of the body. The *yīn wéi* vessel is charged with harmonizing the provision of yin nourishment among multiple channels. This is very significant when considering the broad clinical applications of the PC-6 point, discussed below.

In sum, the *wéi* vessels integrate the provision of yin and yang from multiple channels to the regions of the body beyond the reach of minute vessel circulation. The *yáng wéi* vessel draws its ability to irrigate the areas outside the regular channels from source qi (thus the *shào yáng* collateral point is used) while the *yīn wéi* vessel draws from the yin reservoir of blood (hence the *jué yīn* collateral point).[5]

The *Classic of Difficulties*, written during the second century A.D., was the starting point for the description of the extraordinary vessels. Over the course of nearly two millennia that followed, generations of Chinese physicians interpreted and reinterpreted these passages, all the while developing new clinical approaches.

In effect, a few short passages in the *Classic of Difficulties* regarding the nature of the *wéi* vessels were like seeds planted in the minds of generations of doctors. A statement about one pair of the extraordinary vessels (the *wéi*) led to speculation and clinical exploration regarding the areas in which all the extraordinary vessels are working. For example, later scholars such as Ye Tian-Shi described a process through which chronic disease can enter the extraordinary vessels, and then developed an effective treatment approach that takes this concept into account.[6] Similarly, it was from the phrase "overflows to fill [when areas] are not circulated and irrigated by the various [regular] channels" that the concept, proposed in these pages, of the extraordinary vessels as functioning in the realm of the interstitial fluids was drawn. As always, it is most important to validate these concepts in the crucible of clinical practice[7] (Fig. 11.4).

It was noted earlier that one of the functions of the *wéi* vessels is the irrigation of areas outside of regular channel circulation, but strictly speaking, this could also be said about the extraordinary vessels as a whole. This underlines the inherent difficulty of defining the scope of each of the extraordinary vessels. Each of the eight extraordinary 'vessels' is not as distinct an entity as the regular channels; rather, each represents a particular functional aspect of what might be called the extraordinary vessel *system*.

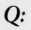

Q:

It is now fairly clear that the eight extraordinary vessels may be associated with the interstitial fluids, but I'm now confused about the relationship of the spleen to all of this. When we discussed tài yīn, you mentioned that the spleen is associated with maintaining the 'cellular bath' and also used the term interstitial fluids in that context. How might I understand spleen function in relation to the extraordinary vessels?

DR. WANG: In general, remember that the regular channels constantly interact with the extraordinary vessels; don't make the mistake of considering them to be closed systems that never touch. However, there is something that should be clarified about the spleen. The spleen is fundamentally associated with maintaining the body's ability to nourish itself. Along with the stomach, it is the root of postnatal

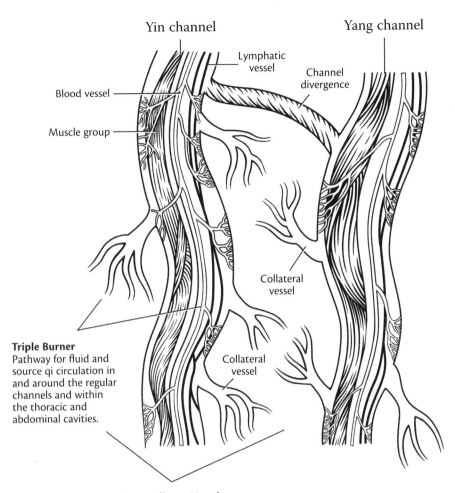

Yin channel

Yang channel

Lymphatic vessel

Channel divergence

Blood vessel

Muscle group

Collateral vessel

Triple Burner
Pathway for fluid and source qi circulation in and around the regular channels and within the thoracic and abdominal cavities.

Collateral vessel

Extraordinary Vessels
Integrate the movement of fluids surrounding the regular channels. There are eight functional categories or vessels (脉 *mài*) within these innumerable channels (奇经 *qì jīng*).

Fig. 11.4
Both the triple burner and the extraordinary vessels are involved with the fluids surrounding the body tissues. In this context, the triple burner is a pathway while the extraordinary vessels represent various functions.

qi. At the specific level that we are calling the interstitial fluids, the spleen is still responsible for maintaining this nutritional aspect. The extraordinary vessels integrate or harmonize the ability of multiple channels to provide nutrition. But the ability of the interstitial fluids to provide cellular nourishment falls within the purview of the spleen. When nutritive qi is abundant, it flows out of the vessels to provide nutrition at a cellular level. Also, as the primary organ involved in the metabolism of dampness, the spleen is involved in the reuptake of fluids back into the vessels.

Remember, however, that a fluid up-take symptom like edema might also be caused by a lack of spleen warmth due to underlying kidney deficiency, or it may be from a lack of blood movement due to heart deficiency. In any case, the most important thing to remember is that I am not saying that the eight extraordinary vessels control everything related to the interstitial fluids. In fact, the complex qi dynamic occurring within those fluids depends on the smooth inter-action of the activities of the regular channels and organs.

THE *Chōng* ('PENETRATING') VESSEL

The *chōng* ('penetrating') vessel is sometimes shown as a collateral of the kidney *shào yīn* channel, or traveling along the pathway of the stomach *yáng míng* channel. A cursory review of the commonly accepted pathway of the vessel reveals that many of the currently used *chōng* confluent points are in fact on the kidney channel, especially along the abdomen. Earlier we noted how *rèn* ('conception') vessel function often overlaps with the *chōng* in clinical applications. The *rèn* vessel is responsible for conception and ovarian function in women, and in general is associated with the yin aspect of reproduction in both sexes. On the other hand, the *chōng* vessel, also described as a 'sea of blood', is associated more with the menstrual cycle. In addition, the *chōng* is an irrigator, especially an irrigator of blood, for the regular channels and the blood vessels associated with their internal pathways.

The Chinese character for *chōng* (沖) means to rush vigorously and thus some modern sources equate the vessel with the vigorous pulsing of the in-ferior vena cava that can be palpated in the abdomen. Classical sources also describe a deep branch of the *chōng* vessel traveling inward from the kidney channel toward the internal organs, and another branch along the kidney (or liver) channel down the leg to the heel. Another collateral on the chest flows outward toward the breasts.

In general, the *chōng* vessel integrates the flow of blood to the internal organs. Integration involves not only large vessels like the aorta and vena cava, but also the smaller vessels entering and leaving the organs, particular-ly the heart, stomach, and intestines. Once again, remember that the *chōng* vessel itself is not equivalent to the blood vessels; rather, it represents the concept of integrating flow among multiple vessels. While one or another vessel might be associated with the internal pathway of one of the regular channels, it is the function of the *chōng* vessel to integrate them all.

The *chōng* vessel is also associated with lactation in women and with beard growth in men. Thus diagrams of the vessel often show small collaterals extending across the chest in women and through the lower face in men.

The *Dài* ('girdle') vessel

The *dài* vessel binds around the waist to integrate the upward and downward movement of qi among the regular channels as they pass through the waist. The vessel is thus particularly associated with those aspects of the regular channels which travel through the waist toward the legs. With a horizontal pathway that arises from the kidneys, the *dài* vessel is unique among the extraordinary vessels in that it does not travel upward in the body. The pathway followed by the *dài* vessel allows it to integrate the circulation of qi to both the back and the lower burner in a transverse flow.

Q: *It seems that you have less to say about the chōng and dài vessels. Why is this?*

DR. WANG: Frankly, I don't feel like I understand the *chōng* and the *dài* vessels well enough to add much to the classical concepts that were just briefly outlined. In the clinic, I certainly use the *chōng* vessel, but less often find conditions that, to my mind, could be categorized as *dài* vessel cases. My understanding of the eight extraordinary vessels is drawn from my readings of classical sources. In the end, however, they must be validated by application in the clinic. In particular, I have yet to reach an understanding of the *dài* vessel that could be used to guide treatment strategies. This is something that we should all consider and try to work towards.

The Extraordinary Vessels in the Clinic

Chapter 29 of the *Classic of Difficulties* provides the earliest example of disease patterns associated with the extraordinary vessels. While the *Inner Classic* mentions the extraordinary vessels in disconnected phrases in both the *Divine Pivot* and *Basic Questions,* it is the *Classic of Difficulties* which lays the foundation for a more systematic understanding of extraordinary vessel pathology. As seen earlier, Chapter 27 introduces the names and general principles of extraordinary vessel theory, while Chapter 28 describes the pathways for six of the eight vessels, and the functions of the *wéi* vessels. It is not until Chapter 29, however, that the disease patterns are finally addressed. Many debates about extraordinary vessel treatment, from the second century A.D. to the present, begin with an analysis of Chapter 29.

This chapter begins with a straightforward question: What happens when the extraordinary vessels are diseased?

The answer involves a description of extraordinary vessel pathology, presented one vessel at a time. The following section will present the descriptions of extraordinary vessel pathology from the *Classic of Difficulties*, followed by a discussion of how these concepts might be applied in the modern clinic.

Integrating the yīn-yáng wéi ('linking') vessels

Chapter 29 begins with the *yīn-yáng wéi* vessels and the concept of integration. Only these vessels are singled out as being prone to problems of integration with one another. In other words, this is the only pathology described that involves two extraordinary vessels as once. The text says that a type of pathology exists in which the *yīn-yáng wéi* "are unable to mutually interlink" (不能自相維 *bù néng zì xiāng wéi).* Recall from the discussion above that the *yīn-yáng wéi* are described in Chapter 28 as acting "to fill [areas] that lack circulation and irrigation from the various [regular] channels." In this type of pathology, there is a lack of communion between yin and yang in the areas beyond the reach of the regular channels. When yin and yang fail to interact, there is a kind of disjointedness in the body.

The *Classic of Difficulties* describes the resulting disease pattern as one involving a type of psychosis. Patients will have a 'loss of will' and be unable to control themselves. This is not the same as the manic loss of will often associated with the fire-type pathodynamic, but involves a lack of control in the sense that a person feels fatigued and unmotivated to get out of bed. There may be fogginess and a lack of clear mental processes. It is a type of depression whereby patients literally cannot pull themselves together.

For this pattern, one might combine treatments using the command points of the *yīn-yáng wéi* (TB-5 and PC-6) with other points that stabilize the qi and blood, such as SP-6 *(sān yīn jiāo)* and CV-6 *(qì hǎi).* Other points could be added based on the symptom presentation and findings of channel palpation.

Yáng wéi disorder

When the function of the *yáng wéi* is compromised, the ability of yang to distribute to the areas outside the twelve regular channels is compromised.

The *Classic of Difficulties* describes the resulting condition as one in which there is a sensation of chills and fever. A lack of yang circulation has led to exterior deficiency. This is a case of lowered resistance in which the patient readily suffers from heat or cold from the external environment, similar to the familiar nutritive-defensive disharmony. Recall that the command point of the *yáng wéi* vessel, located on the *shào yáng* channel, is TB-5 *(wài guān)*, the 'outer gate'. The distribution of yang qi beyond the regular channel collaterals helps maintain the security of the body's defensive gate. Similarly, generalized numbness in the body might also involve problems with *yáng wéi* vessel circulation. In this case, a lack of warming yang qi leads to a sense of lowered sensitivity to external stimulus.

GB-20 *(fēng chí)* Most of the confluent points of the *yáng wéi* vessel are found on the *shào yáng* channel. While GB-20 is the most commonly used— to build up yang qi on the surface and clear external pathogens—it should be noted that GB-13 to GB-24 are all confluent points on the *yáng wéi* vessel.

GB-15 *(tóu lín qì)* Often used in the treatment of wind-cold patterns involving headache with an underlying nutritive-defensive disharmony, the functions of this point are related to those of the *yáng wéi*.

Yīn wéi disorder

Dysfunction in the extraordinary vessels associated with the *yīn wéi* involves a lack of irrigation of yin nourishment to the small spaces outside the twelve regular channels. This lack of yin distribution leads to a symptom pattern that Chapter 29 describes as "suffering from heart pain" (苦心痛 *kǔ xīn tòng*). Recall from the earlier description of *yīn wéi* function that the fundamental yin substance with which this vessel is associated is the nourishing aspect of the blood, and in particular, with the sense of calmness brought about by ample blood flow to even the smallest spaces throughout the body. A *yīn wéi* pattern would not necessarily involve 'pain' in the heart (although it might) but would especially include a sense of emotional angst tied to a feeling of organ discomfort.

This, of course, is a pattern that is commonly treated with PC-6 *(nèi guān)*. As the command point of the *yīn wéi* vessel, PC-6 helps to reestablish *yīn wéi* function to benefit the heart (and thus the emotional state) through improved circulation of yin-blood in the small spaces beyond the channels. Improved harmonization of blood circulation among the blood vessels associated with the regular channels can also help in the treatment of voice loss, stomach pain, epilepsy, and other generalized digestive complaints that include this sense of angst and emotional discomfort.

APPLIED CHANNEL THEORY IN CHINESE MEDICINE

"Suffering from heart pain" might also involve the *yīn qiāo* with a type of generalized anxiety in which the patient shows few symptoms but is quite anxious to search for an identifiable disease that explains their existential discomfort. When this type of *yīn wéi* pattern is suspected, diagnosis should include palpation of the yin channels—particularly the three yin channels of the arm. Anxious patients whose conditions involve the *yīn wéi* vessels will likely have tightness or diffuse nodules throughout the yin surface of the arms.

PC-6 *(nèi guān)* The command point of the *yīn wéi* discussed above is traditionally combined with the *chōng* ('penetrating') vessel command point SP-4 *(gōng sūn)*. This pair acts synergistically to facilitate the distribution of yin-blood. While the *yīn wéi* vessel is charged in particular with integrating the irrigation of yin in areas beyond the reach of the regular vessels, the *chōng* vessel integrates strong movement of blood in vessels associated with multiple channels. The *chōng* vessel, said to be full of both qi and blood, impels strong movement when the two are combined. This pair is often used clinically to treat deficiency-type depression where the accumulation of yin-blood has led to lethargy. It is also used for pain and discomfort in the organs.

KI-9 *(zhú bīn)* The cleft point of the *yīn wéi* vessel may be thought of as a cleft point for all of the yin channels. Because the *yīn wéi* is associated with the irrigation of yin in areas outside the reach of the twelve regular vessels, its cleft point (a moving point) stimulates movement in yin areas throughout the body. In the clinic, this point has been used in the treatment of tumors. As tumors represent an accumulation of yin turbidity in the body, the stimulation of yin fluid circulation is of utmost importance in their treatment. For treating tumors, this point is treated with very strong moxa, usually applied directly on top of 3mm-thick slices of ginger placed on the skin. There should be redness and possibly even mild blisters at the point. A modern explanation for this phenomenon might include consideration of the generalized immune response caused by mild tissue damage to this particular area (Table 11.6).

Yáng qiāo disorder

The *Classic of Difficulties* describes the *yīn-yáng qiāo* as having a kind of balancing function for yin and yang. Because the character for *qiāo* (蹻) carries the meaning of 'walker', most modern clinical applications involve considerations of functional balance between the medial and lateral muscles of the leg. Chapter 29 describes *yáng qiāo* vessel dysfunction as a pattern in which "the yin [*qiāo*] is flaccid while the yang [*qiāo*] is tense." Remember that the pathway of the vessel is associated with all three yang channels on

Vessel	Pathology in *Classic of Difficulties*	Use in Modern Clinic
Yáng wéi and *yīn wéi*	When not 'interlinked', one loses will and thus control	Loss of will, often involving lethargy and depression
Yáng wéi	Cold and heat	Lowered resistance with frequent colds and/or generalized numbness
Yīn wéi	Heart pain	Heart/stomach pain or discomfort due to lack of small vessel circulation; may also involve anxiety with no discernible cause

Table 11.6
Pathologies associated with *yīn* and *yáng wéi* vessels

. . . .

the leg plus the arm *yáng míng* large intestine channel (see Table 11.4). As described earlier, a broader understanding of *qiāo* vessel function involves the idea of integrating motor function among the channel sinews of multiple regular channels. Conditions where the body's ability to execute complex muscle movement is compromised might also involve the *qiāo* vessels. The *yáng qiāo* is likely involved in problems relating to coordination of channel sinew pathways among multiple yang channels (see the case study at the end of this chapter). The pathways of both *qiāo* vessels end in the eyes, thus later sources also associate the *yáng qiāo* vessel with insomnia.

Diagnosis of the *qiāo* vessels should include a determination of whether nodules or muscle tone irregularities are affecting multiple channels. For example, diagnosis of the *yáng qiāo* would involve palpating the yang channels of the leg in an effort to determine whether multiple yang channels present significant patterns of nodules or systemic muscle tightness. This is a difficult skill and requires that one differentiate whether the condition involves multiple channels or just a single channel that later compromised circulation in other channels. Sometimes, of course, a condition that begins with a single channel can later spread to multiple channels, and thus to the extraordinary vessels. Recall again that extraordinary vessel conditions involve problems with integration and communication among multiple regular channels (Fig. 11.5).

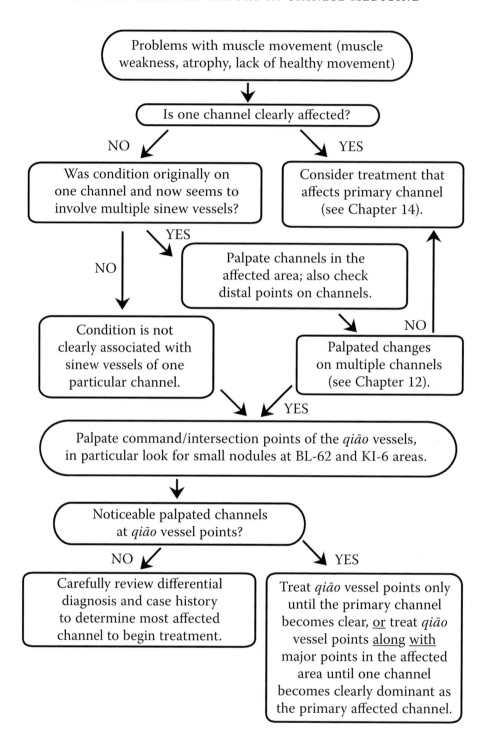

Fig. 11.5

Diagnosis of the *qiāo* vessels

BL-62 (shēn mài) The command point of the *yáng qiāo* is often used for problems with balance and coordination. The *yáng qiāo* in particular is involved in coordination of multiple muscle groups not only for walking, but also for balance. Elderly patients who have problems with coordination, or even younger patients who are clumsy, are often treated with this point. Furthermore, problems in the elderly with maintaining the proper sleep rhythm can also be addressed through the *yáng qiāo*. This isn't exactly insomnia or hypersomnia, but a tendency to sleep and wake repeatedly throughout the day. Finally, the area around BL-62 should be carefully palpated in cases of upper back and shoulder pain, and also facial paralysis, because the pathway of the vessel integrates the channel sinews of the *shào yáng*, *yáng míng*, and *tài yáng* channels.

Yīn qiāo disorder

Like its paired vessel, the *yīn qiāo* involves the coordination of motor movement, specifically among multiple yin channel sinew groups. Chapter 29 of the *Classic of Difficulties* describes a *yīn qiāo* condition as one involving "flaccidity along the yang [*qiāo*] and tension along the yin [*qiāo*]." Thus the most common modern application of the *yīn qiāo* involves treatment of conditions where there is tightness along the muscles of the medial leg and flaccidity of those on the lateral leg. In addition, as previously noted, clinical experience also indicates that there is a relationship of the *yīn qiāo* with the musculature surrounding the internal organs. For example, the peristaltic movement of the GI tract might involve *yīn qiāo* integration of multiple internal channel sinew groups. Specifically, problems with swallowing or digestion following a stroke are responsive to treatment with the *yīn qiāo*.

An effective point pair for dealing with the internal muscle aspect of the *yīn qiāo* involves the combination of the collateral point of the heart, HT-5 (*tōng lǐ*), with the command point of the *yīn qiāo*, KI-6 *(zhào hǎi)*. Recall that HT-5 invigorates circulation of blood in the yin collaterals; it is therefore thought of in conditions involving microcirculation, particularly in the brain. Combining a treatment of the collaterals, associated with microcirculation of blood, with one which benefits coordination of internal muscle movement provides an effective base point pair.

Other conditions traditionally associated with the *yīn qiāo* include hypersomnia (always wanting to sleep) and epilepsy. Another interesting application of *qiāo* vessel theory involves consideration of the patient's circadian rhythm, or the 'movement' of the organs at particular times of day. If a patient presents with symptoms that occur at the same time each day, one might consider treating the *qiāo* vessels. These symptoms might even involve something like recurring cough or abdominal pain.

Symptoms that occur at predictable times may be related to problems with the timing of movement in the organs. Therefore, when one says that the *yīn qiāo* vessel is associated with the 'movement' of the internal organs, this should be understood in the broadest sense. If problems occur at the same time every night, consider the *yīn qiāo*, and if during the daytime, consider the *yáng qiāo*. Similar reasoning would suggest the use of the *qiāo* vessels in the treatment of jet lag, a condition which affects the rhythms of the organs. In all of these cases, careful palpation of the *qiāo* vessel intersection and command points should be performed to verify involvement.

KI-6 *(zhào hǎi)* The very broad clinical application of this point is due in part to its association with the *yīn qiāo* vessel. Used in the treatment of not only regular kidney channel pathodynamics but also problems ranging from GI tract discomfort and heart pain to developmental problems in children, this point has a broad regulatory effect on the movement and healthy integration of the internal organs via the extraordinary vessel system.

KI-8 *(jiāo xìn)* The cleft point of the *yīn qiāo* is effective for treating certain types of depression. Clinically, the point is most effective when depression involves symptom patterns that include pain or dysfunction in the internal organs. This should be contrasted with the types of emotional problems associated above with the *yīn wéi* vessel. In the case of the *yīn qiāo*, there may be actual pain or discomfort that the patient feels in a particular organ, as opposed to a general discomfort or sense that there is an organic problem without clear, consistent pain. These types of depression patterns underline the fundamental concept of the inseparability of emotional conditions from physiology. One should always try to evaluate emotional disorders with the functions and movement of the internal organs in mind.

In conclusion, Fig. 11.5 describes the thought process that is involved when considering *qiāo* vessel treatment. Note the importance of determining the location of disease in diagnosis. This is true with all aspects of Chinese medical diagnostics. In this case, the key is to determine if a regular channel is involved, or if instead it is clearly a lack of integration among multiple channels. This process involves not only clear and logical thinking, but also a degree of experience.

Chōng vessel disorder

Chapter 29 of the *Classic of Difficulties* associates the *chōng* vessel with counterflow qi (逆氣 *nì qì*), which causes urgency or rushing (急 *jí*) in the body. The term 'counterflow' refers to a reversal of normal qi flow. The *chōng* vessel is thus associated with a variety of problems regarding the improper movement of qi in the deep internal environment.

If the *Classic of Difficulties* associates the *chōng* vessel with counterflow qi, then why do the most common clinical applications always involve blood flow? The answer to this question further illuminates the broad regulatory function of the extraordinary vessels. It should first be remembered that the concept of counterflow is quite broad in Chinese medicine. The term might describe vomiting (counterflow of stomach qi) or involve more subtle concepts regarding the proper direction of qi dynamic in specific organs and/or channels. In the case of a *chōng* vessel disorder, there is a generalized counterflow of qi that is less organ or channel specific. Because 'blood is the mother of qi and qi is the commander of blood', a generalized counterflow of qi manifests as a broad disorder in the regular movement of blood. This leads to a physical sense of urgency or rushing—in the wrong direction. Once again, the function of the extraordinary vessels is broad and beyond the normal scope of individual channels or organs.

Clinically, the *chōng* vessel is most closely associated with the integration of blood flow from blood vessels associated with multiple channels in the trunk of the body. Treatment of the *chōng* is considered when counterflow causes a lack of proper blood distribution to the internal organs with such symptoms as abdominal pain and/or cramping. Other symptoms that might also be associated with counterflow of the qi dynamic in the interior include vomiting, asthma, or biomedically-defined problems with organ vasculature, especially when accompanied by strong sensations of odd internal movement felt by the patient.

KI-16 *(huāng shū)* This point is commonly used in *chōng* vessel type cases where there is painful menstruation due to a lack of proper blood distribution to the uterus.

SP-4 *(gōng sūn)* The command point of the *chōng* vessel, this point is especially helpful for resolving counterflow. Not only symptoms such as nausea or stomach pain, but also hypertension leading to a sense of pulsing and fullness, or even pain in the head, respond to treatment with this point.

Dū vessel disorder

Chapter 29 describes problems with the *dū* vessel as involving tightness of the spine and 'reversal' (厥 *jué*). This term is described at some length in the introduction to *jué yīn* (see Chapter 7 of this text). Here, reversal refers to a pattern where the yang qi has become blocked. In the case of deficiency of the *dū* vessel, a 'sea' of yang qi, there is a reverse in yang flow that leads to its failure to reach the extremities. The result is coldness in the hands and/or feet. Reversal might also refer to a condition where tightness along the spine or back creates tension in the body that causes a person to bend the body backward, thus compressing the spinal vertebrae.

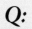 **Q:** *Earlier, when talking about the chōng vessel, you described a pathology of qi counterflow (氣逆 qì nì) while the dū vessel pathology involves reversal (厥 jué). In this case, how do you think about these two seemingly similar terms?*

DR. WANG: Counterflow simply involves movement in the wrong direction. This might be movement of qi or movement of blood. Reversal implies a kind of separation (隔開 gé kāi) as well, but it is more than just that. It is a separation that, in essence, can also cause improper movement. It most often involves a separation of yin and yang. In the case of the *dū* vessel, there is a reversal which has led to cold in the extremities. Yang has separated and is no longer linking outward to the hands and feet. The sensation of cold begins at the tips of the fingers, the furthest point out.

In the clinic, such problems with the distribution of yang qi are common and can lead to a variety of symptoms. Difficulties with body movement, or a systemic lack of warmth, are general examples of how reversal in the *dū* vessel leads to disease and discomfort. There may also be particular areas in the back and/or neck that seem to lack warm circulation. Developmental problems in children, spinal injuries, stroke, and some types of epilepsy also respond well to *dū* vessel points.

GV-1 (*cháng qiáng*) This point should be needled with the patient in a crouching position with head down, sacrum up. For those familiar with yoga positions, this is the 'child's pose' and can easily be done without the removal of undergarments. The technique involves inserting the needle to a depth of just 2 *fen*, then angling it superiorly so that it moves behind the sacrum. You can also needle this point with the patient lying on their side. In either case, the patient should feel a radiating sensation throughout the low back. This technique is helpful in the treatment of rectal prolapse and hemorrhoids, both of which are often associated with the 'bulging disorder' (疝 shàn) described below in relation to the *rèn* vessel.

GV-9 (*zhì yáng*) This point is particularly useful for bringing yang to the chest and stomach. It is an important point in cases of chronic asthma or ulcers due to cold accumulation. The point (or other *dū* points around it) is also often used in cases of digestive discomfort associated with emotional excess. In these types of patients, the spine should be palpated above and below GV-9 to look for nodules, a sense of tightness or discomfort. These areas should then be needled.

GV-12 (*shēn zhù*)   This point is very often used in pediatric cases, particularly those involving developmental issues. It is helpful for children who fail to properly assimilate postnatal qi due to yang deficiency. The point is also often treated with moxa for cold-type asthma.

GV-19 (*hòu dǐng*)   This point is used to stimulate yang so as to reestablish circulation throughout the entire *dū* vessel. Often used in the treatment of back pain, strong stimulation of this point followed by a cough can 'shake out' the *dū* vessel, thus helping to return normal tone to the muscles.

GV-21 (*qián dǐng*)   This point is very often used to bring the clear yang upward to the head in cases of dizziness, mental fogginess, or other conditions involving a lack of yang circulation in the upper body, head, and face.

GV-24 (*shén tíng*)   This point calms anxious patients by bringing clear yang qi to the mind. It is often combined with CV-12 *(zhōng wǎn)*. It can also be helpful in the treatment of poststroke speech problems where the patient cannot 'connect thoughts to words'. In other words, the mouth and tongue appear to function normally, but the patient has difficulty verbalizing words/ideas that are in the mind due to a lack of yang qi stimulus.

Rèn vessel disorders

Problems with the *rèn* vessel lead to knotting (結 *jié*). Chapter 29 of the *Classic of Difficulties* differentiates knotting associated with *rèn* vessel problems that occur in men from those seen in women. In men, knotting is said to lead to the "seven types of bulging disorder," while in women, knotting leads to mobile abdominal masses (瘕 *jiǎ*). Exactly what the text is describing here has been the subject of some debate, but the clinical use of the *rèn* vessel indicates that, in both men and women, it is associated with problems in the lower abdomen and genitals. The term 'bulging disorder', said to occur in men, is likely a reference to hernias affecting the abdominal wall and scrotum, which are also often treated through the *rèn* vessel. In women, mobile abdominal masses involve the various accumulations of qi and/or blood that lead to problems with the uterus and reproduction.[8]

In the clinic, the *rèn* vessel is used most often for problems with development and reproduction. However, the vessel should also be considered for treatment of any condition occurring along its path, including urinary problems, stomach pain, and even sores in the mouth and tongue.

CV-3 (zhōng jí)   As the alarm (front-*mu*) point for the bladder, this point is often used in the treatment of excess-type bladder conditions. However, it is also appropriate for problems with the prostate in men. Both are cases of excess yin accumulation. Remember that the point should not be needled deeply in cases where urinary difficulty has led to an over-filled bladder. It is relatively easy to pierce the organ at this point.

CV-4 (guān yuán)   Accumulation in the *rèn* vessel can be associated with blood stasis. Recall that this is the alarm point of the small intestine, an organ involved in the "transformation of red to maintain blood."[9] In a wide variety of blood-related disorders, this point is combined with SP-6 *(sān yīn jiāo)* to reset blood circulation, and with the 'four gates' (LR-3 and LI-4) to reset the qi dynamic. The needle can be inserted relatively deeply at this point. A 1.5-inch needle is often used with gentle stimulation until a deep radiating sensation is achieved, followed by a return of the needle to a shallow depth (0.5 inches) where it is retained for 25 minutes.

CV-6 (qì hǎi)   This point, called the 'sea of qi' (氣海 *qì hǎi)*, holds particular importance in many types of meditation and *qì gōng* practices. Although the point is located on the yin-natured *rèn* vessel, it has the ability to boost the qi. This is qi coming from the nearby gate of vitality. In cases of channel exhaustion (see discussion in Chapter 20), it is often combined with the 'four gates' points as well. While CV-4 has more of an ability to benefit the yin when combined with the four gates, CV-6 is better able to benefit the qi. In heavier patients, needles of up to 3 inches in length are sometimes used at this point for a strong initial stimulus, followed by returning the needle to a shallower depth (0.5 inches) for retention.

CV-11 (jiàn lǐ)   This point is often used in combination with LI-10 *(shǒu sān lǐ)* and ST-36 *(zú sān lǐ)* to stimulate digestion and postnatal qi. It always has a tonifying effect, and, generally speaking, is not sedated.

CV-12 (zhōng wǎn)   This is a very commonly used point. It can both sedate and tonify the spleen-stomach and is thus used in cases of both middle burner excess *and* deficiency.

CV-17 (tán zhōng)   This point helps to reverse counterflow qi along the *rèn* vessel. It is a favorite of many doctors in cases of counterflow stomach qi (nausea). It is also the alarm point of the pericardium and thus has an ability to harmonize *jué yīn* as well.

Dài vessel disorder

The description of *dài* vessel disease in Chapter 29 of the *Classic of Dif-*

ficulties is brief and to the point. When there are problems with the *dài*, the patient will feel bloating in the abdomen and a "feeling in the lower back as if one were sitting in water." Some modern practitioners use the command point of the *dài* vessel, GB-41 (*zú lín qì*), for back pain accompanied by a sense of heaviness. Alternatively, the vessel is also considered to be involved in low burner accumulation in gynecology leading to abdominal fullness, menstrual irregularity, and vaginal discharge.

Using the Extraordinary Vessel Command Points: New Ideas

Clinical experience has shown that the eight command points, first suggested by Dou Han-Qing (竇漢卿), do have unique effects that can be understood in light of extraordinary vessel theory. The development of applications for these points continues in the modern era. Students of Chinese medicine are likely familiar with the traditional extraordinary vessel command point pairings. While they are often effective, one should not be limited to these traditional point pairs. Creative thinking about the functions of the extraordinary vessels, outlined in this chapter, should lead to innovative combinations of the command and confluent points with regular channel treatment strategies.[10]

When deciding which command point to use, first review the functions of the vessels and the involvement of the regular channels. Always keep in mind the inter-channel effects of the extraordinary vessels. Also remember that four of the eight command points are also collateral points on the regular channels. This is due to the special ability of collateral points to invigorate circulation in the small vessels at the border between the regular channels and the fluids that are so involved in extraordinary vessel function (Table 11.7).

Dr. Wang's clinical experience provides a few new insights and alternate pairings for the extraordinary vessel command points. These alternate pairings can be used for the specific conditions described below, or perhaps for other patterns based on creative thinking (and careful observation of results) regarding extraordinary vessel treatment.

LU-7 (*liè quē*) and SP-4 (*gōng sūn*) This pairing of the *rèn* and *chōng* vessels acts to harmonize blood circulation in the reproductive organs. It is most often used to regulate menstruation when the length of time between periods is irregular. For example, the patient may have a 15-day cycle one month followed by a 35-day cycle the next. It is not appropriate for menorrhagia, amenorrhea, or painful menstruation.

PC-6 *(nèi guān)* and KI-6 *(zhào hǎi)* This pair combines the *yīn wéi* with the *yīn qiāo*. The diffuse irrigation of yin provided by the *yīn wéi* may be likened to the regulating effects of the parasympathetic nervous system. Like that system, the *yīn wéi* acts to stabilize, calm, and nourish the functions among multiple channels. The *yīn qiāo* is associated with muscle movement on the inside of the body and is often used to treat neurological problems affecting the internal organs. Together, the two vessels act to harmonize nourishment and movement in the internal organs. Symptoms may include palpitations or other heart function irregularities that defy conventional cardiovascular diagnosis. Stomach pain or vomiting without discernible organic disorder, or discomfort in the throat without observable changes (including plum-pit qi), are also relevant patterns.

A condition like irritable bowel syndrome (IBS) might also fall within the category of *yīn wéi*/*yīn qiāo* disharmony. For example, in many cases

Point Pair	Vessels with Associated Areas and Common Indications
SP-4* *(gōng sūn)* and PC-6* *(nèi guān)*	*Chōng* and *yīn wéi* vessels AREAS: heart, chest, and stomach INDICATIONS: palpitations, nausea, low appetite, bloating, acid regurgitation
SI-3 *(hòu xī)* and BL-62 *(shēn mài)*	*Dū* and *yáng qiāo* vessels AREAS: neck, shoulder, ear, inner canthus of eye INDICATIONS: back, shoulder pain
TB-5* *(wài guān)* and GB-41 *(zú lín qì)*	*Yáng wéi* and *dài* vessels AREAS: neck, shoulder, cheek, ear, outer canthus of eye INDICATIONS: neck pain, eye problems
LU-7* *(liè quē)* and KI-6 *(zhào hǎi)*	*Rèn* and *yīn qiāo* vessels AREAS: throat, chest, and diaphragm INDICATIONS: sore throat, insomnia, irritability

* These points are also collateral points on their associated channels.

Table 11.7

The classic extraordinary vessel point pairs

there is a psychological aspect to this syndrome whereby symptoms are aggravated by stress and anxiety. As noted earlier, the area around GV-9 *(zhì yáng)* might also reflect palpable changes in these types of patients. Diseases categorized as 'psychosomatic' in modern medicine often include a compromised ability of the body to harmonize nourishment among multiple regular channels. In such cases the calm, regulating functions of the *yīn qiāo* and *yīn wéi* can be therapeutic.

TB-5 *(wài guān)* and BL-62 *(shēn mài)* This is a pairing of the command points associated with the *yáng wéi* and *yáng qiāo* vessels. Together, the vessels act to stimulate yang circulation in cases where there is a lack of inter-channel integration. This point combination has been helpful in the treatment of sudden paralysis (either partial or total) due to emotional/psychological causes. Obviously, this is not a condition encountered often, but two unusual cases in forty years justifies suggesting this as a possible approach. (See the narrative appended to this chapter for an interesting case study of this type of pattern.)

SI-3 *(hòu xī)* and LU-7 *(liè quē)* The *rèn* and *dū* vessels can be paired for another very specific condition. A difficult case led to this application. It involved a patient who, in the course of *qì gōng* practice, had developed a severe, burning back pain that was unresponsive to other treatments. In discussing the case history with the patient, he reported that the pain began after practicing a technique designed to circulate qi around the stomach and back. The back pain appeared one day after practicing the technique for many hours, and then returned, quite severely, every time he began meditating. Because the meditative technique was focused on moving qi along the very pathways of the two vessels, the possibility of blockage in the *rèn* and *dū* vessels came to mind, and this point pair was selected. The results were very good; in fact, for a few years, other *qì gōng* practitioners with this symptom pattern came for treatment. This point pair might therefore be considered in other cases of excess-type back pain in healthy individuals.

When using the eight command points, there are a few things that should be kept in mind about technique. First, the points should be needled less deeply than when using the same points to affect the regular channels. Most of the points are effective at 0.2–0.3 inches and usually aren't needled deeper than 0.5 inches. Second, the points should be located very precisely. This isn't to say that they should be *measured* precisely, but that the practitioner should palpate the channel very carefully. Feel along the course of the appropriate channel for an opening, a softness, a nodule, or an extremely tender spot. That is the location of the point.

■ Case Study

69-year-old male

Chief complaint   Facial paralysis/spasms

History of present illness   Fourteen months previously, during a period of high stress and little rest, the patient developed a severe case of Bell's palsy. Initial symptoms involved relatively severe paralysis and pain on the left side of the face. The patient is an official in a western Chinese province and went immediately to a hospital near his office for consultation. A neurologist diagnosed Bell's palsy and prescribed rest and a one-week course of oral corticosteroids.

Ten days later, the pain had abated to some degree, but the paralysis was unchanged and an uncomfortable facial twitch had begun to develop. He visited a local acupuncture clinic and began a six-week course of acupuncture treatments. The acupuncturist used mainly local points in the face and head on the *yáng míng* and *shào yáng* channels, with additional distal points. Some relief was achieved, and some facial movement was regained. The facial twitch however, continued to be a problem, especially when the patient spoke, ate, or washed his face. Twitching would occasionally lead to spasms around the eye and mouth on the left side.

Over the next nine months, the patient searched for effective treatments in his home city. Although he continued to visit his neurologist and saw other conventional medical specialists, treatment involved mainly acupuncture and Chinese physiotherapy (推拿 *tuī ná*). During this period of time, he consulted with a total of six doctors, using a variety of treatment approaches, but not herbs. The patient reported that "some used just a few needles, some used a great many, some used cups, while others used heat. In the end, I didn't really have significant improvement after the first few weeks." He then traveled to Beijing to seek treatment, arriving at Dr. Wang's clinic fourteen months after initial onset.

The patient had chronic high blood pressure, controlled with a pharmaceutical medication. Bowel movements and digestion were normal. He had difficulty getting to sleep but was generally able to stay asleep. His overall appearance was lively and healthy. His pulse was wiry-fast and his tongue body was red and dry with little coating.

Palpation   Channel palpation revealed soreness and palpable changes mainly on the *yáng míng* and *shào yáng* channels. Specifically, the entire *yáng míng* large intestine channel had a kind of diffuse lumpiness along the forearm, with tenderness and tightness also found below ST-36 *(zú sān lǐ)*. The *shào* *yáng* channel had a large area of diffuse tightness around TB-6 *(zhī gōu)*. On the head and face itself, very careful palpation was done to locate minute nodules. A noticeable nodule was found at ST-7 *(xià guān)*, and smaller nodules were palpated along the gallbladder channel on its pathway over the ears (GB-7 to GB-19).

Diagnosis   Accumulation of phlegm-heat in the *shào yáng* and *yáng míng* channels

The location of paralysis and spasms along the *yáng míng* and *shào yáng* channels on the face was mirrored by palpable changes along the distal course of the channels. The presence of phlegm-heat was due to the chronic nature of stagnation that may or may not have originated in cold (which at this point would be difficult to discern), but now clearly presented as a pattern of heat. The wiry-fast pulse and red, dry tongue condition were also indicative of heat. The fact that the bowel movements were normal indicated that the condition was more likely in the *yáng míng* channel than in the *yáng míng* organs.

The initial diagnosis was one involving the regular channels. To appreciate how treatment eventually involved the extraordinary vessels, it is helpful to look at the results of the first two treatments.

Treatment (first two visits)   Treatment in the initial stage focused on clearing phlegm-heat from the *yáng míng* and *shào yáng* channels. A fairly routine treatment for this type of Bell's palsy pattern was used, which included ST-7 and a needle threaded along the channel from GB-5 *(xuán lú)* to GB-6 *(xuán lí)* locally. The distal points were LI-4 *(hé gǔ)*, the area around ST-36 / ST-37 (an *a-shì* point), and LR-3 *(tài chōng)*. Treatment was performed twice, two days apart, during the first week of treatment.

Technique (first two visits)

A 1-inch needle was used with a shallow insertion at ST-7. A 1.5-inch needle was used to thread GB-5 to GB-6. After initial insertion at GB-5, the needle was moved very slowly through the skin toward GB-6, with minimal twirling, until the patient described a radiating sensation. A 1.5-inch needle was used at the *a-shì* point below ST-36. One-inch needles were used at LI-4 and LR-3.

Results (first two visits)

After the first treatment, the patient reported an immediate reduction in the frequency and intensity of facial spasms. Although the twitches did not disappear, he was able to have conversations in the early part of the day without any noticeable onset. However, by the end of the day, the spasms had returned around the eye, and later in the evening the area around the mouth had spasms when the patient washed his face. There was little added improvement after the second treatment.

Analysis (first two visits)

The initial treatment approach was one that might be used in relatively acute (first six months) cases of Bell's palsy, when it involves stasis in the *yáng míng* and *shào yáng* channels. The selection of local points involves careful palpation of nodules in the areas around and just outside of the affected area. In particular, ST-7 is known as a point where face qi accumulates and should be carefully palpated in any condition involving the face. GB-5 and GB-6 are meeting points for the *shào yáng* and *yáng míng* channels, and are thus particularly indicated in this case. Because of initial indications that these two channels were affected, the area was palpated very carefully to determine a precise location for the 1.5-inch through-and-through needle.

The area one to two inches below ST-36 is often reactive in Bell's palsy cases affecting the *yáng míng* channel. The point should be palpated carefully for tightness and tenderness to determine exact point location.

The use of LI-4 and LR-3 (the 'four gates') in this case represents a classic application of the theory of channel confusion (經絡紊亂 *jīng luò wěn luàn*), discussed further in Chapter 20 of this text. The theory was developed in response to a problem often encountered in China involving patients who have had long, unsuccessful courses of treatment with acupuncture. These types of patients are likened to musical instruments that have been consistently misplayed. Their "strings are out of tune." For such patients, the repeated, unsuccessful acupuncture treatments have reduced their entire channel system to a kind of jumble of mixed messages. Even if a careful, proper diagnosis is made, these patients will still often fail to respond to treatment. Their channels are 'confused' or in disorder. This is a type of presentation that often responds to treatment with the four-gate point pair. This treatment may be likened to a resetting of the channel system before other treatments can go forward.

While the use of the four-gate point pair is often helpful for reestablishing normal channel responsiveness, there is still the important issue of clear and effective diagnosis. The results of the first two treatments with this patient seemed to indicate that the diagnosis left something to be desired. Therefore, upon presentation for the third treatment (one week after the initial visit), the diagnosis was reevaluated. Importantly, channel palpation was performed again and focused on comparing the conditions of the three yang channels relative to one another in an effort to definitively ascertain which of the channels was most affected. However, after careful palpation, it seemed that the *yáng míng* and *shào yáng* channels were equally affected.

This is a very difficult concept to convey and involves some degree of intuition drawn from years of experience. As a general rule, diagnosis should ascertain which of the channels is primarily affected before even considering channels or points for treatment. (This is discussed in later chapters.) There are cases, however, where identifying this channel is impossible because the condition truly does involve multiple channels at once. In such cases, one might still choose a single channel for treatment in an effort to untie the knot. This would involve frequent reevaluations of the diagnosis as symptom patterns change over time, an approach commonly used for complex conditions. On the other hand, there are cases where multiple channels are affected simply because the root lies in a problem with integration among the channels. This falls into the category of 'unusual disease' (奇病 *qí bìng*) and requires treatment with the extraordinary vessels. However, before pursuing this idea further, we should consider the final series of treatments with this patient.

New diagnosis   Lack of integration among the channel sinews of the yang channels: dysfunction of *yáng qiāo* and *yīn qiāo*.

The involvement of the extraordinary vessels is likely due to the fact that the condition is relatively chronic. Also, because of the long course of unsuccessful treatments with other acupuncturists, the condition no longer simply involves the regular channels. Rather, the disease has entered the areas 'outside the twelve channels'. In this case, the inter-communication among yang muscle groups of the face is compromised. As the *yīn-yáng qiāo* are associated with the coordination of muscle groups among multiple channels, this case falls within their scope.

Treatment (later treatments)

The initial treatment of ST-7, GB-5 and GB-6, ST-36/ST-37 *a-shì* point, and the 'four gates' was continued. In addition, the command points of the *yīn-yáng qiāo*, BL-62 *(shēn mài)* and KI-6 *(zhào hǎi)*, and the command point of the *yáng wéi*, TB-5 *(wài guān)*, were added. BL-62 was needled on the side opposite the paralysis, while KI-6 and TB-5 were needled on the same side.

Technique (later treatments)

The same techniques described above were used at the points carried over from the initial diagnosis. A very strong draining technique of quick insertion followed by slow withdrawal of the needle was used at BL-62.

Gentler draining with a similar technique was used at TB-5, while KI-6 was treated with a tonifying technique involving very slow, gradual twirling and a firm grasp, until radiation was felt down the kidney channel on the foot.

Results (later treatments)

The patient returned two days later for the fourth visit and reported very dramatic change in his condition. For the entire day of the treatment and most of the following day, the twitching and spasms were completely abated. He was able to go through the day having conversations and eating without onset. However, at the end of the second day, the spasms around the eye returned while he was washing his face with warm water. He also reported feeling a sense of warmth and some swelling on the left side of his face following the previous treatment, which seemed to have abated by the time of his visit.

The patient came for four more treatments over the next two weeks during which time he went an entire week without symptoms. Because of a need to return home, treatment was discontinued after a total of three weeks, but the patient promised to phone follow-up reports. Three months later, the patient reported that the symptoms of twitching and pain had not returned and that only slight paralysis remained on the left cheek.

Herbal Treatment

Before he returned home, the following modification of Frigid Extremities Powder *(sì nì sǎn)* was prescribed:

Bupleuri Radix *(chái hú)*—6g

Paeoniae Radix alba *(bái sháo)*—11g

Aurantii Fructus immaturus *(zhǐ shí)*—10g

Glycyrrhizae Radix preparata *(zhì gān cǎo)*—10g

Bombyx batryticatus *(bái jiāng cán)*—6g

Cicadae Periostracum *(chán tuì)*—6g

Untreated Magnetitum *(shēng cí shí)*—20g

Fossilia Ossis Mastodi *(lóng gǔ)*—20g

Hordei Fructus germinatus *(mài yá)*—10g

Dry-fried Ziziphi spinosae Semen *(chǎo suān zǎo rén)*—10g

Analysis Ultimately, the success of this case, like any other, depends on precise diagnosis. Precision requires a careful application of the diagnostic tools that Chinese medicine provides, not just the theoretical tools, but also the tools of observation. As the textbooks emphasize, 'observation' in Chinese medicine involves not just the eyes, but also the hands. While it is obviously important to look at the patient's symptoms to determine which channels are affected, it is also very important to palpate the channels in order to ascertain the nature of the change. In this case, the original diagnosis was accumulation of phlegm-heat in the *yáng míng* and *shào yáng*, and the treatment principle arose from this hypothesis. However, because the results were unsatisfactory, the diagnosis was completely reevaluated.

Initially, the goal of reevaluation was to distinguish whether it was mainly a *yáng míng* or a *shào yáng* channel case. If one or the other channel was primarily affected, then the more precise diagnosis might lead to more focused treatment and better results. In other words, the initial goal was to fine-tune the original diagnosis so as to narrow down the number of channels to be treated.

However, after palpating the channels both locally on the head and distally, it seemed that both channels were equally involved. After considering the length of time that the condition had been evolving, it seemed likely that the small spaces 'between the channels' had been affected. A chronic and repeatedly mistreated condition was now affecting the coordination between muscle groups in multiple channel sinews. The next step was to add treatment of the extraordinary vessels.

Although the success of this case was largely due to the inclusion of extraordinary vessel treatment, this may not always be the case. In fact, a problem that often arises involves over-application of the eight extraordinary vessels in the clinic. Many practitioners, unable (or unwilling) to make a precise channel or eight-parameter diagnosis, turn instead to the eight extraordinary vessels as a kind of panacea. While this may be helpful for some conditions, in others it may prove ineffective or possibly even detrimental if channel exhaustion is the result.

In short, if the condition primarily involves the regular channels, treatment should begin with the regular channels. If the extraordinary vessels are used in cases better treated with regular channels, then the effects will likely be too diffuse. One is using the wrong tool for the job. While the extraordinary vessels have the ability to facilitate communication and interaction among regular channels, they have a less direct effect on movement within the regular channels.

In addition, although the diagnosis involved the *yáng qiāo* and *yīn qiāo*, the *yáng wéi* command point (TB-5) was also added in the second treatment phase. This point is appropriate both as a facilitator of yang circulation among multiple channels and as the collateral point on one of the affected channels. Remember that the collateral points are appropriate for improving microcirculation, as the 'collaterals' may be likened to the small, branching, capillary-like vessels. One should think back, for example, to the use of HT-5 in cases involving problems with microcirculation in the brain.

Finally, before the patient returned to his home province, he was prescribed a modification of Frigid Extremities Powder *(sì nì sǎn)*. Frigid Extremities Powder is classically indicated for conditions of yang reversal (陽 厥 *yáng jué)*, where the yang qi is trapped inside, leading to heat. This formula acts to move the *shào yáng* pivot so as to release heat from the deeper levels. Bupleuri Radix *(chái hú)* in particular has a strong moving effect on *shào yáng*, while Aurantii Fructus immaturus *(zhǐ shí)* and Glycyrrhizae Radix preparata *(zhì gān cǎo)* enliven the *yáng míng* and *tài yīn* levels below. The blood-nourishing action of Paeoniae Radix alba *(bái sháo)* roots the formula via internal-external organ pairings *(shào yáng-jué yīn)*.

Bombyx batryticatus *(bái jiāng cán)* and Cicadae Periostracum *(chán tuì)* were used here for their ability to reduce spasms, while Untreated Magnetitum *(shēng cí shí)* and Fossilia Ossis Mastodi *(lóng gǔ)* were used to anchor the liver yang—a cause of the patient's chronic hypertension. Finally, Dry-Fried Ziziphi spinosae Semen *(chǎo suān zǎo rén)* and Hordei Fructus germinatus *(mài yá)* have a calming action, and were prescribed because of an observed tendency in the patient to excitability.

■ Narrative

THE EIGHT EXTRAORDINARY VESSELS IN A CASE OF PARALYSIS

The city of Beijing is surrounded by a series of concentric highways encroaching outward into former farmland like ripples from the splash of a huge stone. The splash in the center of these six-lane loops is the Forbidden City, an exposition in architecture of the classical concept of imperial order. The former throne of the Qing dynasty still sits in the center of the Forbidden City facing southward, the direction formerly reserved for the emperor at official proceedings. In the centuries before the revolution of 1911, the emperor sat surrounded by 9,000 rooms covering 183 acres in this walled city that served as both the literal and figurative center of the Middle Kingdom. Today, the imperial palace is still surrounded by both a 30-foot-high wall and a moat that is 170 feet wide. For the modern city of Beijing, the wall of this ancient palace is the first ring in the series of ringed high-ways.

Formerly, the second ring was the city wall of Beijing, a massive brick structure wide enough at the top for the passage of two horse-drawn carts. After the founding of the Peoples Republic in 1949, the top of the city wall became a two-lane road that carried the city's growing number of automobiles along its 22-kilometer path. By the mid 1950s, the city wall was considered to be a hindrance to traffic through the city center and government planners began to call for its removal. The residents of old Beijing were loath to tear down a structure that had not only protected the city for millennia, but also provided a dramatic entrance and backdrop for their daily lives. Nevertheless, Chairman Mao prevailed and the first bricks were removed from the wall in 1955. The first of the concentric highways, now known as Second Ring Road, was then built on the foundations of the ancient wall. As this is being written, workers in Beijing are completing construction of the Sixth Ring Road, a huge, 200-kilometer ribbon that envelops the city some 40 kilometers out from the ancient imperial throne.

On a sunny winter day, Dr. Wang and I were traveling around the raised six-lane Second Ring Road in his small white car. The slow, precise movements that characterize Dr. Wang in the clinic are mirrored in his careful negotiation of modern highway traffic. Cars whizzed by our windows as he described the huge city gates that once stood in space now spanned by cement bridges bustling with traffic. Each exit off the modern highway bears the name of a city gate dismantled fifty years ago. The names are now in stark contrast to the type of activity that greets the exiting driver. For example, as one takes the Exit of Balanced Peace, a contemporary six-story edifice heaves into view offering 20,000 square feet of restaurant featuring "the most famous Beijing duck in the world." The Gate of Abundant Success does seem to live up to its name, however, as two giant department stores can be found resting upon its ashes. Drivers getting off the highway at an exit named for a Tibetan temple gate now see high-rise condominiums boasting of "temple views." As he drove, Dr. Wang described his memories of those gates and how each gate was reserved for a particular kind of activity...

DR. WANG: "I remember when I was a child, the Yang Facing Gate on the east side of the city was where goods flowed in from farms and the harbors of Tianjin. The north-facing Gate of Virtuous Victory was where troops in the old dynasties would enter the city after successful campaigns. In the south part of the city, there was the Front Gate where families of businessmen kept their trading companies. It is near that gate where you can still find the Tongren Tang (同仁堂 *tóng rén táng*) herb company, in the same location where it's been for hundreds of years. There was quite a bit of unrest here in Beijing when they took down that old wall. I was studying at the Chinese Medicine University at the time and remember that some of the old professors at Beijing University wrote letters to the Communist Party leadership asking that the wall be preserved. It didn't do any good. In the years that followed, there were huge crews of workmen who came to Beijing to help build a modern urban infrastructure. Some of those workmen became my earliest patients.

I remember in particular a young patient who came for treatment in the early 1960s. He was a young man, in his late 30s, and he was quite tall. I remember the strange image of his arrival: this huge guy carried on the back of a much smaller man. He was completely paralyzed from the waist down and had been for a number of weeks. Most interestingly, he hadn't suffered any injury or fall, but had been paralyzed by an emotional shock. As I questioned the patient, a story began to unfold that ultimately led to a greater understanding of the concepts we were discussing earlier regarding the extraordinary vessels.

This patient had experienced a similar episode of paralysis twenty years before (during the 1940s). At that time, he had been working in the northeastern province of Heilongjiang as a factory manager. His factory made uniforms and blankets for the army. You might remember that, during this time, there was a war going on in China. Consequently, the factory he managed came under a great deal of pressure from the central government to produce high volumes of material for the war effort. At one point, the man had just overseen the production of a large shipment of uniforms and blankets that were set to go out to troops fighting the Japanese. However, just days before the shipment was scheduled to be forwarded by train to the front lines, a sudden fire at the factory warehouse destroyed the entire shipment.

As the army at the time was also experiencing a great deal of internal division due to infighting between Communist and Nationalist factions within the government [the People's Republic of China at that point had yet to be formally established], the man was suspected of arson. He was brought in by the military police and held in a military prison. Already under a great deal of pressure, he experienced an emotional crisis that led to a sudden paralysis of his legs. Not long afterwards, the military police determined that enemy agents had sabotaged the warehouse and the man was cleared of all wrongdoing. Unfortunately, despite the fact that his name was cleared and no charges were brought, the man continued to have no movement in his legs. Over the period of a year, he was slowly able to regain movement. Although he eventually returned to normal, the process was very slow and caused him a great deal of suffering. He did eventually return to his duties at the military factory.

Following the war and the establishment of the Peoples Republic, the man was assigned duties in the civil engineering corps for the city of Beijing. During the 1950s, the entire city underwent dramatic changes as the new government strove to modernize the capital. For example, five city blocks in front of the imperial palace were cleared of homes, alleys, and classical architecture in the process of building Tiananmen Square. It was at this time that the city wall was razed and the highway we're driving upon was built.

Being a proven leader from the war effort, the man found himself in the middle of this construction and once again in charge of a government work group. This time, he led a team of workers and engineers charged with building a part of the city's water system. A few years into this work, one of his crew members fell into a ditch and was covered in an avalanche of falling debris. The worker died immediately and the man was held responsible. Once again under the stress of official investigation, his lower limb paralysis returned. As before, there was no specific physical injury, but a paralysis caused by severe emotional strain.

It was at this point that the patient was brought to me on the back of one of his subordinates. He was unable to walk and quite distressed about his condition. He recounted to me the story of his earlier paralysis during the war and expressed fear that it might again take him over a year to recover. Looking at the patient, I began to think of the extraordinary vessels. At that point in my career, I had not developed my understanding and application of the vessels to the point I recently described to you. Instead, I thought more simply about the name of the *yáng qiāo* (yang 'walker') vessel and the name of the *yáng wéi* (yang 'linking') and went from there. His treatment was actually quite simple and basically involved just TB-5 *(wài guān)* and BL-62 *(shēn mài)*, bilaterally. By his third or fourth visit, the man was able to move about slowly and recovered from his paralysis quite quickly.

If I saw this patient today, I might modify the treatment a bit, however. I would still use the extraordinary vessels, but might prefer the *dū* and *yáng qiāo* vessels. A point prescription that comes to mind is GV-21 *(qián dǐng)* with BL-62. The *du* vessel can be used to stimulate yang movement in the whole body, while the *yáng qiāo* integrates muscle movement in multiple channels. In any case, sudden, unusual conditions like this one which are difficult to understand in the context of normal channel or eight-principle diagnosis often fall into the category of extraordinary vessel disorder. The key for me is to remember the idea of integration.

Think about this patient a bit. If he came to me with a similar condition that was instead more chronic and less acute, I might be tempted once again to consider the *yáng wéi* vessel and might still use TB-5. This is because I think of the *wéi* vessels as helping to maintain the distribution of nourishment. Circulation of nourishment is often compromised in chronic cases. Therefore, a patient like this, if he hadn't moved his legs for months and months, would obviously also have a lack of yang nourishment and thus the *yáng wéi* might be appropriate for treatment.

On the other hand, the strong stimulation of yang provided by the *dū* vessel is more appropriate for this patient since his condition is relatively acute. In an acute case, nourishment is less needed than a strong burst of yang to reestablish circulation. Now, as I've said before, the *yáng qiāo* vessel is a vessel of integration for muscle movement and would be appropriate for this patient whether or not his condition was acute. An inability to move the legs at all, in cases without severe spinal damage, very often calls for treatment with the *yáng qiāo*. Multiple meridian muscle groups aren't working together—this is a *qiāo* vessel condition."

By now, the little car had long left the Second Ring Highway and we found ourselves moving through traffic toward lunch. As lunch conversation usually tended to stray away from Chinese medicine, our discussion meandered from the extraordinary vessels. That day, lunch involved a huge plate of sheep stomachs at a restaurant run by Dr. Wang's nephew. The nephew had married a woman from China's Muslim minority and had thus converted from pork to mutton. Because he had just opened the new restaurant, we arrived to show our support and ate multiple plates of his stomach delicacy while dipping cucumbers in bowls of fennel-spiced peppers. Although the meal was delicious at the time, it would be months before I could "stomach" stomach again.

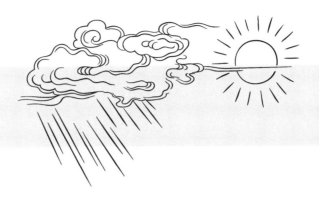

The Terrain So Far

AFTER WORKING TOGETHER in the clinic for a year, conversations with Dr. Wang began to range more freely over subjects that did not always include the theories of Chinese medicine. More often than in the first months of our time together, Dr. Wang would describe important events in his life and his perspective on the dramatic changes that had taken place in China during his lifetime. Most of us who study Chinese medicine outside of China are little aware of how vastly different the lives of those 'modern masters' so diligently translated and discussed in schools around the world are from our own. While he was often at pains to stress to me (and therefore to readers of this text) that the lives of those who wrote the medical classics were vastly different than our own, he was understandably less aware of how different his life had been from mine.

One of the most difficult things about writing this text has been the task of finding ways to convey this fact without veering so far off the subject at hand that the nature of the work becomes more of a biography than a treatise on one person's perspective on medical theory. In fact, at some point one might be tempted to ask me, the translator, what purpose beyond a welcome break from the dense theoretical jungle do these digressions serve. In the introduction, a case was made for trying to put the teachings in context. By placing the reader more closely to the elbow of the doctor in the clinic, the information presumably becomes more interesting, while certain points made can be more clearly illustrated by real life examples. That is the first level.

Another level that should be growing more apparent to the reader is the absolute importance of dialogue to the transmission of a traditional medical system like Chinese medicine. This was also mentioned briefly in the introduction. I myself was only vaguely aware of the historical role of the didactic process when I first began my apprenticeship with Dr. Wang. Of course I was aware that the *Inner Classic*, the earliest book on the subject, was in the form of a dialogue between an emperor and his court physician, but I had failed to note the significance of the choice of literary device. By presenting the information as a conversation, the original compilers of the *Inner Classic* attempted to put in writing what had previously been an oral tradition. In the twenty centuries that have passed since the Han dynasty, the literary wing of Chinese medicine has been forced to struggle with this dilemma. How can one effectively write about a medical system which has at its core a diagnostic approach that is fundamentally subjective? How can one write down what one 'senses,' or describe intuitive leaps based on decades of clinical experience? The *Inner Classic* attempts to bridge part of this gap through the literary device of dialogue. By providing a didactic atmosphere, at least some of the feel of the traditional learning process might be preserved. The same approach was of course utilized a few centuries later in the *Classic of Difficulties* where the dialogue form serves as a template for discussing 'difficult questions' left unanswered by the *Inner Classic*.

A dialogue serves to emphasize the importance of asking the right questions. One might imagine the Yellow Emperor in the *Inner Classic*, the archetype of the diligent student, composing questions that now seem like they were handed down on stone tablets.[1] In many of the questions, the Yellow Emperor takes care to first describe some concept that had been previously discussed. The student-reader of the *Inner Classic* is an eavesdropper in this process. When one reads the questions posed, one immediately notes that they are not the queries of a beginner. Innumerable dialogues begin as if they had already been going on for years. Although some chapters of the text do seem to follow a logical development from question to question, there is often an intuitive leap by the Yellow Emperor before the next question is even asked. Because of the heterogeneous nature of the text, other chapters might take a different approach to a similar subject or even contradict altogether something said elsewhere. There is an inherent acceptance of multiple systems of thought in the *Inner Classic* that in fact continues in Chinese medicine even in the present day.

The process of learning represented by the classical texts is therefore much less linear than that of modern education—it is full of these jumps from idea to idea that is more characteristic of an oral, apprentice-style of teaching. The intuitive leap and the many days, weeks, or years that sometimes transpire before these leaps are made is precisely the most difficult thing to convey in a text such as this. What must appear as a logical, gradual development of ideas in neatly organized chapters was actually conveyed in a radically different way. The process of learning and collecting the information provided in these pages was more like that of painting a picture than taking a course in biology or chemistry. Ideas outlined in fairly typical lecture form in the early months of my work with Dr. Wang would be revisited over and over again during the hundreds of hours in the clinic, eating lunch, driving to my bus stop, or walking down the street. While the early lectures were like the initial brush strokes that a painter might make on a fresh canvas, the months that followed were full of careful detail work. As the years pass and my relationship with Dr. Wang continues to grow, this process continues.

Also reminiscent of working with a visual art was the tendency of Dr. Wang to focus on a subject for a period of time, explaining details and pointing out clinical parallels, before rather suddenly shifting the focus of our discussions to another, equally important, aspect of Chinese medicine. At first this approach was disorienting, especially during the difficult process of trying to categorize and digest all of the information that was discussed. Over time, I became used to the shifts, for example, from the qi transformation of *tài yīn* one week to considerations of what the *Classic of Difficulties* means by the term 'vessel' (脉 *mài*) the next. This is of course the nature of any type of clinical training, but is nevertheless of particular importance in traditional medical systems like Chinese medicine with a strong oral tradition. If the student doesn't ask relevant questions, the teacher often does not provide answers. In order to come up with good questions, sometimes the only method is to wait, watch, and think. In any case, the following section of the book draws more from time spent watching in the clinic than from listening to lectures.

Before turning to the landscape of the next few chapters, it is helpful first to look back at terrain already covered. Initial chapters introduced basic concepts that help define the branch of classical Chinese science termed 'Chinese medicine' and the field of channel theory in particular. In the first chapter, the foundations of Chinese medicine—the three pillars of yin-yang / five-phase theory, organ theory, and channel theory—were described. In Chapter 2, the roots of channel theory were explored and the concepts of the 'six qi' and the 'six channels' were developed. Later in Chapter 2, a short explanation of the interrelationship of the six channels and their tendencies to open, pivot, or close was described. Chapter 3 introduced the concept of channel palpation, a subject that will be broadened considerably in upcoming chapters. Chapters 4 through 11 then undertook the journey through the fairly dense terrain of physiology. In this case, remember that 'physiology' is defined as an understanding of how organ theory and channel theory interrelate to describe a web of metabolic systems.

In this physiological journey, each of the six channels and the functions of the two organs within each channel were considered in turn. Some channels were covered easily without the encumbrance of too many ideas not seen elsewhere, while others involved a complete reevaluation of fundamental concepts. For example, in the last chapter, the physiological role of the extraordinary vessels was addressed and considered in light of more modern concepts regarding interstitial fluids. In all cases, questions were asked and hopefully some satisfactory answers (or starting points) were provided. In short, an entire physiological system has been described which attempts to stay within the bounds of classical theory while offering new ways of understanding ancient ideas.

The ground ahead is new. Many of the ideas in the next six chapters of this book will be familiar, but their application is relatively unique. All of us who have completed programs in Chinese medicine are familiar with the importance of physical contact to the process of diagnosis. Some may have studied with practitioners who have refined their skills at differentiating temperature (or other) changes along the surface of the body, while others may have known mentors, in the Japanese tradition, who place a great deal of emphasis on careful discernment of changes felt on the abdomen. There are also *qì gōng* traditions in which the practitioner attempts to directly ascertain changes in the patient's qi, and, of course, there is the skill of pulse diagnosis. Historically, all of these diagnostic approaches have been shown to improve results. Difficulties have sometimes arisen, however, regarding clear, teachable ways of transmitting these skills without the benefit of extensive one-on-one interface with experienced practitioners. The following chapters will attempt to surmount that difficulty by providing a clear, logical discussion of a very useful diagnostic method.

However, while the skills described in the next section of this text are immediately useful, the depth of insight gained by the reader will vary depending on how well one understands the concepts outlined in the first part of the text. While it is relatively straightforward to understand, for example, that tenderness along the liver channel may indicate a lack of proper coursing by the liver organ, only careful consideration of classical physiology can lead to the most effective clinical treatment approaches. As experienced practitioners have already found from their own patients, one cannot guarantee results in every case by simply treating the channel that is most tender. There is a logical process that one can use, however, and that process involves a sophisticated integration of channel theory, as outlined here, with more commonly discussed organ diagnostic models. This will be the terrain of the following pages.

To that end, the next nine chapters will directly address use of channel theory in the clinic. At this point, it is assumed that the broad outline of classical physiology described in earlier sections of the text is reasonably clear. Complete clarity will grow with time. In order for time to teach its lessons, books must eventually be closed and real patients must be addressed. Consequently, multiple steps in the process of patient treatment will comprise the general framework of upcoming chapters. Before describing these steps, the reader should reconsider a basic point made much earlier in the text in Chapter 3. There, it was asked why one would want to learn about channel palpation as a diagnostic tool in the first place. To answer that question, the traditional approach of exploring what the classics have to say on the subject was followed by some general observations gleaned from modern application of those ancient ideas. The next section of the book will continue to develop those themes. The nine chapters that follow will address these subjects:

CHAPTER 12: **Physiology Under the Fingertips**
How does one actually go about checking the channels?

CHAPTER 13: **Specific Channel Changes**
What are some common changes that one might expect to find along specific channels?

CHAPTER 14: **Selecting Channels for Treatment**
How does one develop treatment strategies based on the information gleaned through channel palpation? What does one do when there are a variety of palpated changes and some confusion as to diagnosis?

CHAPTER 15: **What is an Acupuncture Point?**
Now that a channel has been chosen for treatment, what are some fundamental classical concepts that underlie the concept of acupuncture points?

CHAPTER 16: **The Five Transport Points**
How might the concept that channel qi grows from the fingers to the trunk influence point selection?

CHAPTER 17: **The Source, Cleft, and Collateral Points**
What is the unique role of source qi in acupuncture treatment? How can other traditional point categories help one further understand the nature of individual points?

Thus one can see that the chapters to come will be both interesting and
directly relevant to the clinic. For those who have access to patients, it is
important to begin immediately applying these ideas. Begin by simply palpating the course of the twelve channels in every patient, as described in the
next chapter. Over time, patterns will begin to emerge and much of what is
written in the pages that follow will take on a new life in the mind of the
reader.

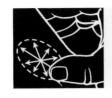

CHAPTER 12

Physiology Under the Fingertips

T HIS CHAPTER WILL introduce the specific palpation techniques used for channel diagnosis. Before considering diagnostic technique, a few concepts should be introduced regarding how the channels are understood in the modern clinic.

The Channels and Disease

From a functional perspective, there are three basic principles regarding the channel system in the presence of disease.

1. The channel system reflects the presence of disease.

If disease is present in the body, there will be changes in the channels. The precise nature of these changes has been a topic of much discussion over the millennia and will be a major focus for us as well in the pages that follow. At this point, it should simply be said that a trained practitioner can objectively discern these changes.

2. The channel system is an important part of the body's defenses.

This is a statement about the role of the channel system in protecting the body from disease. As explained in earlier chapters, the channel system has its own unique role in normal physiology. Part of that role includes a responsibility for providing defense against exterior invasion. The first chapters of this book explained how each of the six channels is associated with one of the 'six qi' of the external environment, which means that it responds to a specific aspect of the external environment. When a person is exposed to cold, for example, it is the *tài yáng* channel that responds as the first level of defense. More specifically, this is not to say that the *pathway* of the *tài yáng* channel is responding to cold, but that the entire physiology of *tài yáng* (including the bladder and small intestine organ functions) resonates and responds when cold is present. One is usually unaware of this process, but palpable changes along the course of the channels can sometimes be ascertained before other signs and symptoms appear.

3. Stimulation of points on the channels can facilitate normal physiology.

If the channels and collaterals are unable to properly carry out their normal physiological functions, the stimulation of appropriately determined points can have predictable effects on the flow within those channels. This is the fundamental principle underlying all acupuncture theory and has been the subject of countless scrolls and books over the past two millennia. The debate lies in the question of *which* channels and points should be stimulated for a particular symptom-pattern in a particular patient. This subject will be addressed in Chapter 14.

The Channels in the Clinic

Now we begin the process of categorizing changes in the channels. First, let's consider the ways that the channel system responds to disease.

In general, palpable changes in the channels may not always directly coincide with the presenting symptom pattern. In this respect, it is not unlike other modern diagnostic techniques. For example, a patient may have headaches and dizziness as the chief complaint, and examination may reveal high blood pressure. Although the high blood pressure may be directly linked to the headaches, they don't always occur at the same time. There may be headaches and dizziness and relatively normal blood pressure at one moment, and then high blood pressure and no symptoms at another. This fact alone does not mean that the headaches are unrelated to the high blood pressure. Similarly, even though channel changes do not always occur at the same time as symptom patterns, they may still be related.

With that in mind, there are four basic patterns used to describe the most common ways that channel change and disease symptoms correlate:

1. Channel changes may occur at the same time as symptoms.

This is a situation where an increase in the intensity of patient symptoms coincides with the development of palpable change along the course of the channel (or channels). This is the most common pattern in the clinic and provides very useful information for the practitioner. Roughly 70 percent of cases are of this type. For example, a patient may present with the pattern of cough and asthma with fatigue, expectoration of clear phlegm, and signs that include a pale face and dry skin. For this type of patient, there may be small, relatively shallow nodules along the lung channel and a corresponding sense of softness and weakness along the kidney channel. The diagnosis might then be a type of *tài yīn / shào yīn* pattern (lung-kidney qi deficiency) and points would be chosen based on this channel diagnosis (Fig. 12.1). (A detailed process for selecting points is described in Chapter 14.)

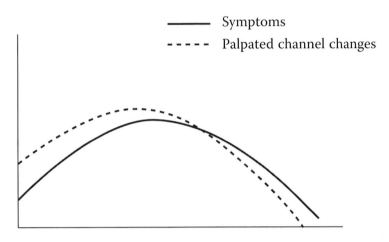

Fig. 12.1
Channel changes occur in a similar time-line with symptom presentation. This is the most common occurrence.

2. Symptoms may precede channel changes.

This is a case where the patient will have signs and symptoms of disease, but no immediately palpable changes along the course of any channel. Usually, changes along the channels will eventually occur, but it may be days or even weeks before the practitioner can find them.

This type of pattern is seen most often in older, weaker, or more deficient patients. A similar situation is that of a patient who has fairly severe symptoms but relatively little channel change. There may be changes in these patients that correspond to current symptoms, but the changes will seem very slight. The channel system is weak in these patients and it is therefore often difficult to get adequate qi sensation (radiation) when needling. These patients also tend to respond more slowly to acupuncture because of their general debility (Fig. 12.2).

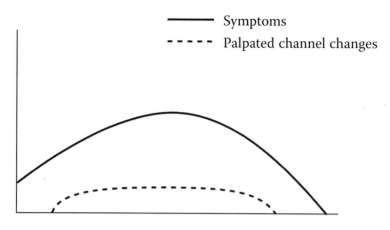

Fig. 12.2
Appearance of symptoms significantly precedes or is much greater than palpable channel changes. Often found in older and/or weaker patients.

3. Channel changes can precede clinical symptoms.

Here there are changes along the course of a particular channel that do not seem to correspond to any current symptom pattern. Yet days or weeks after the channel changes have appeared, a constellation of related signs and symptoms will arise.

This pattern is rarely seen in the clinic, probably because most patients have little reason to see a doctor in the absence of symptoms. Nevertheless, careful channel palpation can sometimes yield this predictive result. These are usually patients who are either generally quite healthy or who have a tendency to allergies or other autoimmune conditions. Because of the healthy (or hypersensitive) state of their immunity, the channels themselves show noticeable change during what might be analogous to the latency period of their condition. The narrative at the end of this chapter provides an interesting example of this pattern (Fig. 12.3).

4. Channel changes may not coincide with clinical symptoms at all.

In this case there are both symptoms and significant changes along the channels, but they don't seem to match. Another example would be a person with a chronic disease who shows no significant palpable changes along their channels. In both cases, there are irregular channel changes (or a lack of change) that provide no real clues for a diagnosis relating to the organs.

These are often patients with unusual diseases, and are relatively rare. Nevertheless, such patients are generally thought to be suffering from 'chan-

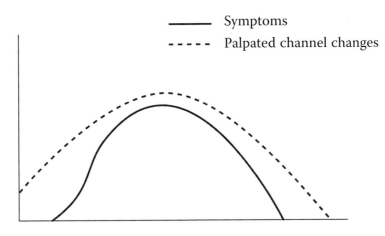

Symptoms

Palpated channel changes

Fig. 12.3

Channel changes may precede onset of symptoms in very healthy patients or those who are hypersensitive.

nel exhaustion' (經絡疲勞 *jīng luò pí láo*) or 'channel confusion' (經絡紊亂 *jīng luò wěn luàn*). A patient with channel exhaustion is deficient and has often had many rounds of unsuccessful treatment with other practitioners (either Western or Chinese medicine). Their channel system has consequently suffered from repeated stimulation that has not led to a healing response. A patient suffering from channel confusion, on the other hand, is not necessarily deficient, but also has a channel system that is not functioning properly due to excessive and unsuccessful treatment. Usually, however, patients with confusion in their channel system eventually suffer from deficiency. In both cases, treatment must focus first on reestablishing regular movement in the channel system as a whole before specific treatment can begin. A common regulating treatment in such cases is the point pair LI-4 *(hé gǔ)* and LR-3 *(tài chōng)* (Fig. 12.4; see also Chapter 20).

Diagnosing via the Channels

Having described the basic tendencies of the channels in the presence of disease, the practitioner is now ready to begin the process of developing skills to observe those tendencies.

When palpating the human body, the practitioner is faced with the question of whether what they feel is normal or abnormal. Patients are in fact variable and a wide variety of things will be discerned when one palpates the channels. Moreover, there are types of nodules and fatty deposits that are unrelated to pathology. Over time, however, common patterns of ir-

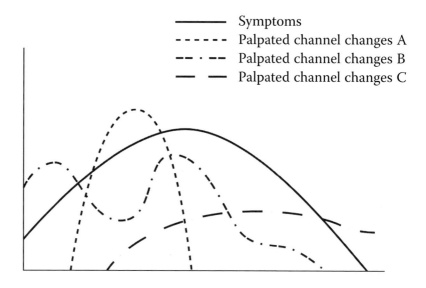

Symptoms
Palpated channel changes A
Palpated channel changes B
Palpated channel changes C

Fig. 12.4
In complex conditions, palpated channel changes may not match or may
contradict the suspected symptom pattern based on other diagnostic input
(from interview, tongue, pulse etc.). In these cases, one must consider the
diagnosis from a variety of angles to determine the most likely scenario.

regularity will begin to emerge, and certain types of noticeable change will
correspond to suspected organ pathologies.

In order to distinguish between changes that are significant and those
that are not, a few criteria should be kept in mind. Changes should generally
meet at least two of the following three criteria in order to be considered
significant for purposes of channel diagnosis:

1. Changes should be in a clear line along specific channel pathways.

2. Changes should have some connection to disease symptoms.

In other words, they should come and go with the ebb and flow of other
symptoms. As noted above, the channel changes may not occur at exactly
the same time as other symptoms, and may appear before or after. For this
reason, careful records should be kept about what palpation reveals at each
patient visit.

3. Changes should be located bilaterally.

One side may, however, be significantly more affected than the other—
especially in those conditions which are situated more in the channels than
in the organs, such as pain.

[336]

Observed changes like lipomas, neuromas, moles, canker sores, pimples, tinea, and melanin irregularities (freckles) that do not meet the above criteria fall outside the scope of channel diagnosis. Changes of this type are better considered in the context of dermatology in Chinese medicine.

THE FIVE METHODS OF CHANNEL DIAGNOSIS

Now we will consider the types of changes that *are* considered relevant to channel diagnosis. It is important to note that there are actually five categories of classical channel diagnosis, of which channel palpation is but one:

- observation of channel pathways (審 *shěn*)
- pulse diagnosis (切 *qiē*)
- palpation of channel pathways (循 *xún*)
- pressing of points (按 *àn*)
- feeling the body surface (捫 *mén*).

The first four of these five methods were mentioned in our discussion of the *Inner Classic* in Chapter 3. In the modern clinic, all five methods are quite important. In this text, however, we will focus on the relatively underutilized technique of palpation of the channel pathways. Discussion of the first two methods can be found in Appendix 4. The other three methods are combined below in a general discussion of manual diagnostic techniques.

Palpation, pressing the points, and feeling the body surface

Although classical sources distinguish three separate techniques of palpating (循 *xún*), pressing (按 *àn*), and feeling (捫 *mén*), in actual practice they overlap. These techniques were first introduced in the *Inner Classic* and discussed further in the *Classic of Difficulties*. The famous Three Kingdoms period text, the *Systematic Classic* (甲乙經 *Jiǎ yǐ jīng*), compiled by Huang-Fu Mi between 215–282 A.D., refines the technique of palpating along the channels and discusses the relationship of channel changes to disease. In Chapter 12, Huang-Fu Mi asserts "where there is disrupted movement [in the channel], there is disease" (是動則病 *shì dòng zé bìng*).[1] From this one could go on to say that when the practitioner discerns disrupted movement or change in a particular channel, it is somehow involved in the disease at hand. (In Chapter 14 of our text, however, we will consider the idea that the channel with palpated changes may *not* actually be the best for treatment.)

The fact that palpable channel changes can be found is one reason why practitioners of Chinese medicine attach such importance to the simple process of taking one's hands and placing them on the patient to understand the condition of the body. This seemingly obvious prerequisite to a clear understanding of a patient's illness is sadly absent from many modern clinics. One often hears about how little physical contact modern physicians have with their patients, but unfortunately, the same is true of modern practitioners of Chinese medicine. To know the condition of the patient's channels, one must begin by laying one's hands on the body.

Taken together, the three manual techniques describe a process of moving along the course of the twelve channels with one's hands.

Palpation Palpation is the process of running one's fingers along the course of the channels. Most often, this involves palpating the channel pathways below the elbows and knees, as discussed in Chapter 13 of the *Classic of Difficulties*. The practitioner should first grasp the patient's hand or foot with the right hand, and use the thumb of the left hand to palpate the lower aspect of the channels. Palpation should follow the course of each of the twelve regular channels from the hands and feet proximally toward the elbows and knees. As one's left hand moves up toward the elbows and knees, one's right hand grip might move to the wrists and ankles (see Fig. 12.1 and 12.5). Especially at first, the practitioner should palpate the channel three times, pressing a bit harder each time to feel for deeper and deeper changes. Some changes may be very clear at the surface but may not be palpable when pressing harder, and vice versa. The goal is to discern structural changes along the course of the channels, which includes not only changes in muscle tension but also nodules, bumpiness, or granularity. The types of changes that one might find are categorized below (Table 12.1).

Pressing Pressing involves the use of the thumb or fingertips to check for tenderness along certain areas of a channel or, more commonly, at particular points. When pressing an area, more severe pain may indicate an accumulation of pathogenic qi (邪氣生 *xié qì shēng),* while a weak and soft feeling (with or without tenderness) indicates that there is qi stagnation in the channel. Tenderness or pain is indicative of an excessive condition, often involving heat or fire. The more slippery-hard the sensation beneath the fingers, the more it tends toward phlegm. The technique of pressing on points is sometimes used to determine proper location as well: When searching an area for the precise location of an acupuncture point, it is often helpful to look for tenderness or pain.

However, it should be noted that a lack of tenderness at a point does not rule out that point for treatment. Especially in cases of deficiency, the fact that the area around a point is not tender should not disqualify it. Furthermore, there is a difference between normal tenderness (which many patients

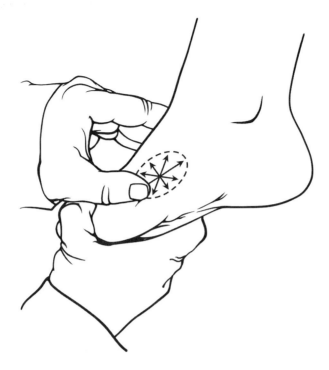

Fig. 12.5
The practitioner should grasp the fingers or toes with the right hand when palpating the most distal aspect of the channel so as to tighten the skin. This facilitates feeling small changes in this area. Later, as the left thumb goes up toward the elbows and knees, the right hand grip might shift to the wrists and ankles (see Fig. 12.9). The idea is to keep both hands in contact with the patient.

will report) and the type of tenderness associated with channel diagnosis. When the practitioner suspects that tenderness has diagnostic significance, it is important to compare the tenderness at that point with tenderness felt in an area nearby. If the change is diagnostically significant, there will be noticeably more tenderness at the point than there is nearby (Table 12.1).

Feeling In feeling, one is attempting to discern noticeable changes in temperature, moisture, and skin texture. Often, the process involves determining if certain areas of the body (as opposed to individual channels) feel different when compared with others. Consequently, the technique of feeling may not always involve channel diagnosis, but may simply be an aspect of diagnosis in general. For example, one may determine that the abdomen around CV-12 is significantly warmer than the area below the umbilicus. This may indicate heat in the *tài yīn* and/or *yáng míng* channels. Extreme warmth

Sensation When Pressing	Possible Diagnostic Significance
Weak and/or slippery-soft	Lack of qi movement in channel (cause may be excess or deficiency)
Slippery-hard sensation	The harder, more fixed the sensation, the more likely that phlegm is in channel and/or organ
Tenderness with pressure	Excess condition in channel and/or organ (often caused by heat)
More severe pain with pressure	Rising accumulation of pathogenic qi (may be heat or cold)

Table 12.1

Significance of common findings from pressing points and channels

in any area is generally a sign of excess. On the other hand, if whole regions of the body are dry, there may be generalized blood deficiency. While this type of feeling certainly aids in diagnosis, it may not help one to differentiate which of the channels are involved.

Specific channels can, however, be differentiated using this technique. For example, cold swelling or dry skin anywhere around the ankles often indicates *shào yīn* qi deficiency while an excessively warm neck reflects excess heat at the *tài yáng* level. In general, dryness in areas associated with particular channels can indicate a deficiency of yin or blood in the channel, which is failing to nourish the skin. The smaller and more specific the area of change (as to channel), the more helpful the changes will be for channel diagnosis (Table 12.2).

In general, to be significant, the changes felt along a particular channel should conform to at least two of the three criteria described above. An exception would be the case of a chronic one-sided condition where qi and blood on a particular limb have been compromised. For example, chronic neck or shoulder pain may lead to dryness further down the channel on the forearm or hand due to qi and blood stasis over a long period of time. In that case, it is unlikely that there would be a corresponding dryness on the opposite side. Also, in chronic cases such as this, multiple channels may readily become involved.

Feeling the channels reveals:	Which may indicate:
Different temperatures on abdomen	Condition of associated burner: sense of heat above umbilicus usually indicates spleen-stomach heat; cold below often indicates kidney deficiency
General dryness	Systemic blood deficiency: often spleen and liver
Local dryness	Blood and/or yin deficiency in channel(s) that pass through area; may be due to stasis in channel
Local temperature variations	Heat: heat, phlegm or fire in the channel(s) Cold: cold, blood stasis, or qi deficiency in channel(s)

Table 12.2

Significance of common findings from feeling points and channels

SPECIFIC TYPES OF CHANNEL CHANGES

In the following section, the term 'channel palpation' refers to all three of the techniques described above. Channel palpation means palpating, pressing, and feeling in turn. As the thumb moves along the course of the channel, one might stop to press or take note of how a particular area feels. As previously noted, channel palpation is usually done below the elbows and knees. In addition, the courses of the *rèn* and *dū* vessels, and the bladder channel, are also often palpated on the head, back, and abdomen. On the abdomen, the front alarm *(mù)* points might also be pressed to determine excess and deficiency. In terms of modern physiology, one might say that the majority of these palpable channel changes are occurring in the connective tissues of the body, just below the surface of the skin. The changes can be found in the various linings that surround all the structures of the body. This is where channel qi moves (Fig. 12.6).

In general, there are three basic types of information to keep in mind: depth, relative hardness, and the size of the changes found. With regard to depth, because these changes are thought to occur within the connective tissues, they are still fairly shallow in a relative sense. Nevertheless, the deepest changes may still require a bit of force to palpate. Hardness refers to the tone of the palpated change. A nodule might be said to be hard if it feels quite turgid, but it might still feel soft when compared to a bone spur, for example. The size of palpated changes varies quite broadly. Sometimes, a series of nodules might be large enough to feel with a fairly perfunctory

[341]

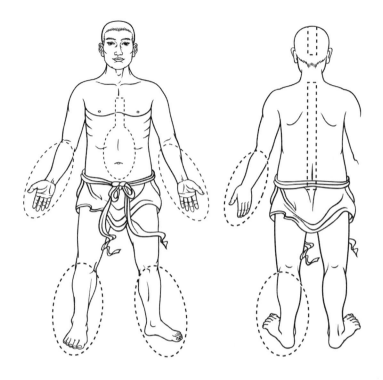

Fig. 12.6
When palpating the channels, the areas below the elbows and knees
are most important for finding diagnostically significant information.
The *rèn* and *dū* vessels, and the bladder channel, are also often palpated.

pass along the channel pathway. More often than not, however, significant
channel change is extremely small and is easily overlooked. For example,
cervical disorders involving *tài yáng* might correspond with an almost sand-
like sensation under the fingers between SI-4 *(wàn gǔ)* and SI-5 *(yáng gǔ).*

Described below are the three general categories of palpable change,
with a few sub-categories (Table 12.3).

Soft-weak areas

When palpating along the course of a channel, there is sometimes a
sense that the muscle or fascia have significantly diminished tone. Certain
channels, or even specific points, have a softness that can be felt when running the fingers along the body surface with mild pressure. This is a sign
of deficiency. In order to fully understand the nature of the deficiency, one
must obviously combine this information with that gleaned from other diagnostic techniques. However, careful channel palpation can help identify

Channel Changes	Likely Indication
Shallow hardness or tightness along channel	Cold, dampness, qi stasis
Deep hardness and/or nodules (can be further subdivided)	Heat, phlegm, blood stasis, chronic condition
Soft-weak areas	Qi or yang deficiency

Table 12.3

The three general categories of commonly-seen palpated changes

the primary organ affected in cases where a patient presents with what looks like generalized qi and/or yang deficiency, or deficiency that seems to involve multiple organs.

For example, one may see a patient with chronic colds, fatigue, a pale face, loose stools, a tendency to pain in the joints and low back, a weak and thin pulse, and a pale, puffy tongue. Organ diagnosis would first be performed through careful differentiation of symptom patterns. There is further clarity when you add the fact that there is softness and very small nodules along the spleen channel, while the lung and kidney channels feel relatively normal. In this case, treatment might proceed with a focus on spleen *tài yīn* (Fig. 12.7).

Generalized hardness and tightness

The second and third types of channel change are sometimes difficult to differentiate, especially for the novice practitioner.

Generalized hardness and tightness is usually felt at a more shallow depth along the course of the channel; it is also usually less hard and covers a broader area than the third type of hardness described below. In many cases, this is a generalized hypertonicity of the tissues along a relatively large portion of a particular channel. Changes that fall into this category are often seen in cold, damp, and/or relatively acute conditions. In such cases, although the channels are affected and movement is compromised, pathogenic qi has yet to lead to a more serious stagnation of blood or accumulation of phlegm.

Slightly hard nodules with borders that are not clearly defined are also included in this category. This type of nodule may even be slightly soft and feel less deep than the nodules discussed below. Often these types of nodules feel as if they are just below the surface or almost attached to the skin.

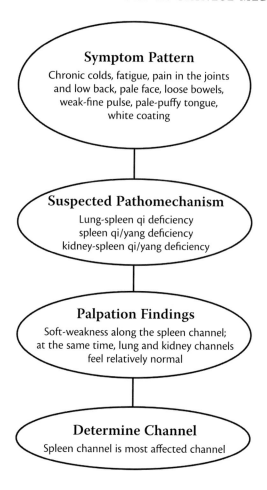

Fig. 12.7
A simple example of how channel palpation can help verify
and refine a diagnostic hypothesis

They are often indicative of a relatively acute situation or one affecting the muscles, tendons, and skin.

Changes that are generalized or relatively shallow and attached to the skin might be thought of as reflecting the 'qi level', while the channel changes discussed below are more likely to reflect the 'blood level'. Qi level changes involve problems with organ function, in contrast to blood level changes that often correspond to more substantial physical changes in the body. The first type is softer and is found in less serious conditions, while deep hardness often has more definition and involves a more serious or chronic pathodynamic (Table 12.4).

	Technique	Significance
Shallow hardness and/or tightness	• Palpate all along the channel • Use mid-level pressure • Carefully determine which channels are involved • Focus on a broad comparison of multiple channels	• Acute condition • Compromised function or circulation in the channel and/or organ • More likely to involve cold
Deep hardness and/or nodules*	• Go along channel stopping to circle noted areas or nodules • Pay attention to shape • Note quality (slippery, soft, fixed, etc.)	• Accumulation of dampness, phlegm-heat, or blood in the channel and/or organ • Chronic condition

* Deep hardness can be subdivided into:
- very hard nodules
- defined hard nodules
- bamboo-like bumpy changes
- stick-like changes

Table 12.4

Techniques for differentiating hardness and tightness in the channels

· ·

Deep hardness

This is the broadest category of channel change. A wide variety of pathomechanisms can lead to changes of this type, but are most often related to stasis of blood, accumulation of phlegm, or the presence of chronic disease. These types of nodules are clearly located below the skin and are less likely to move when the skin moves. Within the category of deep hardness are a few sub-categories:

Very hard nodule that is fairly difficult to move:
   significant cold or blood stasis (Fig. 12.8)

Defined hard nodules that are easily moved and slippery/smooth:
   dampness and phlegm (Fig. 12.9)

Hardness in a line that feels almost like a piece of bamboo:
   chronic condition. These are due to a compromise in the nutritive functions of the fluids and are often more difficult to treat (Fig. 12.10).

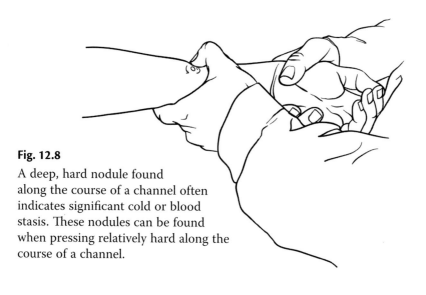

Fig. 12.8
A deep, hard nodule found along the course of a channel often indicates significant cold or blood stasis. These nodules can be found when pressing relatively hard along the course of a channel.

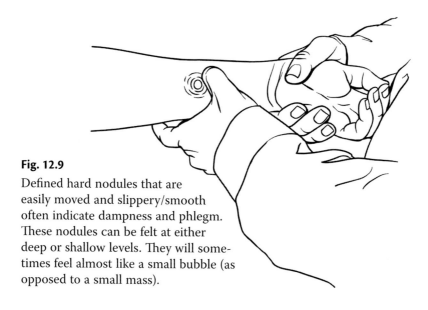

Fig. 12.9
Defined hard nodules that are easily moved and slippery/smooth often indicate dampness and phlegm. These nodules can be felt at either deep or shallow levels. They will sometimes feel almost like a small bubble (as opposed to a small mass).

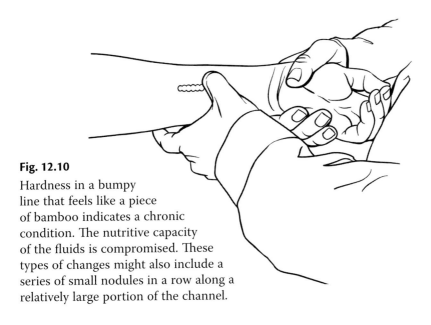

Fig. 12.10
Hardness in a bumpy
line that feels like a piece
of bamboo indicates a chronic
condition. The nutritive capacity
of the fluids is compromised. These
types of changes might also include a
series of small nodules in a row along a
relatively large portion of the channel.

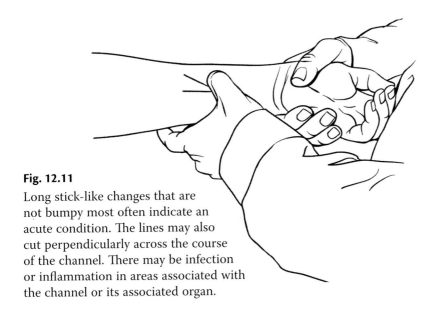

Fig. 12.11
Long stick-like changes that are
not bumpy most often indicate an
acute condition. The lines may also
cut perpendicularly across the course
of the channel. There may be infection
or inflammation in areas associated with
the channel or its associated organ.

Long, stick-like changes that are not bumpy:

acute conditions generally caused by qi stagnation. Stick-like lines may cut perpendicularly across the course of the channel as well. Changes of this type may also arise in the presence of infection in areas associated with the channel (Fig. 12.11).

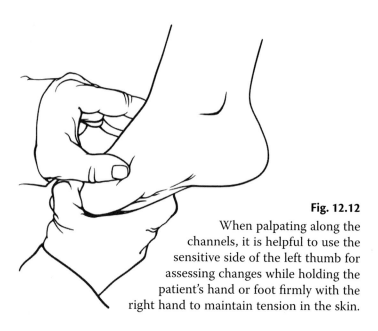

Fig. 12.12
When palpating along the channels, it is helpful to use the sensitive side of the left thumb for assessing changes while holding the patient's hand or foot firmly with the right hand to maintain tension in the skin.

Additional principles that should be kept in mind when palpating the channels are shown in Table 12.5, following page.

··

Case Studies

■ CASE NO. 1

56-year-old male

Chief complaint   Prostatitis

History of present illness   The patient presented with chronic, benign inflammation of the prostate as diagnosed by a urologist, with only slightly elevated (11) prostate-specific antigen (PSA) levels. Symptoms had increased

Softer palpated changes that are less defined are associated with less serious conditions.
The harder, more fixed, and deeper the palpated change, the more serious the condition. These types of changes have generally entered deeper levels.
Generalized roughness of the fascia is often associated with qi deficiency. The patient may also report unusual sensations in these deficient channels such as numbness, hyper-sensitivity, or temperature variability.
Sometimes there will be a generalized sensation of bumpiness all along a channel, like driving a car along a bumpy road. This more likely indicates compromised function in the associated organ (as opposed to channel). There may be an accumulation of cold, heat, blood, or phlegm due to long-term malfunction.

Table 12.5
General principles of channel palpation

during the previous four years. The patient had difficulty initiating urination and complained of a dribbling flow of relatively dark, yellow urine. The patient's pulse was wiry and thin and the tongue was puffy with a dry coat and cracked body.

Palpation The connective tissues on the leg *shào yīn* channel around KI-4 *(dà zhōng)* and KI-5 *(shuǐ quán)* were hard, thick and tender to the touch. The skin in the area was dry and less flexible and seemed to attach to the bone.

Diagnosis Stasis due to underlying kidney deficiency. The root cause of the condition was a deficiency of kidney qi failing to transform (腎氣不化 *shèn qì bù huà)*. Lack of transformation led to stasis of blood, which in turn caused heat.

Point Prescription HT-6 *(yīn xī)* and KI-5, followed by moxa at LR-1 *(dà dūn)*. Later treatments switched to the point pair LU-9 *(tài yuān)* and SP-3 *(tài bái)* combined with KI-3 *(tài xī)*.

Technique Even technique at HT-6 and KI-5 with a gentle, short moxa treatment at LR-1. Later treatment involved tonification of LU-9, SP-3, and KI-3. Treatment was administered weekly for four months.

Results The patient reported improvement in symptoms after three treatments, although a longer course of treatment (3 months) was required to maintain an improved urine flow.

Analysis This was a case of combined excess and deficiency. Initial treatments utilized the cleft *(xī)* points of the *shào yīn* channel (HT-6 and KI-5) to reestablish circulation in the affected (kidney/reproductive) area. Cleft points can be used to reestablish circulation in areas associated with the channel when there is relatively severe stasis.

Once circulation had improved somewhat, later stages focused more on benefiting fluid circulation and made use of the three source points LU-9, SP-3, and KI-3. Although *shào yīn* deficiency is at the root of the condition, the ability of the kidney to transform fluids in urination also depends on the transformation of dampness by *tài yīn*. Both channels were therefore treated in this case.

Channel palpation was important for determining the nature of involvement by the various channels passing through the area of the prostate. In general, prostatitis can have an excess or deficient nature and may involve the *shào yīn, tài yīn, jué yīn,* or *tài yáng* channels. The *shào yīn* and *tài yīn* types often involve qi and yang deficiency; the *jué yīn* and *tài yáng* involve excess. While *jué yīn* involvement usually includes accumulation of cold, *tài yáng* is most affected when problems with urination are severe. This condition, like most, involved aspects of all four. The key is to determine the degree to which each is involved in the initial diagnosis, while reevaluating the condition as it changes over time.

When prostatitis has continued for a relatively long time, the liver channel, which passes through the area, is often affected by cold accumulation. In this case, the addition of a few short moxa treatments at the *jué yīn* well point (LR-1) insured movement and warmth to remove stasis in that channel. Note that moxa was used on the well point to increase movement, even though heat was still involved in the pathodynamic. (The use of well points to promote movement, even in the presence of heat, will be discussed further in Chapter 16.) Nevertheless, the root of the condition was still treated as a *shào yīn / tài yīn* type.

The hardness and thickness of the skin along the *shào yīn* channel at KI-4 and KI-5 indicated that stasis was also a factor in this case, and also underlined the fact that *shào yīn* was primary. Stasis was further confirmed by the presence of tenderness in the area. At the same time, underlying deficiency manifested as dry skin and a sensation that the skin adhered to the bone around the ankle. This was indicative of channel qi deficiency failing to nourish the skin and muscles along its course.

The *tài yáng* bladder was also obviously affected here. When considering the nature of *tài yáng* involvement, one must clearly differentiate excess from deficiency. As stated above, the differential diagnosis and channel palpation in this case indicated deficiency as the primary cause. Deficiency in the paired yin organ (the kidney) had affected the bladder. Often, when there is deficiency in a yang organ or channel, an effective treatment involves tonification of the paired yin channel. Here, *shào yīn* was tonified to support transformation in the paired *tài yáng* organ.

■ CASE NO. 2

60-year-old female

Chief complaint   Asthma with cough

History of present illness   The patient presented with chronic asthma that had worsened during the last three years. She was also very susceptible to colds, with a tendency to develop a chronic cough. Upon presentation, she had been coughing for a week. When the coughing was intense, it usually led to the onset of an asthma attack. The coughing was accompanied by expectoration of foamy white phlegm. In recent days, the patient had been unable to climb flights of stairs or walk long distances without difficulty.

Palpation   A deep, hard nodule was palpated in the area around LU-6 *(kǒng zuì)*, with a line of bamboo-like hard, painful nodules along the course of the lung channel. Another slightly larger and softer nodule was also palpated around LU-5 *(chǐ zé)*. All of the nodules had borders that were relatively undefined and felt slippery under the skin. There was also a narrowing and a tight sensation accompanied by tenderness beneath GV-12 *(shēn zhù)*, and a very tender, soft nodule around BL-12 *(fēng mén)*. All changes (except GV-12) were bilateral.

Diagnosis   *Tài yīn* disharmony with some underlying *tài yáng* deficiency.

Point Prescription   GV-12 and BL-12, together with the point pair LU-5 and SP-9 *(yīn líng quán)*.

Technique   Even technique at all points.

Results   The patient reported improvement in the chronic cough on the day after the first treatment, which gradually improved over the weeks that followed. In the initial stages, the patient came for treatment twice weekly. After three weeks, the patient began to spread treatments out, eventually coming once every three weeks to maintain *tài yīn* function.

Analysis This is a case where palpation revealed both the acute and chronic condition. The line of nodules noted in the area around LU-6 is indicative of chronic inflammation in the respiratory tract (often chronic bronchitis) while the generalized tenderness and hardness around LU-5 is seen more often in acute cases.

The details of the meaning of changes felt at particular points will be explored in greater detail in the following chapter, but it should be noted here that channel palpation often involves careful differentiation of chronic and acute conditions. In other words, changes felt along the course of a channel may not reflect the condition at hand but may instead be a 'memory' of a disease from the past, or an indication of another chronic condition. In this case, the chronic and acute conditions were both found on the same channel. Sometimes this is not the case. Consequently, when palpating the channels, the practitioner should also always ask questions that help contextualize changes that are found. In this case, for example, when the line of nodules was found at LU-6, the patient was asked about her history of lung complaints. Questioning revealed that there had been bouts of pneumonia during young adulthood. The memory of these bouts remained in the channels.

The important thing for the practitioner to remember is that not all felt changes are necessarily related to the patient's chief complaint. This is one of the most difficult aspects of channel diagnosis. The goal of the following chapter is to provide some indication of what specific changes along each channel might mean. After that, the task of channel differentiation, and the selection of channels and points for treatment, will be addressed.

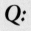 *Q:*

Earlier you mentioned patients who had very strong immunity or even hypersensitive immune systems. You said that these patients might experience changes that can be felt in the channels before symptoms even present. In these types of patients, will they also have a tendency to show stronger and more noticeable changes that can be felt along the course of the channels?

DR. WANG: No. It isn't the case that patients who are strong will have larger or more intense changes along the pathways of the channels. My point here is that stronger or allergic patients will instead have a tendency to have a clear manifestation of disease on the channels. Their channels are healthy, so they are actively participating in the immune response. That third general category of channel change serves to highlight the role of the channel system in immune response. In other words, because, in some cases, the channels have this almost predictive tendency in healthy patients, one can see that they are responding as the first line of defense. In fact, in weak patients with chronic disease, the changes one can feel along the course of the channels are actually often more noticeable, especially to the novice. This is because the fluid movement in the channels is particularly compromised in these patients and thus shows more noticeable change.

Palpation is subtle and takes awhile to get used to. There are a lot of things you can feel when you start to palpate along the course of the channels. Sometimes things that feel 'unusual' are actually quite normal, and sometimes it's the tiniest nodule or area of fascial thickening that is very important. The most important thing is to start palpating all patients and looking for patterns.

▪ Narrative

PALPATION ON THE TRAIN

Another aspect of my time with Dr. Wang involved helping to arrange for other practitioners to come study with him for a few weeks. With help from friends and teachers back home, we were able to arrange for groups to come to China and spend time at the Ping Xin Tang and other Beijing hospitals. We would generally see patients all morning, and then spend the afternoon listening to Dr. Wang lecture about physiology or channel palpation. I was able to learn quite a bit myself in my capacity as translator for these groups. In fact, much of the information in this text draws from recordings of these lectures and the insightful questions other students asked him. I am much in debt to practitioners with more clinical experience than I who asked questions I would never have thought to ask.

The following story is one that Dr. Wang told to a visiting group of acupuncturists and teachers from New York. It was a fairly hot day in August and we had given up on the air conditioner, not, as one might expect, because it wasn't working, but because it worked all too well. Every time we turned it on the room would become unbearably cold and the pace of the lecture would be broken as one student or another struggled with the confusion of the remote control device that all Chinese air conditioners require. There are no simple thermo-stats on a Chinese air conditioner. In any case, by this time the heat had returned and the sound of crickets outside the room in the hot Beijing afternoon had lulled everyone beyond the point of listening to yet more information about the *Inner Classic* or channel theory. We had been talking about channel palpation, and then Dr. Wang changed gears...

DR. WANG: This brings to mind an experience I had in 1972. At that point in my career, I was extremely busy, treating upwards of eighty patients a day with the assistance of three nurses at a large hospital in Beijing. I've told you many times how the sheer volume of patients in the early decades of my work served as my greatest teacher. At that point, I had been seeing patients for twelve years or so and had begun to explore the process of chan-nel palpation. Having found the fundamental ideas and techniques in various classical sources, I began checking the channels of all of my new patients. I had begun to notice that there was a cor-respondence between changes that I could feel along the channels and the symptoms patients described. I saw that some patients had changes that were roughly in line with the symptoms they were having, while others didn't show channel changes until days or even weeks after the onset of the condition. In other words, I was in the process of categorizing the types of patterns that I was seeing. Significantly, at that point I hadn't really run into any cases that showed me the ability of the channels to predict diseases for which no symptoms had appeared. It was a train trip in those last chaotic years of the Cultural Revolution that brought home to me, in a very real way, the fact that the channels are the body's first line of defense.

In those days, groups of doctors were sent by the Ministry of Health to other provinces to review ongoing clinical research. I went on a few of these trips. In 1972, word came down that I was to go with a group of doctors to Shandong province to review an ongoing study of the use of acupuncture in the treatment of gall-stones. The central government in Beijing was always receiving claims describing studies where Chinese medicine was shown to cure this or that disease, and it was our job to verify the results as best we could. If the research seemed promising, then the larger universities might consider doing studies of their own. In any case, this particular trip in 1972 involved six doctors: three doctors of Western medicine and three doctors of Chinese medicine.

For some reason, the trip was arranged fairly suddenly. We were told one day that we had to leave the following morning. As you may know, taking trains in China is often a chaotic affair. In the 1970s it was especially so. There were fewer sleeper cars and 'soft seats' than there are now, and most people rode in the crowded 'hard-seat' cars with wooden seats and open windows. It was usually very difficult to get tickets on the coveted 'soft sleeper' cars that featured private four-bunk rooms. Because of the last-minute nature of our trip, we were only able to get two soft-sleeper beds. Among the doctors in our group, there were two who were Communist Party members and government officials. Naturally, they got the two sleeper beds while the other four of us ended up sitting on the hard seats in a crowded car. I was young at the time and didn't really mind. The officials were older than we were and it was better that they were able to lie down anyway.

Not all of the doctors I was with were so resigned to our fate, however. One of the doctors, a surgeon I think, was often irritable and this kind of situation irked him to no end. Following some encouragement from this surgeon, we all went to the young man who was taking tickets in our car and asked if we might up-grade to some soft sleeper beds. Not surprisingly, he replied that he couldn't help since we had obviously bought the hard-seat tickets—he could see them there in our hands. Undeterred, the surgeon demanded that we speak with the head conductor of the train. The man was eventually brought before us and the surgeon buttoned his blazer and said, "Comrade, we are on a mission from the central Department of Health and are all famous doctors. We must be given better seats than this. It is an outrage that doctors of our stature should be forced to cram ourselves into these seats. There's hardly any room in this car!" Space was almost always tight in the train cars of the 1970s. Obviously affronted, the conductor replied, "You venerable doctors must have great connections at the Department of Health. I'm surprised that the department was unable to secure better seats for you on this train. Unfortunately, if they can't help you, then neither can I!" Train conductors in those days were figures of some power. They could make or break you on a long trip, since most long trips involved days and days on the train.

After some time on the hard seats, the surgeon stood up and began to make his way through the back of the car toward the soft-sleeper beds in the car behind us. A few minutes later he returned and once again accosted the conductor who had remained in our car idly sipping tea. "I've just returned from the sleeper cars and I must point out that there are many open beds back there. How is it that you can't give us a bed then? What is the meaning of this?" yelled the surgeon. Now, to appreciate the situation I have just described, you also have to understand the culture of train life at that time. As I said, the conductor of the train was a kind of despot in his traveling kingdom and didn't necessarily have to answer to anyone. In general, it was the policy of the conductors to keep as many of the soft-sleeper beds empty as possible so that they and their subordinates would have less clean-up work at the end of the line. Any money that they collected for the beds was strictly managed by the train system. They didn't make any more money if people got into those soft sleepers. They just had to do more work. It was much easier for them if they kept everyone crowded into a few cars so that there was less mess. In fact, a familiar sight on trains at the time was that of the conductor and his cronies sipping tea and smoking cigarettes with their feet up in the soft sleepers at night while passengers crowded three to a seat in the regular cars. Thus they had a strong incentive to maintain the status quo in our case.

I was surprised to see that the surgeon had not given up. Instead, he tried another tack. As I said, the Cultural Revolution was still a real presence in our lives at this time, and allusions to political ideology came up in all sorts of conversations. So the surgeon turned to the man with a voice that somehow combined authority with a sense of proletarian duty: "Comrade, we are members of the people's Department of Health and are on a mission to serve the people in the countryside. You can help to serve the people by preparing those rooms for us and allowing us some rest before we begin our arduous duties among the proletariat." The conductor took a sip of tea before replying: "Comrade, I also serve the people, just not you people in particular. I cannot turn over those rooms to you."

At this point, other passengers on the train, having nothing to do, began to crowd around to watch the unfolding struggle. The surgeon made a final attempt to scale the fortress of the conductor's indifference by again angrily denouncing the way doctors of such fame and skill were being treated. The thing is, this surgeon was in fact a doctor of some fame. He was one of the leading specialists on gallbladder and liver surgery and was responsible for innovations in acupuncture anesthesia. Imagine: a liver doctor with anger problems! In any case, he began to see that his pleas were futile and that they had begun to degrade his importance. He returned to the seats where the three of us were trying to stifle our amusement.

The surgeon's remonstrance did have some effects, however. Passengers in the car around us began to offer more comfortable seating arrangements. Where before, four of us had been crowded onto a seat designed for two, we suddenly found that we each had our own bench. Once again, you have to understand something about that time in China in order to appreciate why this might happen. In those days, it was still very difficult for the average person to get quality medical care. The best most people could hope for was a few minutes at the ear of one of the highly over-worked general practitioners in the few public hospitals. The following decade would see a lot of new building of hospital facilities and the training of new doctors, but in the early 1970s there were still very great limits on health care—especially given some of the chaos wrought by the Cultural Revolution. In any case, the generosity of our fellow passengers didn't come without a price. After providing us with the comfort of their seats, many passengers began to crowd around us asking for medical advice on a whole host of complaints. We didn't have anything else to do and so obliged their requests. Tables were cleared of tea and sunflower seeds and we began doing intakes as best we could, while the grey-brown forests of north China passed by in windows behind our heads.

We began writing formulas that our impromptu patients might fill in their hometowns. We treated some with small ear-pellets on auricular points, and did full acupuncture treatments on others while they sat in their seats. After an hour or so, word began to spread through the train and passengers from nearby cars began to make their way to our mobile clinic. Other passengers, getting in the spirit, acted as nurses and helped manage the crowd while keeping the 'treatment area' open. We weren't charging any money, and were actually having a pretty good time.

At one point, it got so crowded in our car that movement through the corridor virtually stopped. This kind of irritated the young man who was in charge of carrying food and hot water from one car to another, and he stood at the door staring at us with some annoyance. We could occasionally hear him muttering to those around him, "These 'famous' doctors think they are so great. I think that they're just getting in the way!" We had gotten so busy, however, that he was forced to just stand there fuming.

Now, throughout this time, I was doing channel palpation on all of the passengers that I saw. I would begin before even asking the patient about their chief complaint. I was having a good time trying to guess the chief complaint by the nature of the changes I could feel along the course of the channels. The young man who had been fuming as he watched finally stepped forward and said, "OK, you famous doctors should diagnose me then and tell me if there's anything wrong. Give me a turn!" He sat before a young doctor who had studied channel palpation with me in Beijing. Knowing that the young man had been so critical over the last few hours, the young doctor was very thorough in palpating all of the man's channels. When he palpated the large intestine channel, he found a very tender spot in the area around LI-10 *(shǒu sān lǐ)* and another on the stomach channel at ST-37 *(shàng jù xū)*. He then even checked the large intestine and stomach points on the ears and found the large intestine area to be very tender.

The young doctor turned to the man and said with a smile, "You have some stomach pain don't you?" The man shook his head "no." Unperturbed, the doctor then asked, "Okay, then you have some problems with digestion, maybe bloating or gas when you eat?" Again, the man shook his head "no." The doctor scratched his head and touched the very tender point on the man's arm. "Ow!" said the train employee, "you are pressing very hard!" "No," said the young doctor, "I'm just touching the area. Look, if I press here it doesn't hurt at all." The train attendant agreed that other areas were not nearly as sore. "Okay," said the doctor again, "you have constipation, dry stools, or maybe hemorrhoids, don't you?" Again the young man said no, and now began to snicker, "See, I told you guys that you are just sitting here playing with everyone's mind with your silly 'channel palpation'. That stuff doesn't work and I actually feel totally fine! In fact, my digestion is so good that I could eat rocks and feel normal!" At this point, the young doctor turned to me and asked, "Teacher Wang, can you take a moment and come here to check this patient? See if you don't feel these changes I'm noticing on the *yáng míng* channels."

I went over to where the young doctor and the attendant were sitting, surrounded by the curious eyes of the other passengers. When I palpated the young man's channels I did notice the same changes. In fact, the area around LI-10 in particular was unusual. There was an area the size of a large coin that was very hard and kind of warm to the touch, and another hard nodule at ST-37. I don't exactly know why now, but I suddenly heard myself saying to the young man, "Well, you know that sometimes there will be changes on the channel without symptoms in the case of a disease that has just entered the vessels and not yet developed. You may actually develop symptoms in the next day or so." The man nodded reluctantly. I could see that he wasn't satisfied with that answer, so I added, "Also, there are cases where a healthy person like yourself might have changes on the channels and never actually get any disease at all because your body manages to keep it away." He looked at me and I could tell that he thought I was pulling his leg or trying to cover my own tracks. What could I do? He obviously felt fine and we had told him everything we knew. The attendant left the car, once again muttering under his breath that we were there wasting everyone's time. The other patients in the car, many of whom had already been helped by our treatments, continued to crowd around us clamoring for advice. At that point, we assumed that he was just one of those cases you can't figure out and left it at that.

A few hours later, however, we were still treating patients in our rolling clinic when the young man came running to the car saying, "You guys really are amazing! I've been on the toilet the last half-hour with severe diarrhea. I never get hit with anything like that. It's pretty stunning that you knew before I even did that there was something wrong with my intestines!" The man sat down next to us and we palpated his large intestine channel again. This time, the nodule on his arm was less large and he reported less tenderness.

It was then time for us to break for lunch and, as we waited to get in line for a box of rice and vegetables, we saw the train conductor making his way toward us. His demeanor had changed and he was now all smiles. "I saw your clinic this morning on the train and heard about how you diagnosed my employee before he was even sick! Look, it turns out that we had an unexpected opening in the soft-sleeper car. It seems we have four beds for you doctors to take a rest. In fact, if you ever find yourselves in need of soft sleepers on trains in the future, please give me a call. Here's my office number." We were then escorted into the welcome silence of the clean room where lunch was brought to us. We kept the conductor's number and he was able to arrange for us to have soft-sleepers on the way back from Shandong as well. I kept in touch with the conductor and he has helped me quite a few times over the years with train tickets.

Now, I want all of you to remember that there are cases where one will find palpable changes along the course of a channel before disease shows up. And, although rarely seen, there are patients who will have significant changes along the course of their channels and have no disease at all. Again, patients who have significant change (especially tender pain) along the channels without disease are usually younger patients, or ones with very sensitive immune systems."

By this time the heat in the room had cooled a bit, as the afternoon was coming to an end. It was nearly time for dinner and we all began to talk about a walk around the Forbidden City before heading out for some Beijing duck.

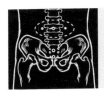

Specific Channel Changes

HAVING DISCUSSED TECHNIQUES for palpating the channels, this chapter will outline some of the most common changes found along the fourteen main channels (twelve regular channels plus the *rèn* and *dū* vessels). Of course, we cannot list *all* of the possible changes that might be found; that would be impossible. Moreover, there are more details provided for some channels than for others. This is not meant to imply that the channels with less information tend to show less change. Rather, the apparent gaps in discussion represent areas where the variety of changes that might be felt is especially broad. For example, the discussion of the liver channel is fairly brief, but in the clinic, soft nodules are often found all along that channel—especially on the lower leg and foot. In the clinic, these distinct lines of general bumpiness do not represent a specific pathodynamic, but rather a general lack of dredging and draining by the liver.

The goal of this chapter is to describe consistent patterns of change at specific points and how they might indicate a particular pathodynamic. For example, while a generalized bumpiness along the liver channel is not discussed, the tendency of soft, painful nodules to appear at LR-5 (*lǐ gōu*) in certain types of carpal tunnel patterns is described.

In general, when there are dispersed nodules, lines of bumpiness, weakness, or increased muscle tone along any of the channels, one might infer that there are problems with qi transformation in that organ. Just as often, however, dispersed changes along the course of a single channel may indicate a lack of circulation in the associated muscles and tendons (as opposed to the organs themselves). This is particularly true for chronic pain conditions.

In the end, the first goal is still to determine which channel has the most significant change. Once that channel has been identified, the practitioner can combine this information with the other vital clues provided by the patient's symptom-pattern to create a more accurate diagnosis and treatment plan.

Tài Yīn Lung Channel

The discussion of qi circulation in the channels generally begins with the lung. This is largely because of the function of the lung to 'command qi'. As the organ of breath, the lung is responsible for bringing the qi of the external environment into the body. Many texts state that the lung 'rules the hundred vessels'. This expresses an understanding that external qi, brought into the body by the lung, is present in all the vessels of the body. It also reflects the belief that the rhythms of the body can be controlled with the breath. In short, this is a statement about the importance of breathing to movement in the blood. Because of the vital role that the lung plays in moving qi, many types of problems associated with qi circulation will be reflected as palpable change along the lung channel.

This frequency of palpable change on the lung *tài yīn* was also mentioned in the *Inner Classic*. Chapter 74 of the *Divine Pivot* describes a technique by which disease can be diagnosed through evaluation of the "thickness, slipperiness, roughness, and muscle condition" of the lung channel in the forearm. Singling out the lung channel for a discussion of palpation serves to highlight its unique importance in both physiology and diagnosis. It is likely that this passage inspired the compilers of the *Classic of Difficulties*, in Chapter 13, to take up palpation of the forearm as a general diagnostic technique.

Novice practitioners of channel palpation are often confused by the apparent preponderance of change that can be felt along the lung channel in a wide variety of patients. But when you remember that the breath from the lung is associated with all movement of qi, one can begin to see how the qi dynamic of that organ would be involved in a wide range of pathodynamics. For example, a patient with dampness and heat affecting the gallbladder might have a series of soft nodules along the triple burner *shào yáng* channel, indicating dampness, while also presenting with tenderness and puffiness at GB-40 (*qiū xū*). The practitioner may be confused by the concurrent presence of soft bumpiness along the course of the lung channel. In this case, a compromised qi dynamic in the pivot of *shào yáng* has led to a more generalized stagnation of qi. Sometimes, in patients of this type, it is helpful to first regulate the qi in a general way before proceeding to the primary channel. In fact, many conditions that involve qi stagnation also involve the

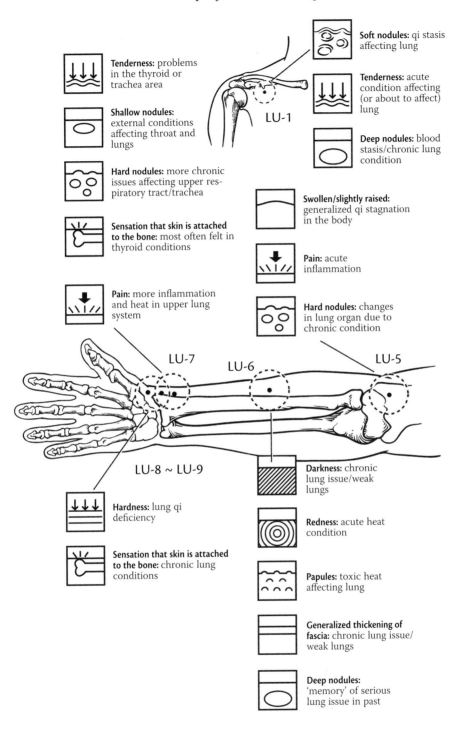

Soft nodules: qi stasis affecting lung

Tenderness: problems in the thyroid or trachea area

Tenderness: acute condition affecting (or about to affect) lung

Shallow nodules: external conditions affecting throat and lungs

Deep nodules: blood stasis/chronic lung condition

Hard nodules: more chronic issues affecting upper respiratory tract/trachea

LU-1

Swollen/slightly raised: generalized qi stagnation in the body

Sensation that skin is attached to the bone: most often felt in thyroid conditions

Pain: acute inflammation

Pain: more inflammation and heat in upper lung system

Hard nodules: changes in lung organ due to chronic condition

LU-7   LU-6   LU-5

LU-8 ~ LU-9

Darkness: chronic lung issue/weak lungs

Hardness: lung qi deficiency

Redness: acute heat condition

Sensation that skin is attached to the bone: chronic lung conditions

Papules: toxic heat affecting lung

Generalized thickening of fascia: chronic lung issue/weak lungs

Deep nodules: 'memory' of serious lung issue in past

Fig. 13.1
Tài yīn lung channel

lung. This helps explain why, in the clinic, it is often helpful to first regulate a new patient using the uniting (*hé*-sea) point pair LU-5 *(chǐ zé)* and SP-9 *(yīn líng quán)*. After one or two regulating treatments, you can then proceed to treat the primary channel.

In any case, changes along the lung channel are common and a careful in-take will help the practitioner identify whether or not the lung *tài yīn* is primary in a particular patient.

Physiological significance of channel changes

Observation of areas related to *tài yīn* lung

The presence of papules at LU-1 *(zhōng fǔ)* and LU-2 *(yún mén)* will often be found when there is heat in the lung channel. Papules or other changes at LU-7 *(liè quē)* or LU-9 *(tài yuān)* will sometimes be found when there is heat in the lung or acute bronchitis.

There may be darkening of the skin, redness, or papules in the area around LU-6 *(kǒng zuì)* in the case of bleeding in the lung organ. Most often, this indicates bleeding or other problems in the bronchioles, or the deepest levels of the lung.

Look at the lung associated point BL-13 *(fèi shū)* or LU-1 for weakness, softness of the muscles, or dry skin as a sign of lung qi deficiency. Red papules may also be seen in the area in cases of acute infection in the lung (lung heat). Thick, dry skin in the area may indicate chronic phlegm-type accumulation in the lung.

Pulse palpation of areas related to *tài yīn* lung

Although it is not a lung channel point, palpation of the pulse around LI-5 *(yáng xī)* may reflect the condition of *tài yīn*. An especially strong pulse in the area reflects the presence of external disease, while a very deep pulse often indicates *tài yīn* deficiency leading to diarrhea. If the pulse is particularly weak, it may also indicate deficiency of lung qi.

Palpating the channel, pressing the points, and feeling the body surface

Tenderness at LU-1 *(zhōng fǔ)* generally indicates an acute condition in the lung organ, usually a cold or cough. If soft nodules are palpated in this area, the lung qi is stagnant, often due to chronic disease or blood stasis. In cases of general qi stagnation in the body, this front alarm point may be quite tender (without nodules). There may also be a relatively deep nodule at LU-1 in a patient who has recovered from a rather serious lung problem in the past; this represents the physical 'memory' of that disease.

Changes are often palpated at LU-5 *(chǐ zé)*. A soft, slightly puffy tenderness in the area is indicative of relatively mild, systemic qi stagnation. Many patients react to the general stressors of modern life with changes at this point, and regulation of *tài yīn* is often a necessary first step when treating such patients. Pain with light pressure indicates acute inflammatory disease, while nodules indicate a chronic issue. The harder the nodule, the more likely it is that there is actual physical changes in the lung organ or respiratory tract. Hard nodules or pain around LU-5 are often seen in chronic asthma patients where compromise in the qi dynamic of the lung organ is the root cause. This type of asthma is often characterized by relatively severe inflammation of the bronchioles.

There will often be a large area of hardening or deep nodules around LU-6 *(kǒng zuì)* in the case of chronic disease in the lung organ or a 'memory' of lung disease from the past. For long-standing lung conditions, the area may also be slightly darker than the surrounding skin. On the other hand, if the area is slightly reddish, this indicates a more acute condition, often involving heat. Slight, raised papules indicate more heat (possibly toxic heat). Severe tenderness may indicate lung heat and is seen sometimes in pneumonia.

LU-7 *(liè quē)* and the area proximal to this point are also important. Relatively shallow nodules generally indicate external conditions affecting the throat or lungs. Hardness, inflexibility, and/or pain in the skin around the point are often seen in chronic tracheitis or in growths in the trachea. If the area is very painful with a sensation that the skin has adhered to the fascia below, this can be indicative of thyroid problems. Classically, this could be seen as a problem with circulation in the collaterals of the lung channel, an explanation sometimes used by Chinese doctors when describing goiter. Most often, changes of this type are found when there is also noticeable enlargement of the actual thyroid gland in the patient. Remember that changes observed at collateral points are not only indicative of pathology in the paired yin or yang channel, but may instead indicate a pathodynamic associated with any of the small collaterals or microcirculation along the path of the palpated channel.

Hardening or inflexibility of the skin in the area between LU-8 *(jīng qú)* and LU-9 *(tài yuān)* is often seen in lung qi deficiency. There may even be a sensation that the skin is attached to the bone as well, which also indicates chronic lung conditions.

BL-13 *(fèi shū)*, while not a lung channel point, is the back associated point of the lung. Tenderness in the area represents an acute condition, and a sense of weakness or dry skin represents a chronic or deficient condition. Actual nodules are indicative of more chronic conditions.

In summary, points that most often exhibit change are LU-9, LU-6, LU-5, and LU-1. The most common point pairs used in treating conditions involving the lung are LU-9 and SP-3 *(tài bái)* and LU-5 and SP-9 *(yīn líng quán)*. The LU-5 and SP-9 combination, both *hé*-sea points, is used to regulate the channel; it is often used as a first-line treatment for generalized qi stagnation. By contrast, the LU-9 and SP-3 combination, both source points, is used to strengthen when there is a deficiency of *tài yīn* qi dynamic. While these are the two most common pairs, there are many other points used for treating the commonly-seen case of lung disharmony.

Yáng Míng Large Intestine Channel

Physiological significance of channel changes

Observation of areas related to *yáng míng* large intestine

Redness around the nostrils may indicate heat-toxins in the large intestine.

Pulse palpation of areas related to *yáng míng* large intestine

Check the area around LI-5 *(yáng xī)*, also mentioned in relation to the lung channel. A large (even visible) pulse in this area may indicate an external disorder. This may even be seen in early cases of Bell's palsy where the *yáng míng* channel is primarily affected. A deep, tight pulse in the area may indicate *yáng míng* excess constipation or severe pain in the face. Sometimes, this pulse will also be especially weak in the case of *yáng míng* (or *tài yīn)* deficient cold-type diarrhea or constipation.

Palpating the channel, pressing the points, and feeling the body surface

Palpating the *yáng míng* channel may sometimes reveal weakness or softness along the entire path of the channel on the forearm. This indicates deficiency. Bowel movements will most likely be loose, with visible fecal pieces mixed with fluids. In this type of patient, deficiency of the large intestine has led to a lack of proper reabsorption of fluids. Hardness along the channel is often seen in tooth pain, gum inflammation, or certain types of external headache.

If there are shallow nodules or tenderness in the area of LI-4 *(hé gǔ)* and LI-6 *(piān lì)*, this often indicates the presence of an external condition, pain in the face (Bell's palsy), tooth pain, or other types of inflammation along the *yáng míng* channel.

Nodules (generally hard, movable, and tender) between LI-7 *(wēn liū)* and LI-10 *(shǒu sān lǐ)* are often noticeable when there is colitis or polyps in the large intestine. The area between LI-7 and LI-10 may also present with a line of nodules in chronic throat conditions. This can be understood

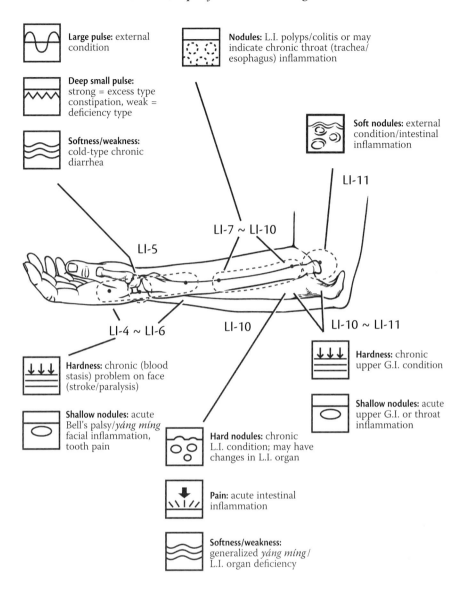

Fig. 13.2

Yáng míng large intestine channel

by thinking of the *yáng míng* channel as reflective of not just the stomach and intestines, but also other aspects of the entire G.I. tract and the areas nearby. In this case, the throat is passing right alongside the upper aspect of the esophagus.

If there is pain with pressure and some swelling at LI-10, this often indicates an acute intestinal inflammation. Often in *yáng míng* deficiency cases, there will be softness or even a 'drop' in the fascia around the point and along the surrounding channel. Deficiency palpated along the channel in this area may be accompanied by an aching at LI-10 that is relieved by pressure. Chronic large intestine deficiency is associated with malabsorption and/or chronic low-grade intestinal inflammation. Harder nodules may also be found in the presence of constipation or physical changes in the organ.

LI-11 *(qū chí)* will often have a soft, tender nodule in the presence of an external condition. Acute large intestine inflammation may also correspond with tenderness in this area. The area between LI-10 and LI-11 may also have tenderness or shallow nodules when there are problems with the upper digestive tract. Note that this is an area below the upper esophagus and throat. Clinical experience has shown that as one moves proximally along the large intestine channel, conditions further and further down the G.I. tract begin to manifest. In other words, while the area between LI-7 and LI-10 often reflects problems in the throat (or nearby upper esophagus), the area around LI-11 tends to reflect more the lower esophagus.

Yáng Míng Stomach Channel

Physiological significance of channel changes

Observation of areas related to *yáng míng* stomach

Redness or heat on the forehead or around the eyebrows reflects stomach heat. A red nose (not the same as the nostrils in large intestine heat) can indicate an acute accumulation of heat in the stomach. Swelling or sores on the face, as well as some types of acne, can be reflective of heat-toxin in the *yáng míng*. Swollen gums and tooth grinding at night may also indicate *yáng míng* heat or fire.

Pulse palpation of areas related to *yáng míng* stomach

A noticeable, fast pulse at the ST-8 *(tóu wéi)* area indicates rising *yáng míng* heat—this could be associated with headaches or stomach problems.

Palpating the channel, pressing the points, and feeling the body surface

Tenderness or very small nodules found between ST-44 *(nèi tíng)* and ST-43 *(xiàn gǔ)* indicate constraint, heat, and blockage in *yáng míng*. If there is heat trapped in the *yáng míng*, the patient will also often present with thirst, bad breath, and nausea.

Severe tenderness between ST-41 *(jiě xī)* and ST-42 *(chōng yáng)* is often seen with severely painful *yáng míng*-type headache, toothache, high blood

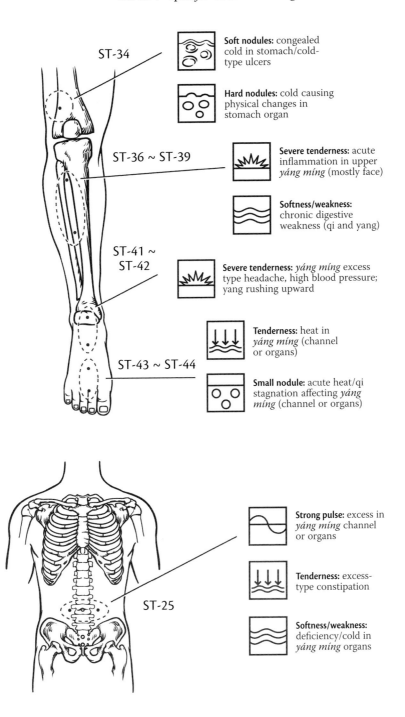

ST-34

Soft nodules: congealed cold in stomach/cold-type ulcers

Hard nodules: cold causing physical changes in stomach organ

ST-36 ~ ST-39

Severe tenderness: acute inflammation in upper *yáng míng* (mostly face)

Softness/weakness: chronic digestive weakness (qi and yang)

ST-41 ~ ST-42

Severe tenderness: *yáng míng* excess type headache, high blood pressure; yang rushing upward

Tenderness: heat in *yáng míng* (channel or organs)

ST-43 ~ ST-44

Small nodule: acute heat/qi stagnation affecting *yáng míng* (channel or organs)

Strong pulse: excess in *yáng míng* channel or organs

Tenderness: excess-type constipation

ST-25

Softness/weakness: deficiency/cold in *yáng míng* organs

Fig. 13.3
Yáng míng stomach channel

pressure, or nausea. This is due to *yáng míng* heat rushing to the head.

The area between ST-36 *(zú sān lǐ)* and ST-39 *(xià jù xū)* can be especially informative. Its general quality is helpful for assessing overall digestive function. In addition, cases of *yáng míng* type facial pain or numbness due to accumulation and stagnation (積滯 *jī zhì*) in the *yáng míng* will present with severe tenderness in this area; bleeding can be curative. Weakness or softness indicates *yáng míng* deficiency or possibly cold congealing (寒凝 *hán níng*) in the channel. This may include chronic gastritis or deficiency-type ulcers.

A soft nodule in the area around ST-34 *(liáng qiū)* indicates congealed cold in the *yáng míng,* causing stasis. This is often associated with patterns involving stomach pain or gastric spasms. Chronic cold stagnation in the channel can also lead to ulcers or growths in the stomach, which might present as a hard, tender nodule at ST-34.

ST-25 *(tiān shū)* will show strong pulsing in cases of excess accumulation in the *yáng míng* channel or organ. If there is softness or a sense of weakness in the area around ST-25, this might indicate a deficiency of *yáng míng* channel qi. Deficiency-type constipation may also manifest as softness in this area, while tightness and tenderness generally indicates excess.

Tenderness or nodules at the stomach back-associated point BL-21 *(wèi shū)* indicates chronic stomach problems due to long-term stagnation in the channel. This may include ulcers.

Tài Yīn Spleen Channel

Physiological significance of channel changes

Observation of areas related to *tài yīn* spleen

Observation of the spleen channel does not involve any special considerations. Nevertheless, observed changes along the skin surface such as redness, papules, or swelling are possible indicators of abnormal spleen function.

Pulse palpation of areas related to *tài yīn* spleen

Similarly, there are no special pulses palpated along the spleen channel. However, it should be remembered that the nature of pulsing along the abdomen on the *rèn* vessel (see discussion of the *rèn* below) may reflect the health of the spleen.

Palpating the channel, pressing the points, and feeling the body surface

A sense of mild pain with pressure at SP-2 *(dà dū)* or SP-3 *(tài bái)* indicates spleen deficiency.

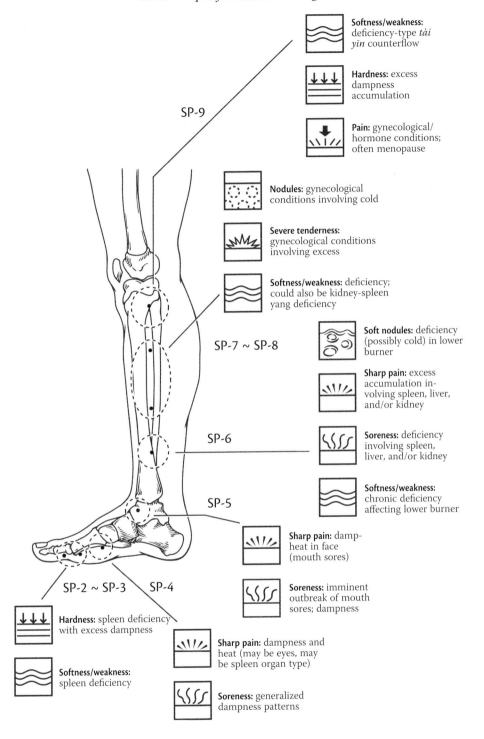

Softness/weakness: deficiency-type *tài yīn* counterflow

Hardness: excess dampness accumulation

Pain: gynecological/ hormone conditions; often menopause

SP-9

Nodules: gynecological conditions involving cold

Severe tenderness: gynecological conditions involving excess

Softness/weakness: deficiency; could also be kidney-spleen yang deficiency

SP-7 ~ SP-8

Soft nodules: deficiency (possibly cold) in lower burner

Sharp pain: excess accumulation involving spleen, liver, and/or kidney

SP-6

Soreness: deficiency involving spleen, liver, and/or kidney

Softness/weakness: chronic deficiency affecting lower burner

SP-5

Sharp pain: damp-heat in face (mouth sores)

Soreness: imminent outbreak of mouth sores; dampness

SP-2 ~ SP-3   SP-4

Hardness: spleen deficiency with excess dampness

Sharp pain: dampness and heat (may be eyes, may be spleen organ type)

Softness/weakness: spleen deficiency

Soreness: generalized dampness patterns

Fig. 13.4
Tài yīn spleen channel

Sharp pain at SP-4 *(gōng sūn)* indicates dampness and heat in the channel. Heat accumulation of this type often manifests as swelling, pain, and possibly itching in and around the eyes. In fact, many types of eye disorders (such as sties) can be due to spleen-stomach heat-toxin. Treatment with SP-4, bilaterally, will often be very helpful. If the eye swelling is severe, one might also consider bleeding the tip of the ear. The area may also be just slightly sore in patterns of spleen deficiency that also involve dampness.

Sharp pain with pressure at SP-5 *(shāng qiū)* may also be indicative of damp-heat encumbering the spleen, especially when there is a corresponding symptom of mouth ulcers or sores on the lips. This point can be treated to help with the pain of an acute outbreak, but long-term treatment must address the underlying spleen deficiency. Milder pain in the area is also sometimes palpated when there is an imminent outbreak of chronic mouth sores.

SP-6 *(sān yīn jiāo)* is an area that will show changes in the presence of both excess and deficiency. Conditions of excess will generally manifest with a sharper pain in the area, while deficiency is more often reflected in a soreness that is relieved with pressure. Deficiency may also lead to a soft, swollen nodule at SP-6, especially in gynecological conditions. However, because the area is also associated with the liver and kidney channels, it is sometimes difficult to know which channel or condition is involved when a change is palpated. Other symptoms must be taken into account. In general, SP-6 is associated more with the lower abdomen than with specific indications involving qi transformation of the spleen. Therefore, tenderness in the area may reflect a variety of infections or inflammations in the lower burner.

The area around SP-7 *(lòu gǔ)* and SP-8 *(dì jī)* will also show changes in patients with gynecological conditions. In particular, this includes painful menstruation and irregular menstrual cycles. The nature of palpated change will vary based on the underlying pathodynamic. For example, there may be weakness or softness in the area in the case of deficiency, nodules if there is stagnation or cold, or severe tenderness where there is excess. Nodules may also be found in cases of uterine fibroids, ovarian cysts, and endometriosis. In men, changes in this area are relatively rare. However, as the cleft *(xì)* point of the spleen channel, SP-8 will often be tender in cases of acute pain that involve the pathway of the spleen channel.

The area around SP-9 *(yīn líng quán)* will often show changes where there is deficiency. In particular, there will often be a soft tenderness where deficiency has led to dampness or a counterflow of *tài yīn* qi transformation. Recall that counterflow, the irregular movement of qi, is often treated with the uniting points. The area around SP-9 will also often be very tender in gynecological conditions. In particular, it is often extremely tender in women before and during menopause. In such cases, the area can be treated with a relatively strong draining technique. SP-9 is also often painfully tender in the presence of urinary tract infections.

Shào Yīn Heart Channel

Physiological significance of channel changes

Observation of areas related to *shào yīn* heart
Redness at the inner canthus of the eyes, or irritated eyes, may indicate wind or fire in the heart channel. Remember as well that swollen and deep red vessels under the tongue may also indicate heat toxin in the heart channel. Also, raised red papules (丘疹 *qiū zhěn)* in the area around T_5 (GV-11) on the back may indicate toxic heat in the heart.

Pulse palpation of areas related to *shào yīn* heart
Palpate the pulse in the area around HT-6 *(yīn xī)* and HT-7 *(shén mén)* for excess and deficiency. It is easiest to feel a strong pulse in this area when excess affects the heart.

Palpating the channel, pressing the points, and feeling the body surface
Tenderness and some puffiness in the area around HT-3 *(shào hǎi)* may indicate a dermatological condition that involves heat in the heart. However, significant change in this area is relatively rare.

Tightness or thickening of the fascia in the forearm, or nodules along the heart channel for a few inches proximal to HT-4 *(líng dào),* may be associated with memory problems or a chronic mental fogginess. Thickening in this area is also seen sometimes in angina or valve problems associated with rheumatic heart disease (rare in the West). Some types of skin disease may also correspond to changes in this area.

The area between HT-4 and HT-7 *(shén mén)* is quite important. In cases where the skin feels thin and/or rough with very small, grainy nodules, there are often conductivity problems in the heart leading to irregular heartbeat. There may also be nodules in the case of heart-type insomnia or heart yin/blood deficiency-type memory problems (especially in the elderly). One may therefore think of this area as generally reflecting the condition of microcirculation in the brain (腦絡 *nǎo luò).* It may also be very tender where there are dermatological problems involving heat in the heart.

Tenderness or small, soft nodules around HT-8 *(shào fǔ)* is associated with excess heat in the heart channel. Changes in this area are often seen

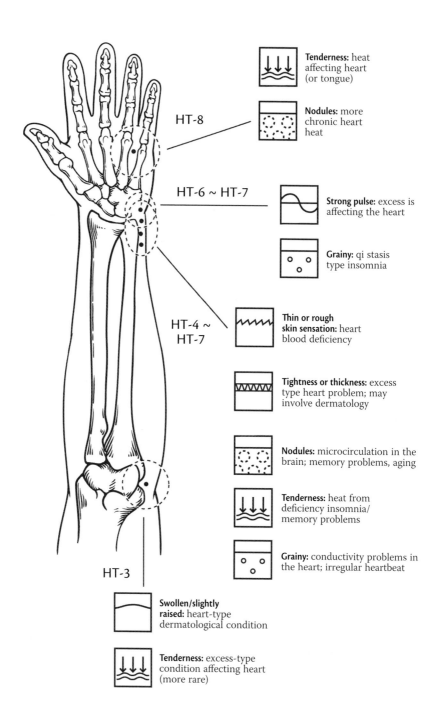

Fig. 13.5
Shào yīn heart channel

in sleep-related pathodynamics. Insomnia of this type often involves waking easily throughout the night. There may also be changes palpated around HT-8 in conditions involving the tongue when the heart channel or organ is involved.

Tài Yáng Small Intestine Channel

Physiological significance of channel changes

Observation of areas related to *tài yáng* small intestine

Redness in the outer canthus of the eye is associated with wind-heat affecting the small intestine channel. Sties are often due to toxic heat in the small intestine channel. Tenderness and redness around the area in front of the ears is also regarded as excess heat in the small intestine channel. Papules inside the ear may indicate damp-heat in the channel. However, changes around the ear are also often related to the gallbladder channel and therefore should be considered in the context of other signs and symptoms.

Pulse palpation of areas related to *tài yáng* small intestine

There are no particular pulses that can be palpated along the path of the small intestine channel.

Palpating the channel, pressing the points, and feeling the body surface

The whole lower aspect of the small intestine channel often shows a variety of changes in the presence of musculoskeletal problems involving the neck and shoulders.

For musculoskeletal problems in the neck, shoulders, and scapula, the area from SI-3 *(hòu xī)* to SI-4 *(wàn gǔ)* most often will present with small nodules, and will also feel slightly tight. The area is generally tight (without nodules) in acute exterior conditions that involve blockage in the *tài yáng* channel. Finally, this area may actually feel soft and weak where there is chronic yang deficiency-type immunity problems (e.g., easily catching colds).

Nodules, pain, or tenderness in the area from SI-4 to SI-6 *(yǎng lǎo)* often indicates the presence of the fire pathogen (inflammation) in the upper aspect of the *tài yáng* channel. This area should be examined very carefully in any patient who presents with neck problems. The area begins distal to SI-4, and then continues to the area proximal to the styloid process of the radius (above SI-6). In the most distal section, a tendency to headaches along the bladder channel or apex of the *dū* vessel (around GV-21 [*qián dǐng*]) is most prominent; then, moving proximally, cervical/neck issues are

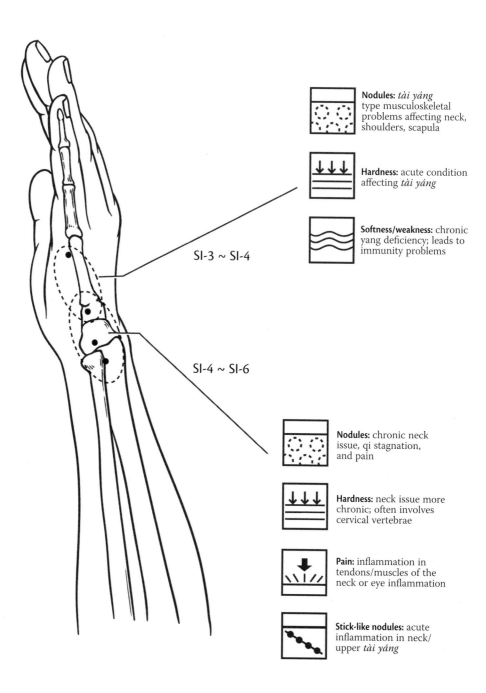

SI-3 ~ SI-4

Nodules: *tài yáng* type musculoskeletal problems affecting neck, shoulders, scapula

Hardness: acute condition affecting *tài yáng*

Softness/weakness: chronic yang deficiency; leads to immunity problems

SI-4 ~ SI-6

Nodules: chronic neck issue, qi stagnation, and pain

Hardness: neck issue more chronic; often involves cervical vertebrae

Pain: inflammation in tendons/muscles of the neck or eye inflammation

Stick-like nodules: acute inflammation in neck/ upper *tài yáng*

Fig. 13.6
Tài yáng small intestine channel

also more likely to manifest. Eye problems are often reflected in palpable changes in this area. In general, tenderness or a generalized increase in muscle tone over the entire area is associated more with muscle and tendon injuries, while nodules are more likely to indicate changes in the cervical vertebrae. Finally, because SI-6 is the cleft point of the channel, there may be a very thin nodule cutting across the channel here in acute low-back spasms (*tài yáng* channel affected).

The small intestine channel on the face and in front of the ears is often affected in cases of facial pain, Bell's palsy, or trigeminal neuralgia. Carefully palpate to determine the affected area for treatment. In acute cases of any of these conditions, it is best not to needle the face at all; only distal points should be used. Only after the initial inflammation has subsided (5–7 days) is it considered safe to lightly needle around the affected areas. In general, the small interweaving channels on the face are regarded as collaterals. Therefore, collateral *(luò)* points on all the channels passing through the area should be considered for treatment (in this case, SI-7) in both acute and chronic cases.

Tài Yáng Bladder Channel

Physiological significance of channel changes

Observation of areas related to *tài yáng* bladder

If the patient has fairly severe tightness in the neck or back that greatly inhibits movement, this is often due to excess cold or dampness in the channel. Redness and boils, on the other hand, generally indicate heat and blood congealing due to a lack of lively bladder qi transformation.

The presence of visible capillaries behind the knees at BL-40 *(wěi zhōng)* indicates blood stasis in the bladder channel or *dū* vessel. However, observable signs along the channel do not always mean that the bladder is an important part of the pathodynamic. For instance, the presence of small reddish papules or cysts along the bladder channel in the area between T_3 and T_7 might be indicative of heat from constraint in the upper burner (lungs and heart). Similarly, small red papules on the lower back may indicate heat in the large intestine—a sign often seen in patients with chronic inflammation or hemorrhoids.

Pulse palpation of areas related to *tài yáng* bladder

There are no special areas for palpating pulses along this channel.

Palpating the channel, pressing the points, and feeling the body surface

Any nodules, tenderness, weakness or increased muscle tone on the back transport points is indicative of some sort of dysfunction in the associated organs. Because of the warm, yang nature of the *tài yáng* channel, it is more likely to involve yang or qi deficiency. Because the area is also in close proximity to the yang-natured *dū* vessel and its collateral vessel along the important M-BW-35 (*Huá Tuō jiá jǐ*) points, a wide variety of palpable changes can be found in the area. In general, it is most helpful to keep the organs associated with each of the back transport points in mind when you find changes along the bladder channel on the back.

Tenderness at BL-64 *(jīng gǔ)*, the source point of the bladder, indicates qi deficiency of the channel. This is often seen in chronic back pain. Also, in cases of chronic back pain where blood stasis is involved, there may be a series of small, relatively hard nodules in this area.

On the other hand, the cleft *(xī)* point of the channel, BL-63 *(jīn mén)*, is reactive and very tender in cases of excess. Palpable change at the point is indicative of stagnation in the channel. Common symptoms include acute back pain, *tài yáng* channel headaches, and urinary or kidney stones.

Weakness or tenderness at BL-62 often indicates accumulation of cold-dampness in the sinew channels of the bladder. Because this point is also the command point of the *yáng qiāo* vessel, tenderness may indicate the involvement of the sinew channels of multiple channels.

Sinew problems may involve increased tightness or thickening of the fascia in the area between BL-57 and BL-58. This may include acute low back or neck spasms and/or tightness.

For acute back sprain, BL-40 *(wěi zhōng)*, the command point of the back, will show nodules, distended vessels, or a tightening of the surrounding tendons. In patients with chronic back problems, the area will look puffy and will usually feel quite soft when cold accumulation in the bladder channel is part of the pathodynamic. Nodules may also be found in this area in bladder-type (occipital) headaches. Because this is a uniting point on the channel, there may be palpable changes (or small, visible blood collaterals) here in the case of counterflow in the bladder channel. Commonly, counterflow in the bladder channel is seen in cases of summerheat that include nausea, vomiting, and headaches. In such cases, a few drops of blood should be directly removed from any visible blood collaterals. Finally, there may also be visible blood collaterals (that should be bled) in cases of hemorrhoids.

When there is a tumor or enlargement in one of the internal organs, the area between BL-36 *(chéng fú)* and BL-37 *(yīn mén)* may have deep nodules or tenderness when pressing deeply.

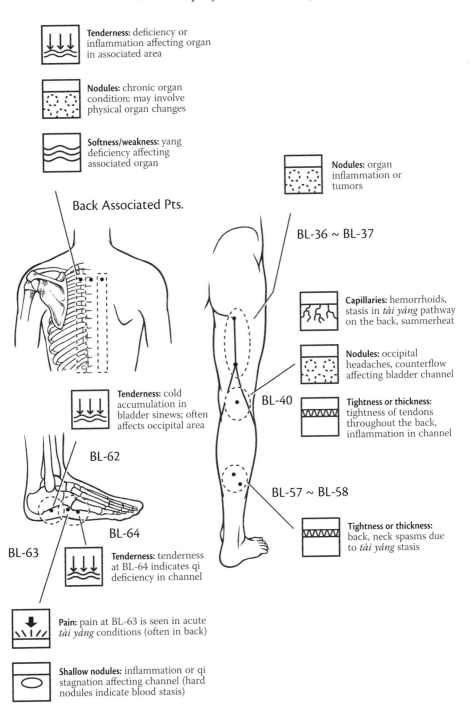

Tenderness: deficiency or inflammation affecting organ in associated area

Nodules: chronic organ condition; may involve physical organ changes

Softness/weakness: yang deficiency affecting associated organ

Nodules: organ inflammation or tumors

Back Associated Pts.

BL-36 ~ BL-37

Capillaries: hemorrhoids, stasis in *tài yáng* pathway on the back, summerheat

Nodules: occipital headaches, counterflow affecting bladder channel

BL-40

Tightness or thickness: tightness of tendons throughout the back, inflammation in channel

Tenderness: cold accumulation in bladder sinews; often affects occipital area

BL-62

BL-57 ~ BL-58

BL-64

BL-63

Tenderness: tenderness at BL-64 indicates qi deficiency in channel

Tightness or thickness: back, neck spasms due to *tài yáng* stasis

Pain: pain at BL-63 is seen in acute *tài yáng* conditions (often in back)

Shallow nodules: inflammation or qi stagnation affecting channel (hard nodules indicate blood stasis)

Fig. 13.7
Tài yáng bladder channel

Shào Yīn Kidney Channel

Channel changes and physiological significance

Observation of areas related to *shào yīn* kidney

The area along the channel between KI-3 *(tài xī)* and KI-7 *(fù liū)* will often present with dryness in cases of kidney yin deficiency. The skin in the area may also appear slightly scaly and a bit red in these cases.

Pulse palpation of areas related to *shào yīn* kidney

Palpation of the pulse at KI-3 can give an impression of the condition of kidney qi. In cases of kidney qi deficiency, the pulse at KI-3 will most often be deep and fine. The KI-3 pulse is also very helpful in diagnosing the cause of high blood pressure. Often, high blood pressure is caused by an underlying deficiency of kidney qi, leading to hyperactive yang. In cases where deficiency predominates—a weak, fine pulse at KI-3 can verify this diagnosis—the use of strong heat-clearing and downward-directing herbs might actually lead to a rise in blood pressure. In such cases, the treatment principle should therefore focus instead on strengthening the kidney. Tooth pain may also be caused by a similar kidney qi deficiency. In these cases, the deep, fine pulse at KI-3 might be combined with tenderness in the area. A strong pulsing at KI-16 *(huāng shū)* indicates a combination of kidney deficiency and strong pathogens. In such cases, the pathogen might be water, qi stagnation, or even blood stasis.

Palpating the channel, pressing the points, and feeling the body surface

Tenderness or small painful nodules in the area around KI-4 *(dà zhōng)* and KI-5 *(shuǐ quán)* is often found in the presence of kidney or urinary stones. This may also indicate urinary tract infection or prostatitis. Tenderness in this area (or around KI-3) may also indicate general kidney deficiency.

Tenderness around KI-6 *(zhào hǎi)* indicates swelling or inflammation in the throat or larynx. Recall that KI-6 is the meeting point of the *yīn qiāo* vessel, which travels through the throat. Because the *yīn qiāo* is also responsible for integrating muscle movement among multiple channel sinews, this area may also show small nodules in chronic conditions affecting multiple channels on the leg.

Weakness, softness, and/or tenderness around KI-7 and KI-8 *(jiāo xìn)* is often indicative of fire due to yin deficiency. Symptoms may include tooth pain, mouth sores, or even such emotional signs as irritability, restlessness, prone to crying, or insomnia. Because this area reflects the quality of kidney yin, there is often also tenderness in the presence of allergic and autoim-

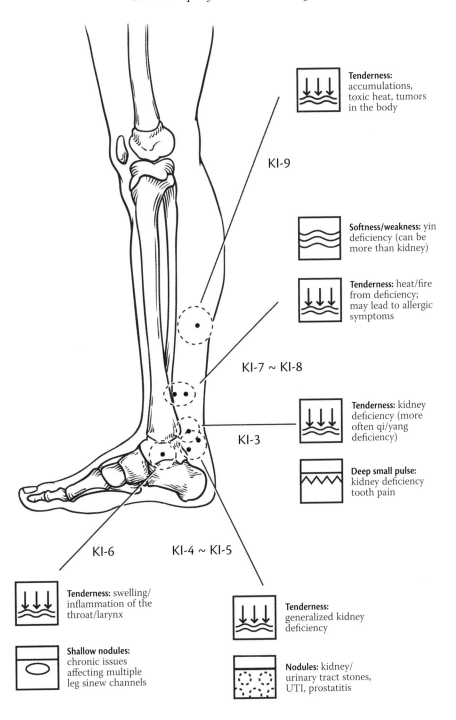

Tenderness:
accumulations,
toxic heat, tumors
in the body

KI-9

Softness/weakness: yin
deficiency (can be
more than kidney)

Tenderness: heat/fire
from deficiency;
may lead to allergic
symptoms

KI-7 ~ KI-8

Tenderness: kidney
deficiency (more
often qi/yang
deficiency)

KI-3

Deep small pulse:
kidney deficiency
tooth pain

KI-6   KI-4 ~ KI-5

Tenderness: swelling/
inflammation of the
throat/larynx

Tenderness:
generalized kidney
deficiency

Shallow nodules:
chronic issues
affecting multiple
leg sinew channels

Nodules: kidney/
urinary tract stones,
UTI, prostatitis

Fig. 13.8
Shào yīn kidney channel

mune conditions (including allergic rhinitis and asthma) when the pathodynamic includes a deficiency of kidney yin.

The area around KI-9 *(zhú bīn)* may be tender when there are tumors in the body. KI-9 is the cleft point of the *yīn wéi* vessel, the integrator of yin circulation to the areas beyond the flow of the regular channels. Because some types of tumors may be thought of as accumulations of phlegm, the cleft point of the channel can be indicative of problems of this type. This area may also be tender in autoimmune conditions similar to the ones described above.

Jué Yīn Pericardium Channel

Physiological significance of channel changes

Observation of areas related to *jué yīn* pericardium

The pericardium channel has no areas of unique significance for observation.

Pulse palpation of areas related to *jué yīn* pericardium

There are no special considerations for palpating the pulse along the pericardium channel.

Palpating the channel, pressing the points, and feeling the body surface

Pain in the area between PC-7 *(dà líng)* and PC-6 *(nèi guān)*, often sharp and distended, may indicate heat from constraint in the upper burner, and often corresponds to such symptoms as irritability, insomnia, and/or headaches. There may also be graininess in this area when there are stomach problems *(yīn wéi* vessel-type problems with internal organ nourishment).

Tenderness or pain around PC-5 *(jiān shǐ)* often coincides with chest pain or distention around CV-12 *(zhōng wǎn)* that can also lead to irritability or restlessness. This is considered to be stagnation of phlegm. In fact, many psychological conditions will coincide with palpable changes in this area—especially when the pressures of life are the cause. This point is often used in treatment. The area rarely has nodules, but instead may show tenderness or a change in the quality of the subcutaneous fascia that involves a sense of 'crunchiness.'

The area around and above PC-4 *(xī mén)* will often be tight or inflexible when there is blood stasis in the collateral vessels of the pericardium. This often involves problems with circulation of blood to the heart organ. In more severe cases, there may even be a deep, hard nodule in the area. If there is only a general swelling and/or thickening of the fascia, it is easier to treat. Deep, hard nodules indicate a more serious condition, which is often

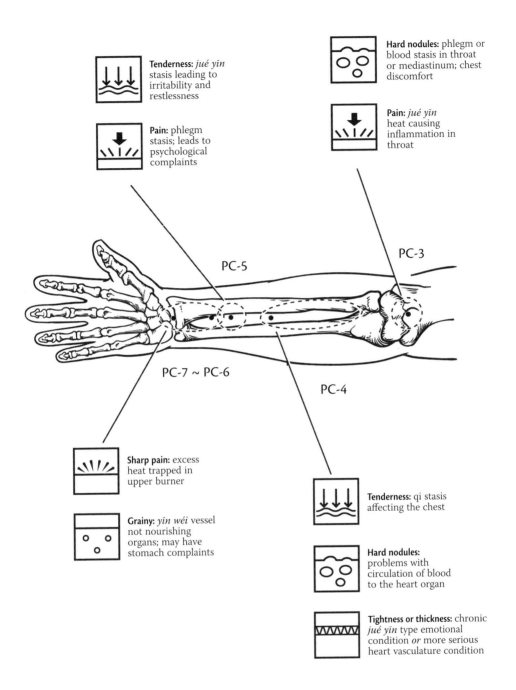

Tenderness: *jué yīn* stasis leading to irritability and restlessness

Pain: phlegm stasis; leads to psychological complaints

Hard nodules: phlegm or blood stasis in throat or mediastinum; chest discomfort

Pain: *jué yīn* heat causing inflammation in throat

PC-5

PC-3

PC-7 ~ PC-6

PC-4

Sharp pain: excess heat trapped in upper burner

Grainy: *yīn wéi* vessel not nourishing organs; may have stomach complaints

Tenderness: qi stasis affecting the chest

Hard nodules: problems with circulation of blood to the heart organ

Tightness or thickness: chronic *jué yīn* type emotional condition *or* more serious heart vasculature condition

Fig. 13.9
Jué yīn pericardium channel

unresponsive to treatment with acupuncture and herbs.

Pain or hard nodules around PC-3 *(qū zé)* often indicates phlegm or blood stasis in the throat or mediastinum; this is often accompanied by chest discomfort. If the nodule is quite hard, this may indicate the presence of growths or other physical changes in the throat.

Shào Yáng Triple Burner Channel

Physiological significance of channel changes

Observation of areas related to *shào yáng* triple burner

In general, because the *shào yáng* channel has "an abundance of qi but a dearth of blood," it tends to generate heat. When observing the channel, especially on the neck and shoulders around TB-15 *(tiān liáo)* to TB-17 *(yì fēng)*, one should look for redness, small papules, or acne, which indicates an accumulation of heat in the channel.

Pulse palpation of areas related to *shào yáng* triple burner

There are no special considerations for palpating the pulse along this channel.

Palpating the channel, pressing the points, and feeling the body surface

In many patients there may be a generalized bumpiness all along the triple burner channel on the forearm. The channel will feel somewhat like one is bouncing along an unpaved road. This sensation is indicative of generalized heat accumulation in the triple burner (ministerial fire). Clinically, it often coincides with conditions of chronic, systemic inflammation and/or some type of autoimmune condition. The pathways of the triple burner have been blocked by stagnation of qi and/or accumulation of phlegm. Alternatively, very soft nodules all along the forearm may indicate a deficiency of source qi and an accumulation of cold in the triple burner pathways.

Tenderness in the area around TB-2 *(yè mén)* and TB-3 *(zhōng zhǔ)* indicates qi stagnation leading to compromised dispersion of warmth from the *shào yáng*. Although many types of qi stagnation may produce changes in this area, the changes most often appear when there is back pain, especially pain due to cold accumulation in the muscles of the low back. This is due to compromised circulation of source qi affecting the gate of vitality area on the back. The area may also be tender in the presence of heat in the *shào yáng* channel affecting the ears. Symptoms may include earache, excessive wax, or a sensation that the ears are clogged.

There will often be a deep aching sensation with pressure at TB-4 *(yáng chí)* in the presence of yang qi deficiency. This often involves deficiency of

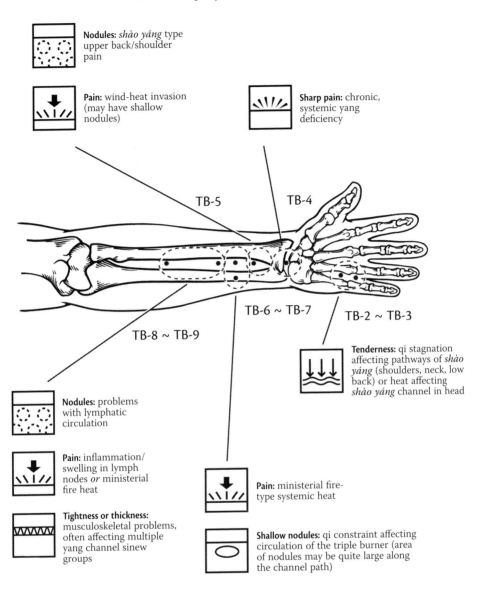

Nodules: *shào yáng* type upper back/shoulder pain

Pain: wind-heat invasion (may have shallow nodules)

Sharp pain: chronic, systemic yang deficiency

TB-5   TB-4

TB-8 ~ TB-9

TB-6 ~ TB-7

TB-2 ~ TB-3

Tenderness: qi stagnation affecting pathways of *shào yáng* (shoulders, neck, low back) or heat affecting *shào yáng* channel in head

Nodules: problems with lymphatic circulation

Pain: inflammation/ swelling in lymph nodes *or* ministerial fire heat

Tightness or thickness: musculoskeletal problems, often affecting multiple yang channel sinew groups

Pain: ministerial fire-type systemic heat

Shallow nodules: qi constraint affecting circulation of the triple burner (area of nodules may be quite large along the channel path)

Fig. 13.10
Shào yáng triple burner channel

yang qi in the extremities—typically spleen-kidney yang deficiency—with symptoms of coldness and/or numbness. Moxa or needles may be used in treatment.

Pain, tightness, or nodules around TB-5 *(wài guān)* may indicate invasion by external wind-heat in the *shào yáng* channel. Symptoms may include wind-heat exterior patterns, headache, redness in the eyes (including pink eye), tinnitus, or even sudden deafness. Nodules can often be found around TB-5 in cases of upper shoulder or back pain involving the *shào yáng* channel.

The area around TB-6 *(zhī gōu)* and TB-7 *(huì zōng)* is important in diagnosis. Chronic conditions that involve triple burner function begin to show as one moves up the channel. Pain or shallow nodules in this area indicate qi constraint (氣鬱 *qì yù*) in the *shào yáng;* this is a more serious condition than qi stagnation (氣滯 *qì zhì*), which is reflected diagnostically around TB-2 and TB-3. Symptoms may include pain throughout the body, constipation, irregular or painful menses, vaginal discharge, or the variety of symptoms associated with ministerial fire described in Chapter 6.

TB-8 *(sān yáng luò)* and TB-9 *(sì dú)* will often show tenderness and/or nodules when there are problems with lymph circulation. This may include infection or swelling in nodes in the armpit, neck, or throat. In addition, because TB-8 is a meeting point for the sinew channels of the three arm yang channels, there may be notable tightness in this area when a musculoskeletal condition is affecting all three arm yang channels. This may be seen, for example, in some types of facial paralysis or problems with numbness, weakness, or pain in the upper extremities.

Shào Yáng Gallbladder Channel

Physiological significance of channel changes

Observation of areas related to *shào yáng* gallbladder

The outer canthus of the eye is often red and/or swollen in the presence of wind-heat in the gallbladder channel.

Pulse palpation of areas related to *shào yáng* gallbladder

There are no special considerations for palpating pulses along this channel.

Palpating the channel, pressing the points, and feeling the body surface

Tenderness in the area between GB-41 *(zú lín qì)* and GB-43 *(xiá xī)* often indicates gallbladder channel or organ heat (ministerial fire). The more prevalent the nodules in the area, the more likely that dampness is also a significant factor.

Nodules or tightness in the fascia around GB-40 *(qiū xū)* is often indicative of gallbladder fire counterflow (膽火逆 *dǎn huǒ nì*). The area will also be severely tender in the presence of stones in the gallbladder or an inflam-

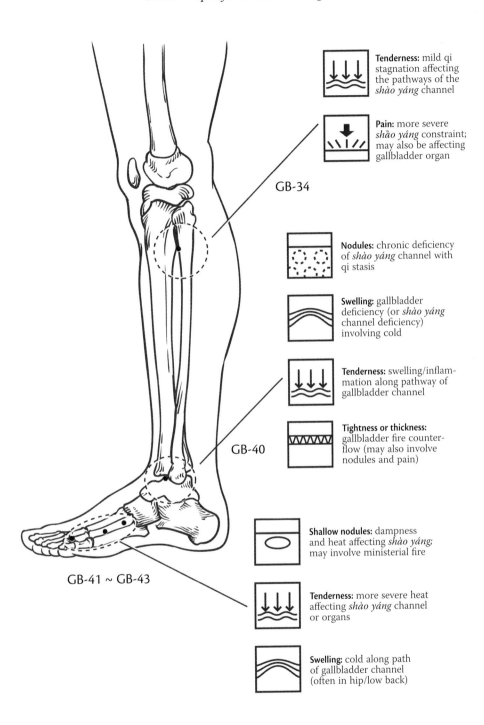

Tenderness: mild qi stagnation affecting the pathways of the *shào yáng* channel

Pain: more severe *shào yáng* constraint; may also be affecting gallbladder organ

GB-34

Nodules: chronic deficiency of *shào yáng* channel with qi stasis

Swelling: gallbladder deficiency (or *shào yáng* channel deficiency) involving cold

Tenderness: swelling/inflammation along pathway of gallbladder channel

Tightness or thickness: gallbladder fire counterflow (may also involve nodules and pain)

GB-40

Shallow nodules: dampness and heat affecting *shào yáng;* may involve ministerial fire

Tenderness: more severe heat affecting *shào yáng* channel or organs

Swelling: cold along path of gallbladder channel (often in hip/low back)

GB-41 ~ GB-43

Fig. 13.11
Shào yáng gallbladder channel

mation of the gallbladder organ (cholecystitis). GB-40 can also become puffy and slightly swollen in the presence of *shào yáng* qi deficiency or accumulation of cold in the gallbladder. Because GB-40 is the source point, conditions that manifest with changes in this area are most often rooted in deficiency.

Qi constraint in the gallbladder channel often manifests as tenderness or pain at GB-34 *(yáng líng quán)*. This can lead to a wide variety of problems ranging from shoulder pain, neck stiffness, and sciatica to internal conditions such as hepatitis, irritable bowel syndrome (when the liver overacting on the spleen is primary), or gallstones. *Shào yáng* type constipation also may coincide with tenderness in this area.

Jué Yīn Liver Channel

Physiological significance of channel changes

Observation of areas related to *jué yīn* liver

If the eyes experience problems with movement or are crossed, this may indicate a lack of proper nourishment of the tendons of the eye from the liver.

Pulse palpation of areas related to *jué yīn* liver

There are no special considerations for palpating pulses along this channel.

Palpating the channel, pressing the points, and feeling the body surface

Pain or tenderness at LR-2 *(xíng jiān)* can be found in the presence of liver heat, especially when related to eye conditions; if it is tender, this point may be used in the treatment of the condition. Increased interocular pressure may also manifest as tenderness in this area. Note that eye conditions may be reflected in palpable change on not just the liver channel, but also often on the spleen and small intestine channels as well. Graininess felt in the area of LR-2 may indicate qi stagnation and/or blood stasis in the liver channel.

Nodules around LR-3 *(tài chōng)* often indicate qi stagnation in the liver channel. In some cases, instead of clearly-defined, larger nodules one might instead find multiple smaller nodules. In such cases, this represents more of a deficiency of liver function in not properly directing qi. This type of change often coincides with spleen dysfunction brought about by liver-spleen disharmony, and is a type of combined excess and deficiency. If there is generalized tightness in the area around LR-3, this is a less serious case of liver qi stagnation.

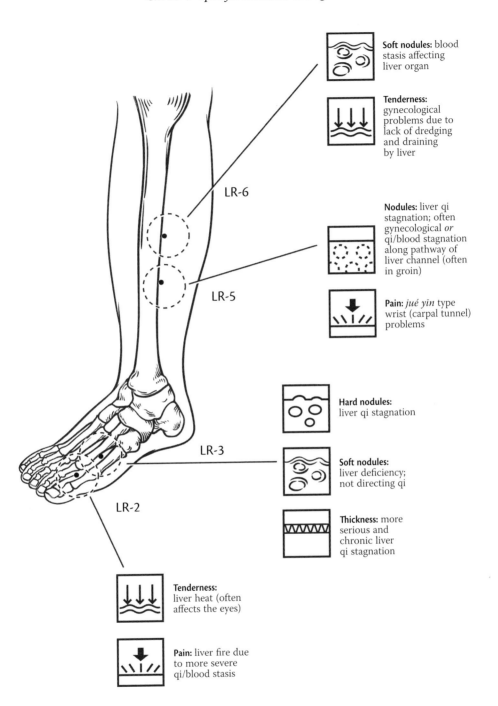

Soft nodules: blood stasis affecting liver organ

Tenderness: gynecological problems due to lack of dredging and draining by liver

Nodules: liver qi stagnation; often gynecological *or* qi/blood stagnation along pathway of liver channel (often in groin)

Pain: *jué yīn* type wrist (carpal tunnel) problems

Hard nodules: liver qi stagnation

Soft nodules: liver deficiency; not directing qi

Thickness: more serious and chronic liver qi stagnation

Tenderness: liver heat (often affects the eyes)

Pain: liver fire due to more severe qi/blood stasis

LR-6

LR-5

LR-3

LR-2

Fig. 13.12
Jué yīn liver channel

If nodules or tenderness with pressure is noted in the area around LR-5 *(lǐ gōu)*, this indicates qi stagnation and is often associated with *jué yīn* type menstrual irregularities, especially during menopause. In addition, in carpal tunnel patterns where the *jué yīn* pericardium channel is involved, there will be extreme tenderness in this area. When this occurs, the point should be needled as part of the treatment.

Small, soft nodules around LR-6 *(zhōng dū)* often indicate blood stasis in the collaterals of the liver. Changes in this area are often seen in conjunction with cirrhosis of the liver.

The area will also often show severe tenderness in cases of painful menstruation due to lack of proper dredging and draining by the liver.

Dū Vessel

Considerations of the *dū* vessel also involve the region associated with the M-BW-35 *(Huá Tuō jiá jǐ)* points. As noted earlier, these points are actually located on a collateral of the *dū* vessel.

Observation of areas related to the *dū*

Observation of the condition of the skin over the spine at the level of each back transport point can provide clues to the condition of the qi dynamic in the organs. In general, dryness indicates deficiency while small red macules or raised papules indicate heat or stasis of blood.

Pulse palpation of areas related to the *dū*

There are no special pulse considerations for palpating pulses along this vessel.

Palpating the channel, pressing the points, and feeling the body surface

In considering the twelve regular channels, palpation was discussed only on the distal limbs. For the *rèn* and *dū* vessels, however, palpation of the pathways on the body trunk can provide important diagnostic information. In general, changes found at *dū* vessel points should also be considered in the context of the organ associations indicated by the nearby back transport points. For example, tenderness or a thickening between the vertebrae found at GV-12 *(shēn zhù)* might indicate a pathodynamic of the upper burner in general or, alternatively, a specific condition affecting the lung organ. (BL-13, *[fèi shū]* is also found at the level of T₃.)

The first area to consider when palpating along the *dū* vessel is the head. If tenderness or pain is found when palpating the area between GV-19 *(qián dǐng)* and GV-21 *(hòu dǐng)*, this indicates an overall lack of smooth circulation in the *dū* vessel. The cause may be stagnation, deficiency, or cold. Symptoms might include low back pain, neck pain, headaches, dizziness, emotional conditions, or even insomnia.

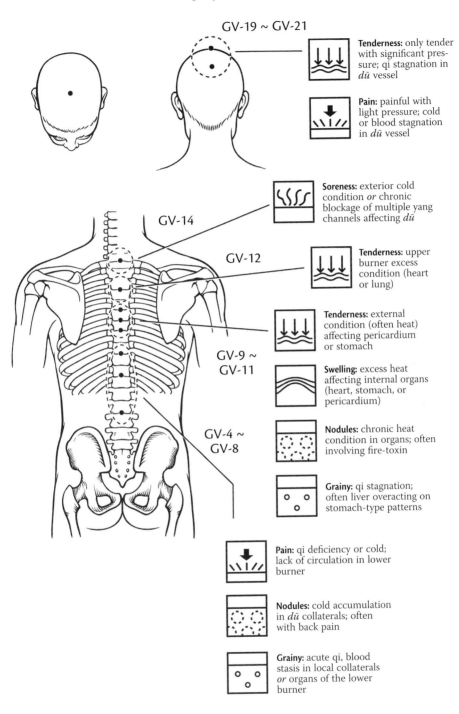

GV-19 ~ GV-21

Tenderness: only tender with significant pressure; qi stagnation in *dū* vessel

Pain: painful with light pressure; cold or blood stagnation in *dū* vessel

GV-14

Soreness: exterior cold condition *or* chronic blockage of multiple yang channels affecting *dū*

GV-12

Tenderness: upper burner excess condition (heart or lung)

Tenderness: external condition (often heat) affecting pericardium or stomach

GV-9 ~ GV-11

Swelling: excess heat affecting internal organs (heart, stomach, or pericardium)

Nodules: chronic heat condition in organs; often involving fire-toxin

GV-4 ~ GV-8

Grainy: qi stagnation; often liver overacting on stomach-type patterns

Pain: qi deficiency or cold; lack of circulation in lower burner

Nodules: cold accumulation in *dū* collaterals; often with back pain

Grainy: acute qi, blood stasis in local collaterals *or* organs of the lower burner

Fig. 13.13
Dū vessel

Soreness or a thickening of the intervertebral space around GV-14 *(dà zhuī)* indicates blockage of the yang channels. While this is most commonly seen in exterior wind-cold patterns, there is also a tendency for this area to become tender in cases of chronic cold accumulation in the collaterals of the *dū* vessel. Symptoms associated with this pattern may include back pain, stiffness, or a cold sensation in the body.

Tenderness at GV-12 *(shēn zhù)* often indicates qi deficiency in the upper burner, which includes both the lung qi and the gathering qi (宗氣 *zōng qì)*.

Palpated changes around GV-11 *(shén dào)*, GV-10 *(líng tái)*, and GV-9 *(zhì yáng)* generally follow two patterns. If there is tenderness in the area, this generally indicates external heat or a combination of heat and cold, usually in the heart, pericardium, or stomach. If, on the other hand, the area is swollen or has nodules (not necessarily red), this indicates a more severe case involving fire toxin in the internal organs. Note that the nodules may be along the top of the vertebrae when palpating the *dū* vessel, while tenderness is generally found between the vertebrae.

The area around GV-8 *(jīn suō)*, GV-6 *(jǐ zhōng)*, or GV-4 *(mìng mén)* will have pain or very small nodules along the top of the vertebrae in the presence of back pain due to cold or blood stasis in the *dū* vessel.

The sacrum will present with a variety of palpable changes in the presence of gynecological problems or emotional conditions (including insomnia) due to constraint (鬱 *yù)*. These patterns often involve a deficiency of yang.

Rèn Vessel

Observation of areas related to the *rèn*

There are no special considerations for observing the *rèn*.

Pulse palpation of areas related to the *rèn*

On the *rèn* vessel, the first pulse to consider is CV-12 *(zhōng wǎn)*. Deep to this point, one can find the descending aorta. When palpating this area the pulse should generally be difficult to find. Strong pulsing at CV-12, known classically as pulsing beneath the heart (心下動脈 *xīn xià dòng mài)*, most often indicates a condition of excess in the spleen-stomach. Another pulse of significance can be found at CV-6 *(qì hǎi)*. This pulse should not be felt at all on the surface, and should be flexible but noticeable at the middle and deep levels. A very firm and strong pulse at CV-6 generally indicates cold or stagnation in the lower burner. Weakness at the CV-6 pulse indicates kidney deficiency.

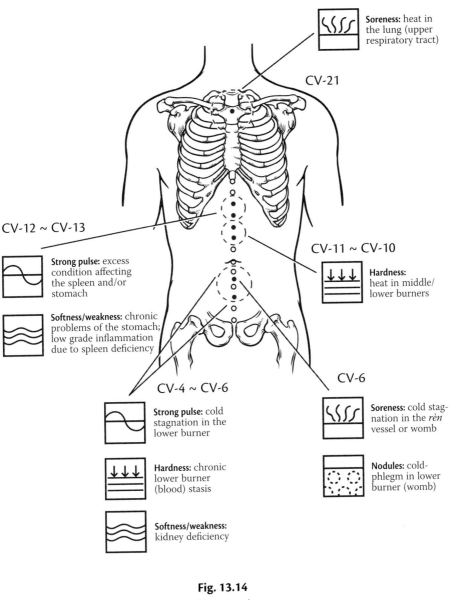

Soreness: heat in the lung (upper respiratory tract)

CV-21

CV-12 ~ CV-13

Strong pulse: excess condition affecting the spleen and/or stomach

Softness/weakness: chronic problems of the stomach; low grade inflammation due to spleen deficiency

CV-11 ~ CV-10

Hardness: heat in middle/ lower burners

CV-4 ~ CV-6

Strong pulse: cold stagnation in the lower burner

Hardness: chronic lower burner (blood) stasis

Softness/weakness: kidney deficiency

CV-6

Soreness: cold stagnation in the *rèn* vessel or womb

Nodules: cold-phlegm in lower burner (womb)

Fig. 13.14
Rèn vessel

Palpating the channel, pressing the points, and feeling the body surface

Tenderness is often found at CV-21 *(xuán jī)* when there is inflammation in the upper respiratory tract.

If there is tightness or a tendency to spasms around CV-14 *(jù què)*, this may indicate problems with the diaphragm that can present as heart-type pain.

Softness or tender nodules found in the area of CV-13 *(shàng wǎn)* or CV-12 *(zhōng wǎn)* may indicate chronic stomach problems (often gastritis). In such cases there is often a lack of proper ascending and descending by the spleen. Lack of proper transformation, over time, leads to dampness and possibly heat accumulation that can be palpated in the area.

Hardness felt around CV-11 *(jiàn lǐ)* and CV-10 *(xià wǎn)* may indicate heat in the middle and lower burners. Symptoms might include a stomach or duodenal ulcer, or inflammation of the intestines (colitis, diverticulitis, or Crohn's disease).

Tenderness or mild swelling around CV-6 *(qì hǎi)* or CV-4 *(guān yuán)* is often seen in gynecological, bowel, or urinary problems caused by accumulation of cold in the *rèn* vessel or womb.

If pain is very severe at any of the *rèn* vessel points, it is not advisable to needle in the area. Instead, one should consider 'downstream' points on the three yin channels of the legs, especially the cleft points, to help drain accumulation in the channel.

Conclusion

In this chapter we have sketched some broad outlines of channel diagnosis. Because the details vary quite significantly from patient to patient, there is still much more that careful palpation can reveal. Over time, the practitioner will begin to discern patterns in palpation. In fact, more extensive experience with palpation will likely lead to a sense of which point prescriptions are best for treating certain types of palpated channel change. Because changes in the channels fundamentally reflect changes in the qi dynamic, experience will gradually reveal that these channel changes actually represent physiology at the level of subtle perception. In the next chapter we will begin to explore the process by which an experienced practitioner can choose a channel for treatment based on the findings of palpation.

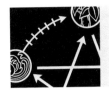

CHAPTER 14

Selecting Channels for Treatment

AFTER THE CHANNELS have been palpated, the next step is to determine which channel is most involved in the chief complaint. This means evaluating the palpated changes in the channels in the context of the patient's presenting symptom pattern. Only then can one choose the best channel on which to focus treatment.

In this chapter we will describe a two-step process. The first step is to determine the affected channel in a given complaint, known as channel differentiation (經絡診斷 *jīng luò zhěn duàn*). The second step is to select the primary channel for treatment, known as channel selection (選經 *xuǎn jīng*). Before describing these steps, a few general issues should be addressed regarding channel therapy in the clinic.

Integrating Palpable Changes in the Clinic

As noted in the previous chapter, one often finds in the clinic that many channels will present with palpable changes. Usually, the channel with the most obvious changes will be most directly involved in the patient's chief complaint. Quite frequently, however, the practitioner is faced with a group of channels with palpable changes, and the trick is to determine which among them is most likely to be involved in the symptom pattern at hand.

The process of ascertaining which of the channels is most affected in a particular complaint is like doing detective work. By combining classical concepts of channel and organ physiology with information gleaned through differential diagnosis (primarily by asking questions), the practitioner can narrow the selection down to a few primary suspects. Palpation along the course of these channels then serves to validate or modify the initial hypothesis. Once the case is clearer and the primarily affected channel has been identified, the focus can then turn to considerations of selecting channels for treatment and, eventually, to the selection of specific points.

In order to determine the main organs that are involved, the first step is traditional organ pattern differentiation. In other words, the patient interview (and radial pulse palpation) should precede channel palpation. The organ diagnosis will lead to a hypothesis of the likely pathodynamic. The next step involves the evaluation of suspected channels to verify the hypothesis. If the channels and/or organs identified through organ diagnosis match the changes discerned along the course of the channels, then one can fairly easily identify the affected channel(s). Selection of channels and points for treatment can then proceed. In most cases, careful palpation of three or four channels is sufficient to determine the affected channel. However, with new patients, or for novice practitioners, the process may go more slowly. For practitioners who are just beginning to integrate channel palpation into their diagnostic approach, the more thoroughly the channel system is evaluated, the better. Again, one often finds that it takes awhile to begin to know which changes are normal and which may be indicative of channel pathology. Moreover, sometimes the channel diagnosis does not match the organ diagnosis. This will be discussed below.

The 'clinical encounter' first mentioned in Chapter 3 describes the sevenpart process that may be said to constitute an acupuncture visit (Fig. 14.1).

In earlier chapters we introduced the concept of channel diagnosis and discussed palpation techniques. In this chapter we will describe techniques for both channel differentiation and the selection of channels for treatment. Channel differentiation involves developing strategies to analyze the sometimes confusing findings that were gleaned from channel palpation. This helps us identify which channel is primarily involved in a given pathodynamic at the time the patient presents at the clinic. Selecting the appropriate channel for treatment then follows.

One may be tempted to think that channel 'differentiation' and channel 'selection' are one and the same. In fact, it does seem reasonable to assume that, once one has identified the affected channel(s), treatment would involve little more than choosing points from those channels based on their ability to affect qi transformation. However, clinical application often requires more complex considerations. In order to get the best results, the practitioner must bring to bear an understanding of qi transformation and other aspects of classical physiology. For example, consider a patient who presents with symptoms indicating a lack of dredging and draining by the

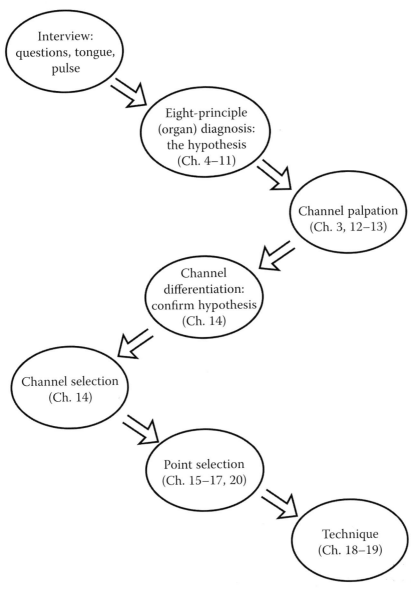

Fig. 14.1
The clinical encounter and related chapters in this book

liver (肝不疏瀉 *gān bù shū xiè*) such as irritability, hypochondriac discomfort, and digestive complaints associated with an emotional state. In the clinic, the most effective channel to treat this type of yin channel excess is not the *jué yīn* liver channel. Instead, effective treatment would most often mean choosing points from the paired *shào yáng* triple burner and gallbladder channels, discussed in Chapter 7. This is just one fairly simple example of what is often a rather complex mental process. Once one becomes used to the process, however, it is quite natural and interesting.

Again, the affected channel is not always the best one for treatment because effective point selection requires that one consider the qi transformation of the channel system as a whole. This is what is meant in the *Divine Pivot* when it says that a great doctor treats disease by using needles with an elegance that is like "wiping dirt off the skin or untying a knot"[1] (Fig. 14.2).

Step 1: Channel Differentiation

Integrate the information gleaned from the patient interview with subjective information from pulse and channel palpation. You are looking for the channel most affected at the current time.

Step 2: Channel Selection

After identifying the most affected channel, consider qi transformation in the channels to select a primary channel for treatment. You are now selecting a channel that will help change the pathodynamic in the future.

Fig. 14.2
Two steps in channel treatment

Step One: Channel Differentiation

Channel differentiation is the process of identifying the primary channel(s) that is affected in a particular pattern. The need to differentiate arises from the fact that not all channels with palpable change are necessarily involved.

To differentiate among the channels, one must first note the nature of the changes on the channels and how changes on one channel contrast with changes on others. This is the process that was followed in the last chapter, where the significance of changes along each of the channels was considered. The specific conditions and the likely reflection areas along the channels described in the previous chapter represents the ideal scenario. In other words, if one has ascertained a particular chief complaint and/or symptom pattern and then finds palpable changes in the areas associated with that pattern (as described in Chapter 13), one can then be fairly confident that the most affected channel has been found. As often as not, however, diagnosis will be somewhat more complex than this. Nevertheless, when palpation has revealed a variety of changes, possibly along multiple channel pathways, other steps can be taken to narrow down the likely location of disease. The next step in this process involves the evaluation of changes in the context of the channel system as a whole.

Let us consider a few of the common difficulties which are encountered when looking at the larger picture.

A channel may hold 'memories'.

Analogous to scars left over from a long-ago injury, the channel system may contain significant palpable changes that reflect a condition from the past. This may be a disease from which the patient has only recently recovered, or signs of a fairly severe disease from many years before. These 'memories' should be kept in mind when palpating the channels, especially on a new patient, and a careful history should be taken so as to rule them in or out of the chief complaint at hand.

Some channel changes may reflect an unrelated but ongoing condition.

Like the 'memories' of past conditions, other palpated changes in a patient may be related to an ongoing condition that is less directly involved in the patient's chief complaint. For example, the patient may not have recovered from a chronic condition that is now woven into the current channel presentation.

The channel reflecting the chronic condition may not be the primary channel in the patient's chief complaint. Patients with chronic lung problems, for example, may show changes along the lung channel even when there are no clear lung symptoms as part of the current chief complaint. In such cases, a patient may appear to have two separate channel disharmonies at the same time. It is the practitioner's responsibility to determine which channel is most closely associated with the symptom pattern of the chief complaint. Once again, carefully taking the patient's history is crucial to correct diagnosis.

When multiple channels are actually involved in the chief complaint, it may be difficult to determine which is the most important channel.

This is the most challenging type of case. As all practitioners are aware, a patient's chief complaint is rarely so simple as to involve only one channel or organ. Unlike the situation described just above, this represents the common situation of a complex pathodynamic involving multiple channels. This next section will discuss the most commonly used approach for untying these difficult clinical knots.

DIFFERENTIATING WHEN MULTIPLE CHANNELS ARE INVOLVED

Because the channels are interconnected, a problem in one channel can spill over into others. Acute or relatively recent disorders may generally stay within the confines of a particular organ or same-name channel pair. When disease lingers or develops slowly, however, the physiology of multiple organs and channels is readily affected. Nevertheless, even with a complex pathodynamic it is often possible to identify the primary channel; differentiation requires the practitioner to do so.

The process of differentiation in such cases is a combination of logic and the insight born of experience. As noted above, it involves consideration of the results of channel palpation in the context of a suspected disease pattern based on differential diagnosis. The following case study provides a concrete example of this process.

■ Case Study

51-year-old female

Chief complaint   Weight gain/lethargy

Presentation   The patient was a military nurse with both an active career and a high school-aged child. In recent years, she felt her energy decline significantly and, although her life was busy, she felt that the decline in energy involved more than a lack of rest. Even rest and exercise had failed to relieve her lethargy. The patient started to become perimenopausal three years earlier, without severe symptoms. She had continued to have very irregular periods (2–3 times over the previous 12 months) when she came to the clinic. In addition, she had gained approximately 6 kg (13 lbs) over the previous 16 months.

The patient also reported that her sleep was sometimes "not deep enough" and that she occasionally woke early in the morning and was unable to get back to sleep. While her digestion was normal (no bloating or gas after eating, and a normal appetite), she did have a tendency toward constipation. This tendency was kept in check by eating plenty of fruit and leafy vegetables and the occasional use of mild laxatives. She reported frequent urination during the day (4–6 times/day). Some years ago, a complete physical exam revealed a mild atrial tachycardia, but she reported feeling no symptoms of this condition. In addition, a recent medical exam revealed elevated LDL cholesterol levels (numbers not available).

Upon presentation, the patient appeared fairly healthy, slightly overweight, and with a slightly dark complexion. Her pulse was generally wiry, submerged, and slightly thin. Her tongue was regular in size, with some tooth marks, and a slight darkening of the tongue body on the sides.

Channel palpation Thorough channel palpation revealed notable changes on five channels:

Tài yīn lung

Palpating along the lung channel, a deep, hard, slightly mobile nodule was found in the area around LU-6 *(kǒng zuì)*. When this nodule was found, the patient was asked about the condition of her lungs. She reported having no shortness of breath or difficulty with breathing, allergies, or with the nose. However, she did report a very severe case of pneumonia in her high school years that had required more than a month for recovery.

Shào yīn heart

A small, soft, bubble-like nodule was found in the area around HT-7 *(shén mén)* while a longer stick-like nodule was palpated cutting across the channel in the area around HT-5 *(tōng lǐ)*.

Shào yīn kidney

The kidney channel in the area between KI-3 *(tài xī)* and KI-5 *(shuǐ quán)* was slightly puffy and tender when pressed.

Jué yīn liver

The area around LR-3 *(tài chōng)* revealed a region of small, soft nodules throughout (possibly 10 small nodules in the area). The liver channel along the anterior edge of the tibia was also tender.

Shào yáng gallbladder

There was a generalized puffiness in the area between GB-40 *(qiū xū)* and GB-41 *(zú lín qì)*. The area felt as if there was slight edema.

Analysis The patient presented with a constellation of signs and symptoms and palpable changes on five channels. The following discussion will consider the palpated changes in groups.

Group 1: lung channel

The palpated change in the area around LU-6 is a memory of a past condition—possibly the childhood pneumonia. Although the change is deep and hard, it is still relatively movable and not painful when pressed. Because the palpated change is quite deep and not tender, it is more likely related to her past condition and was therefore not considered to be relevant to the current condition.

GROUP 1: **lung channel**

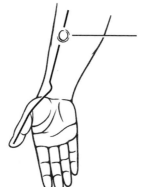

A deep nodule, relatively mobile, palpated at LU-6 *(kǒng zuì)* is indicative of a chronic condition less directly related to the current chief complaint.

GROUP 2: **heart and kidney channels**

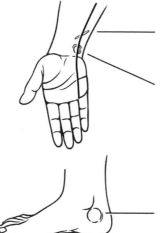

A stick-like nodule cutting across the channel near HT-5 *(tōng lǐ)* is likely related to sleep problems.

Softer bubble-like nodule at HT-7 *(shén mén)* is likely related to the chronic irregular heartbeat.

Soft puffiness in the area of KI-3 *(tài xī)* ~ KI-5 *(shuǐ quán)* indicates mild kidney deficiency and relates to the frequent urination.

GROUP 3: **liver and gallbladder channels**

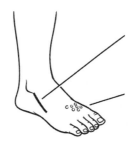

Puffiness in the area of GB-40 *(qiū xū)* ~ GB-41 *(zú lín qì)* suggests gallbladder qi stagnation.

Multiple diffuse small, soft nodules in the area of LR-3 *(tài chōng)* indicate (liver qi) deficiency.

Fig. 14.3
Notable changes in channel palpation, considered in three groups

Group 2: heart and kidney channels

A variety of information is conveyed by the changes felt on these two channels. There are two significant areas of change on the heart channel. The first, at HT-7, is most often associated with more chronic or congenital problems with the heart conduction system (or chronic heart-type emotional conditions). Therefore, it was concluded that the changes in this area likely reflect the tendency to tachycardia, a more chronic 'source point-type' condition. On the other hand, the thin, stick-like change cutting across the heart channel in the area of HT-6 is more related to the patient's tendency to have problems with sleep (recall that stick-like changes are often related to stagnation of qi, usually a less serious condition). At the same time, a puffy tenderness was noted in the area between KI-3 and KI-5. Here, this reflects a deficiency of kidney qi (the patient did not report feeling cold, a possible indicator of kidney yang deficiency).

The overall condition of the heart and kidney channels, together with the symptoms of frequent urination and a tendency to mild sleep problems, indicates a condition of heart-kidney not communicating (心肾不交 *xīn shèn bù jiāo*). Although this can often be an important primary diagnosis, in this case it is a less important aspect of the patient's chief complaint. Obviously, in a perimenopausal woman, there may be an aspect of kidney deficiency when the chief complaint is lethargy (more likely to be spleen, however). In addition, in this patient, the absence of strong kidney symptoms and a relatively strong kidney pulse seem to place the *shào yīn* condition more in the background—at least for the initial treatments.

Group 3: liver and gallbladder channels

The changes on the liver and gallbladder channels were considered together, given the internal-external pairing of the two organs. Changes on both channels involved a sense of relative softness/puffiness. In general, these are signs of deficiency.

After considering the interaction of symptoms and palpated changes in this case, an initial diagnosis was given of liver-gallbladder disharmony. More specifically, the condition was thought to most clearly involve a weakening of the dredging and draining (疏瀉 *shū xiè*) function of the liver that led to compromised gallbladder function. Over time, the deficiency in the yin organ (liver) led to a kind of accumulation in the yang organ (gallbladder). The puffiness along the GB-41 area often indicates an accumulation of gallbladder qi.

As described in Chapter 9, the gallbladder is involved in 'making decisions' about what is absorbed during the process of digestion. In this case, the underlying pathodynamic involved a problem with the dredging and draining of qi function of the liver that affected the gallbladder in its role of regulating proper absorption. The patient had experienced a rather sudden onset of weight gain and fatigue along with more chronic constipation due to this dysfunction.

An example of using modern diagnostic testing to inform Chinese medical diagnosis would be to consider the recent revelation of high serum cholesterol levels, which would indicate that the gallbladder was not effectively 'choosing' the best constituents in its pivotal role in the digestive process. It is important to recall that the gallbladder is not just a yang organ, it is also one of the miscellaneous organs (奇恒之腑 *qí héng zhī fǔ)* that are thought to have unique substantive functions of their own. In other words, it is a yang organ that not only moves substances through the digestive system, but also has a role of its own in its 'choosing' function.

Channel differentiation

In conclusion, the channels that were most affected in this condition were identified as the internally-externally paired liver-gallbladder.

Later in this chapter, this case will be reconsidered in the context of selecting the channel for treatment. Before doing so, however, recall that one must first go through the careful process of considering the entire picture in the context of patient history, presenting signs/symptom pattern, and palpated findings.

Sometimes, the importance of this type of diagnostic process gets lost in the rush to start thinking about treatment. A common sight is that of a practitioner who immediately asks the patient, "What's going on?" then follows with a wave toward the treatment table. These are practitioners who are quickly thinking through 'experience points' for the condition at hand rather than undertaking the careful process of differential diagnosis and channel differentiation. The results will reflect their effort. This is an unfortunate tendency which has led to the commonly held belief that acupuncture is appropriate for only a narrow range of complaints. It is not that there is a paucity of acupuncture approaches for the complaint, but rather a lack of thoroughness on the part of the practitioner.

In any case, the technique of differentiating the most affected channel is often under-utilized. In the most basic sense, this is another example of the common admonition to always identify the location of the disease before beginning treatment.

Now, having determined where the disease is, the time has come to select the most appropriate channel for treatment.

Step Two: Channel Selection

When selecting channels for needling, always keep in mind the basic principle that the primary channel identified during differentiation isn't necessarily the best channel for treatment. This is a difficult concept to grasp at first.

One of the most important considerations in selecting a channel for treatment involves the concept of time. Channel differentiation looks backward in time and helps the practitioner figure out how the condition has evolved up to that point. Channel selection, on the other hand, is forward looking, with the goal of steering the condition into the future. In other words, channel differentiation shows where the condition is, while channel selection determines where the condition will be.

Once again, considerations of classical physiology are helpful. Here is where an understanding of ideas developed in the earlier chapters of the book becomes relevant. Of particular importance are the concepts of 'opening', 'closing', and 'pivoting', first described in Chapter 5 of the *Divine Pivot* (discussed in Chapter 2 of our text). In selecting channels for treatment, the practitioner must consider where the affected channel is within the matrix of the six levels. This is not, by the way, a simple process of considering its relative 'depth'. Rather, the goal is to determine the overall effect of inducing movement (tonification) or relaxation (draining) in one channel on a number of other channels. (The concepts of tonification and draining will be addressed more thoroughly in Chapters 18 and 19 on technique.) The important thing to remember is that treatment always occurs in the context of the overall physiology of the patient. This is why treating the channel with disease is not necessarily the best way to get results.

Considerations of time also involve thinking backward to where a disease may have originated. Consider the common clinical pattern of the 'liver overacting on spleen' or 'wood overacting on earth'. In this pattern, the presenting symptoms may be of a spleen-stomach type, while the root cause is actually a condition of excess in the liver. To complicate matters further, the liver may have since returned to what appears to be normal function (very few liver symptoms). That is to say, when the patient presents at the clinic, the liver *jué yīn* or even the gallbladder *shào yáng* channels (excess condition affecting the paired yang channel) may show fewer significant palpable changes and the patient may not even mention liver-type complaints. Only careful questioning might reveal that a liver-type pattern of stress/anxiety with vertex headaches, for example, preceded the initial onset of diarrhea. In this case, in order to return spleen-stomach function to normal, liver (and/or gallbladder) treatment strategies would have to be included. Thus the process of unwinding a disorder also involves thinking back to how it may have begun. But in the end, the goal is still to think of channel selection in terms of where the condition is headed in the future, even if going ahead means returning to the original cause.

Fundamentally, resolving the pathodynamic depends on reestablishing normal channel flow. Acupuncture is an effective method for doing this.

Six approaches to channel selection

In the clinic, the methods of selecting a channel for treatment may be divided into six general categories.

1. Selecting the channel where the disease is located

This approach is fairly well understood by most practitioners. For example, in the case of lung symptoms like cough or asthma, the lung *tài yīn* channel would be chosen for treatment. This approach is usually most effective when channel diagnosis also reveals the most significant change to be along the course of the channel associated with the presenting organ pattern indicated by differential diagnosis. This is a fairly cut-and-dried case of directly modifying qi transformation in the channel which is most affected by the disease. While this treatment approach is popular, it is not always particularly effective. There are certain criteria that must be met for it to work.

This approach is only effective in cases where at least one of the following conditions exists:

- Where the onset of disease is relatively recent and the condition has not yet begun to affect other channels.

- Where the other organs and channels are generally healthy.

- Where the disorder is primarily located in the muscles or tendons, such as acute injuries and pain.

When a patient's condition does not meet at least one of these prerequisites, treatment using only the affected channel is often less than satisfactory. On the other hand, if more than one of these prerequisites is met, it is more likely that a single-channel treatment will not only be enough, but will actually be more effective than adding other, unnecessary points.

Unfortunately, it is at this point that the thought process sometimes stops, thus limiting the scope for acupuncture. Even the 'bread and butter' of an acupuncturist's practice—the treatment of pain—can often be limited by an over-dependence on this approach. Conditions as seemingly simple as shoulder and back pain often stubbornly refuse to improve. This is often due to the fact that the condition has entered other channels, or even the internal organs, and thus requires a more sophisticated treatment strategy. In order to increase effectiveness in these cases, qi transformation and the interplay of the channel system must also be taken into account.

2. Selecting the internal-external paired channel

In this approach, rather than selecting the channel most involved in a given pathodynamic, its paired yin/yang channel is chosen instead. Once again, certain criteria are required for this method.

Basic yin-yang theory will help to explain this approach. Yin is the solid material foundation for the yang function of moving qi transformation upward and outward. In general, yang is thus more appropriate for draining while yin is more appropriate for tonifying. The active nature of yang promotes movement through areas of stagnation. Yin material is used to build yang movement and warmth.

Consequently, when a yang channel is affected, it is most appropriate to choose the paired yin channel for treatment in cases of deficiency and/or cold. Digestive disorders provide a clear example of this concept. Ulcers and stomach prolapse are often deficient-type digestive disorders that may also involve cold. In these cases, tonification techniques on the spleen channel are most often effective. This is so even if differential diagnosis and channel palpation have indicated that the condition is in the stomach.

Similarly, where the yin channel is affected, it is most appropriate to choose the yang channel for treatment in cases of excess, heat, and stasis. A common clinical example of this approach is the use of the point pair TB-5 (*wài guān*) and GB-41 (*zú lín qì*) when there is heat and excess in the liver channel and/or organ. Here, a clearing treatment is used on *shào yáng* to clear *jué yīn* excess. Note that points from both aspects of the yang channel—both the gallbladder and triple burner *shào yáng*—are being used to treat a condition in just one *jué yīn* organ, the liver. The same treatment strategy might be applied in the case of heat, excess, or stagnation in the *tài yīn* organs (choose *yáng míng*) or *shào yīn* organs (choose *tài yáng*).

Finally, it should be pointed out that in cases where there is deficiency, cold, or insufficiency in the yin channels or organs, it is most appropriate to choose the yin channel for treatment. Similarly, when there is excess, heat, or stagnation in the yang, it is most appropriate to treat yang channels (Tables 14.1 ~ 14.3).

Palpated Change	Likely Significance
EITHER: • both yin and yang channels have relatively similar intensity of channel change OR: • yang channel change is relatively greater	Excess condition; the primary channel is most likely a yang channel
Changes most clearly noted on the yin channel(s)	Deficiency condition
Both yin and yang channels have significant palpable change, but yin channel change seems more significant	Combined excess and deficiency

Table 14.1

General patterns when both yin and yang channels present with palpable change

· ·

Channel differentiation determines that:	Channel selection might include:
Yin channel is primary; deficiency pattern	Yin channel for treatment
Yin channel is primary; excess pattern	Internal-external paired yang channel
Yang channel is primary; deficiency pattern	Internal-external paired yin channel
Yang channel is primary; excess pattern	Yang channel for treatment

Table 14.2

Relationship between channel findings and channel selection

· ·

3. Using both yin and yang channels together for treatment

In a condition where either a yin or yang channel is determined to be primary, the practitioner may decide to use both a yin and a yang channel for treatment. This is appropriate in the commonly encountered situation where both excess and deficiency are combined in the pathodynamic. An example would be the common presentation of spleen deficiency with accumulation of dampness. The fundamental condition is a yin channel condition of deficiency, but where excess dampness is also clearly a factor. In this

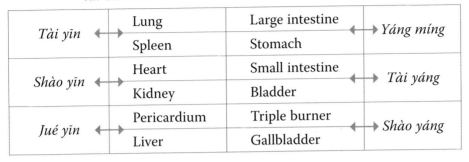

	Yin Channels		**Yang Channels**		
Tài yīn ↔	Lung		Large intestine	↔	*Yáng míng*
	Spleen		Stomach		
Shào yīn ↔	Heart		Small intestine	↔	*Tài yáng*
	Kidney		Bladder		
Jué yīn ↔	Pericardium		Triple burner	↔	*Shào yáng*
	Liver		Gallbladder		

Table 14.3
The internal-external paired channels

case, stomach *yáng míng* channel points can be combined with spleen *tài yīn* points (e.g., SP-3 [*tài bái*] and ST-36 [*zú sān lǐ*]). The classics are full of examples of this treatment strategy, and many of the point pairs described in Chapter 20 of this text are also of this type.

In Chapter 7 of the *Systematic Classic* (甲乙經 *Jiǎ yǐ jīng*, ca. 270 A.D.) there are extensive lists of diseases and pathodynamics followed by recommended treatment strategies. This text emphasizes the combination of yin and yang channels, especially for conditions where there is heat in the yin organs. This would include the condition described above where there is a combination of excess and deficiency in yin and yang channels. Another example would be cases where heat from deficiency in the liver is treated with both *jué yīn* and *shào yáng* points. The combination of yin-yang channels is not limited to internally-externally paired channels, however. Consider, for example, the use of the point pair PC-6 (*nèi guān*) and ST-44 (*nèi tíng*) to clear heat trapped in the pericardium with summerheat symptoms (Chapter 20).

4. Selecting the associated leg-arm aspect of the affected channel

This approach involves selecting the channel with the 'same name' as the affected channel. For example, one might choose the spleen *tài yīn* channel for treatment in cases of dysfunction in lung *tài yīn*. In most cases, this means using points from both the affected channel and its same-name counterpart. As described in earlier chapters on qi transformation in the six levels, organs associated with channels of the same name have a relationship of mutual regulation and/or synergy. Consequently, this treatment strategy can help harmonize organs linked by the same channel. For example, the spleen organ governs transportation and transformation. This includes the transformation of dampness and the transportation of the nutritive aspect generated by the middle burner. However, the spleen does not act alone. As described in Chapter 5 on the *tài yīn* organs, the spleen depends on lung function to provide qi for the distribution of nutrition around the body. As a result of this functional integration, the transformation of dampness by the spleen can be facilitated by a treatment that benefits the lung. A similar approach can be used when the descending function of the lung is compromised, with symptoms of fullness in the chest and cough. By combining lung channel points with appropriate tonifying points from the spleen channel, increased upward movement (升 *shēng*) of qi from the spleen synergistically benefits the downward movement (降 *jiàng*) of lung qi.

This physiological principle is generally true for all same-name paired organs. However, remember that, although organs of the same channel can benefit each other's qi transformation, the nature of that relationship is different at each level. In other words, while the lung and spleen have the synergistic relationship described above, the relationship between the heart and kidney, for example, is more one of balance (see Chapter 6). The unique qi transformation which occurs at each level should be considered when selecting channels and points on those channels. Many of the point pairs used in the clinic, and even herb pairs within common formulas, are based on the treatment strategy of combining organs from same-name pairs.

5. Selection based on five-phase relationships

This approach is especially applicable to the more complex conditions of internal medicine. Fundamentally, this is because of the implicit understanding of interrelationship that the theory represents. An understanding of interrelationship arises from the origins of five-phase theory in careful observation of the natural world. The controlling/overacting (相克 *xiāng kè*) relationship likely draws from observations of predators and prey. Specifically, there is an appreciation of the fact that organisms limit and are limited by the activities of other living organisms in their environment. Similarly, the generating (相生 *xiāng shēng*) or 'mother-child' relationship represents a parallel observation that nature also has a corresponding set of mutually beneficial relationships. Animals, plants, and even the organs within the body depend on each other for nourishment and support. At the same time, predators and their prey maintain the balance of the system as a whole (Fig. 14.4).

The analysis of internal disease benefits from the appreciation of complexity in relationships that is reflected in five-phase theory. This is especially true of five-phase approaches that have passed the test of clinical

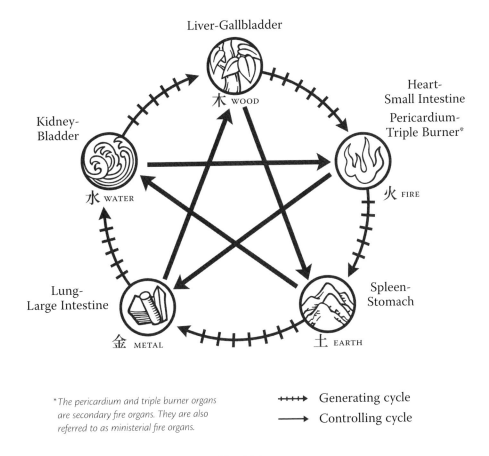

*The pericardium and triple burner organs
are secondary fire organs. They are also
referred to as ministerial fire organs.*

+++▶ Generating cycle

──▶ Controlling cycle

Fig. 14.4

An understanding of interrelationship arises from the origins of
five-phase theory in careful observation of the natural world.

application over time. In the process of channel selection, five-phase theory
also has an important role to play.

For example, there is the common involvement of the five-phase overacting relationship in the physiology of the spleen and the liver. Much has been
said about spleen-type conditions involving diarrhea due to liver overacting
on the spleen. Another common spleen-liver condition is similar to that
seen in the case described above involving certain types of constipation. In
these cases, lack of qi dredging by the liver can lead to a corresponding lack
of proper transformation by the spleen. Many readers may be aware of the
use of TB-6 (*zhī gōu*) in the treatment of constipation. It is more precise
to say that TB-6 is appropriate for conditions where *jué yīn* dredging is

compromised and has impaired the transformative function of the spleen. In this case of yin channel excess stagnation, one uses a yang channel (here *shào yáng*) for treatment. Clinically, an effective point pair for this presentation would be TB-6 and GB-34 (*yáng líng quán*). In this example, one is combining the method of using a yang channel for treating a yin condition with the method of five-phase theory. When the diagnosis is correct, the result is a clinically effective treatment.

To extend the previous example a bit, in a case where spleen deficiency is primary leading to 'opportunistic' overacting by the liver, the emphasis in treatment might shift to tonifying the spleen. The use of the pair SP-3 (*tài bái*) and ST-36 (*zú sān lǐ*), with the addition of LR-2 (*xíng jiān*), might be more appropriate. This is still a type of five-phase treatment, but with a shift in emphasis based on a different organ diagnosis of spleen deficiency rather than liver excess (Fig. 14.5).

Now let's consider the five-phase mother-child concept. In general, this approach involves tonifying a deficient channel by using the 'mother' channel in five-phase theory. For example, when presented with a patient showing clear signs of liver blood deficiency, treatment could involve tonifying the kidney—water gives birth to wood in the generating cycle, so the kidney is the 'mother' of the liver. Specifically, kidney yin supports the liver, and one might combine the kidney source point (KI-3 *[tài xī]*) with the liver source point (LR-3 *[tài chōng]*).[2] (Fig. 14.6)

Q: *This discussion brings to mind a difficult subject for many students of Chinese medicine, namely, how do you integrate on a day-to-day basis the concept of the five phases with organ theory? Sometimes they seem to be contradictory, or, at the very least, inconsistent with each other.*

DR. WANG: Yes, I know what you mean, and so do thousands of practitioners over the centuries! For me, as I've said many times, the most important thing for any theory is its ability to withstand the test of clinical efficacy. In certain periods of Chinese history, five-phase theory has been a kind of calcified, intellectually inflexible system, with armies dressed in red rushing to 'conquer' armies dressed in white and the like. The easiest way for me to answer your question is to provide a clinical example of how I use five-phase theory in my own practice.

In the late 1950s during my first years in the clinic, I had already found that, in some cases, mother-child theory would lead to channel

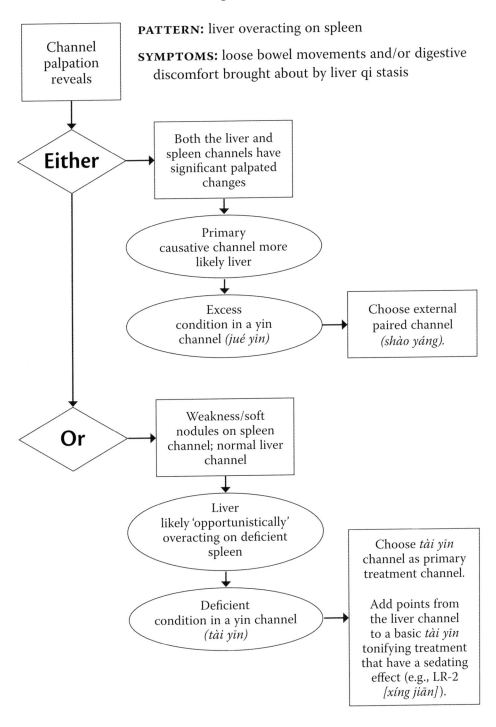

Fig. 14.5

An algorithm for integration of channel palpation into treatment

EITHER: There is a problem in the controlling cycle...

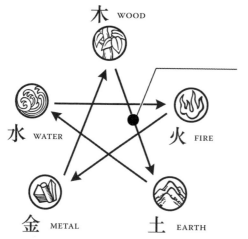

For example, the liver might "overact" on the spleen.

OR: There is a deficiency caused by problems in the generating cycle.

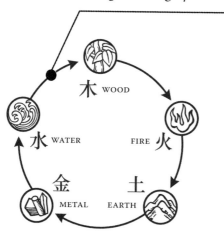

The water phase (kidney) may fail to nourish wood (liver) leading to a deficiency of liver blood.

Fig. 14.6

Comparison of two of the most common five-phase disharmonies

and point choices that produced good effects, but that in other cases, much was left to be desired. Eventually, I began to question whether this theory was going to be helpful as a guide to appropriate treatment strategies. After some years I concluded that although the five-phase approach is certainly helpful in the clinic, it does have limitations. Basically, for me it must always be considered in the context of organ and channel theory.

For example, in the approach that was just described of treating liver blood deficiency with the 'mother' kidney channel, it is actually only effective in conditions where the deficiency of the child is directly due to a lack of nourishment from the mother organ. In other words, it is inappropriate to always choose kidney points in cases of liver blood deficiency. Instead, the *shào yīn* kidney channel should only be used for situations where the root of liver blood deficiency lies in a lack of sufficient kidney essence to help engender blood. By contrast, in cases of liver blood deficiency caused by excessive blood loss, the use of kidney points will be less beneficial, while spleen-stomach tonification will be more appropriate. I therefore like to integrate five-phase theory with my understanding of organ and channel theory. On its own, five-phase theory is sometimes too inflexible for the demands of the clinic.

This is another one of those concepts that is difficult to adequately describe in words. In very complex and/or chronic cases, I often step back and evaluate the pattern in the context of five-phase theory. Often, when other approaches have proven ineffective, I find clarity and good results from five-phase treatment strategies. Consider again the kidney-liver situation described above. Notice that an analysis of symptom patterns (such as low back pain, chronic nature, puffiness around KI-3 [*tài xī*]) might lead one to infer a coinciding deficiency of kidney essence in the presence of liver blood symptoms. In this case, by considering the five-phase relationship of the kidney and the liver, I can develop a treatment strategy that gets results. I combine organ and channel diagnosis with the five-phase generation concept. I don't blindly use five-phase theory, but rather consider it in the context of the symptoms at hand. This is the kind of thinking that can bring five-phase theory to life.

6. Selection using points on the eight extraordinary vessels

Extraordinary vessel points are unique because most of the vessels themselves do not have direct connections to the yin and yang organs. While there is often a general association of the *rèn* vessel with the yin of the whole body and the *dū* vessel with the yang, the other six extraordinary vessels serve to regulate the interactions of groups of regular channels. Recall, for example, how the *yīn wéi* was described in Chapter 11 as a regulator of the interaction of nourishment from small vessels among multiple yin channels. The *yīn wéi* is therefore appropriate for conditions that affect the ability of multiple yin channels to nourish the interior. An example would be systemic gastrointestinal complaints involving weakness or atrophy in multiple organs. In this type of condition, the familiar point pair PC-6 (*nèi guān*) and SP-4 (*gōng sūn*), pairing the *yīn wéi* vessel with the *chōng* vessel, is helpful.

To better understand this approach, compare the type of case where one of the twelve regular channels might be chosen with the type of case that is appropriate for extraordinary vessel treatment. Regular channel treatment would still be appropriate in the relatively common case of a condition in which a particular channel has, over the course of time, begun to affect the functions of other channels and/or organs. In this type of case, where multiple channels are affected, choosing from among the treatment strategies above would still likely be appropriate. This is because, in most cases where a single channel condition has begun to affect other channels, the condition has not spread into the realm of the extraordinary vessels. In other words, the ability of multiple channels to interact is still intact; the channel system itself is still relatively healthy. On the other hand, there may be certain conditions which have begun to affect the way that multiple channels interact. When this is suspected, one should carefully consider the course of the disease at hand.

A metaphor might be helpful. Consider the types of problems that might affect an irrigation system which depended on natural rivers and streams. The simplest problem might involve blockage or change in the flow of a single stream. When this happens, other streams, rivers, lakes, and reservoirs may be affected in relatively predictable ways. On the other hand, if there were a dramatic change over an entire environment due, for example, to a chronic change in rainfall or severe, chronic blockage of a major stream, then the entire water system must readjust. In this more serious situation, an entire region would be affected and coordination across larger areas would have been compromised. Old waterways linking areas of abundant rainfall may need to be dredged to reinvigorate flow, or altogether new channels may need to be forged. Of course, the environment might adjust naturally over time, but the overall health of the region would be more quickly regained by balancing the excess and deficiency in flow. In the clinic, the role of the extraordinary vessels is similar to this. When a condition reaches a level of imbalance that begins to affect the way that multiple channels interact, then single or paired channel treatments are simply not enough (Fig. 14.7 and 14.8).

In the clinic, these types of cases involve conditions that are very large and systemic, or are so chronic that it is impossible to identify a primary

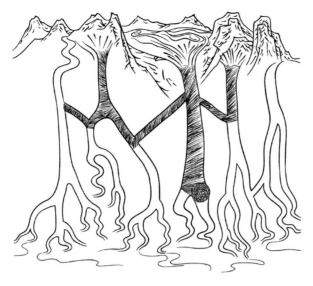

Fig. 14.7
In regular channel pathology, a blockage of flow can cause stasis or flooding in more than one channel. Treatment may involve consideration of qi transformation in multiple channels, but the condition is still not considered to involve the extraordinary vessels.

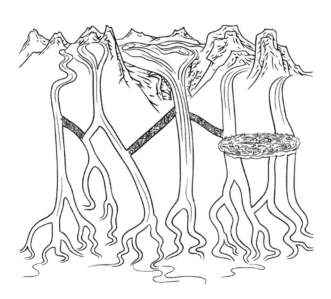

Fig. 14.8
In chronic conditions or severe illness, the nature of the internal environment may change dramatically and/or the normal integration of multiple channels may be blocked. In these cases, it is often more appropriate to choose the extraordinary vessels for treatment.

[417]

channel. In such cases, using the eight extraordinary vessels helps to clear the air. The eight extraordinary vessels can reestablish proper regulation among groups of regular channels. The concept of the extraordinary vessels was discussed in some detail in Chapter 11. It might be helpful to review that chapter now, together with the case study at the end of that chapter.

The important thing to remember is that the eight extraordinary vessels are most effectively used in situations that are beyond the scope of clear explanation using organ, five-phase, or regular channel qi transformation theories. In these cases, it might be assumed that the condition is at a high level of complexity or that the channel system is in disarray. This may include conditions such as epilepsy, spasms, or muscle problems involving the sinews of a group of channels. In addition, problems associated with the spinal and/or cranial nerves, as well as conditions associated with brain dysfunction in modern medicine, often fall within the category of extraordinary vessel dysfunction. In each case, the condition defies normal Chinese medicine classification, and the classical texts may even disagree about the pathodynamics.

It should be remembered that, in cases where involvement of the extraordinary vessels is suspected, channel palpation can provide important corroborative evidence. This will often include palpated changes on multiple channels that confound explanation through considerations of normal qi transformation. One should not simply palpate the area around BL-62 (shēn mài), for example, when considering whether the yáng qiāo vessel is involved in a particular condition. Rather, given the function of the yáng qiāo as described in this text, one should palpate multiple channel sinew pathways and consider the case history as a whole so as to carefully determine both the cause and current location of the disease.

A case reconsidered

Having now described the six most common approaches to applying channel-style thinking in the clinic, it is time to return to the clinical example described earlier in the chapter. The example had been evaluated up through the process of channel differentiation. What about channel and point selection? Remember that channel differentiation had determined the primary affected channels to be shào yáng and jué yīn.

This case illustrates the oft-encountered clinical picture of combined disease in yin and yang channels. This calls for the third treatment approach listed above, namely, a combination of yin and yang channels due to intertwined excess and deficiency. In the clinic, however, this principle is often divided into stages of treatment. Other case studies in this book have broken down the course of treatment into a series of steps—like the untying of a knot.

In this particular case, the first step in treatment involves clearing excess from the yang channel. The point pair TB-6 *(zhī gōu)* and GB-34 *(yáng líng quán)* was chosen as most appropriate. After three treatments and an improvement in bowel function (less constipation), the treatment focus then changed to the yin organ. The second series of three treatments included the pair PC-7 *(dà líng)* and LR-2 *(xíng jiān)*. This second pair is also often used to clear excess but, because it is now on the yin channel, might be considered as the second step in untying the clinical knot. Finally, a third point pair, LU-5 *(chǐ zé)* and KI-7 *(fù liū)*, was used in later treatments to regulate the underlying heart-kidney and lung deficiencies. At the first visit, a series of nine treatments were thus recommended to the patient with the goal of first clearing and then regulating the liver-gallbladder, and finally supporting the underlying disharmony of heart-kidney-lung. An herbal formula like Minor Bupleurum Decoction *(xiǎo chái hú tāng)* was used to begin, followed by Spiny Zizyphus Decoction *(suān zǎo rén tāng)* in later visits.

There are some general tendencies in this pattern that offer useful clinical guidelines. In cases of deficiency, the yang channels often show relatively less change. In cases of combined excess and deficiency, although both the yin and yang channels will likely show palpable changes, those on the yin channels are usually greater than those on the yang channels. In this case, the diffuse palpated changes on the liver channel were in fact more notable than the generalized puffiness along the gallbladder channel. This indicates that the root of the patient's chief complaint was in the liver.

Summary

The clinical application of channel theory has now been considered up through the stage of choosing points for treatment. The following chapter will explore this process further. As indicated throughout the text, a helpful way to approach point selection is to consider them in prescriptions of point pairs. Later, in Chapter 20, we will describe some commonly used point pairs. However, for readers who are relatively new to channel style approaches, it is important to first take a fresh look at the meaning of the term 'acupuncture point'. A reexamination of what is actually happening at an acupuncture point will comprise the general theme of the next three chapters.

Before proceeding, however, the reader should again review the basic seven-part process of treatment illustrated in Fig. 14.1. The next three chapters discuss Step 6 in that process, while Chapters 18 and 19 take up Step 7.

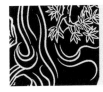

CHAPTER 15

WHAT IS AN ACUPUNCTURE POINT?

BEFORE EXPLORING, IN the chapters to come, the ways that points are traditionally categorized and understood, we will first briefly address a few basic questions. Most importantly, what exactly is an acupuncture point? In Chinese, the most commonly used term is comprised of the two characters 俞 and 穴 *(shū and xué)*. The first of these characters (俞) describes water-like movement and activity. The second (穴) describes a kind of dug-out open space (空隙 *kōng xi)* which serves as a place of protection—not unlike the cellars or basements found in many homes. Thus within the Chinese term are two concepts which, taken together, describe points as unique places on the body where significant movement and activity is occurring. The movement and activity is that of qi and blood. The places are small openings within the connective tissue matrix of the body.

The first of these characters describes the nature of points (they are moving and active) while the second implies that they have a discernible, physical structure (an opening). In modern terms, the nature of the points involves considerations of point categories, functions, and indications (what the points are thought to do). The location of points, on the other hand, involves anatomical measurement and palpation skills (where the points are thought to be). Modern acupuncture education emphasizes point location while failing to explore the implications of the concept, in the Chinese model, that the points themselves are active participants in physiology. Of course, there is discussion of the *uses* of the acupuncture points in the form of lists of diseases and 'which points to choose', but less often is there a careful analysis of what classical texts may have been asserting is actually taking place at these points on the body.

In fact, the very use of the English term 'point' to describe places of needle insertion has already taken us quite a distance from the meaning of the Chinese term *shū xué*. The English term might actually be a translation of the commonly used modern Chinese term *xué wèi* (穴位). The first character in this pair is the same *xué* seen above, but the second, significantly, describes a fixed place or point. This term, often used in modern Chinese medical textbooks, implies that the points are relatively fixed, measurable anatomical locations. However, by thinking of acupuncture points as static sites to be found on the surface of the body, while failing to consider the dynamic activity implied by more traditional Chinese terminology, means that we are literally missing half of the picture.

Having considered these basic terms, a clear definition of an acupuncture point might be advanced:

> ▶ Points are places on the body surface from which there
> is transformation and transportation (轉輸 *zhuǎn shū*)
> of information, regulation (調節 *tiáo jié*) of channel and
> organ function, irrigation (灌滲 *guàn shèn*) of surrounding
> tissues, and connectivity (聯繫 *lián xì*) to the channel
> system as a whole.

These points, via the circulation of qi and blood, are unified in a channel system which ultimately links the organs of the body to the distal appendages. Through this system, not just the channels, but also the points themselves play an active role in both the physiology and pathology of the organs. By inserting a needle into a point, one is not only affecting local tissue, but the entire associated channel and organs. In addition, because the system constantly interacts, the points and channels can also reflect outwardly the status of the internal organs with which they are linked. Thus channel palpation involves actually feeling this physiology.

Chapter 29 of the *Divine Pivot*, in describing the relationship of the channels to the organs, introduces another concept that influences our understanding of acupuncture points when it says that "the articulations of the body are the [external] cover for the organs."[1] In this case, the 'articulations' (支節 *zhī jié*) are those places along the channels, far above the level of the internal organs, where changes in the flow of channel qi occur. They 'cover' the internal organs much like the branches of a tree cover its trunk. In fact, in this chapter of the *Inner Classic* the term for points is a word that is also used to describe the distinctive joints along a bamboo stem. By using this term, a different aspect of the nature of the acupuncture points is emphasized, namely, that besides being a specific place where the movement of qi and blood occur, an acupuncture point is also an important piece of a larger whole.

One of the characters translated here as 'articulation' (節 *jié*) has historically had meanings as diverse as knot, chapter, rhythm, and holiday. In each case, there is the common suggestion of an important interval along a course. Thus the points are literally 'turning points', places where there is great potential for changing the nature of channel circulation in both the channels and the organs.

The same character (節 *jié*) is also used in the first chapter of the *Divine Pivot* to describe the points:

> [Among] the intersections of [these] articulations, there are 365 meetings. The knowledge of their importance can be spoken in [just] a few words. [Nevertheless,] to be ignorant of their importance is to invite endless confusion. These articulations [節 *jié*] are where the spirit qi moves, exits, and enters. They are not [the same as] skin, flesh, sinews, and bones.[2]

Here, the *Divine Pivot* introduces a few more ideas regarding the points:

▶ They are places where 'spirit qi' moves.

When classical texts describe the points as containing the movement of spirit qi, they are describing the very real ability of acupuncture points to convey information about physiology. As noted in Chapter 5, spirit (神 *shén*) is the intelligence of existence. Broadly speaking, when the term spirit is used in Chinese, it is often in reference to something that cannot normally be seen or felt. In Chinese physiology, the subtle activities of the qi dynamic occur within the points, beyond the realm of vision with the naked eye. These are the interactions of qi and blood within the interstitial spaces, described often in this text.

▶ The points "are not [the same as] skin, flesh, sinews, and bones."

At first, it seems counterintuitive to assert that needling acupuncture points does not affect these fundamental structures. If we are not going through the skin and flesh and affecting the tendons and bones, then what is going on? If we remove these structures, then what is left? In short, what is left are the articulations or open spaces described earlier: spaces *between* the muscles, vessels, tendons, and bones. Once again, these are not empty, hollow spaces, but places of interchange. By stimulating a point with a needle, a change is produced in the imperceptible qi transformation in that important area of interchange. The point is not in the belly of a muscle or any other structure, but in the empty areas surrounding them. Acupuncture thus creates movement through the open spaces along the course of the channel to initiate a cascade of physiological change through the organs.

These articulations are also, of course, quite important to the normal functioning of the areas in which they are found. Locally, the points are places of irrigation (灌溉 *guàn gài*) of the tissues in the immediate area surrounding the points. Each point radiates small collaterals like roads fanning off a central hub. The points are thus vital to healthy local qi and blood circulation and, when injuries occur, become important for helping to re-establish normal function in the area.

Two Sides of the Coin: Theory and Practice in the Concept of an Acupuncture Point

Having considered the nature of points in general, it is helpful to take a look at the ways that the individual points are understood. To broaden a concept introduced above, one might consider the idea of an acupuncture point from two aspects: the first involves the nature of points, and the second involves practical considerations for finding the points in the clinic. Channel theory and the point categories described in upcoming chapters might be thought to represent the mental processes that bring one's hands to the proper areas of the body during diagnosis and treatment. These are considerations about the 'nature' of the points (what they do). Once one has thought through the desired effects of a particular treatment *in theory*, the next step involves finding the precise location where needle insertion can be most effective. In other words, the manual skills of acupuncture practice are just as important as theory.

The next section will very briefly review what, for some, may be the basics. However, because this chapter is setting the stage for upcoming chapters, the basic context for that information is nevertheless pertinent.

The nature of the points

An understanding of the nature of an individual point is shaped by the following considerations:

The channel on which the point is found

This is the most familiar delineation of the acupuncture points into fourteen channels (twelve regular channels plus the *rèn* and *dū* vessels). In this type of categorization, most points on the channels (especially those below the elbows and knees on the twelve regular channels) have specific effects on qi transformation in the organs and along the pathways of the channels with which they are associated. This concept also includes the idea that the actual physical location of a point (where it is on the body) often affects its nature and clinical use.

The categories to which the points belong

These are the point categories: transport (輸 *shū*), source (原 *yuán*), cleft (郄 *xī*), etc. Point categories help the practitioner to differentiate likely effects on qi transformation of the various points on a particular channel.

Empirical uses

These are uses for individual points that seem to defy categorization under channel theory and point categories. In some cases, a kind of channel theory logic can be imposed on the function of the point to help conceptualize its nature, but the reality is that in the clinic, some points simply have special uses of their own. For example, consider the use of ST-38 *(tiáo kǒu)* in the treatment of frozen shoulder or shoulder pain. While the *yáng míng* channel does in fact traverse the shoulder, this point has an effect on all types of shoulder pain. Another example would be the use of GV-19 *(hòu dǐng)* for acute muscle spasms along the back of the body. Of course the *dū* vessel does travel through these areas, but this particular point is uniquely effective. There are points of this type throughout the body. Nevertheless, the functions of the majority of points can be conceptualized by carefully considering channel theory[3] (Fig. 15.1).

ACUPUNCTURE POINTS ARE PLACES OF:

Transformation and transportation	Regulation
Irrigation	Connectivity

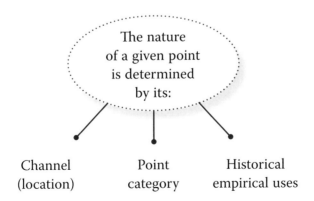

The nature of a given point is determined by its:

Channel (location) Point category Historical empirical uses

Fig. 15.1
The nature of acupuncture points

The location of the points

The second major aspect of a point involves finding the precise location for a given point at a given time. Location is the key to both avoiding discomfort and attaining the best results in the clinic. Throughout the history of acupuncture, a variety of techniques have been advocated for helping the practitioner properly locate the points.

Proportional measurement

One of the most common means of location involves the familiar delineation of the body into zones that can be measured in Chinese anatomical units or inches (寸 *cùn*). In practice, different distances on the body are said to have fixed lengths that often correspond to those of major bones. This type of measurement has therefore been known as 'bone units' (骨度 *gǔ dù*).

Special location techniques

This encompasses all of the location tricks that are taught in the process of learning acupuncture points. The methods are many and varied. For example, SP-10 *(xuè hǎi)* is often found by laying the palm on the patella and then finding the point with the thumb on the medial aspect of the lower thigh. LU-3 *(tiān fǔ)* can be found by raising the arm to the nose then looking for the place where the bicep muscle meets the tip of the nose. Experiential location also includes the use of landmarks on the body to find points. For example, a common technique for finding ST-36 *(zú sān lǐ)* involves measuring one thumb-width out from a ridge found on the tibia beneath the patella. Techniques of this type can often be more helpful than proportional measurement for finding certain points.

The goal of all location methods is to make the finding of points more precise. However, as noted above, precision is not determined solely by measurements in units or distances from palpable or visible landmarks on the surface of the body. Rather, it is absolutely imperative that the points be palpated so as to find those places within which the 'spirit qi' is said to be moving. When openings or divisions are found with the hands along the landscape of the body, one need not use excessively strong technique to achieve the desired results. Too often, substandard results are not due to flawed understanding of point functions, indications, or technique, but to imprecise location and perfunctory palpation.

Consider Fig. 15.2 below. In this image, one sees a stream flowing quickly through a valley. The stream has a major channel, which is determined by the topography of the landscape. Rocks along the way and trees beside the stream affect the nature and direction of flow. Areas where flow is concentrated and moving in the stream can be likened to the acupuncture points.

A sudden blockage caused by the felling of a tree may have dramatic effects on the flow both above and below the blockage. Alternately, if one were to put a huge bag of fresh black tea leaves at one of these points, then a large area downstream would quickly darken. In other words, these are points along the flow with great potential for transformation. If one were to put the tea leaves in a place not far from the point, but with significantly less concentration of flow, the downstream effects would be measurably less. Similarly, the acupuncture points are sites on the body with this tendency to have both intersection with and broad effects on systemic flow. Other sites on the body that do not have this potential are not acupuncture points. The precise location of these points varies from person to person, just as the flow in a stream or river will vary with time and place (Fig. 15.2).

If the body is viewed simply as static flesh, then one runs the risk of missing the subtle nature of the acupuncture points. If a rote learning of point location that fails to take variability into account becomes the norm, the very heart of acupuncture therapy is at risk. When palpating the channels to find points, one should not move along the body like a truck barreling through and alley, but instead move slowly and carefully with the most sensitive part of the fingertips.

This discussion of points will close with one final comment from the *Divine Pivot*. Chapter 10 of that text includes a discussion of the development of the body from conception and the "establishment of essence" (成精 *chéng jīng)*. It says that once the essence has arisen, then the marrow is created and the bones become the trunk, the (blood) vessels become the nutritive (aspect), the sinews become the firmness of the body, and the muscles become the defining structure. The skin then binds the body together and produces hair. Upon hearing this, the questioner (the court physician Lei Gong) persists in wondering how the channels fit into this theory. He says, "Let me finally ask what it is that the channels and vessels bring about?" The Yellow Emperor replies: "The channels are determiners of life and death. They treat the hundred types of disease by regulating excess and deficiency. They cannot be allowed to not be open! [they must not become congested]"

This passage from the *Inner Classic* highlights the importance of maintaining regular movement in the vessels. The points are the places where movement has a potential to change. They are also places of possible stagnation. It is stasis of qi, blood, fluids, and phlegm that creates the chain reactions of pathology that Chinese medicine describes as a pathodynamic. In classical physiology, it is the channels, and the acupuncture points that make up the intervals and spaces along their course, which regulate the entire body. If they do not function properly, they fail in their role as determiners of life.

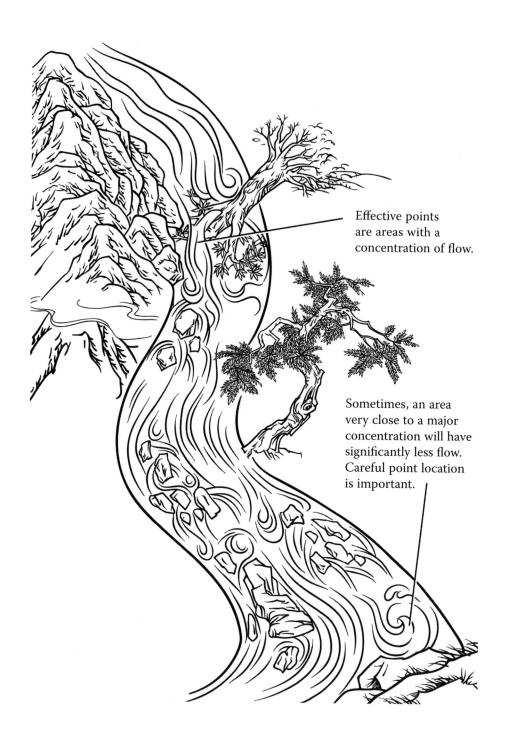

Effective points
are areas with a
concentration of flow.

Sometimes, an area
very close to a major
concentration will have
significantly less flow.
Careful point location
is important.

Fig. 15.2
The precise location of these points varies from person to person,
just as the flow in a stream or river will vary with time and place.

Q: *How did you think about the points when you began practicing acupuncture?*

DR. WANG: When I first began studying, I believed that points were just measured places on the body that might be located on a cadaver or in an anatomy text. Also, I believed that all points on the body were roughly the same: that they are all openings between the various structures in the body. Later, I began to appreciate subtle differences among the points. Some have more qi or more blood, some have less. In some places the type of qi is different than in others. Importantly, the exact nature of qi sensation that should be generated from each point varies, and should be varied depending on the desired effect. Each point actually has its own nature or personality. Once I began to truly note these differences among the points on my patients, I became more and more interested in the classical point categorizations. It is from here that I began my exploration of the source, collateral, and five transport points.

In fact, after many years, I now think of many of the points on the body as old friends. I know what they are like, what their strengths and weaknesses are, and when to call on them for help. When you get to know the points in this way, treating in the clinic is kind of like waking good friends from a slumber—gently prodding the points to wake them up and send them on their way. Also, as I've said before, some of the points are like jacks-of-all-trades, friends that you might call on to help with a wide variety of projects. Other points have very specific strengths and should be used in more specific cases. The points, to me, really do seem to have these different personalities.

■ Narrative

PROFESSOR ZHU ZONG-XIANG

On a rainy September morning, my wife and I met Dr. Wang on the street in front of the Ping Xin Tang. Sharing an umbrella, we walked south down tree-lined Tai Ji Chang Avenue in central Beijing. The street had been at the heart of the embassy section of the city during the final decades of the Qing dynasty (1644–1911) and still retained architectural memories. We walked along a sidewalk next to an old brick wall that wouldn't have looked out of place in a European city. The wall had once defined the border of the Italian embassy and flourishes of glass and carved wood could be glimpsed inside the compound. We passed a small Catholic church as we searched for the alley that would eventually lead us deeper into an area once filled with the merchants and shops that supported the 19th century foreign community. Through openings in an old iron gate we glanced into the churchyard to see framed paintings of religious scenes and a small rock garden. I later discovered that this church had been the heart of the expatriate French community a hundred years ago, and I toured the neighboring state guest house that was once home to the French legation. Even today, it is still possible to imagine the ambassador standing at the top of a huge sweeping oak staircase flooded with hues of light filtered through stained glass. That grand chamber is now home to offices of party officials but retains a distinctly non-communist bright yellow trim on the exterior moldings.

We finally found the alley that Dr. Wang was looking for and turned away from the past into the sharp intensity of the hutong alleys. Stepping over puddles in the growing downpour, we negotiated a chaotic stream of bicycles, yellow-capped students, three-wheeled truck-like bicycles filled with vegetables, and slow-moving elderly Beijingers. As we neared our destination, I began to notice that the number of older pedestrians was increasing and that many of them were walking with slow determination toward a group of about thirty retirees standing around a gate in a grey wall. Older Beijing residents are much more likely to wear the head to toe blue suits and 'Mao caps' that young Chinese might only wear at art shows with a strained sense of irony. This gathering was a lively reunion of the old guard. Smiling, aged faces turned toward us as we came to the gate where an older man in a blue cap handed each of us a plastic folder that held a small book, a CD-ROM, and a few sheets of paper on which there appeared to be printed musical lyrics.

A few days before, Dr. Wang had given me a red envelope which held a very formally printed invitation from his friend, Professor Zhu Zong-Xiang (祝总骧) of the Beijing Channel Research Association (北京經絡研究協會 *Běi jīng jīng luò yán jiū xié huì)*. As he passed me the envelope Dr. Wang had said, "He is having a conference to introduce his '3-1-2 channel exercise system' next week and would like us to come. Maybe you could say a few words." I had met Professor Zhu the month before when I translated a lecture he gave to a group of visiting foreign acupuncturists. During his lecture, he had described his research into ways that modern science might explain the concept of acupuncture channels. Now 86 years old, Professor Zhu is a kind of institution within the Beijing acupuncture community. Dr. Wang told me how he had continued his research for fifty years, often despite official indifference to his work and a chronic lack of adequate funding. Before the lecture to the foreign students, Dr. Wang had told me that, "I have the greatest respect for Dr. Zhu, not only because I think that his approach represents a promising direction for scientific research into the source of channel theory, but also because of his personal integrity. I will never forget the bitterly cold winter night when I found Professor Zhu carefully looking after the conditions of the rabbits that he used for his research. He was determined that their cages be kept clean and warm during a time when all of us were living in less than luxurious surroundings. He has a very good heart."

Dr. Zhu's lifetime of research has included a variety of experiments conducted on both animal and human subjects that show increased light, sound, and electrical conductivity along channel pathways. Avoiding the approach of many Western researchers whose experiments emphasize nerve pathways or the unique anatomical/physiological nature of specific acupuncture points, Dr. Zhu has focused on looking at the unique properties of the tissues along channel pathways as a whole. In the process, he has found that there is a measurable difference between conductivity in the tissues along channel pathways and those tissues a few centimeters away which aren't associated with the acupuncture channels. During his lecture to the visiting doctors, he showed a series of slides and video recordings of his work followed by demonstrations on the visiting doctors themselves.

Dr. Zhu had also developed a very simple program designed to invigorate circulation in the channel system. This was the reason for our early morning walk that day. His program, the '3-1-2 channel exercise system', involved stimulating twice daily 'three' acupuncture points (ST-36, PC-6, and LI-4) in conjunction with focus on unified 'one' breathing and daily use of 'two' legs to exercise. Despite (or due to) the apparent simplicity of his regimen, it had attracted a huge following—especially among retirees. As Dr. Wang and I were led past a busy anteroom in which older women sat behind tables selling books, CDs, and videotapes, my wife was escorted to another door. A few moments later, I was surprised to find that Dr. Wang and I were to be seated at a table on stage in the front of a large auditorium filled to the walls with elderly Beijingers, many of whom were jostling with each other for better seats or spaces under the chairs for canes and purses. We were seated at one end of the stage while Professor Zhu and an assistant were seated at another raised table behind which a huge screen showed a photograph of a bronze statue upon which one could see the familiar lines of the acupuncture channels. I watched as an elderly man in a blue blazer showed my wife to a seat in the front row. There was a bit of complaining as she sat down, but feathers were smoothed just before the lights began to dim.

A young woman came to the center of the stage and, with a wave of her hand, indicated that the assembly should stand. A few minutes of clutter followed while a sea of white heads swayed to attention. Behind me a speaker crackled to life as the marching-band sounds of 1950s era Chinese political music strained the capacity of the auditorium's antiquated sound system. Dr. Wang, sitting beside me, indicated that I should remove the sheet of lyrics from my plastic folder. I picked it up, watched the woman holding the microphone in front of me for a cue, then began singing with the chorus of reedy voices:

> Aged friends, let's get together to collectively,
> happily study 3-1-2.
> Just press *nèi guān* (PC-6), rub *hé gǔ* (LI-4),
> and tap *zú sān lǐ* (ST-36).
> Breathe in the belly and calm your heart AHH!...
> Beloved friends, a hundred years of health depends on who?
> Depends on you, depends on me,
> depends on us all practicing faithfully!

There were three full verses, all of which were sung.

Following the song and a brief introduction of Dr. Zhu and other honored attendees seated in the first row, another slow marching song accompanied a procession of octogenarians onto the stage. One by one, they stepped forward, took the microphone, and described how the '3-1-2 channel exercise system' had helped them to recover from a wide variety of afflictions. One old woman spoke of her battle with breast cancer, while a particularly spry gentleman demonstrated that he had "the legs of a thirty-year-old" by doing a short dance across the stage. The crowd ate it up. There were peals of laughter or moans of commiseration as each speaker told of how daily acupressure, breathing, and exercise had helped them make often miraculous recoveries. Professor Zhu would often nod in agreement as each speaker told their story, or interrupt the particularly long-winded in an effort to give everyone a chance at the microphone. During this section of the program, Dr. Wang and I sat on stage occasionally sipping from bottles of spring water that had been given to us by the man in the blue blazer.

After an hour or so, the final speaker took her seat and Professor Zhu introduced Dr. Wang who slowly walked to the microphone and gave a three minute speech congratulating Professor Zhu on his work and the assembled crowd on their health and dedication. He then took his seat and I was introduced. Although I don't mind public speaking, the size of the crowd and the fact that I would be speaking in Chinese (not to mention the long wait) had made me a bit nervous. Nevertheless, I managed to make a fairly anemic joke about how the elderly dancing man would make an excellent skier followed by a passable digression into how the '3-1-2 channel exercise system' might be well received by my North American patients. With great relief, I returned to my seat next to Dr. Wang. Five minutes later, Dr. Wang indicated that we could step down, and we watched the last fifteen minutes of the presentation from the safety of an alcove.

After a series of handshakes and a diversion to the front row to meet my wife, the three of us made our way back onto the busy streets in search of lunch. As we ate a bowl of noodles, Dr. Wang told us more about Professor Zhu and the period of his life when he saw him most often:

> **DR. WANG:** In the late 1970s and 80s, I saw Zhu Zong-Xiang almost every day. He was doing his research in the same area where I was working. Do you remember where we went that day when you translated his lecture? That is where we both worked in those days. As you know, those buildings are right next to the Forbidden

City and were in fact part of the imperial government during the Qing dynasty. They were originally a temple complex dedicated to the God of Wind. There were temples like that on each of the four corners of the Forbidden City. The God of Wind protected the city from storms. I also remember older people when I was young talking about the other temple at the end of the street that was dedicated to the God of Fire. In those days, people burned incense at that temple to ask for protection of wooden buildings from disaster.

In any case, by the 1970s, the former temple to the God of Wind had become a large acupuncture clinic. We moved over there in 1975 when construction began on the new Dong Zhi Men Hospital. I ended up working there for ten years. It was one of the busiest periods in my life. There were forty doctors in my department and twenty of us would see patients at a time. The old wooden temple buildings had been sub-divided into six large treatment rooms with two to four doctors in each room. I remember once that the twenty of us saw six-hundred patients in one morning alone. We had a lot of beds. I actually ended up living in a small room there on weekdays, as it was easier than going all the way home then coming back. We would cook meals in a courtyard in front of the clinic. Professor Zhu would come to ask questions about our treatments and I sometimes gave lectures on channel theory to the groups of Western scientists that he worked with.

Finally, in the mid 1980s, they finished work on the new hospital and we moved out. Professor Zhu and his group stayed there, however, and continued using the old buildings. Of course, he's still there now. These days, all of the buildings around him have come under the control of the Museum of the Forbidden City but he has refused to leave. Because he's fairly famous, I suspect that he'll be there until he decides to retire. As he's still working at the age of 86, I'm not sure when that will be! He is fiercely dedicated to his work. I hope that we can all be that dedicated. I believe that the key to understanding channels in the Western scientific system will eventually be found in the direction that Professor Zhu has taken. After forty years of clinical work, my intuition is that a deeper understanding of what modern biology terms 'interstitial fluids' may prove fruitful. I believe that there is an under-appreciation of the role of those fluids and their circulation in basic physiology.

Acupuncture channels are not ancient models of nerve, lymph, or blood vessel pathways but are instead something altogether different. After all these years and all of my work, I still find that there are many questions that I want to ask. I sometimes feel that if I just keep studying and seeing patients, eventually I'll get to a place of even greater clarity. I'm not quite there yet, and I sometimes feel as if I'm looking out a window and can see the broad outlines of shapes, but some of the details aren't filled in yet. It is this sense that makes me so excited about my work. The things that I talk with you about are the things that are clear in my mind. I try to stay away from the subjects that I myself don't understand completely. Hopefully with time...

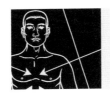

THE FIVE TRANSPORT POINTS
(五輸穴 *wǔ shū xué*)

THE FIRST AND second chapters of the *Divine Pivot* in the *Inner Classic* compress a staggering amount of basic theory into a very short space. Chapter 1 introduces the following concepts:

- needling
- nine types of needles
- needling techniques, including an introduction to 'tonifying and draining'
- radial pulse diagnosis
- observation of the skin color in diagnosis
- discerning the state of the environment before treating disease
- determining excess and deficiency in pathodynamic
- names, locations, and uses of the source points
- introduction to the five transport points and their locations below the elbows and knees (Table 16.1).

Readers of modern English textbooks should keep in mind that the history of medicine in China involves century upon century of nuanced interpretation of the ancient texts. Interpretation begins with the broad brush strokes drawn with concise economy, as in the first chapter of the *Divine Pivot*. While the characters used in the writing of the ancient text are basically the same as those used in modern Chinese newspapers, the concepts arise from a culture in a stage of early history that is still relatively opaque to us today. As many modern scholars have pointed out, the *Inner Classic* represents both a survey and a standardization of prehistorical medical tradi-

Channel	Well (井 jǐng) WOOD/METAL*	Spring (滎 yíng) FIRE/WATER	Stream (輸 shū) EARTH/WOOD	River (經 jīng) METAL/FIRE	Sea (合 hé) WATER/EARTH
Lung	LU-11 (shào shāng)	LU-10 (yú jì)	LU-9 (tài yuān)	LU-8 (jīng qú)	LU-5 (chǐ zé)
Spleen	SP-1 (yǐn bái)	SP-2 (dà dū)	SP-3 (tài bái)	SP-5 (shāng qiū)	SP-9 (yīn líng quán)
Heart	HT-9 (shào chōng)	HT-8 (shào fǔ)	HT-7 (shén mén)	HT-4 (líng dào)	HT-3 (shào hǎi)
Kidney	KI-1 (yǒng quán)	KI-2 (rán gǔ)	KI-3 (tài xī)	KI-7 (fù liū)	KI-10 (yīn gǔ)
Pericardium	PC-9 (zhōng chōng)	PC-8 (láo gōng)	PC-7 (dà líng)	PC-5 (jiān shǐ)	PC-3 (qū zé)
Liver	LR-1 (dà dūn)	LR-2 (xíng jiān)	LR-3 (tài chōng)	LR-4 (zhōng fēng)	LR-8 (qū quán)
Large Intestine	LI-1 (shāng yáng)	LI-2 (èr jiān)	LI-3 (sān jiān)	LI-5 (yáng xī)	LI-11 (qū chí)
Stomach	ST-45 (lì duì)	ST-44 (nèi tíng)	ST-43 (xiàn gǔ)	ST-41 (jiě xī)	ST-36 (zú sān lǐ)
Small Intestine	SI-1 (shào zé)	SI-2 (qián gǔ)	SI-3 (hòu xī)	SI-5 (yáng gǔ)	SI-8 (xiǎo hǎi)
Bladder	BL-67 (zhì yīn)	BL-66 (zú tōng gǔ)	BL-65 (shù gǔ)	BL-60 (kūn lún)	BL-40 (wěi zhōng)
Triple Burner	TB-1 (guān chōng)	TB-2 (yè mén)	TB-3 (zhōng zhǔ)	TB-6 (zhī gōu)	TB-10 (tiān jǐng)
Gallbladder	GB-44 (zú qiào yīn)	GB-43 (xiá xī)	GB-41 (zú lín qì)	GB-38 (yáng fǔ)	GB-34 (yáng líng quán)

Table 16.1
The five transport points

*Yin channels begin with wood while yang channels begin with metal.

[438]

tions.[1] Over time, and even in the modern era, these concepts are revisited and reinterpreted. Consequently, for example, the acupuncture points now referred to as the five transport points, like the source points discussed in the next chapter, represent a concept that was first transmitted by the *Inner Classic* and then interpreted and modified over the many centuries that followed.

The second chapter of the *Divine Pivot* delves into much greater detail about the five transport points: well, spring, stream, river, and sea. It describes the nature and the quality of channel flow at each of these points, their names, and (most) of their locations on each of the twelve main channels. There are differences between the points described in this chapter and those commonly used today. Most notably, the transport points for the heart channel described in the *Inner Classic* are the pericardium channel points in modern textbooks. Only in later centuries was the channel now associated with heart *shào yīn* actually needled. Earlier traditions used the heart's 'envoy' (臣使 *chén shǐ*), the pericardium, as a substitute for treating the emperor (heart) directly.

A widely debated subject, related to early descriptions of the five transport points, involves the direction of flow in the channel system. Chapter 2 of the *Divine Pivot* describes the flow of qi along *all* of the channels as moving along the five transport points from the hands and feet inward toward the body.[2] However, there are discrepancies elsewhere. For example, Chapter 10 of the *Divine Pivot* describes a circuit of channel flow moving up and down the appendages from the yin to the yang channels. Channel qi is said to move in a circuit from the lung to the large intestine, stomach, spleen, heart, small intestine, bladder, kidney, pericardium, triple burner, gallbladder, and liver.

In other words, while the early chapters of the *Divine Pivot* describe the flow of channel qi from the extremities toward the body in all of the channels, later chapters seem to contradict this and instead describe the channel flow in a kind of closed circuit. This closed-circuit flow moves outward from the trunk and then inward toward the heart and head as it travels from yin to yang paired channels (Fig. 16.1 and 16.2).

What can be made of this apparent conflict? One answer is that they actually represent two simultaneously occurring phenomena. The five transport point flow represents the gradual development of channel qi from its inception, where "yin and yang meet" in the extremities. The closed circuit flow, on the other hand, describes a circuit of nutrition.

This is a difficult concept to grasp at first. It is helpful to consider that, in the five transport point model, channel qi is growing in volume while mov-

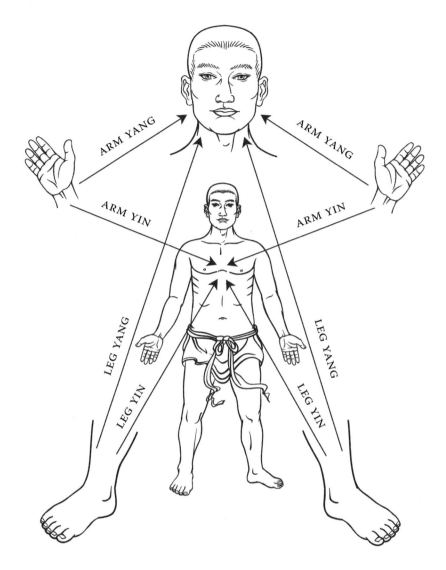

Fig. 16.1

Chapter 2 of the *Divine Pivot* describes a flow of all channels
from the arms and legs toward the head and trunk.

ing deeper into the body along the path from the well points near the finger
and toenails to the sea points around the elbows and knees (Fig. 16.3). At
the same time, there is a circular flow of nutritive and source qi occurring
along the pathways of the twelve channels. There is an almost multidimen-
sional aspect to these two movements. On the one hand, the five transport
point circuit represents the development of function along the channels

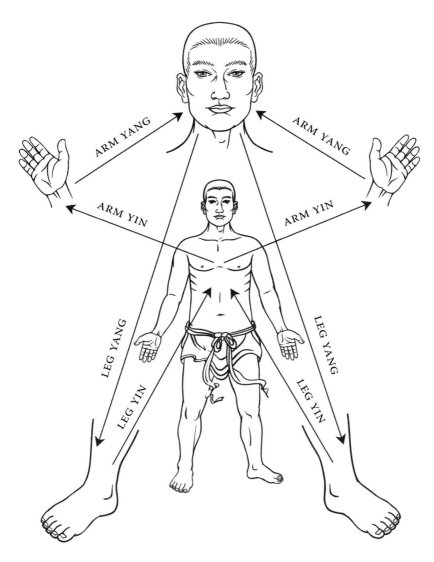

Fig. 16.2
Chapter 10 of the *Divine Pivot* seems to describe a different
direction for channel flow. Now a circuit is being described.

from their roots in the fingers and toes toward their accumulation in the
organs. On the other hand, as described in the section on the triple burner,
there is a simultaneous movement of the nutritive-protective aspect in the
trunk and along the extremities that carries nutrition and prenatal stimulus
to where it is needed (Fig. 16.4). Both of these systems interact in the hands
and feet.

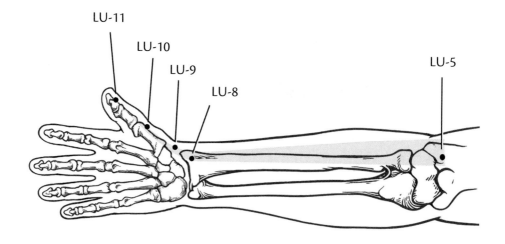

Fig. 16.3
Channel qi comes out at the well points, flows at the
spring points, pours at the stream points, moves (with
force) at the river points, and then enters the body more
deeply at the uniting points.

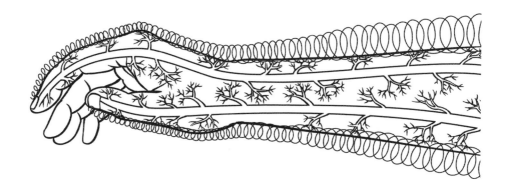

Fig. 16.4
The circuit of nutritive-protective flow provides the nutritive
support for the gradual growth of channel qi. Both are
happening at the same time.

Q: *I almost understand what you are saying at this point, but don't quite see what you mean by 'function' being developed along the course of the five transport points.*

DR. WANG: This is sometimes the hardest thing for students to understand. It has certainly been difficult for me to reconcile these two systems of circulation in my own mind. At first, I was tempted to think of them as simply representing two different theoretical traditions. Certainly, some scholars have asserted just this. The problem, however, is that they both seem to be true at the same time. When one thinks about the conveyance of nutrition and source qi into the fluids of the body, as described in my understanding of triple burner theory, it fits very well with a lot of classical concepts regarding channel qi as a closed circuit. On the other hand, there is still the very real clinical fact that points below the elbows and knees have quite profound effects when compared with other points on the body. In the end, I concluded that, in this case at least, the *Inner Classic* is not contradicting itself but is describing two simultaneous physiological processes.

Now, your question arose because of the use of the term 'function' (功能 *gōng néng*). I'm talking here specifically about the development of the qi that drives and defines the individual organs. For example, as the lung channel progresses from LU-11 *(shào shāng)* inward toward the sea point LU-5 *(chǐ zé)*, there is a slow growth of channel qi. Channel qi is different from the circulation of the nutritive-protective aspects and source qi that is simultaneously occurring in the triple burner. Channel qi is *functional*, while the qi of the twelve-channel circuit in the triple burner is *nutritive*. The development of channel qi involves those 'functions' we memorize for the organs in Chinese medicine. The ability of the lung, for example, to be 'responsible for the skin and small hairs', or the ability of the heart to be 'responsible for the spirit', derives from this interesting concept of channel qi. This is where function begins.

A metaphor might be helpful. Consider the workings of a large city like Beijing. The city requires roads and lines of communication to supply the multitude of activities engaged in by its population. There are systems for delivering all types of food, building supplies, and water through the various gates of the city, while other systems act to remove waste. In fact, I mentioned to you during one of our drives around the city how the different gates in old Beijing were associated with particular products based on how the lines of supply converged. These supply systems may be likened to the closed-circuit flow of the twelve regular channels occurring within the larger environment of the triple burner.

At the same time, within the city, there is a growth of 'human function'. People consume the raw materials that come through the city's supply lines and transform them into refined, specific actions. A city has cooks, bankers, policemen, and factory workers all drawing their nourishment from the circuits of supply and transport. This metaphor may not be perfect, but it might open a door to seeing how two movements of qi can occur at once. There is a circuit of nutrition and, at the same time, a gradual development of function along the course of the transport points.

As long as the supply lines are open and coming through the city gates, people will be moving about doing their normal daily work. If, for example, a policeman doesn't show up to work on a particular day, you might suspect that his supply lines (carrying his salary and/or food) have somehow been cut. In the body, normal organ function is dependent on both the circuit of general nutrition and the specific development of organ qi through the five transport points. Again, these points represent the process of developing function. They depend on the circuit of nutrition provided by the twelve regular channels for their material foundation. Of course, these points are part of those channels, but they represent another aspect of them that is occurring at the same time. Keep thinking about this and turning it over in your mind. You may not completely get it the first time you hear it.

We should also take note of the concept of *transformation* that is described as occurring along the course of the five transport points. As channel qi grows, it consumes qi and blood (nutritive-protective aspect) through the medium of fluids in a transformation to 'channel qi'. The nutritive aspect within the closed circuit of the twelve channels thus provides the material foundation (yin) for the growth of channel qi (yang). Many texts describe channel qi as somehow starting with a gradual, slow flow at the well points, and then growing in strength as it moves toward the elbows and knees. However, there is no conceptual explanation of how this might occur. How can a flow that is gradual and slow at the fingers and toes become full and deep at the elbows and knees? The answer lies in the concept of the closed twelve-channel circuit. As qi grows along the course of the five transport points, it is consuming nutrition from the twelve-channel circuit. The resulting channel qi is then conveyed inward to the organs. Channel qi grows by consuming nutrition in what amounts to a kind of snowball effect (Fig. 16.5).

Chapter 2 of the *Divine Pivot* describes the distal limbs as the 'roots' of the channels. Like roots in the plant kingdom, these channel roots absorb what is specifically needed by their associated organs. Actually, the image of a root *system* might be more appropriate, if one keeps in mind that the

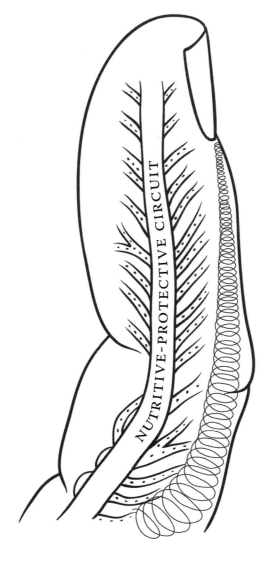

Fig. 16.5

Channel qi builds from the fingers and toes by consuming nutritive qi as it rises to the surface with protective qi.

channels continue to absorb all along their courses as they move through the five transport points toward the elbows and knees. From their inception at the well points where yin and yang meet in a flash of qi creation, the channels develop form and heft. As they grow in volume, they selectively take in information from the rest of the body and from the surrounding environment. This occurs at a particularly brisk rate in the multitude of interactions that take place around the stream points (also source points on the yin channels). The process continues as the flow in the channels moves proximally. In addition to information, the channels are also developing a strong flow of qi which, eventually, becomes the qi of the organs themselves.

One of the most confusing aspects of these concepts is that the term 'channel' is used for both types of flow. This is necessary because both the flow of nutrition in the circuit and the development of qi along the course of the five transport points occur at the same time in the channels. This may be further clarified by reviewing the general functions of the channel system first described in Chapter 2. There we said that the channels are an interwoven network with two broad functions: pathway and communication system. Here, we might consider the twelve-channel circuit as an expression of the pathway concept—moving the raw materials of nutrition around the body. The five transport points, on the other hand, represent the channel system as a network through which various parts of the body are connected in a physiological system of communication and function. The pathway carries material substance, while the network conveys the qi.

While the channel qi grows as it moves along the course of the five transport points, it should not be thought of as transporting 'nutrition' to the internal organs. In other words, it should not be thought that the raw materials for physiology mysteriously spring forth from the fingers and toes. Instead, it is a process of growth in the *action potential* that Chinese medicine calls 'channel qi'. The growth of channel qi does depend on the transformation of nutrition as it increases in depth and volume. By absorbing nutrition, it generates the qi that helps to drive the organs. This is where Chinese medicine and modern Western medicine begin to diverge. The theory of the five transport points asserts that organic function is fundamentally affected by the quality of circulation far away in the extremities.

Returning to the less philosophical realm of the clinic, one should keep in mind that the best use of the distal points takes into account the physiological process of channel qi development, as described in five-transport point theory. Because channel qi is developing and deepening along the forearms and lower legs, the stimulation of these points can initiate change in the qi dynamic of the organs. Different changes will occur from stimulating different points. When crafting treatment strategies, one must therefore consider the movement and development of channel qi at each of the transport points. With that in mind, the traditional categories of well, spring, stream, river, and sea are the best place to start.

The Five Transport Points in the Clinic

Chapter 68 of the *Classic of Difficulties* addresses the uses of the five transport points. It was here that the most common applications of the transport points were first introduced:

- The well points treat fullness below the heart.
- The spring points treat heat in the body.
- The stream points treat heaviness in the body and pain in the joints.
- The river points treat wheezing, coughing, heat, and cold.
- The sea points treat qi counterflow and diarrhea.

In the nearly twenty centuries that have passed since publication of the *Classic of Difficulties*, an enormous amount of commentary has been written about these short passages. Yet in the end, while helpful, this information is incomplete. The *Classic of Difficulties* provides hints about the general nature of the transport points, but not the level of detail that consistent clinical application requires. It is of course possible that portions of the ancient text were lost over time. In any event, the modern understanding of the five transport points draws from layer upon layer of well-documented clinical experience. Debate about the precise nature and uses of the transport points continues to this day, but one thing remains largely undisputed: the five transport points on each channel have unique clinical efficacy.

1. WELL POINTS (井穴 *jǐng xué*)

The well points have the following primary clinical uses:

- Drain excess and dispel stagnation (瀉實祛滯 *xiè shí qū zhì*)
- Disband obstruction and open up clumps (宣痺開結 *xuān bì kāi jié*)

In order to understand the clinical applications of the well points, it is necessary to consider the nature of the channel qi at these points. Often described as places where the channel qi arises from the interaction of yin and yang, the well points are located near the nails of the fingers and toes, where the nutritive-protective aspect from the twelve-channel circuit first begins its transformation to channel qi. As previously noted, the nutritive circuit in the twelve channels is the yin substance to the yang function of channel qi. The well points are therefore regarded as the place where the yin and yang first meet.

Thus the well points are thought to represent the inception of qi transformation by the organs. At these initial points in the growth of the channels, the volume of channel qi is smallest and the rate of movement slowest. The nature of channel qi at the well points is described as seeping and dripping like a spring from the side of a mountain. The flow is not continuous like a stream, but is characterized by gradual accumulation. The term used in Chapter 68 of the *Classic of Difficulties* to describe movement at the well points is 出 *chū*, which means to emerge or come out. The appropriate image is that of the nutritive-protective aspect and source qi from the twelve-channel circuit slowly being transformed into channel qi at the well points (Fig. 16.6).

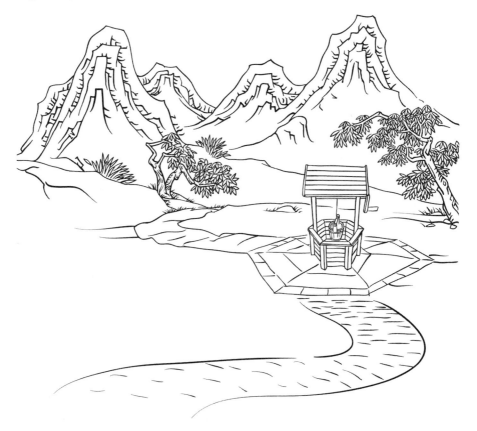

Fig. 16.6
The well points are places where the qi of the channel
comes out and makes its appearance on the body surface.

Q: *What is the initial spark that gets channel qi going at this point?*

DR. WANG: Like everywhere in the body, the spark that initiates the qi dynamic comes ultimately from source qi. Here, at this place of slow, initial development of channel qi, source qi activates the process of transforming nutrition into channel qi. Now, I know you'll want to know why these points wouldn't then be called 'source points'. My understanding of this apparent contradiction is that the source qi is not yet abundant enough at these early points. There is much more circulatory activity at the source points further along the channel.

This is not to say that all channel qi ultimately comes from the well points. It simply begins here at the meeting point of yin and yang. Not only do the yin and yang channels meet at the well points, they are also the places where the nutritive-protective aspect first transforms to the yang function that drives the qi dynamic of the organs. Because the well points are places where channel qi originates, their stimulation can have a strong effect along the entire course of the channel.

This image of the slow and gradual accumulation of channel qi should be kept in mind when thinking about how to use the well points. The two primary uses of the well points in the clinic will now be considered:

1. Drain excess and dispel stagnation

Using the well points to clear and move stagnation of qi and/or blood is often the most familiar to practitioners. Although the nature of qi and blood movement at these points is described as being gradual and dripping, draining the points by removing 8–12 drops of blood can initiate an effect that may be likened to shaking the branch of a tree. The actions of the well points can also be understood by considering the physiological effects of 'draining' an area where channel qi begins. Puncturing the well points and removing a little fluid and blood is like taking some of the pressure out of the channel. When fluids and blood are taken from the starting point of the channel, this begins a chain reaction of relaxation that has the effect of draining excess and eliminating stasis all along the course of the channel.

In modern textbooks, the most common indication for well points is cases where excess and stasis have led to distention and pain. In these cases, heat and/or swelling are often observed along the course of the channel. The type of excess and stasis that can be treated with the well points is not limited to cases involving swelling and pain however. Well point patterns might also include irritability. This is hinted at in the *Classic of Difficulties* when it advises using the points for 'fullness below the heart'. This symptom pattern may involve an irritable restlessness that is rooted in excess. Other well point patterns can include insomnia, tooth grinding, Bell's palsy, headaches, or even stomach disorders that are characterized by excess and heat. For example, tooth grinding, certain types of insomnia, and even herpes zoster can be caused by *yáng míng* excess heat. This type of pattern responds to bleeding of LI-1 *(shāng yáng)* and ST-45 *(lì duì)*. As always, the appropriate channel for treatment is determined through careful differential diagnosis and channel palpation.

2. Disband obstruction and open up clumps

This clinical application is similar to the first, but there are some differences in the diagnosis which require a different treatment technique. Here, the points are used to loosen stagnation in the channels where excess may not be involved. Rather than stasis, there may be a slowness of movement in the channel—a type of deficiency.

A metaphor may be helpful in explaining the difference. The use of well points in cases of excess and stasis may be likened to restoring movement to a river that is blocked by debris. In such cases, strongly bleeding the points stimulates strong movement that breaks apart excess in the channel. This is the type of movement that was compared earlier to shaking the limb of a tree. On the other hand, in the case of obstruction and clumps, the channel is more like a river that has slowed because of a lack of water. In these cases, the qi in the channel slows and congeals, but there will be no signs of stasis and heat. Instead of the healthy movement that is characteristic of a normal channel, there is a kind of stickiness that is referred to classically as 'obstruction' or, when more serious, 'clumps' in the channel. Here, you can generate a tonifying effect at the well points—and thereby improve the flow—by bleeding just three or four drops of blood, or by using needles or moxa (Fig. 16.7).

The term obstruction here is translated elsewhere as painful obstruction, bi (syndrome), or impediment. In other words, the well points can be used in treating various arthritic-type patterns associated with this category of disease. When an obstruction persists, it may become a 'clump'—a more severe case in which the channel qi becomes congealed. When there is obstruction, qi and blood cannot move freely in the channel (氣血失常 *qì xuè shī cháng*). By contrast, a clump is more like a knot in the qi dynamic of the channel (氣機閉結 *qì jī bì jié*). It may also be compared to a vapor lock in which the water in a full bottle turned upside down will not flow out be-

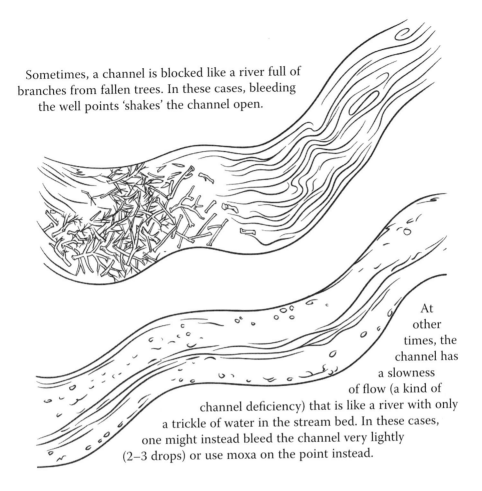

Sometimes, a channel is blocked like a river full of branches from fallen trees. In these cases, bleeding the well points 'shakes' the channel open.

At other times, the channel has a slowness of flow (a kind of channel deficiency) that is like a river with only a trickle of water in the stream bed. In these cases, one might instead bleed the channel very lightly (2–3 drops) or use moxa on the point instead.

Fig. 16.7
The use of well points in cases of excess and stasis may be likened to restoring movement to a river that is blocked by debris.

cause air cannot get in. In both cases, although sluggish, the flow of channel qi doesn't necessarily cause overt signs of excess and/or heat. Clinically, this pathodynamic might manifest in sudden fainting, shock, or psychosis—conditions which are also classically treated with the well points (Fig. 16.8).

Other common symptoms associated with well points can also be explained in terms of obstruction and clumps in the channels. For example, consider the use of SI-1 *(shào zé)* in the treatment of insufficient lactation. It is indicated for this purpose when the pathodynamic involves clumped qi—most often caused by sudden, violent anger or some other emotional disturbance, including many types of postpartum depression. The well points

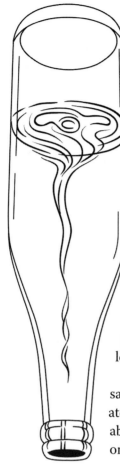

Fig. 16.8
When a channel has a very slow flow due to an impediment, it is like a vapor lock in an overturned bottle. Moxa or mild bleeding (2–3 drops) at the well point reactivates flow throughout the channel.

are also often used to treat generalized numbness around the hands and feet, not because of their ability to break up excess stasis, but because of their ability to stimulate movement and thereby disperse obstruction in the channels.

Other examples of using well points to initiate a tonifying movement include the use of SP-1 *(yǐn bái)* to treat spotting between periods (漏 *lòu;* see Chapter 5 for a discussion of spleen-type uterine bleeding) or KI-1 *(yōng quán)* to treat asthma associated with kidney deficiency. In both cases, the well points have a tonifying effect largely drawn from their location at the very inception of channel qi.

The *Systematic Classic of Acupuncture and Moxibustion* says that the well points on the yin channels are appropriate for many types of deficiency patterns because of their ability to stimulate the qi dynamic, while the well points on the yang channels are better for treating excess. This general principle holds true in the modern clinic. The main idea to keep in mind is that the well points can be used both to drain excess and to create a kind of mild tonification in the channel, depending on the technique used for stimulation.

Techniques for treating well points

When using the well points to treat excess, at least 8–12 drops of blood should be drawn from the point with a lancet needle to truly shake out the channel. In severe cases, as much as 40 drops of blood may be drawn. When drawing more drops of blood, the technique involves squeezing the area around the point, then quickly removing small drops of blood with a few cotton balls while counting. The goal is not necessarily to remove a large volume of blood from the point but to generate a very small trickle that is counted off by the practitioner. When bleeding to drain excess, it is important that the color of blood drawn turn from dark to light. When the drops become pale or even clear, enough blood has been drawn.

On the other hand, when the well points are used to treat obstructions and clumps, one is more likely to use moxa or low stimulation needle techniques. Often, needles can create gentle movement in the channel, in contrast to the strong draining achieved by bleeding. Sometimes a similar effect can be achieved by bleeding only 4–5 drops of blood from the point. Bleeding in this manner may be thought of as a 'neutral' (as opposed to tonifying or draining) technique to create movement. Also, because obstructions and clumps are not often rooted in excess or heat, the blood will generally be pale or even clear. This is in contrast to the bright-red blood seen in presentations of more excess, or the dark blood seen in cases of more severe blood stagnation.

In summary, the use of well points described in the *Classic of Difficulties* for treating 'fullness below the heart' should be viewed as an example of a pattern type, rather than as an exclusive indication. In other words, fullness and tightness in the epigastrium is just one manifestation of the types of channel excess that can be eliminated by stimulating the well points. But, as explained above, the points can also be quite effective in treating conditions that don't present with clear symptoms of excess. The actual symptom presentation will obviously vary depending on which of the channels is involved.

Point	Treatment Goal	Indication
SI-1 *(shào zé)*	Open bindings	Binding from emotional excess leads to insufficient lactation
ST-45 *(lì duì)*	Drain excess stasis	*Yáng míng* heat causing tooth grinding at night or insomnia
LI-1 *(shāng yáng)*	Drain excess stasis	*Yáng míng* heat insomnia
SP-1 *(yǐn bái)*	Diffuse impediments	Spleen deficiency causing spotting between periods
LR-1 *(dà dūn)*	Diffuse impediments	Liver deficiency leading to heavy uterine bleeding
KI-1 *(yǒng quán)*	Diffuse impediments	Kidney deficiency causing asthma

Table 16.2
Representative uses for selected well points

2. Spring points (榮穴 *yíng xué*)

Also known as the gushing points, the spring points have the following primary clinical uses:

- Clear heat from deficiency (清虛熱 *qīng xū rè*)
- Foster yin-blood (育陰血 *yù yīn xuè*)

The spring points are generally found around the distal metacarpal and metatarsal joints. In these areas, flesh begins to accumulate and the development of channel qi undergoes a change. There is increased circulation of qi and blood. Channel qi is said to be moving at a faster rate at the spring points, although its nature is still dripping and the flow is not yet strong. Nevertheless, the *Inner Classic* describes the qi here as flowing (流 *liú*) and conveys the idea that channel qi begins to move at these points. Specifically, this is the first movement inward. While channel qi emerges at the well points, it begins to move in a particular direction at the spring points (Fig. 16.9).

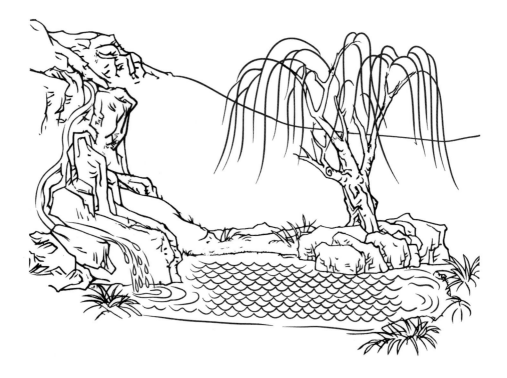

Fig. 16.9

Spring points are where channel qi collects and begins to slowly flow in a particular direction. They generally have cooling, yin-nourishing natures.

Chapter 68 of the *Classic of Difficulties* says that the spring points are appropriate for treating heat in the body. For this reason, most modern texts list the spring points for cases of fever. Once again, although true, the clinical application of the spring points is broader than this. A review of such classical sources as *Gathering of the Blossoms of Acupuncture* (針灸聚 英 *Zhēn jiǔ jù yīng*, 1529), *Classic of Nourishing Life with Acupuncture and Moxibustion* (針灸資生經 *Zhēn jiǔ zī shēng jīng*, 1220) and the *Great Compendium of Acupuncture and Moxibustion* (針灸大成 *Zhēn jiǔ dà chéng*, 1601) reveals some general patterns that help refine our understanding. The applications identified below are drawn from these sources.

The classical texts suggest that the heat-clearing function of the spring points should be narrowed to mostly those cases where heat is caused by a deficiency of yin and/or blood. Because of the slow initial movement of channel qi at the spring points, stimulation in this area has an effect of generating yin fluids. The next transport point up the line, the stream point, integrates the more yang-natured source qi into the process.

In the clinic, the pathodynamic of the spring points often involves patients with low-grade fevers. The use of spring points in cases of heat from deficiency is hinted at in Chapter 44 of the *Divine Pivot* where it prescribes their use in "diseases that cause changes in the patient's complexion." This is the commonly-used phrase for the flushing of the cheeks associated with yin-blood deficiency. For other types of fever, the spring points are often less effective.

For example, in the fairly common case of lung heat due to yin deficiency causing sore throat, LU-10 *(yú jì)* can be quite effective. Heat caused by yin-blood deficiency is also often present in cases of pelvic inflammatory disease. In these cases, the spring points of the spleen, liver, and kidney channels (SP-2, LR-2 and KI-2) may be appropriate. LR-2 *(xíng jiān)* is commonly listed in modern texts for clearing liver fire. In fact, while the point does have the ability to help clear excess-type liver patterns, it is most appropriate when liver (blood) deficiency is also part of the pattern. In cases of true liver fire excess, it is often more effective to choose points on the paired *shào yáng* channel to clear heat upward and outward.

The spring points are also used for many patterns that involve chronic inflammation with an element of deficiency. Acute inflammation, on the other hand, is usually better treated by bleeding the well points. For example, when using LU-10 for throat inflammation, the inflammation should be of a relatively chronic and deficient nature. If a patient presents with acute tonsillitis, the well point LU-11 *(shào shāng)* is much more likely to be effective. Similar principles hold true for most of the other channels.

An obvious exception to the deficiency-heat theme is ST-44 *(nèi tíng)*. This point is, in fact, very useful for clearing excess-type *yáng míng* heat. There are always exceptions.

Techniques for treating spring points

When needling, keep the nature of channel qi at the spring points in mind. The movement here is said to 'flow' in a very thin, broken line in contrast to the dripping nature of channel qi at the well points. Consequently, qi sensation for the patient should also involve a light and gentle movement down the channel. By facilitating the natural tendency of the point, the production of yin-blood in the channel can begin. Specifically, needle insertion should be shallow and the stimulus should be a gentle, twirling technique. The result of spring point stimulation is not a large burst of yin-blood, but gradual growth (Table 16.3).

Point	Pathodynamic
LU-10 (*yú jì*)	Deficiency of lung yin leading to sore throat
SP-2 (*dà dū*)	Fluid deficiency combined with exterior condition; patient unable to sweat
LR-2 (*xíng jiān*)	Liver blood deficiency leading to heat
ST-44 (*nèi tíng*)	Strong heat in the *yáng míng* channel and/or organ; yin often damaged

Table 16.3

Representative uses for selected spring points

3. STREAM POINTS (輸穴 *shū xué*)

Also known as the transport points, the stream points have the following primary clinical uses:

- Augment the qi and warm the yang (益氣溫陽 *yì qì wēn yáng*)
- Transform dampness (化濕 *huà shī*)

The stream points are generally found around the wrists and ankles, areas of high mobility on the limbs. The *Classic of Difficulties* describes the movement of the channel qi at the stream points as 'pouring' (注 *zhù*). The qi now moves through the channel in a steady, natural stream like water poured from a flask. Here, at the wrists and ankles, the channels are active. This type of active qi circulation marks the beginning of a brisk interaction between qi and blood. Consider the fact that the blood vessels in these areas tend to be numerous and relatively thin-walled. These small vessels have the flexibility and permeability needed to provide abundant nutrition for the active joints in the area. In fact, it is because of this interaction of qi and blood that the stream points also serve as the source points on the yin channels. See Fig. 16.10. (This will be discussed further in the next chapter.)

Earlier it was noted how source qi provides the spark that initiates the development of channel qi at the well points. Here at the stream points, the source qi enters the channel in force. The concept of source qi and the use of the source points will be discussed further in the next chapter, but a few of the concepts are especially important when considering the role of source qi in the system of the five transport points.

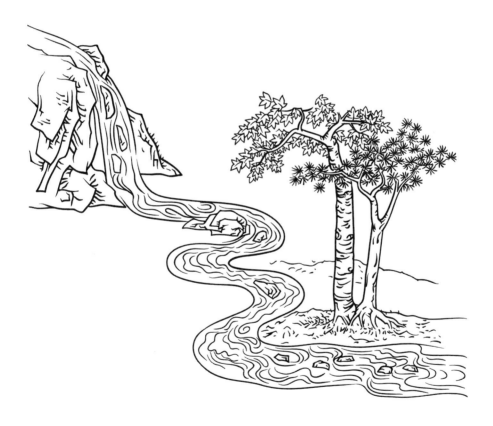

Fig. 16.10
The stream points are areas of lively qi circulation. Here, channel qi begins to truly pour along with great activity—but still without large volume.

In particular, it is important to remember that the source qi plays an active role in the entire process of channel qi development. All along the channel pathways, source qi acts as a primary stimulus. Earlier in the chapter, the question was posed as to how transformation could occur at the well and spring points when the source qi only enters the channel at the stream points (or the next point up the line on the yang channels). The answer was that source qi is in fact present even at the finger tips. This is because of the pervasive reach of the passageways of the triple burner. Thus the source qi is present not only at the source points, but also in the fluids around all acupuncture points.

However, in the development of channel qi, it is at the stream points that the source qi begins to strengthen the flow in the channels, which becomes quicker and deeper as it approaches the sea points. Again, remember that the influx of source qi here in particular stems from increased blood circulation and joint movement. Higher turnover of qi and blood brings about this first significant draw of source qi.

Clinically, the *Classic of Difficulties* advises using the stream points in the treatment of heaviness in the body and pain in the joints. This indication can be attributed to the same physiological characteristic that causes the stream points to double as source points on the yin channels: the diverse circulation that draws source qi to the area makes the stream points especially useful for building yang movement in the channels. As most practitioners know, a deficiency of yang leading to an accumulation of dampness is at the root of many chronic patterns involving heaviness and pain not only in the joints, but throughout the body. Ultimately then, the ability to treat these conditions at the stream points depends on strengthening yang transformation along the course of the channel. In short, by generating yang through increased source qi circulation, dampness and cold are transformed and pain is reduced.

The major difference between healthy and pathogenic fluids can be found in their ability to deliver nutrition. Without the stimulus of yang qi, not only will dampness linger in the channels, but the fluids will also lose their ability to nourish the muscles and joints. Thus a cycle is created in which lack of transformation leads to inadequate nutrition; in turn, the absence of proper nutrition leads to heaviness and a sense of weakness causing lethargy that further inhibits movement and the development of yang qi. Eventually, the joints themselves may be affected. Thus the joints require both abundant yang qi for active movement and a constant supply of fluids to moisten and carry nourishment to the spaces between the bones. Once this cycle reaches the point of pain in the joints, there is likely to be significant accumulation of pathogenic dampness with swelling that, if allowed to linger, may become phlegm.

In any case, while heaviness and joint pain are most likely due to pathogenic dampness caused by stagnant fluids, the ultimate cause is a lack of yang transformation from source qi. Thus the general function of the stream points is to boost the qi and warm the yang. The effect of boosting the qi and warming the yang will be the transformation of dampness and cold.

Techniques for treating the stream points

Like the spring points above, the goal of needle technique for the stream points should be to obtain a gentle moving sensation along the channel. As the stream points are often located near relatively large vessels, insertion should be slow so as to allow the vessels to move out of the way. The practitioner shouldn't try to push the vessel out of the way with the thumb, as is sometimes advised, for example, when inserting at LU-9 *(tài yuān)*. Instead, a slow, gradual insertion will accomplish this while also facilitating the best qi response. Once the proper depth has been attained, a rapid twirling technique should be used. Twirling helps to facilitate the proper sense of radiation (Table 16.4).

Point	Mechanism and Indications
TB-3 *(zhōng zhǔ)*	Brings warmth to the *shào yáng* channel; appropriate for lateral low back/hip stiffness due to cold stasis
BL-65 *(shù gǔ)*	Warms *tài yáng* channel; appropriate for low back pain due to cold in channels
SP-3 *(tài bái)*	Heaviness throughout the body can be treated by strengthening spleen (yang) qi.
SI-3 *(hòu xī)*	Treats neck and upper back stiffness caused by cold in the *tài yáng* channel
KI-3 *(tài xī)*	Treats chronic deficiency/cold-type low back pain by strengthening kidney yang qi

Table 16.4

Representative uses for selected stream points

4. River points (經穴 *jīng xué*)

Also known as the traversing points, the river points have the following primary clinical use:

• Promote proper movement of channel qi (行經氣 *xíng jīng qì*)

The river points are found in areas of relatively deeper flesh than the previous three transport points. Here, there are fairly clear separations between tendons and muscles that are large enough to accommodate the steady, large, and deepening flow of qi in the channels, which classical physiologists compared to a river. The term 行 *xíng*, used classically to describe the movement of qi at the river points, conveys an image of strong, constant movement. The qi here is even and full though not yet moving with the depth seen at the sea points (Fig. 16.11).

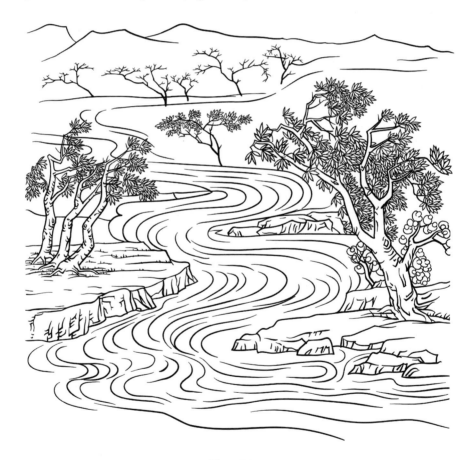

Fig. 16.11
The strong channel flow of the river points can be used
to forcefully clear the surface.

Chapter 68 of the *Classic of Difficulties* recommends the river points in cases of wheezing, coughing, heat, and cold—often symptoms of external pathogenic invasion. Because the qi is truly moving at the river points, their stimulation provides a burst of channel qi that can help force exterior pathogens out of the body. It is the sheer force of the movement of qi at these points that accounts for their effectiveness in clearing the surface of external pathogens. Again, the force here is still along the relatively superficial layers of the muscles. In general, the clinical applications of river points reflect their ability to promote proper movement.

An example of promoting movement to release the exterior is the use of LU-8 *(jīng qú)* to treat invasion of wind-cold with symptoms of coughing, body pain, and fever accompanied by a lack of sweating (excess exterior condition). The effects of the point are slightly modified when combined with the spring point SP-2 *(dà dū)*. This point pair can be likened to the formula Combined Cinnamon Twig and Ephedra Decoction *(guì zhī má huáng gé bàn tāng)*. Like the formula, stimulation of these points acts to release an exterior pathogen outward where there is a slight underlying *tài yīn* deficiency—a fairly common situation. The river point LU-8 moves the channel qi to force the external pathogen out of the body, while the spring point of the spleen channel (SP-2) helps to clear heat from deficiency. Together, LU-8 releases the *tài yīn* lung while SP-2 acts to clear heat from deficiency by gently supporting the *tài yīn* spleen. Each of the points clears a different type of heat, and together they are quite effective in helping deficient patients get over a persistent, unrelenting fever. Note that while the spring points are sometimes used on their own to treat low-grade fever due to heat from deficiency, this pair is effective in cases where a high fever refuses to break. The important diagnostic marker is that the patient is unable to sweat. The effectiveness of this point pair lies in its ability to initiate the removal of pathogens by inducing sweating. The treatment technique in such cases should be fairly strong twirling of the needles.

Some of the river points are hard to fit into the *Classic of Difficulties* mold of treating wheezing, coughing, heat, and cold. For example, a commonly used point like TB-6 *(zhī gōu)* does not have the same ability to release the exterior as the nearby TB-5 *(wài guān)*. In general, TB-6 is a point for clearing heat in the channel. This function is based on its ability to move qi in the channel. The point is also familiar to many as useful in treating constipation, specifically the type associated with stasis of qi combined with heat in the liver and gallbladder. The river point on the *shào yáng* channel clears this constrained heat from all three burners. In the clinic, TB-6 is often paired with GB-34 *(yáng líng quán)* to dredge and drain the *shào yáng* channel. By combining the regulating action of a sea point (discussed below) with the moving action of a river point, the net result is to dredge (疏 *shū*) the *shào yáng*.

By contrast, KI-7 *(fù liū)*, another river point, largely acts to strengthen the yin. Unlike KI-3 *(tài xī)*, which stimulates the qi dynamic of the kidney organ by facilitating the flow of source qi, KI-7 strengthens by moving. In the case of the kidney (a yin-water organ), the provision of yin sometimes requires an extra boost of movement. Note as well that the five-phase categorization of KI-7 associates the point with metal, the 'mother' of water in the generating cycle. It therefore has a slightly more tonifying effect than other river points.

In summary, for the river points in particular, it is important to consider the net effects of moving the channel qi on the qi dynamic of the organ and/or channel. Because these effects are quite varied, the indications for the river points may be quite different from channel to channel. As always, the functions of the points described in the *Classic of Difficulties* must be considered in context (Table 16.5).

Point	Moves channel qi to cause...
LU-8 *(jīng qú)*	external pathogens to clear by strengthening movement of lung channel; pathogens forced outward
KI-7 *(fù liū)*	benefits to kidney yin by moving channel and organ qi
TB-6 *(zhī gōu)*	'shaking out' the sinews of the *shào yáng* channel for pain due to qi stasis
BL-60 *(kūn lún)*	strong clearing of excess from the bladder channel by moving downwards; most clearly affects the upper end of the channel (head)

Table 16.5

Representative uses for selected river points

Techniques for treating river points

Technique should reflect the fact that the qi and blood are moving more rapidly at the river points. Specifically, slightly stronger techniques are indicated. To obtain qi at a river point, one might utilize the scratching or flying techniques (see Chapter 19). The goal should now be focused on initiating movement in the channel, and less on creating the gentle radiation that is important at more distal points. To that end, longer needles can be used where appropriate, with less twirling and more lifting and thrusting.

5. Sea points (合穴 *hé xué*)

Also known as the uniting points, the sea points have the following primary clinical uses:

- Treat counterflow (治逆氣 *zhì nì qì*)
- Regulate organ qi transformation (調理臟腑氣化 *tiáo lǐ zàng fǔ qì huà*)

At the sea points, the channel qi dives inward toward the organs themselves. The flow is full, wide, and deep at these points around the elbows and knees. The *Classic of Difficulties* says that the qi enters (入 *rù*) at the sea points. The strong, deepening flow of channel qi here makes these points some of the most widely used in the clinic. Note also that not only are the points located near the elbows and knees, but also near large blood vessels. There is no longer the dispersed exchange of microcirculation that characterized the stream points in particular. Here, the channel qi is united, solid, and fast (Fig. 16.12).

The *Classic of Difficulties* recommends sea points in the treatment of qi counterflow and diarrhea. In the modern clinic, the points are used to regulate the organs and benefit the channel qi. Specifically, these are cases where qi transformation is somehow chaotic or disordered. The term 'counterflow' refers to just this type of situation. The symptoms of qi counterflow can vary, based on which organ is affected. For example, in the stomach, qi counterflow often involves vomiting, since the normal direction of stomach qi is to descend. In the lungs, symptoms might include cough, while liver qi counterflow might manifest with emotional symptoms or signs of heat. Because diarrhea may be caused by counterflow involving a variety of organs, the *Classic of Difficulties* lists it as a representative symptom. Often, diarrhea is a symptom of spleen channel counterflow. Problems with fluid metabolism may be due to qi counterflow in the bladder, spleen, kidney, or even lung channels and are thus often treated with point pairs that include the sea points.

The term 'qi counterflow' is sometimes misunderstood. Simply put, it implies that there is a type of problem with the organ at a functional level that involves a disordered movement of qi. This type of complaint often responds quite quickly to acupuncture treatment. For example, consider the use of the sea-point pair LU-5 *(chǐ zé)* and SP-9 *(yīn líng quán)*. This pair

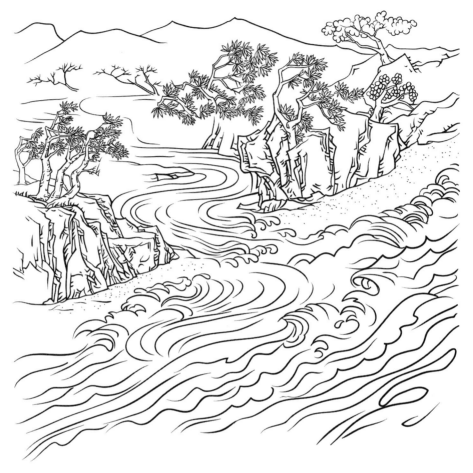

Fig. 16.12
The ability of the sea points to regulate comes from their location at
places where deep, strong channel qi enters the sea of the internal organs.
The place of intersection can regulate large-scale counterflow.

regulates the *tài yīn* qi dynamic and is effective in treating a wide variety of
pathodynamics. Symptoms as varied as cough, chronic colds, shortness of
breath, diarrhea, low appetite, fatigue, edema, skin problems, or even grief
and/or lack of concentration might all indicate a root cause of dysfunction
in the *tài yīn* qi dynamic. The sea points of the other channels have similarly
broad effects on the organs by virtue of their ability to broadly regulate the
proper movement of qi transformation.

Another type of qi counterflow treated with sea points might not involve
a chaotic qi dynamic in the organs, but instead might be rooted in stasis and
clumping (瘀結 *yū jié*) in the channels. Most often, this type of stasis leads

to symptoms of excess. Consider, for example, the use of BL-40 *(wěi zhōng)* in the case of relatively acute low back pain, GB-34 *(yáng líng quán)* for *shào yáng* channel leg pain, or ST-36 *(zú sān lǐ)* for excess type stomach conditions. In these cases, the sea points (especially on the yang channels) act to release stasis in the channel by stimulating strong movement. In that sense, they have some similarity to the river points.

In general, the sea points regulate by moving. While they can be used, like the river points, to move the qi in the channels, they can also have broader effects because of their ability to regulate organ function. Their ability to both reestablish proper movement of qi in the channels as well as the qi dynamic in the organs is attributed to their nature as places where the channel flows deep and strong (Table 16.6).

Point	Counterflow reversal with sea points...
LU-5 *(chǐ zé)*	creates harmonized qi movement throughout the body; the lung commands the body's qi
SP-9 *(yīn líng quán)*	regulates transformation of dampness and transportation of nutritive qi by the spleen
ST-36 *(zú sān lǐ)*	benefits qi and blood of the whole body by optimizing movement of the yang aspect of digestion *(yáng míng)*
GB-34 *(yáng líng quán)*	benefits muscles and sinews by harmonizing movement of the pivot; harmonized movement also clears heat and qi stagnation
BL-40 *(wěi zhōng)*	improves circulation to the low back by stimulating proper movement of qi and blood through the broad pathway of *tài yáng*

Table 16.6

Representative uses for selected sea points

· ·

Techniques for treating sea points

When needling the sea points, bear in mind that the channel flow here is not only strong, but deep. The goal is therefore to obtain qi at a relatively deep level. In addition, lifting and thrusting is used to obtain a strong sense of radiation down the entire channel. Practitioners should consider the commonly reported qi sensations at points like ST-36 *(zú sān lǐ)*, GB-34 *(yáng líng quán)*, and LI-11 *(qū chí)* as representative.

Examples of Five Transport Point Pairs

In general, there are three ways that the five transport points are paired:

1. STRENGTHENING THE MOTHER OR DRAINING THE CHILD

This is a traditional application of the five transport points. In this approach, points are chosen based on their five-phase associations. One common method is to choose the point associated with the 'mother' or 'child' phase of the channel on which it is found. The mother phase is the one before the affected phase in the generative cycle, while the child phase follows the affected phase. Mother points tonify while child points drain. For example, one might choose SP-2 *(dà dū)*, the fire point on an earth channel, to tonify the spleen and SP-5, the metal point on the earth channel, to drain spleen excess.

Another approach is to choose five-phase points on one channel to treat a different channel. Continuing with the example of the spleen, one would choose HT-8 *(shào fǔ)*, the fire point on the fire channel (mother of earth), in cases of spleen deficiency, and LU-8 *(jīng qú)*, the metal point on the metal channel (child of earth), in cases of excess. This approach is generally familiar to most students of Chinese medicine. Modern 'five-element' acupuncture traditions also explore in greater detail the complexities of the five-phase associations and the use of the controlling cycle points as well (Fig. 16.13).[3]

2. OPEN POINT TREATMENT

The second approach to using the five transport points involves chrono-acupuncture and similar traditions that emphasize certain 'open' points based on the circulation of qi in the channels throughout the day. This approach involves considerations of classical Chinese astrology, *Yì jīng* (I-Ching) studies, and Daoist traditions. These systems have been used extensively both in the past and in the modern era. The idea that there is more qi and blood in a particular channel at a particular time of day is one that deserves further research. In any case, the subject is beyond the scope of this book and will be left to more specialized texts.

3. TREATMENT BASED ON TRANSPORT POINT PHYSIOLOGY

The third approach involves considerations of qi development in the channels and the nature of qi movement through the five transport points

IN METHOD ONE, the 'mother' fire point is tonified while the 'son' metal point is sedated. In cases of spleen deficiency, choose SP-2 (*dà dū*), and in cases of excess, SP-5 (*shāng qiū*).

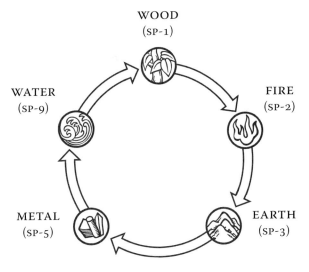

IN METHOD TWO, tonifying the spleen involves choosing the mother point on the mother channel (HT-8 [*shào fǔ*]). This is often combined with the point on the affected channel that is associated with the channel's element (SP-3 [*tài bái*] in this case). To sedate the spleen, one would choose the son point from the son channel (LU-8 [*jīng qú*]). This might be combined with the son point (metal) on the spleen channel (SP-5 [*shāng qiū*]).

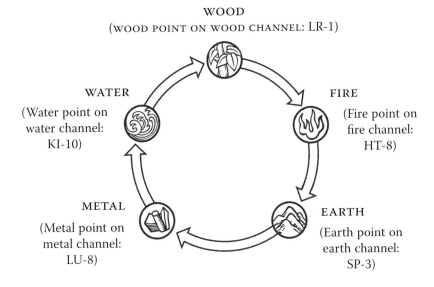

Fig. 16.13

Two methods for sedating and tonifying the spleen using
transport points in 'mother-son' treatment

as conceived in the physiological model of the *Classic of Difficulties*. This is the model described in this chapter. The functions of the points are considered in the context of overall channel qi development, from the 'roots' in the fingers and toes to 'junctions' in the organs of the trunk.

In reality, the use of point pairs in the clinic often involves both the first and third approaches, sometimes at the same time. This is mostly because the nature of the points suggested by their five-phase associations is often in tandem with the development of channel qi as envisaged by the *Classic of Difficulties*. However, because the nature and functions of the organs differ, the ability of their five transport points to clear heat, transform dampness, move qi, tonify or drain also differ slightly from channel to channel. In the end, the ultimate determinant of which points to use is the impartial standard of clinical efficacy. If the treatment works, then it will be used. Fortunately, the model outlined by five-transport point theory and, to some degree, the indications of five-phase theory, help to give structure to the process of point selection.

A survey of classical texts, as well as the acupuncture point 'odes' memorized by students of Chinese medicine over the millennia, reveals that the majority of classical acupuncture prescriptions incorporate the five transport or source points of the twelve channels. Similarly, in the modern clinic, most acupuncture treatments involve at least one of these important points. A helpful way to conceptualize their use in the clinic is to combine the points into functional pairs. Chapter 20 addresses point pairs in detail, but a few examples will be discussed here to illustrate the concepts described above.

SP-3 (tài bái) and SP-9 (yīn líng quán)

The combination of the stream (source) and sea points on the spleen *tài yīn* channel has the ability to warm the yang and benefit the spleen qi to transform dampness. In the clinic, the pair is effective in cases of abdominal swelling caused by qi deficiency. It is less effective in cases where swelling is of an excess, water-dampness accumulation type. Qi deficiency can lead to diffuse swelling that feels soft to the touch and gives way easily to pressure. On the other hand, the accumulation of water-dampness causes the abdomen to feel hard when pressed, indicating substantial build-up of fluids. Diarrhea and/or abdominal distention due to spleen deficiency are also often treated with this point pair.

In analyzing the pair, remember that the *Classic of Difficulties* says that the stream point is used to treat heaviness in the body while the sea point acts to regulate the qi transformation of the spleen. As the source point, SP-3 also guides the source qi into the channel to strengthen spleen function.

The net result is to effectively benefit and regulate the spleen qi with the specific goal of transforming dampness caused by deficiency. This point pair can also be used for swelling related to spleen qi deficiency in other areas of the body, and in cases of leg swelling during menstruation as well. Sometimes, the pair is combined with other similar pairs for greater emphasis, for example, with ST-36 *(zú sān lǐ)* and CV-12 *(zhōng wǎn)* to further benefit the qi of the middle burner.

LU-11 *(shào shāng)* and LU-5 *(chǐ zé)*

This pair is used clinically to clear heat and benefit the throat. It is indicated not only for the common sore throat, but also for tonsillitis and laryngitis. The pair can also nourish the yin and stop coughing. Patients who present with loss of voice secondary to external invasion are often treated at these points when the primary pathogen is heat. In such cases, LU-11 is usually needled shallowly and gently twirled for a moment after insertion to disperse the area. By contrast, the technique at LU-5 generally involves more lifting and thrusting of the needle.

This is a well-sea point pair. Heat is cleared by 'shaking' the channel out with the well point, while the sea point facilitates strong movement. The net effect is to clear and open both the organ and its divergent channel through the throat. The ability of the pair to benefit the yin is a secondary effect of clearing the heat by moving the channel qi. It is the heat that damages the yin.

This pair should be contrasted with the pair LU-8 *(jīng qú)* and SP-2 *(dà dū)*, described above in the river points section. In the LU-5 and LU-11 pair, the case is more strictly one of excess and heat and rarely involves deficiency. The apparent 'yin deficiency' in the throat is actually just a side effect of excess heat in the internal pathway of the lung channel. Thus, while the pair LU-5 and LU-11 benefits the throat by clearing heat, the pair LU-8 and SP-2 releases the exterior by virtue of its ability to move and also protect the yin. Consequently, in the clinic, LU-5 and LU-11 are most often used in treating acute excess cases where the dominant symptom is sore throat. The LU-8 and SP-2 pair is used in more lingering cases of external invasion where deficiency is also present.

TB-6 *(zhī gōu)* and GB-34 *(yáng líng quán)*

This pair combines a river point with a sea point, both on *shào yáng* channels. Both points can strongly move the qi. Together, the pair is used in the clinic to strongly dredge and drain (疏瀉 *shū xiè*) the *shào yáng*. Because yang channels are often used to clear excess in their paired yin channels, these points can also clear excess from the *jué yīn*.

Clinical manifestations of this pathodynamic are varied and may include abdominal distention, premenstrual syndrome, dysmenorrhea, constipation, hypochondriac pain, or inflammation of the gallbladder. Most importantly, the underlying cause should be stasis in the *shào yáng* or *jué yīn*. In Chapter 20, the functions of this pair are compared and contrasted with a similar *shào yáng* pair, TB-5 *(wài guān)* and GB-41 *(zú lín qì)*.

ST-36 *(zú sān lǐ)* and SP-3 *(tài bái)*

The first two pairs above were of transport points on the same channel, while the third pair involved two same-name channels. In this fourth pair, there are transport points from internally-externally paired channels. The sea point on the yang channel regulates movement while the stream (source) point on the yin channel tonifies. Together, they move the yang qi. In this case, because of the addition of a yang channel point, the spleen yang is stimulated, which strengthens the middle.

Like the pair SP-3 and SP-9 introduced above, this pair is used to strengthen the spleen. However, while the ST-36 and SP-3 pair has a stronger ability to tonify the spleen, the former pair acts more upon dampness. This pair is therefore used in chronic cases with more serious deficiency that is likely to involve the yang. The pathodynamic may lead to such medical diagnoses as chronic colitis, chronic gastritis, some types of anemia, or Crohn's disease.

KI-7 *(fù liū)* and LR-2 *(xíng jiān)*

This is a variation on the theme of mother-child treatment. In this case, the metal (river) point of the water channel (mother point) is combined with the fire (spring) point on the wood channel (child point), with the net effect of 'benefiting water and calming wood'. Here, one is tonifying the mother and draining the child at the same time. Also reminiscent of the pair LU-8 and SP-2, described earlier, the moving, heat-clearing actions of a river point are combined with the ability of the spring point to calm heat from deficiency. This case is different, however, because, instead of combining two points on channels of the same name *(tài yīn)*, this pair combines points on mother-child five-phase channels. The net effect is different. With this pair, tonification is combined with draining in a mother-child channel pair.

The underlying pathodynamic indicated for this pair is kidney deficiency that leads to liver yang rising. Symptoms may include dizziness, irritability, ear ringing, high blood pressure, or Ménière's disease.

Note that this pair involves the combination of five-phase concepts with the *Classic of Difficulties* five-transport point theory. The same logic regarding the use of river and spring points that was used in conceiving the LU-8 and SP-2 point pair is combined with a consideration of five-phase channel relationships. This is the kind of integrative thinking which, when combined with an understanding of organ theory, leads to innovation and flexibility in the clinic (Fig. 16.14 and 16.15).

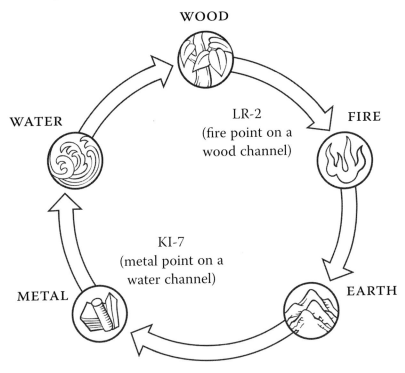

Fig. 16.14

In the KI-7 and LR-2 point pair, the liver is both cleared and benefitted by combining mother-child theory in a slightly different way.

Five-Transport Point Theory and Classical Physiology

At this point, we would like to revisit and expand upon some concepts introduced at the beginning of this chapter regarding the physiological role of the channels and the concept of 'channel qi'. It was pointed out above that the *Inner Classic* seems to describe two different models of qi movement. On the one hand, Chapter 2 of the *Divine Pivot* describes a movement of qi beginning at all of the fingers and toes that moves inward toward the trunk of the body. This is the basis for the model described above that we have called five-transport point circulation. The second model of qi flow, described in Chapter 10 of the *Divine Pivot*, is a kind of closed circuit from

LU-8: river point strongly moves channel qi
to give forceful clearing of external pathogens

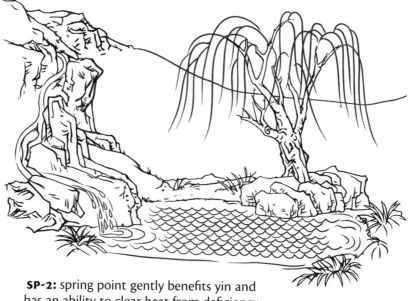

SP-2: spring point gently benefits yin and
has an ability to clear heat from deficiency

Fig. 16.15
The LU-8 and SP-2 point pair is best understood by considering
the different types of qi flow at spring and river points. In this case,
five-phase theory is less helpful for conceptualizing function.

yin to yang channels that moves alternately outward to the extremities then
inward toward the trunk.

As described above, these two circuits occur at the same time and can
be thought of as involving two distinct and interdependent aspects of physiology. The first involves the growth of stimulus for organ function known
as 'channel qi' while the second is the circuit of the nutritive and protective aspect. The first is function while the second is form. The next section
will consider how this approach to circulation theory can help to shape an
understanding of the different natures of points on different areas of the

body. In a later section, we will turn to a final synthesis of the interaction of qi circulation and organic function as it may have been understood by the compilers of the *Inner Classic*.

FIVE-TRANSPORT POINT THEORY AND THE NATURE OF DISTAL VERSUS TRUNK POINTS

Descriptions in the early chapters of the *Divine Pivot* of five transport point circulation describe the distal extremities as the 'roots' (根 *gēn*) and the linking of channels to the internal organs as 'accumulations' (結 *jié*). To the modern mind, this theory of circulation may still seem a bit strange. Nevertheless, five-transport point theory represents a very fundamental principle within the larger concept of channel theory. Early in the evolution of Chinese science, it was understood that the movement of qi and blood in the extremities was of a different nature than that in the trunk. The idea that something called 'channel qi' is developing in the extremities is one of the most novel claims made in Chinese medicine. And the fact that patients have for centuries attested to improved health because of treatment based on these theories suggests that they are worthy of our consideration.

In particular, consider the fact that the metaphors of classical texts describe an ongoing process that is occurring along the course of the five transport points. While the description uses images of gradually increasing water flow, the process involves qi. When one says that channel qi is growing along the course of the five transport points, it should be pointed out that, once the qi 'enters' (入 *rù*) deeply at the sea points, multiple channels begin to interact with each other in a different way than they had on the distal extremities. Consider exactly what this might mean. Like the flow of water down the side of a mountain, the channels within the trunk of the body have both picked up speed and breadth while also intermingling with broader and broader sources as small vessels meet to create large. While it is thus said that there is greater volume to the channels as they move inward, there is also a kind of intermixing which, paradoxically, renders stimulation of these more proximal points less and less specific to the qi dynamic of the individual organs with which they are associated. Nevertheless, even though the channels interact quite a bit on the trunk and abdomen, the specific channel qi that began far out on the limbs still continues to home to its associated organ. In other words, the channels themselves do not lose their relationship to particular organs because of this intermixing. The effect of stimulating individual points, however, does become more localized. This is a complex idea that should be considered and reconsidered slowly.

Fundamentally, this has to do with the concept of diffusion. At the more distal transport points, far away from the organs, there is an interplay of a relatively even sampling of qi and blood from all over the body. From this great diversity comes the spark that begins the process of channel qi development that stimulates organ function. Then, consuming the nutritive qi of the body (the second circuit), organ qi begins to grow in volume as it approaches the elbows and knees. As it moves beyond the transport points, however, it also loses some of the specificity of its qi in relation to an individual organ that one finds early in the development of channel qi growth.

In order to appreciate how this manifests in the clinic, consider how the applications for points on the trunk contrast with those on the distal limbs. Take, for example, the points ST-25 *(tiān shū)* and KI-16 *(huāng shū)*. Although on two different channels, both points have significant functional overlap. Both points might be indicated for stomach pain, abdominal distention, diarrhea, or poor appetite. In short, both points, located very close to each other, not only treat stomach-type patterns but also those associated with the stomach, spleen, kidney, or even liver in classical physiology. While they are excellent and often-used points, their effects are considered to be more general in nature, and they are less often used as lead points when trying to effect specific changes in individual organs. Instead, they often serve as important secondary points that guide or move qi in a particular area.

In fact, as many practitioners have surely noticed, most of the points on the abdomen can be effective to some degree in the treatment of various types of gastrointestinal pain. Some are obviously better than others, depending on the diagnosis and location of disease, but there is nevertheless a general tendency to be beneficial mainly for conditions that originate in the abdomen. Consequently, one would rarely use a point like ST-25 as a lead point for toe pain. Conversely, classical texts abound with prescriptions using SP-3 *(tài bái)* on the lower leg for spleen disorders. It is the broad interplay of the collaterals and small vessels of multiple channels on the body trunk that account for these differences. To be clear, this is not an assertion that point location on the abdomen is not important. It is still crucial that one carefully locate the point on the channel through measurement and palpation. The various abdominal points may be similar but they are still distinct from both one another and the surrounding 'non-point' areas.

Of course, there are certainly well-known points on the extremities where multiple channels also meet (e.g., SP-6 [*sān yīn jiāo*]). The interactions represented by these points have a different effect, however, because of their location in an area of growing channel qi. Nevertheless, distal intersection points such as SP-6 do often tend to have broader and less specific effects than some of their nearby transport points. For example, while a point like SP-3 is an excellent point for facilitating spleen qi, one would be less likely to use SP-6 as the primary point for a specific case of spleen qi deficiency. On the other hand, SP-6 is appropriate as a general stimulator of qi in the middle and lower burners. The net result of stimulating the liver, spleen, and kidney channels, at a distal intersection in this case, is often to benefit blood. In sum, while SP-3 can serve as a very specific and powerful point in a particular case, SP-6 is more of a jack-of-all-trades with broader, but less precise, effects. In a similar (but more localized) manner, the points on the abdomen and chest have broad effects on the circulation of qi and blood in the areas in which they are found.

Of course, the different functions of the five transport points arise from the unique qi dynamic of each of the organs. Simply put, the channel points in the distal extremities have fairly specific effects on the organs with which they are associated. In general, this becomes less and less so as the channels approach the trunk. On the trunk, the points may still be quite powerful, but they are less specific in action. Remember, we are describing the most appropriate clinical applications for points on the body trunk, and are not suggesting that the channels somehow become murky or unfocused in these areas. In the end, the theories are honed in the field of clinical application (Fig. 16.16).

Points on the head provide yet a different case. In the clinic, scalp acupuncture is particularly effective for musculoskeletal problems of the extremities. In fact, while points on the extremities can have very profound effects on the qi dynamic of the internal organs, it is often important to combine points from the scalp when treating musculoskeletal problems affecting the limbs. The interesting subject of scalp acupuncture must be set aside for a different text, however.[4]

Synthesis of qi circulation theories: a summary

In many ways, five-transport point theory fills an important missing link in some basic concepts of Chinese physiology. The physiology of organ theory describes the process by which prenatal qi interacts with postnatal qi to create the nutritive-protective aspect and source qi that nourishes the body. Organ theory also describes how excess, waste, pathogenic qi, and fluids are removed from the body in an effort to maintain balance. What is missing from the picture, however, is a discussion of how the organs actually get their qi. In other words, how does the body ultimately metabolize the nutritive-protective aspect and source qi? The missing link in modern descriptions of classical physiology actually comes from the unlikely direction of five-transport point theory.

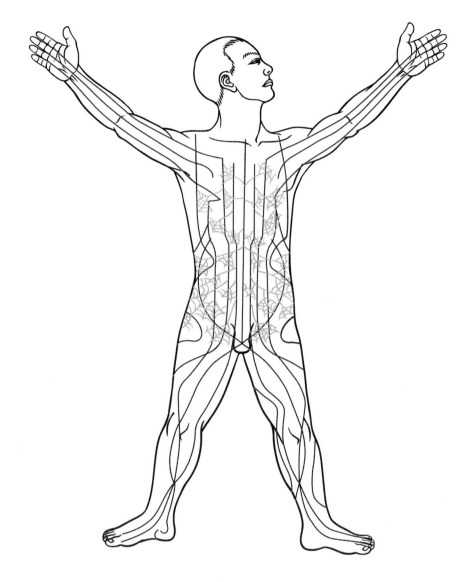

Fig. 16.16
The channel points on the distal extremities have fairly specific effects
on the organs with which they are associated. In general, this
becomes less and less so as the channels approach the trunk.

Chapter 9 of the *Divine Pivot,* entitled "On Endings and Beginnings"
(終始 *zhōng shǐ),* provides insight into how classical physicians might have
understood the process of metabolizing nutrition and source qi. It says that
"yang receives its qi in the four extremities while yin receives qi from the
five yin organs." Here, the *Inner Classic* is outlining the general physiological

principle that the organs generate yin substance, namely, the nutritive-protective aspect (see description of nutritive-protective aspect production in Chapter 5). At the same time, far away from the organs, at the smallest levels of circulation, there is a transformation to yang function. The nutritive-protective aspect travels in the vessels from the yin organs out to the areas of microcirculation. The cells of the body are nourished in the interstitial fluids, bathed in nutrition from the arteries, and cleansed by the reuptake of waste by lymphatic and venous circulation. Or, in other words, yin comes from the inside and goes outward, while yang comes from the outside and travels inward.

Chapter 62 of the *Divine Pivot* describes what happens: "The four extremities are where yin and yang meet; it is here that one finds the large connections of qi." In other words, the *Inner Classic* conceives of a kind of transformation from yin to yang that occurs at the 'ends' of the body and gives rise to qi. Strictly speaking, these areas can be found throughout the body, wherever microcirculation invigorates the cellular bath. However, the *Divine Pivot*, in the first and second chapters described earlier, asserts that the furthest areas from the organs, out at the ends of the appendages, are particularly important. The appendages provide the proper environment for the development of channel qi; a process that grows from the fingers and toes inward. In the process (yang), it consumes the nutritive-protective aspect (yin).

What exactly is being developed? It has been stated that there is a development of organ qi. Because the channels can be regarded as extensions of the organs themselves, these places along the distal appendages are where organ function begins. Here is where the 'lung qi' or 'heart qi' arises. The ability of the organs to have the wide systemic functions described in the Chinese model (the liver holding the blood, the spleen transforming fluids, etc.) depends, somewhat surprisingly, on the quality of movement in the connective tissue spaces in areas below the elbows and knees. As unusual as it may seem, this is the vision of the *Inner Classic*.

Simply put, the growth of channel qi along the course of the five transport points depends first on source qi for stimulus, then on nutritive-protective qi traveling in the twelve-channel circuit for its material foundation. At the same time, the nutritive-protective qi is dependent on channel qi because channel qi stimulates the qi dynamic of the organs which are its source (Fig. 16.17).

Now, the obvious question arises as to why this happens in the first place. One may be inclined to accept the theories described above in a general way, but still not appreciate exactly why the qi of the organs needs

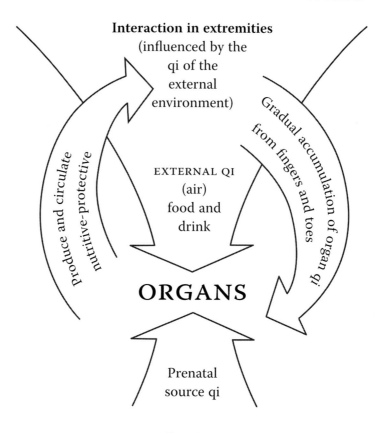

Fig. 16.17

Synthesis of qi circulation. In this image, one can see both of the circuits described in Figs. 16.1 and 16.2 happening at the same time.

to build from the outside in. The physiological model described by modern science provides some helpful perspective. The model of blood vessel circulation found in contemporary medical textbooks describes a system in which blood is pumped out to the extremities by the heart and returns inward via venous return. The veins, having one-way valves, depend on four general forces to bring blood back to the heart:

- osmotic pressure to bring fluids into the capillaries
- an increase in velocity as venules concentrate into larger veins
- 'milking' along the veins by muscle contractions, and
- changes in pressure brought about by the movement of the diaphragm in breathing.

The model described by modern physiologists of blood circulation has antecedents in some of the Chinese texts, and, as mentioned earlier, is roughly analogous to the twelve-channel circuit of the nutritive-protective aspect.[5] However, classical Chinese physiology seems to posit that there is another important type of circulation (channel qi) which depends as well on the forces generated by muscle movement in the extremities to stimulate its growth and development. Because of the active movement of the limbs of the body, there is a strong draw of qi and blood to these areas of abundant microcirculation. It is the abundance of microcirculation in these areas, combined with the variety of qi and blood from the rest of the body that mixes there, that provides the perfect environment for transformation. It is in these areas far away from the organs that the nutritive-protective aspect reaches its apex and is completely transformed from yin-substance to yang-function. The muscles of the four limbs move. The nutritional needs that are required by this movement stimulate the internal organs to produce.

In addition, like the concept of venous return in modern physiology, the development of channel qi (and eventually organ qi) is facilitated by muscle movement and the increased velocity gained as it moves inward with a faster and heavier flow at what are called the sea points. Of course, the concept of 'velocity' in classical Chinese science wasn't understood in the same way as that described by modern physics. Nevertheless, there are clear assertions in classical texts that channel qi begins to move more quickly as it travels toward the elbows and knees. The most famous example, noted above, is the statement in the *Classic of Difficulties* that qi pours (注 *zhù*) at the spring points and really moves (行 *xíng*) at the river points. The question of whether or not classical physiologists understood that the increased speed created a draw of qi and blood from the hands and feet will certainly remain unanswered.

The next chapter, on the source points, explains how qi in the extremities is a kind of 'average' of the qi in the rest of the body, because of the lively interaction of microcirculation in the limbs far away from the organs. Because of the mixture of qi and blood from all over the body in the hands and feet, there is also 'information' in these areas about all the organs of the body. It is here, at the roots of the channels in the extremities, that the nutritive-protective aspect from the blood and prenatal source qi from the kidneys begins to undergo transformation to the specific channel qi that makes the very specific and systemic functions of the organs in Chinese medicine. It is also in these areas of qi development that the six qi of the external environment are added to the informational mix.

In a repeating and interdependent cycle, the organs depend on qi while qi depends on the nutritive substance that the organs produce. This is the unification of the two seemingly contradictory circulation theories advanced in Chapters 2 and 10 of the *Divine Pivot*. In fact, this unification goes right to the heart of the meaning of classical assertions that "qi is the commander of blood and blood is the mother of qi." In the clinic, the functions of acupuncture points should be considered in the context of this ongoing process of transformation. It is a process that involves channel qi first coming into existence at the wells, then beginning to flow and later to pour and travel before finally entering toward the sea of the organs.

 Q: *One question comes to mind now, after thinking about the five transport points. Given that the theory says that there is more qi/blood flow at the sea points, why wouldn't one simply always use those points for deficiency? I know that the source points, for example, are often used for tonification, but I'd like to hear how you understand the mechanisms of the other points.*

DR. WANG: I understand your question. Simply put, the answer lies in the concept that there is *interchange* at the source points and *concentration* at the sea points. A metaphor might be helpful. If, for example, you wanted to buy food for dinner, you would go to a market that had as many of the raw materials needed as possible. If you needed bread, vegetables, fruit and meat, you wouldn't go to four different warehouses that specialized in each of these individual items. They might only sell carrots in 100 kg bags! Instead, you would go to a variety store or a large market with many vendors. The source points are like a large market where a wide variety of 'information' about the rest of the body is exchanged. This is because of the diverse microcirculation required to nourish those active, precise joints and also because of the simple fact that they are farther away from the internal organs than the sea points.

For example, consider a source point like LU-9 *(tài yuān)*. At this point near the wrist joint, there is diverse capillary microcirculation. One might contrast this with the much larger blood vessels near LU-5 *(chǐ zé)*. Because of the abundant microcirculation and its distance from the internal organs, the LU-9 area contains a fairly even mix of qi and blood from everywhere else in the body. Here, in this lively interchange of qi and blood, the source points of the six channels interact. The so-called 'information' that is needed to modify lung channel metabolism enters the channel here, while information about the condition of the lung also travels from this area to inform the other organs. It is truly an area of interchange. Needling the source points then can both initiate the in-flow of source qi and also facilitate proper uptake of what I call 'information' in the area. I will talk more about these ideas later when we discuss the source points.

In other words, stimulating the more distal transport points helps to draw exactly what is needed to the channel in question. On the other hand, the sea points are areas where the channels have become focused, strong and deeper. At the sea points, there is relatively more qi and blood, but, at the same time, there is less of the variety of interaction and specificity of function that gives source points their unique power.

Of course, there are many times when one might rather tap into that powerful volume of qi and blood from the sea points in the clinic. Remember that the sea points are said to be effective for 'reversing counterflow'. This refers to problems with qi transformation in an organ. For example, this might be stomach qi going upward and causing belching, spleen qi sinking downward as diarrhea, lung qi counterflow in coughing, or other problems where qi seems to be moving in the wrong direction. In these cases, one needs to tap into places where a strong effect can be had on the movement of qi in a broader sense. These are the sea points. This is why they are used much more often for regulation than for tonification.

The Five-Phase Associations of the Five Transport Points

Many of the clinical applications of the five transport points take into account the five-phase associations of the points. This concept was briefly touched upon earlier in the discussion of clinical application. Here, a few things will be said about the theoretical underpinnings of the five-phase assignments for each of the transport points.

Most acupuncture texts describe how the transport points on the yin channels begin with wood while the yang channels begin with metal. This categorization then proceeds through the five-phase cycle of wood-fire-earth-metal-water. As most practitioners already know, point prescriptions derived from many classical texts are based on the five-phase relationships of the points to each other and/or the five-phase associations of the organs. These concepts are fully elaborated in five-phase acupuncture traditions (Table 16.7).

In some texts, there are lengthy philosophical discourses on why exactly

	Well	**Spring**	**Stream**	**River**	**Sea**
Yin channels	Wood	Fire	Earth	Metal	Water
Yang channels	Metal	Water	Wood	Fire	Earth

Table 16.7

The five-phase associations of the transport points
is different on the yin and yang channels.

the yin channels begin with the wood phase points while the yang channels begin with the metal phase. They often involve complex and arcane dissertations on traditional Chinese numerology, heavenly stems/earthly branches, and *Yì jīng* theory. But this concept might be more readily summarized in one aspect of the yin-yang relationship, that of the 'material foundation' from yin supporting the 'action/movement' from yang. This is the idea that yin provides the material basis for yang action.

This simple concept sheds a great deal of light on the five-phase associations of the transport points on the yin/yang channels. For example, the well points on the yin channels are associated with wood. Among the five phases, wood represents the concept of beginnings. Wood is associated with spring and the east, from which the sun arises. In nature, wood and the leaves of the plant kingdom begin the cycle of life by photosynthesizing the energy of the sun. Similarly, the body depends on the physiology of the yin channels to get its start. The yin channels therefore start with wood, the phase of beginnings.

The yang channels begin with the phase of metal. Metal is the phase of consumption and endings. It is associated with the season of fall and the descent of the sun in the west. Metal swords and axes fell men and trees, and its associated color (white) is the Chinese color of mourning. In the five-phase system, metal is thus said to 'control' (克 *kè*) wood. In cases of need, metal can 'consume' or 'over-act' on wood. The yang channels depend on the yin channels for material foundation. Yang draws sustenance from yin. The yang channels thus begin with the consuming phase of metal.

Consider now the progression of the five phases as one moves along the course of the five transport points. The yin channels move from wood-fire-earth-metal-water while the yang channels move from metal-water-wood-fire-earth. If one sets a prototypical yin channel next to a prototypical yang channel, it will be seen that the yang channel is 'over-acting' at each point along the way (Fig. 16.18).

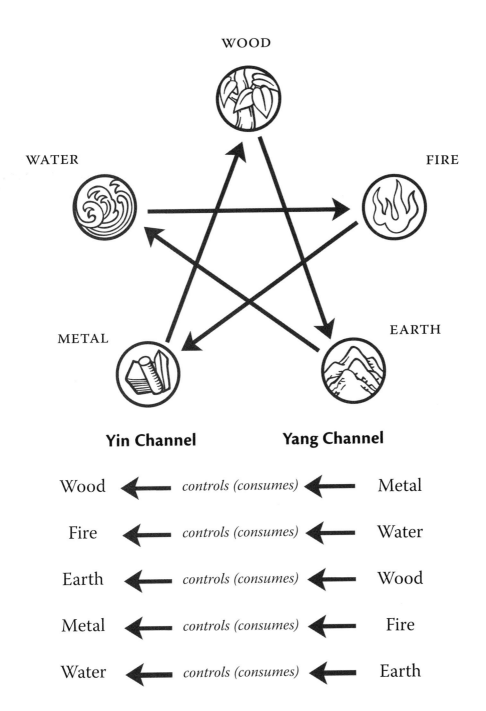

Fig. 16.18

The five-phase associations of the transport points on the yin/yang channels

Thus, the five-phase nature of the transport points and the relationship of the transport points of the yin and yang channels to each other provide yet another insight into how channel qi develops. That is, as the yang channels progress toward the interior of the body, there is a constant consumption of material support from the yin channels. The ability of the yang organs to move and transport ultimately depends on the nutritive foundation provided by yin organ physiology. On the distal extremities, the pathways of the yang channels therefore closely follow their paired yin channels.

Before going on it should be emphasized that here, as elsewhere, theory is dependent on application in the clinic, not the other way around. The points do not conform to five-phase theory; rather, five-phase theory represents an attempt to categorize the points based on their natural function. In other words, the five transport points have inherent effects on the qi dynamic which were observed and then later categorized according to one or another of the five phases. For this reason, some of the points do not fit neatly into their respective categories.

For example, on the heart channel, strict five-phase theory would suggest that one could use HT-9 *(shào chōng)*, the wood point on a fire channel, in cases of deficiency to 'tonify the child using the mother point'. Clinical application suggests otherwise. In fact, experience indicates that heart qi/blood deficiency patterns respond better to HT-7 *(shén mén)*. Although five-phase theory would assert that HT-7 is the 'child' point on the channel (the earth point on a fire channel) and thus better for draining, it is also the source point. There are other examples where clinical approaches seem to contradict strict five-phase application. In the end, the five-phase associations provide a helpful starting place for categorizing inherent point functions. But they should not be used inflexibly when clinical reality suggests otherwise.

To review, two types of flow in the channels have been explored in this chapter. The five transport points are part of a flow that moves from the fingers and toes inward toward the trunk. At the same time, another flow involves circulation through the twelve main channels in a circuit of nutrition along the commonly seen internally-externally paired channel pathways. While both types of flow occur at the same time and through essentially the same areas, they have fundamentally different natures and physiological functions. The twelve-channel circulation is associated with providing the nutritive-protective aspect, and the five-transport point circulation is associated with channel qi. Channel qi is the qi transformation or 'function' of the organs themselves. At the well, spring, and stream points, the channels have very specific effects on the organs with which each is associated. However, as they advance beyond the sea points, they begin to interact with each other via the myriad collaterals, and their effects become broader and more generalized. Once the channels have entered the trunk, stimulating points along their paths have effects which are thought to be more localized.

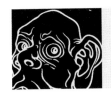

THE SOURCE (原 *yuán*), CLEFT (郄 *xī*), AND COLLATERAL (絡 *luò*) POINTS

IN THIS CHAPTER we will explore some of the categories of points used by classical acupuncturists to organize the acupuncture points. In general, an understanding of the point categories helps an acupuncturist to conceptualize other ways that the nature of qi circulation will vary at different places along the pathway of a given channel. The source (原 *yuán*), cleft (郄 *xī*), and collateral (絡 *luò*) point categories will be considered in this chapter.

In the previous chapter we discussed the theory of the five transport points, one of the primary ways of understanding the nature of channel flow. But, as is typical of Chinese medicine, there are other understandings as well. In other words, while the theory of five transport points describes a rather orderly building of qi in the channels as it approaches the elbows and knees, other point categories describe different types of change in the channel qi, sometimes in the same areas as the transport points. The trick is in holding multiple concepts in the mind at the same time.

This is one of the difficulties in studying Chinese medicine, namely, that one must consider multiple theories when interpreting a given patient presentation or developing a viable treatment strategy. When considering the nature of an acupuncture point, one must view it through different theoretical prisms. This is largely because the structure of Chinese medicine was built over many centuries, and new ideas were often incorporated within an older structure. Like the five transport points discussed in Chapter 16, the clinical applications of the point categories described below have evolved over the millennia.

Source Points (原穴 *yuán xué*)

The first acupuncture points cited in the *Inner Classic* are what we now call the source points. Discussed in the first lines of the *Divine Pivot*, source points have likely been used for nearly two millennia. A passage in Chapter 66 of the *Classic of Difficulties* says that they can be used "whenever there is disease in the yin and yang organs." While their application has been refined over the centuries, they are nevertheless still used in the treatment of a wide variety of disease patterns (Table 17.1).

Channel	Source point
Lung	LU-9 (*tài yuān*)
Spleen	SP-3 (*tài bái*)
Heart	HT-7 (*shén mén*)
Kidney	KI-3 (*tài xī*)
Pericardium	PC-7 (*dà líng*)
Liver	LR-3 (*tài chōng*)
Large intestine	LI-4 (*hé gǔ*)
Stomach	ST-42 (*chōng yáng*)
Small intestine	SI-4 (*wàn gǔ*)
Bladder	BL-64 (*jīng gǔ*)
Triple burner	TB-4 (*yáng chí*)
Gallbladder	GB-40 (*qiū xū*)

Table 17.1
The source points

Other chapters of the *Inner Classic* describe the relationship of the triple burner organ to 'source qi' (see discussion of the *shào yáng* in Chapter 9). The use of the same term to describe the type of qi associated with the triple burner as well as the name for these important points on each of the twelve regular channels is significant. This is highlighted in Chapter 66 of the *Classic of Difficulties* where a list of the twelve source points is followed by a description of the role of the triple burner.[1] The text says that the source qi moving in the triple burner arises from the fire at the gate of vitality in the kidney, and that the source points are associated in particular with this type of qi in the channels. Thus, the source points are related to the triple burner function of irrigating the channels with fire from the gate of vitality. In modern texts, one often reads that the source points "connect with the triple burner" and are used clinically to increase the circulation of source qi in the twelve channels.

But how, exactly, does this happen? For example, how can a point like KI-3 *(tài xī)* on the leg be related to the functions of a channel like the triple burner, which passes through the arm and to the 'three burners' of the trunk? The first step in answering this question is to return to the concept of the triple burner organ described in Chapter 9. There, the triple burner was broadly defined to include the movement of fluids through empty spaces outside the vascular system—beyond the level of capillary circulation. These interstitial spaces are found throughout the body around muscles, joints, and bones. Therefore, the ability of source points to access source qi arises not from direct connections to the triple burner channel, but from the pervasive presence of the triple burner organ in the fluids that suffuse the connective tissues of the entire body.

In fact, strictly speaking, it could be said that all of the channels have a connection to the fluids within the triple burner, as described in this text. Each of the twelve channels represents a circuit of fluid movement along a definable course of muscles, nerves, and vessels that has a particular relationship to one or another of the internal organs. Therefore, when one thinks, for example, of the pathway of the spleen channel, it might be helpful to think of that channel as being part of the triple burner system that has a particular relationship to the spleen (see related question in Chapter 9). Remember that the triple burner is described as an "environment" that surrounds the organs and other tissues of the body. The relationship of the acupuncture points to the triple burner is also described in Chapter 66 of the *Classic of Difficulties* where it says that "the points of the five yin organs are places where the movements within the triple burner pause in their qi flow" (五藏俞者, 三焦之所行, 氣之所留止也 *Wǔ zàng shū zhě, sān jiāo zhī suǒ xíng, qì zhī suǒ liú zhǐ yě).*

Nonetheless, the question is still not fully answered. One might understand that the triple burner organ has broad effects due to the pervasiveness of these spaces throughout the body, but the question of why the source points in particular have this ability to provide abundant source qi remains unanswered. The answer lies in a combination of classical theory, basic anatomy, and clinical experience. Five-transport point theory describes the slow growth of channel qi as it moves from the hands and feet toward the elbows and knees. Source points, the third transport point on the yin channels and the point proximal to the third transport point on the yang channels, are in the area where channel qi is said to begin to pour (注 *zhù*) into a connected stream. Thus, while channel qi is growing at the well and spring points, it does not have a smooth, even flow until it reaches the area around the source points. In other words, the location of the source points corresponds to the place on the channels where the flow of qi is like that of the stream points in five-transport point theory.[2]

Before proceeding, it will be helpful to briefly review what has been said up to this point. First, the triple burner, through its pervasive presence in the fluids and connective tissues of the body, is directly connected not only to points contiguous to the three burners of the abdomen, but to points on the extremities as well. Second, classical theories describe the gradual growth of channel qi as it moves from the fingers/toes to the elbows/knees. However, this begs the question of why these places in particular, and not other points along the course of the channels, are said to draw source qi from the spaces of the triple burner. For example, one might assume that the uniting (*hé*-sea) points, with their strong, deep flow of channel qi, would draw source qi. It would also seem to be logical to consider points on the trunk of the body, within the traditional scope of the three-part triple burner organ, as possible locations from which to draw source qi toward the yin and yang organs. Moreover, because the model of the triple burner presented in this text posits that all channel movement in fact occurs within the spaces of the triple burner, one might assert that all acupuncture points could be termed 'source points'. The heart of the answer to these questions lies in the anatomy.

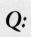 **Q:** *In the same vein, another question comes to mind: Why the stream points and not the well or spring points?*

> **DR. WANG:** Remember from our earlier discussion of the five transport points that the qi only begins to move strongly in a particular direction at the stream points. The well points are where channel qi emerges and the spring points are where it begins to flow in a particular direction. It is at the stream points, however, that channel qi gains the momentum necessary to draw source qi into its flow. The classical description of qi movement at the stream points is that qi begins to 'pour' in these areas. You might think of the pouring as creating a kind of draw that brings in source qi.
>
> So, while there are points on each of the channels that precede the source/stream points, they do not as yet have the strength of flow to act as source points by drawing in source qi from the triple burner.

Now, don't forget that all of this is ultimately based on clinical observation and empirical results. There may have been a time when doctors thought of the well points as being appropriate for tonification because they were the first points on the channels. Over time, however, actual clinical experience began to indicate that tonification was more effective at the source points, and theory then developed from there. In the end, when you think of channel flow as being slower and less substantial at the well and spring points, it makes sense that they are less able to provide strong tonification.

As many texts point out, the source points are found around the wrist and ankle joints. The range of motion and the sheer frequency of movement in these small joints are among the greatest in the body. The movement of the ankles and the myriad fine motor adjustments of the wrist and hand coordinate the acts of walking, balancing, grasping, gesturing, and lifting. This requires a great deal of qi and blood. In modern physiology, these areas are described as having a high rate of cellular metabolism, hence the warmth of the hands and feet. When there is a lack of abundant qi and blood in the body, these areas are often the first to feel cold or exhibit obvious changes due to compromised circulation. The locations of the twelve source points are found in the heart of these areas of increased qi transformation.

One might also note that the source points are located in areas very close to the most distal palpable pulse on each of the twelve regular channels. This is not an accident. It is precisely because of the heightened qi and blood circulation at these points that they have a particularly strong need for source qi. While movement of larger joints like the shoulder and hip may require higher volumes of qi and blood, there is a unique circulation around the wrists and ankles which creates the particular environment that gives rise to the source points (Fig. 17.1 and 17.2).

Because of the nature of circulation in these areas, the source points may be likened to a great market. In these concentrations of heightened activity, there is a brisk trade in information from the body as a whole. In the distal appendages of the arms and legs, far from the internal organs, nutritive circulation reaches its apogee, just like the branches at the top of a tree or trading posts at the far corners of an empire. Like bazaars where many cultures meet, the source points bustle with activity. The abundant supply of qi and blood here requires not only adequate capillary supply, but, just as importantly, the ability to reabsorb fluids back into the circulatory system in an area with lower blood pressure. In other words, just as blood comes far from the heart to the ankles and wrists to facilitate movement, it must also

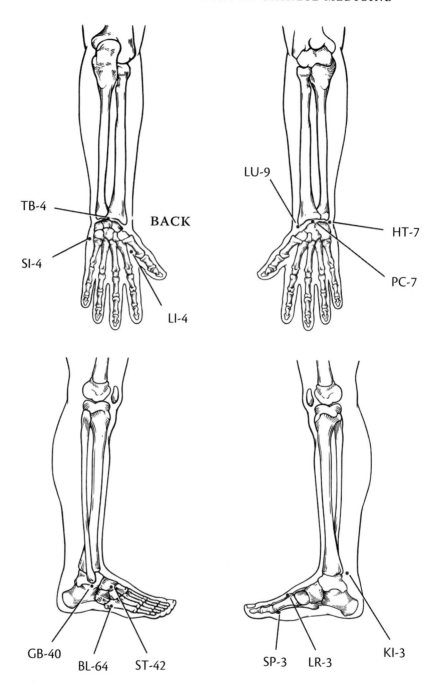

Fig. 17.1
The source points are located in areas where there is a high degree
of precise mobility in the human body. These areas undergo
a high turnover of qi and blood.

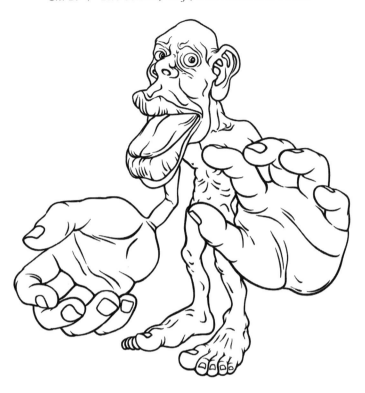

Fig. 17.2
The homunculus exaggerates those areas of the body where there is a higher
degree of nerve and blood concentration. Many of the source points can be
found at the borders of these more vascularized and innervated areas.

be quickly carried away and replaced to prevent swelling that might compromise the range of motion. Again, when circulation is compromised, it is
at the wrists, and particularly the ankles, where the fluids build up. Thus the
arms and legs experience a rapid turnover of blood from other parts of the
body. One might also say that the areas around the source points receive
constant communication from a wide variety of distant organs. Therefore,
despite (or because of) their distance from the internal organs, the source
points have a unique clinical value that is associated with the diversity of
information that they receive from elsewhere in the body.

Consider again the model of the triple burner presented in Chapter 9.
The concept of the triple burner, a hollow yang organ, was linked to the
spaces between the muscles and surrounding the connective tissues. While
these spaces exist in all muscles and in the lining around the organs of the
abdomen, the substances within those linings will vary in different areas
of the body. In fact, it is most varied in areas furthest from the trunk. This

seems counterintuitive at first: How can areas so far from the primary metabolism of the internal organs be filled with a diversity of qi and blood? One would expect that the areas around the organs themselves might have more of the various types of qi in the body. But in fact, while the organs of the trunk may have more qi and/or blood, the nature of that qi and blood is quite specific to that organ. For example, while the lung is filled with qi, it is a particular type of qi classically termed 'lung qi' (a component of ancestral qi). Similarly, the liver is filled with blood, but of a type called 'liver blood' in Chinese medicine. By contrast, at the source points, there is a fairly even mix of qi and blood from every corner of the body. Combine this with the high nutritional requirements of the joint spaces, and one can begin to appreciate how movement and diversity of all qi in the body combines at the source points around the ankles and wrists (Fig. 17.3).

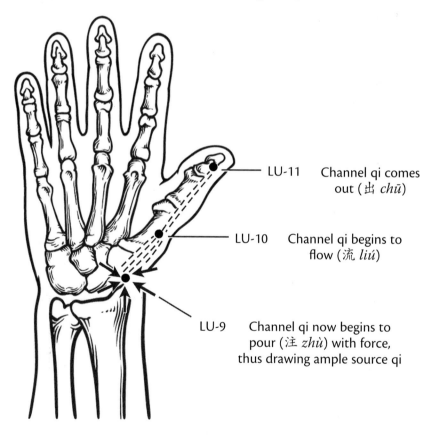

LU-11 — Channel qi comes out (出 *chū*)

LU-10 — Channel qi begins to flow (流 *liú*)

LU-9 — Channel qi now begins to pour (注 *zhù*) with force, thus drawing ample source qi

Fig. 17.3
At a source point like LU-9 (*tài yuān*), the increasing flow of channel qi at the highly active joint on the wrist creates the lively interplay which brings source qi from the fluids of the triple burner into the qi dynamic of the channel.

It is important to note how the mixing of the various types of qi is vital to normal physiology. Ultimately, this involves an aspect of the role of the channels as a communication system (途徑 *tú jìng*), one of the three general functions of the channels described in Chapter 2. Communication occurs through the medium of fluids. Consider the following example from the clinic. If there is a deficiency of heart qi, this information enters the spaces of the triple burner in the chest as a change in the environment of the other organs. This environmental shift travels through the fluids of the body to points of highly active transfer at the source points. There, information regarding the heart might enter other channels very quickly. Also, as has been shown in clinical experience, stimulating a point like HT-7 *(shén mén)*, the heart's source point, has a noticeable effect which, in Chinese medicine, corresponds to a benefit to heart qi. In other words, stimulating the heart source point sends a precise signal to the channel system as a whole which initiates a chain reaction that benefits heart qi.

Obviously, the brain is another area of increased circulation and communication that classical theory tends to underemphasize. It is quite possible that modern research will reveal that the way information is processed in the brain is influenced more profoundly than previously expected by changes in connective tissues and the fluids associated with them. This would involve an acknowledgment that there is a kind of 'intelligence' in the body itself that is in constant interplay with the brain. While modern physiologists often (correctly) point out that classical Chinese physiology tends to underemphasize the role of the brain, there may very well be a similar lack of appreciation on the part of physiologists of the importance of the 'non-organ' tissues in regulating metabolism and consciousness. The experience of Chinese medicine would seem to point in this direction.[3]

Careful observation does reveal inconsistencies in certain aspects of the theory outlined above. For example, why are the source points of the liver, spleen, large intestine, and bladder not located on the ankle and wrist joints? Once again, the answer lies in considerations of form and function. The areas around the large toes, thumbs, and lateral surfaces of the foot use a relatively greater amount of qi and blood than the proximal areas on those channels near the ankles and wrists. In other words, because the joints around LR-3 *(tài chōng)*, SP-3 *(tài bái)*, LI-4 *(hé gǔ)*, and BL-64 *(jīng gǔ)* use more qi and blood than the areas on those same channels near the wrists and ankles, the source points have 'migrated'. As evolution may have changed the structure of the human body, so has the movement of qi and blood changed over time. The important thing to remember here is that clinical efficacy guides theory. If the theories can't provide appreciable benefits in treatment, they should be reconsidered. The use of these points in the clinic over time indicates that they have the ability to stimulate source qi on their respective channels. Observation of the importance of the large toes, thumbs, and lateral surfaces of the feet in walking and grasping is one way that this clinically relevant theory might be conceptualized (Fig. 17.4).

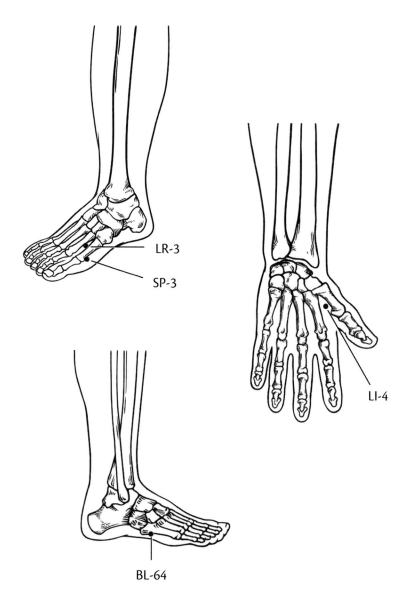

Fig. 17.4
Four source points are away from the wrist and ankle joints,
in areas more distal on the channel where mobility is even greater.

Using the source points

In the clinic, the source points are used almost exclusively for tonification. They have an ability to augment the qi and warm the yang (益氣溫陽 *yì qì wēn yáng)*. This is particularly true of the yin channels. In the clinic, the source points of the yang channels have less of a strictly tonifying effect on their respective organs. Instead, the source points of these channels strengthen by virtue of their ability to unblock circulation and increase movement. Some yang source points are more useful than others. For example, ST-42 *(chōng yáng)* is sometimes more difficult to use because needling the point often causes pain. On the other hand, TB-4 *(yáng chí)* has a broader application than might be suspected. This point is used very often in some traditions of Japanese acupuncture, particularly the school of Sawada Ken (澤田建),[4] who advocated the use of moxa on TB-4 and CV-12 *(zhōng wǎn)* for severe deficiency. In the clinic, TB-4 is in fact effective in the treatment of yang deficiency patterns including tinnitus and cold-type shoulder and upper back pain. This is because, as the source point of the triple burner channel, the point has a particularly strong stimulating effect on the circulation of yang.

By considering the nature of the source points one can begin to answer the question of why certain source points seem to have such a wide variety of apparently contrasting clinical applications. For example, while it is relatively easy to understand how a point like LU-9 *(tài yuān)* is indicated for lung qi deficiency, it is more difficult to appreciate the mechanism underlying its ability to also tonify yin. Thus, while the point is often used in cases of chronic weakness to treat lung qi deficiency, it is also helpful in relatively acute cases of dry throat or dry cough. The ability of the point to both tonify qi and benefit yin is best appreciated by thinking of the qi dynamic of the lung organ, outlined in Chapter 5. There, the metabolism of the *tài yīn* system was characterized as fundamentally involving the metabolism of dampness and the generation of nutrition. In particular, the lung organ provides qi from the external environment to facilitate the transformation of dampness and to invigorate the nutritive aspect of blood produced by the spleen. The ability of the lung to benefit yin arises from its capacity to work synergistically with the spleen to produce the yin-nourishing nutritive aspect of blood. By strengthening lung qi with the source point of the channel, a physiological chain reaction is initiated which has an indirect ability to benefit yin.

The dynamic functions of the other source points should be considered in a similar light. For example, the source point of the kidney channel, KI-3 *(tài xī)*, enriches kidney yin and invigorates original yang. The best way to fathom the precise meaning of these traditional functions is to consider the qi dynamic of not just the kidney, but also of the *shào yīn* channel as a whole. This channel is a pivot between the depth of blood storage at *jué yīn* and the outward opening of *tài yīn*. The movement of the *shào yīn* pivot provides the stimulus of original yin and original yang to the body. By stimulating a point like KI-3, one is not actually generating new prenatal qi in the body.[5] Rather, the source point on the kidney *shào yīn* channel is used for regulating vital, prenatal substances. This means that it is enriching the yin and invigorating the yang by optimizing their metabolism. Thus KI-3 can strengthen the kidneys only insofar as it helps to reestablish healthy flow of channel qi to the organ, thereby normalizing its qi dynamic.

In this way, the ineffable fine-tuning of understanding that must come from considering the unique qi dynamic of each channel when evaluating the effects of its points begins to take form. The powerful ability of source points to benefit the organs might then be summarized as arising from the ability of source qi to 'jump start' the normal metabolism of the organs themselves. This is also why source points must be used in cases of deficiency. When the qi dynamic of the organs becomes so compromised that normal metabolism is impossible, it may be difficult to obtain qi at other points on the channel. It is sometimes therefore necessary to first build metabolism with the source points before going on to regulate the qi dynamic with other points.

Later in this chapter, each of the individual collateral and cleft points will be discussed in turn. However, the individual source points will not be discussed in this manner largely because of the breadth of their applications. These are points that might be likened to 'jacks-of-all-trades' in that any condition involving qi deficiency in a particular organ may call for the use of the source points. By contrast, points in the other categories listed below tend to have more specific applications.

When stimulating the source points, technique should be gentle and radiation down the channel should be gradual. For source points in particular, light stimulation and a slow arrival of qi leads to better results in cases of deficiency. Achieving this sensation requires skill and practice. When using the points for pathodynamics that also involve excess and/or heat, one might stimulate the points a bit more.

Cleft Points (郄穴 *xī xué*)

The character 郄 *(xī)* generally refers to a narrow opening or pathway. Consequently, many modern texts describe the cleft points as being in areas where the channel pathway narrows and has a tendency to blockage and an accumulation of qi and blood. A more clinically useful conception would be areas where channel qi is filtered and flow is controlled. The cleft points are like sluice gates or toll booths regulating the nature and rate of channel flow.

As might be expected, these points are often found in areas along the body surface where an opening or clear separation can be readily palpated. Sometimes, these palpable openings are between the bodies of muscles, or, in many cases, between small bones. There are a total of sixteen cleft points, one for each of the twelve regular channels plus the yin-yang *qiāo* vessels and the yin-yang *wéi* vessels (Table 17.2).

Channel	Cleft Point
Lung	LU-6 *(kǒng zuì)*
Spleen	SP-8 *(dì jī)*
Heart	HT-6 *(yīn xī)*
Kidney	KI-5 *(shuǐ quán)*
Pericardium	PC-4 *(xī mén)*
Liver	LR-6 *(zhōng dū)*
Large intestine	LI-7 *(wēn liū)*
Stomach	ST-34 *(liáng qiū)*
Small intestine	SI-6 *(yǎng lǎo)*
Bladder	BL-63 *(jīn mén)*
Triple burner	TB-7 *(huì zōng)*
Gallbladder	GB-36 *(wài qiū)*

Table 17.2
The cleft points

While the cleft points have the ability to regulate the flow of qi in the channels, it is important to remember that they are by no means the only points with this ability. The type of flow regulation thought to be occurring at different points along the channel varies. Understanding the nature of that variability comes from considering the point categories. For example, the source points are where the prenatal source qi enters the channels. If the cleft points are likened to stoplights along the highways of the channels, then the source points may be likened to gas stations. To extend the metaphor, the collateral points (discussed below) may be likened to regulators along the small side roads of a complex road system, while the growth of qi transformation among the five transport points may be represented by ever-increasing speed-limit signs along increasingly wide highways. While this metaphor may be helpful, it is important to remember that changes in the nature and rate of channel flow can be effected to some degree at all acupuncture points. The value of point categories lies in the ability of these general groupings to help direct the practitioner to some of the most useful points on the body and to describe ways of visualizing how to creatively use these points in the clinic to affect physiology (Fig. 17.5).

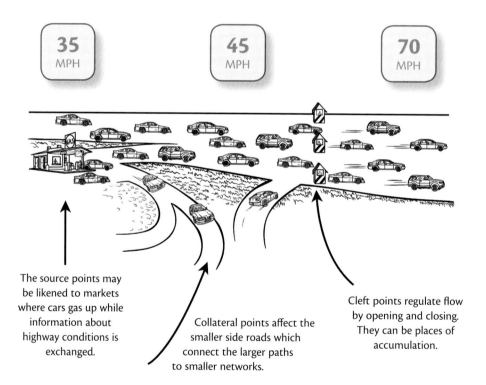

Fig. 17.5
The five transport points describe a process of
growing movement that is different at each stage.

The cleft points have two general functions, both of which are most applicable in relatively acute cases in which pain is part of the symptom pattern:

1. Facilitate the movement of qi to alleviate pain and eliminate swelling (利氣止痛消腫 *lì qì zhǐ tòng xiāo zhǒng*)

This is the most common use of the cleft points and refers to unblocking channel circulation in cases where lack of free and open circulation has led to pain (不通則痛 *bù tōng zé tòng*). This function of the cleft points is especially relevant on the yang channels, as these channels and their associated organs require constant movement for optimum function.

2. Redirect counterflow to stop bleeding (降逆止血 *jiàng nì zhǐ xuè*)

These are cases where counterflow qi in the channel has led to a kind of stagnation. The stagnation, in turn, has built up in the channel and has led to bleeding or bruising. The cleft points can be used to unblock the circulation, reduce stasis, and slow the rate of bleeding. The net result, somewhat counterintuitively, is an increase in channel circulation that actually reduces bleeding or bruising. This function often applies to the cleft points of the yin channels, as these are the ones which tend to produce, direct, and nourish the blood.

Our discussion of the source points did not consider specific indications for each of the twelve points. This is largely because the functions and uses of those points can be broadly understood by considering the effects of the improved qi dynamic in their associated organs. In the case of the cleft points, however, indications tend to vary idiosyncratically and they should therefore be considered individually. Yet the effects listed below should still be considered in the context of the general cleft point function described above. In other words, the ability of the points to treat specific indications stems primarily from the regulation of channel flow that occurs in these areas of narrowed circulation—the clefts.

INDIVIDUAL CLEFT POINTS

LU-6 (*kǒng zuì*) This point is used to clear heat from the lung and to stop bleeding. It also benefits the fluids of the lung by removing heat. The point is often used in cases where there is swelling of the throat (tonsillitis) or upper respiratory tract due to infections such as bronchitis or pneumonia. Traditionally, the point is often used in cases where lung heat has led to coughing of blood. Interestingly, this point is also sometimes used for headaches due to deficiency when there is reduced absorption of oxygen due to compromised lung function. These patients often have headaches accompanied by severe cough. The point is also sometimes used for hemorrhoids, as it can clear heat from the large intestine through its paired yin organ.

LI-7 (wēn liū)   This point is used to clear heat and regulate the stomach and intestines. Most commonly, it is used for painful disorders of the head including toothache, headache, nosebleed, inflammation of the nasal cavity, facial paralysis, and trigeminal neuralgia. LI-7 is also sometimes used for spasmodic pain in the abdomen (often large intestine) and sudden-onset abdominal pain with diarrhea.

ST-34 (liáng qiū)   This point is used very often for stomach pain and spasms. It is also useful for acute swelling in and around the breasts and for swelling of the knees. In both of these cases, the point is used in treating the branch of the disease; the root should be carefully discerned to prevent recurrence of the condition.

SP-8 (dì jī)   This point is used primarily in the treatment of lower abdominal pain. Most often, this includes dysmenorrhea with severe, cramping pain. The treatment of bladder pain is also appropriate for this point. SP-8 is also used to reduce swelling in the lower leg.

HT-6 (yīn xī)   This point is used to clear heat from deficiency and to stabilize the spirit. The point has a kind of astringent action that both restrains and calms. Clinically, this involves symptom patterns that include a stifling discomfort in the chest, palpitations, mild agitation, or disconnected speech with an underlying pathodynamic of deficiency. (This is not an excess-type mania or agitation.) In addition, the point is often used in protective qi disorders including either excess sweating or an inability to sweat.

SI-6 (yǎng lǎo)   This point is used to clear the head and brighten the eyes. It can treat acute neck or lumbar pain. For the eyes, this involves cases where older people begin to develop nearsightedness.

BL-63 (jīn mén)   This point clears the orifices and reduces pain by unblocking channel circulation. It is often used for acute lumbar pain, occipital headaches, and to reduce the intensity of epileptic seizures. In the modern clinic, BL-63 is also used for hyperactive disorder (ADD/ADHD). In recent decades, this point has been a favorite for use in acupuncture anesthesia, especially for cranial surgery. Consequently, it is often chosen for patients with head pain that feels as if it is deep within the bones of the head.

KI-5 (shuǐ quán)   This point is often used for pain in the lower abdomen, especially in cases of painful urination due to urinary tract infections, cystitis, bladder spasms, and kidney stones. The point can also be used for painful or delayed menstruation, especially in cases where the point is also tender.

PC-4 (xī mén) This very useful point is used to clear the nutritive level of heat and to stop bleeding. The point also has the ability to calm the spirit. It is used clinically for a variety of conditions involving the organs of the upper abdomen and chest, especially those that also involve bleeding. Clinical examples include coughing, vomiting or spitting blood, and nosebleeds. To be appropriate for these conditions, they should also involve heat in the nutritive level. Other symptoms of nutritive level heat that often respond to treatment with PC-4 include inflammation of the mesenteric linings of the upper burner (e.g., pleuritis, pericarditis) and inflammation of the mammary glands. This point frees and unblocks the flow of blood in the upper burner and is thus also appropriate for a variety of conditions involving blockage of the coronary arteries (especially when heat is present).

Here it would be helpful to pause and note the differences among the three cleft points of the arm yin channels. While it is relatively easy to conceptualize LU-6 (kǒng zuì) as a point that is useful for pain in the chest and lungs with coughing of blood, how does one differentiate the pericardium and heart cleft points? PC-4 (xī mén) is more useful for problems with flow in the coronary arteries—a more substantial problem in the blood of the heart. By contrast, HT-6 (yīn xì) is more often used for night sweats, a problem often caused by a deficiency of heart blood. The deficiency of heart blood that leads to night sweats can be thought of as involving blockage in the channel causing problems with the qi transformation of the heart. As noted in an earlier discussion about the heart and pericardium, the heart is often involved more in the functions of the heartbeat and blood movement while the pericardium is more often associated with problems in the physical muscle and blood supply of the heart organ.

LR-6 (zhōng dū) This point is used to clear heat and regulate qi. Related symptoms include hypochondriac pain and abdominal distention. This type of qi level heat is often associated with recovery from acute hepatitis. Other qi level heat conditions that can be addressed with this point include tonsillitis, abdominal infections, and inflammation in the joints. It is also often used in treating premenstrual syndrome and dysmenorrhea of the type where the patient feels abdominal discomfort after the period has finished. All of these symptoms involve a compromise of the liver function of directing the flow of blood. When adequate blood flow is not maintained, heat can develop. By unblocking the flow of channel qi with the cleft point, this function of the organ is stimulated.

Pause again to note the differences among the three cleft points of the yin channels of the leg. All three points are used to treat pain in the abdomen. Both SP-8 and KI-5 treat pain in the lower abdomen. SP-8 treats menstrual pain due to a relatively excess-type stagnation of qi and blood, while KI-5 similarly treats excess-type stagnation in the kidney or bladder (often stones). By contrast, the effects on the qi dynamic that arise from stimulating LR-6 tend to affect the middle burner and blood distribution in general. For all three points, the movement of channel qi that occurs from stimulating the cleft points serves to clear stagnation and heat.

Cleft points of the extraordinary vessels

BL-59 (*fù yáng*)   The cleft point of the *yáng qiáo* vessel is most often used to clear the head (清頭 *qīng tóu*). Clinically, this often involves patterns involving headache and dizziness. Also, because of the association of the *qiáo* vessels with the coordination of muscle movement, the point is used for trigeminal neuralgia and problems with movement of the musculature of the face (such as Bell's palsy).

GB-35 (*yáng jiāo*)   This cleft point of the *yáng wéi* vessel is often used to clarify consciousness (清神志 *qīng shén zhì*) in cases where yang circulation is failing to reach the head. Consequently, traditional indications for this point often include mania and withdrawal (癲狂 *diān kuáng*). As might be expected, the point also benefits qi circulation in the liver and gallbladder and is thus often seen in cases of hypochondriac or chest pain.

KI-9 (*zhú bīn*)   One interesting use of this *yīn wéi* cleft point that is not commonly listed is for clearing deep-seated toxic phlegm. Recall that the *yīn wéi* is associated with coordinating the provision of yin nourishment in the internal environment; one may therefore consider toxic accumulations such as tumors to involve a blockage in *yīn wéi* function. A few clinical experiences indicate that using strong, scarring moxa at this point may create a kind of immune response which stimulates the body's anti-tumor reserves.

KI-8 (*jiāo xìn*)   The *yīn qiáo* cleft point is often used for emotional disharmonies which also involve discomfort in the abdominal cavity. Recall that the *yīn qiáo* vessel has a function of coordinating multiple channel internal muscle movement. KI-8 helps to regulate the musculature around the internal organs and thus calm patients who have a feeling of disquietude that is associated with a sense of organic discomfort. Note as well how close KI-8 is to SP-6, another point often used for discomfort of the organs, in particular the organs of the lower abdomen.

Collateral Points (絡穴 *luò xué*)

NATURE OF THE COLLATERAL VESSELS

The collateral vessels were first discussed in Chapter 10 of the *Divine Pivot*. This chapter, entitled "On Channels and Vessels" (經脈篇 *jīng mài piān)*, includes a description of the pathways of the regular channels. The chapter also mentions, in varying degrees of detail, the collateral pathways which connect interior-exterior paired regular channels to each other and the specific points at which these collaterals are thought to leave the regular channels. Thus the most common understanding of the collateral vessels, as first outlined in the *Inner Classic*, describes a mechanism for facilitating connections between the regular yin and yang channels (Table 17.3).

Channel	Collateral Point
Lung	LU-7 *(liè quē)*
Spleen	SP-4 *(gōng sūn)*
Heart	HT-5 *(tōng lǐ)*
Kidney	KI-4 *(dà zhōng)*
Pericardium	PC-6 *(nèi guān)*
Liver	LR-5 *(lǐ gōu)*
Large intestine	LI-6 *(piān lì)*
Stomach	ST-40 *(fēng lóng)*
Small intestine	SI-7 *(zhī zhèng)*
Bladder	BL-58 *(fēi yáng)*
Triple burner	TB-5 *(wài guān)*
Gallbladder	GB-37 *(guāng míng)*

Table 17.3

The collateral points

However, another use of the term collateral (絡 *luò)* in the *Inner Classic* involves the smaller, sometimes visible vessels closer to the surface of the body. Later, in Chapter 10, the *Divine Pivot* poses a question to help clarify how the collateral vessels differ from the regular channels:

Lei Gong asks: How does [one] know the difference [between the] channels (經脈 *jīng mài)* and the collaterals (絡脈 *luò mài)?*

The Yellow Emperor states: The channels are generally not seen; [instead] their relative excess and deficiency is [ascertained at the] qi opening [radial pulse]. [Those] vessels that are visible are the collateral vessels.

Thus these surface vessels, now often associated with the visible blood capillaries that can be seen on the skin, have also been known as 'collaterals' throughout the history of Chinese medicine. Here the text is asserting that, while the regular channels connect to each other deep in the body, there are also aspects of the channel system which must come up to the surface. This superficial aspect is also often associated with the term 'collateral'. Because these collaterals are often found at the surface of the body, the vessels are often mentioned as being places where the removal of a few drops of blood can be beneficial in cases of stasis.

In addition, the collateral vessels have been traditionally thought to run perpendicular (across) to the pathways of the regular channels. In fact, the very term used to describe the channels in Chinese, 經絡 (jing luò), contains both the character for the main channels (經) and the character for the collaterals (絡). For this reason, one sometimes sees this two-character term translated as 'warp and woof', an allusion to the crossing threads seen on a weaver's loom. While the channels are the pathways from the head and trunk to the appendages, the collaterals represent a crisscrossing of microcirculation which completes the web. The channels are relatively deep to the surface; the crossing collaterals are thought to be more shallow. The collaterals are also branches from the main channels in the same way that the branches of a tree come up and out from the trunk (Fig. 17.6).

To extend the metaphor of the tree, the collaterals themselves are also thought to divide into branch collaterals (支絡 zhī luò) and ever-smaller minute collaterals (孙絡 sūn luò). To be more specific, the aspect of the collaterals which comes up to the surface of the skin (but is not visible) is traditionally described with the term 'floating collaterals' (浮絡 fú luò). By contrast, the collaterals which can be seen (tiny visible capillaries) are termed blood collaterals (血絡 xuè luò). Collateral vessels are thus found all over the body. In fact, the presence of tender or a-shi points on the body away from the major acupuncture points can be understood by considering the innumerable branches of the collaterals which spread to areas all around the regular channels.

When discussing the collaterals, many sources say that there are fifteen major collaterals. It is the major collaterals that are described in modern textbooks as facilitating connection of paired yin and yang channels. For example, the collateral vessel which leaves the lung channel at the collateral

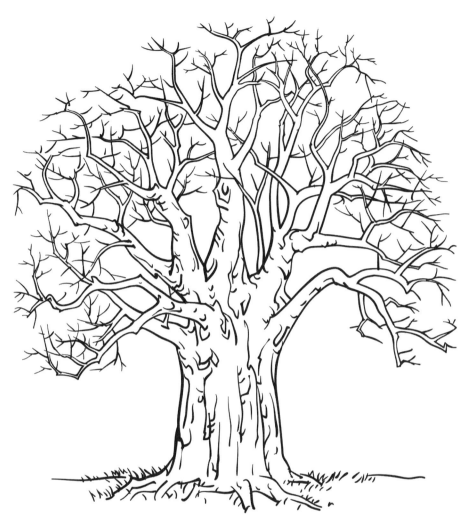

Fig. 17.6
Like the ever-dividing branches of a tree, the collaterals branch off the main
channels and move outward from the main channels while interweaving.

. . . .

point LU-7 *(liè quē)* is described as traveling to the yin-yang paired large
intestine channel. In addition to the collaterals that connect the paired yin
and yang regular channels to each other, the *rèn* and *dū* vessels also have
collaterals. Completing the group of fifteen major collaterals is a secondary
collateral of the spleen channel which is called the 'great collateral of the
spleen' (脾大絡 *pí dà luò*; see the question below).

As might be surmised from the broad nature of these vessels, the important exterior-interior connection function of the collateral vessels is

only part of the picture. When the collateral points are used in the clinic, the practitioner is also often thinking about the small vessel circulation implied by the original Chinese term. Collaterals, by their very nature, are also working at the level of microcirculation. In fact, the ability of the collateral points to facilitate connection between yin and yang channels draws from the fact that these points are thought to be influencing circulation at the places of intersection—where microcirculation of one channel meets the microcirculation of another nearby channel.

The reader should resist the temptation to make an absolute association of this concept of collateral vessels with the modern understanding of capillary circulation. The concepts are obviously similar and must necessarily overlap. However, within the context of classical channel theory, the collaterals are thought of as branches of the regular channels (經 *jing*). As previously noted, the concept of the channels is larger than that of blood vessel circulation. The channels are integrated regions of flow within the connective tissues of the body. They integrate groups of blood vessels, nerves, and muscles into areas with common effects on the larger physiology of the body. When taken together, the groups of structures said to be within the influence of each channel also have effects far away on specific organs or other larger functions of the body. Conversely, the internal organs affect the far-away channel pathways. The collateral vessels represent the smaller and smaller, ever-dividing branches of the channel system. The capillary system of modern physiology is one part of this idea, but is not equivalent to the traditional concept of collateral vessels.

USES OF THE COLLATERAL POINTS

While the body has innumerable small collaterals, there are certain points along the channels that are more directly associated with the larger branch collaterals thought to facilitate interconnection between yin and yang channels. By this we don't mean to suggest thick or substantial 'collateral pathways' going between LU-7 and the large intestine channel, for example. Rather, the collaterals are small vessels, branching out from the major channels from the area around the collateral points out to the level of microcirculation, where they meet the microcirculation of their paired channel (Fig. 17.7).

The collateral points are areas along the channels where one can induce a fairly quick and dramatic effect on this interplay of yin and yang. By using the collateral points to affect paired channels, the result is a kind of regulation of yin and yang—a balancing between the often-contrasting functions of the two paired organs. For example, consider the use of a stomach chan-

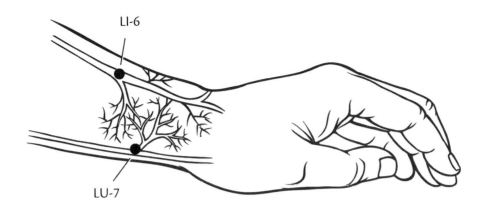

Fig. 17.7
A point such as LI-6 *(piān lì)* describes an area of
small vessel interplay between the lung and large intestine channels.

. . . .

nel point like ST-40 *(fēng lóng)* as a collateral point to affect the interior-exterior paired spleen channel. Modern functions for this point most often describe transformation of phlegm and stagnant fluids. To be precise, the effects of the point draw from its ability to balance the yin-yang natures of the spleen and stomach organs. In this case, the spleen organ has become encumbered by phlegm (excessive yin) and thus needs a boost of yang movement from the stomach. The collateral point is a place from which this goal can be pursued rather quickly.

Another way to describe the function of the collateral points might therefore be to say that they are balancing excess and deficiency. If 'pressure' is high in the yin channel, then the collateral point of the yang channel might be used to reduce the excess. If there is 'low pressure' in the yang channel, the collateral point of the yin channel might facilitate a filling-in of the deficiency.

To restate, collateral circulation is by no means limited to the connection of interior-exterior paired channels. The concept also represents microcirculation of small vessels along the paths of the associated channels. Taking both of these concepts into account, one might identify two major uses of the collateral points:

Treat interior-exterior paired channel disease

This use of the collateral points involves the use of yin channel collateral points to treat yang channel conditions and vice versa, as described above.

[509]

Treat collateral disease

Here, the collateral point is used to affect microcirculation along the pathway of the selected channel. For example, one might use LI-6 *(piān lì)* in the treatment of chronic facial paralysis when one suspects that the ability of the channel to bring nourishing qi and blood into the collaterals on the face has been affected. This concept has very broad clinical application.[6]

Treatment technique for the collateral points

Treatment technique should reflect the fact that, within the channel system, the collaterals are relatively shallow. When stimulating any of these points, whether to treat interior-exterior paired channel disease or collateral disease, the depth of insertion should accordingly be shallow. In addition, the best manual technique for these points involves either very low-intensity lifting and thrusting, or rapid twirling.

INDIVIDUAL COLLATERAL POINTS

LU-7 *(liè quē)* Traditional considerations of the channel collaterals involve the division of symptom patterns into categories of excess and deficiency. For example, on the lung *tài yīn* channel, excess in the collaterals involves redness, heat, and inflammation on the forearm; deficiency includes both frequent yawning and frequent urination. In the discussion that follows, the traditional symptoms of excess and deficiency will be mentioned only in cases where the author's clinical experience in using the point can be illuminated by these concepts. This is not meant to suggest that the traditional collateral vessel patterns should be ignored.

The collaterals of the lung channel service the throat and upper respiratory tract, and LU-7 is appropriate for many conditions involving this area. When the point is stimulated at a very shallow depth (0.1–0.2 inches), it is effective for treating throat discomfort and cough. Needling at this shallow depth is also appropriate for treating a narrowing or blockage in the upper respiratory tract or spasms in the smooth muscles of the throat that has led to difficult or shallow breathing. When needled slightly more deeply, the point is more effective for treating headaches, often those involving external patterns. Finally, at the deepest level (approaching the bone), the point is sometimes used for problems with the cervical vertebrae.[7]

LU-7 is also used to release the exterior in cases of external invasion and cough. This function of the point and its traditional use for treating urinary problems are not unrelated. Recalling that *tài yīn* opens (開 *kāi*) to the external aspect of the internal environment, one can imagine how the collaterals of *tài yīn* reach up to the border of the skin. By facilitating circulation at these outward-opening collaterals, one can resolve problems affecting the surface. Similarly, the *tài yáng* channel opens to the external aspect of the external environment. Because both channels have an outward-opening movement, their functions can overlap. The sweating of the skin and the passage of urine are both means of releasing fluids and waste. When there are problems releasing upward due to dysfunction of the *tài yīn* collaterals, the symptom of frequent urination might arise. In the clinic, not only frequent urination, but other types of urinary problems where the lung is also involved respond to treatment with this point.

Because of the interior-exterior pairing of the lung-large intestine, the point can also be used to unblock collateral circulation on the large intestine channel on the face in cases of facial paralysis from stroke, Bell's palsy, and trigeminal neuralgia.

Finally, the point is used in those cases of high blood pressure where lung function is also compromised, or palpation reveals significant changes along the lung channel.

LI-6 (*piān lì*)   In general, the effects of this point are in the upper aspect of the body. Deficiency of the large intestine collaterals is most commonly associated with tooth pain (including sensitivity to cold). Deficiency in the *yáng míng* collaterals might also involve discomfort in the chest or an uncomfortable feeling in the esophagus.

LI-6 is often used to clear heat from the *yáng míng* collaterals. This includes symptoms such as frequent nosebleeds, red eyes, toothache, tinnitus, swelling in the throat, and/or face or facial paralysis. In fact, LI-6 is one of the most common points used for trigeminal neuralgia or facial paralysis. In addition, when there is heat trapped in the *yáng míng* collaterals, the ability of *tài yáng* to open outward might be compromised, leading to a lack of warmth on the exterior. The net result of this pathodynamic might involve a tendency to be easily affected by exterior invasion or, alternatively, difficult urination.

ST-40 (*fēng lóng*)   As noted above, ST-40 is indicated for a variety of conditions involving dampness and the accumulation of phlegm. This draws from the ability of the point to provide a yin-yang balance with the functions of the paired *tài yīn* spleen channel. It is important to remember that the type of phlegm and damp conditions that respond best to treatment with ST-40 involve excess-type accumulation that is encumbering the spleen. In these cases, the spleen is overwhelmed and requires stimulus from the yang of the stomach channel.

In addition, ST-40 is also an excellent point for treating *yáng míng* channel type facial problems. When there is heat in the face, there will occasionally be more pronounced palpable change at ST-40 than one might find at LI-6. In these cases, ST-40 is more appropriate.

SP-4 *(gōng sūn)* Not only is SP-4 the collateral point of the spleen, it is also the command point of the *chōng* vessel. The functions of the point thus reflect not only the spleen-stomach but also the strong blood flow of the *chōng*.

This point is used to regulate the spleen-stomach in a wide variety of conditions which, like those associated with the collateral point of the stomach, also often involve pathogenic dampness. The collaterals of the spleen are associated with the face, in particular the area around the eyes. Swelling around the eyes is therefore often thought to reflect an accumulation of dampness in the collaterals of the spleen. The collaterals also travel through the chest and, in some cases where there is also tenderness in the area, SP-4 can be used in the treatment of pleuritis.

Because the *chōng* vessel brings a strong flow of blood to the organs of the abdomen, SP-4 is also often used for digestive problems involving deficiency. Symptoms may include an inability to digest food and abdominal distention. These conditions may be due to a lack of proper acid production in the stomach. In addition, because of the relationship of the *chōng* vessel to blood, this point is often used in the treatment of irregular menstruation and pelvic inflammatory disease.

On the other hand, SP-4 also has an ability to clear the collaterals of the paired *yáng míng* stomach channel; in these cases, it is actually used to clear heat. Symptoms of this type of *yáng míng* heat may include nausea/vomiting, stomach pain, insomnia, and irritability. Note that in such cases the trapped *yáng míng* heat is moving upward to affect the heart. (This is similar to the pattern for which Pinellia and Millet Decoction *[bàn xià shú mǐ tāng]* is indicated in Chapter 71 of the *Divine Pivot*.[8])

HT-5 *(tōng lǐ)* The collateral vessels of the heart are described in the *Inner Classic* as traveling to the root of the tongue and then upward to the brain and back of the eyes. HT-5 is used in the treatment of a wide variety of conditions affecting the tongue (speech) and brain. When there is excess accumulation in the collateral vessels of the heart, a sensation of distention in the chest may arise. Deficiency in these collaterals is traditionally associated with speech problems.

The types of speech problems associated with the heart collaterals involve a slowed rate of speech, low speech volume, or an unwillingness to speak at all. In all cases, there is also a sense of compromised clarity of mind in which ideas and concepts are often not clearly described. (See further discussion of the tongue in Appendix 2.)

This very useful point has four main clinical applications:

• *Unblocking the collaterals of the heart* (通心絡 *tōng xīn luò*)

HT-5 is used to regulate the beating of the heart (electrical conduction system of the heart) and to treat chest pain.

• *Unblocking the collaterals of the tongue* (通舌絡 *tōng shé luò*)

This function encompasses treatment of a wide variety of problems involving movement of the tongue, including acute paralysis of the tongue, sudden loss of speech due to severe emotional stress, or even chronic tongue sores.

• *Unblocking the collaterals of the brain* (通腦絡 *tōng nǎo luò*)

This very common use of HT-5 involves the treatment of patients who have had a stroke. Because the heart collaterals travel through the brain, this point is often a lead point in the treatment of many types of poststroke sequelae.

• *Clearing heart fire* (清心火 *qīng xīn huǒ*)

HT-5 does not clear heart fire directly, but it does effectively clear the fire by unblocking microcirculation. It can be useful for heavy menstruation and other types of heat and inflammation in the uterus, especially when the symptom pattern also involves the heart. This should be contrasted with other types of heat in the uterus. For example, it was noted above that SP-4 can be used for inflammation in the abdomen (including uterine inflammation) when there is a damp-heat pattern involving the spleen. HT-5 is more appropriate for inflammation involving heat and toxins in the blood.

SI-7 (*zhī zhèng*) This point is traditionally said to unblock the collaterals and transform stasis (通絡化瘀 *tōng luò huà yū*). SI-7 is also described as having the ability to generate yin-fluids (液 *yè*). The qi dynamic of the small intestine is often associated with the generation of these thicker, more viscous fluids in the body.

This point has been clinically useful in the treatment of headaches, dizziness, stiff neck, sties, or other small growths in and around the eyes (often related to liver fire). For dizziness, it is appropriate in cases where an external hot-type pathodynamic has led to fever and a rush of blood to the head. Although the *Great Compendium of Acupuncture and Moxibustion* (針灸大成 *Zhēn jiǔ dà chéng*) states that SI-7 is a useful point for treating warts related to deficiency in the collaterals of the small intestine channel,

Dr. Wang's clinical experience would indicate that it is not helpful for this type of condition.

BL-58 (*fēi yáng*) This point has an ability to unblock the collaterals and awaken the brain (通絡醒腦 *tōng luò xǐng nǎo*). It is therefore useful in the treatment of headaches, dizziness, nosebleeds, and nasal congestion due to external invasion.

BL-58 also facilitates nourishment of the sinews by stimulating the movement of moistening yang-fluids (津 *jīn*). This would make the point an appropriate choice in the treatment of low back, thigh, and leg conditions involving spasms or a lack of moistening of the sinews. The point is also often used in the treatment of hemorrhoids and cystitis.

KI-4 (*dà zhōng*) This point unblocks the collaterals, calms the spirit, and clears *tài yáng* heat. When using the point, the two collateral pathways leading from KI-4 should be considered. The first travels upward to the tongue and then connects with the bladder channel. The second collateral travels shallow to the regular kidney channel up through the kidney and pericardium organs, then around the chest to the spine and back. KI-4 is therefore often considered in the treatment of lumbar pain when there is concurrent irritability and/or a stifling sensation in the chest. This condition is said to arise from deficiency in the kidney collaterals. By contrast, excess in the kidney collaterals is associated with combined constipation and difficult urination.

Because of its collateral pathway connections, this point is also helpful in the treatment of dry mouth, mouth ulcers, difficult urination, and irregular menstruation. And because of the effects of this point on the spirit, it is also helpful in the treatment of panic (驚恐 *jīng kǒng*), slow development in children, or dementia in the elderly.

When needling the point, the sensation will rarely travel up or down the channel. Instead, the goal should be to achieve an aching sensation that radiates in all directions from the point.

PC-6 (*nèi guān*) The association of this important point with the *yīn wéi* vessel was discussed at some length in Chapter 11. The clinical uses of PC-6 are broad. In general, the point has three functions: to regulate the qi, calm the spirit, and harmonize the stomach (by directing counterflow downward) (理氣, 安神, 和胃 *lǐ qì, ān shén, hé wèi*). The ability of the point to regulate the qi is helpful in cases where there is pain in the internal organs due to deficiency or qi constraint, a mechanism that is also at work when one uses the point to harmonize the stomach in cases of gastritis or stomach spasms. The ability of the point to harmonize the stomach makes it a favorite in many point prescriptions for nausea as well. Besides the stomach, however, the point is often used for angina, carditis, pleuritis, and intercostal neuralgia.

The effects of the point on the spirit are most pronounced in cases of constraint or depression. These patterns may be combined with an irregular heartbeat or other symptoms due to lack of yin nourishment to the heart organ.

When considering PC-6 in the context of the pathway of the pericardium collaterals, it is sometimes helpful to remember that deficiency in the collaterals is associated with weakness or numbness of the elbow, while collateral excess is associated with spasms of the elbow or surrounding muscles. These are conditions for which PC-6 is less often considered, but may nonetheless be beneficial.

TB-5 (*wài guān*) This point has the ability to unblock the collaterals, clear heat, and resolve toxicity (通絡, 清熱, 解毒 *tōng luò, qīng rè, jiě dú*). In particular, the point is used to unblock the more superficial floating collaterals to vent heat from the body.

Like PC-6, LU-7, and SP-4, TB-5 is another collateral point that is also a command point of the extraordinary vessels. All of the collateral points that also relate to the extraordinary vessels have broader uses than their regular channel association might suggest. In this case, the relationship with the *yáng wéi* vessel means that TB-5 is often used to benefit circulation of yang to areas beyond the pathways of the regular channels. This concept would explain the mechanism through which TB-5 is able to vent heat from the body. By linking the yang circulation in multiple yang channels, the point has a decidedly upward-and-outward-directed function.

This upward-and-outward motion also allows the point to promote movement of qi and to open the orifices (行氣開竅 *xíng qì kāi qiào)* in cases of external invasion of either a warm or cold nature. Symptoms may include fever, cough, headache, or even bronchitis. Heat trapped in the body may lead to red painful eyes or conjunctiva, tinnitus, insomnia, or high blood pressure. Finally, conditions associated with triple burner dysfunction affecting the digestive system such as diarrhea, abdominal pain, or constipation may also be treated with TB-5.

GB-37 (*guāng míng*) The Chinese name for this point, 光明 *guāng míng,* literally means light or brightness and is a hint to the point's particular affinity for the eyes. As other texts often point out, it is used clinically for a wide variety of eye disorders. GB-37 is used to slow the process of cataract development; it can be helpful in less severe cases. It is most effective, however, in cases where the eyes are affected by heat coming from the liver-gallbladder which involve redness, itching, or swelling. Chronic allergies or conjunctivitis are particularly responsive.

LR-5 (*lǐ gōu*)   The collateral point of the liver is used primarily to regulate the circulation of qi and blood. The liver organ is charged with maintaining the pathways and supply of qi and blood throughout the body, and it is from the collaterals of *jué yīn* that circulation reaches out.

The collaterals of the liver channel are especially related to the lower abdomen and genitals. Consequently, LR-5 is often used in the treatment of excess-type menstrual disorders (frequently involving stasis of qi). In addition, the point is used in many classical prescriptions for a variety of problems in the groin and genitals including herpes zoster, testicular pain, uterine inflammation, and leucorrhea.

In addition, because of the commonly seen relationship of the musculature of the groin to low back pain, this point can be helpful in treating lumbar pain, especially when there is also tenderness at the point. Because the pathway of the *jué yīn* pericardium passes through the forearm and wrist, there will also often be tenderness in this area in cases of carpal tunnel syndrome. In such cases, LR-5 can be an effective distal point.

CV-15 (*jiū wéi*)   Many sources list this point as contraindicated for needling. In fact, it can be safely needled at a shallow depth (0.5–1 inches) if the patient raises their hands above the head. Nevertheless, because of the presence of the heart organ nearby, care should be taken and the technique should be gentle and slow.

This collateral point of the *rèn* vessel is used to transform blood stasis (especially in the pericardium), transform phlegm, and redirect counterflow downward (化血瘀,化痰,降逆 *huà xuè yū, huà tán, jiàng nì*) to benefit the stomach. For transforming blood stasis, the point is used when stasis leads to symptoms such as angina or intercostal neuralgia. The ability of the point to transform phlegm can be brought to bear by using moxa; this technique is utilized in cases of pericarditis, childhood epilepsy, and heart-type mania. For chronic belching and asthma, the point is used to direct qi downward.

GV-1 (*cháng qiáng*)   For those familiar with yoga positions, this point is best needled in the crouching 'child's pose' position (knees bent, head down, hips up). In this position, the point can often be needled without requiring the patient to completely remove their undergarments. The point is generally needled to a depth of 1–1.5 inches until a deep radiating sensation is achieved, which may radiate to the back.

GV-1 can also unblock the collaterals to resolve dampness (通絡利濕 *tōng luò lì shī*) and clear heat to resolve toxins (清熱解毒 *qīng rè jiě dú*).

The point is clinically effective for removing damp-heat accumulations that affect the genitals, including itchy, painful sores or herpetic outbreaks. It is also used for treating hemorrhoids, pain of the sacrum, and prolapse of the anus.

Q: *What is your understanding of the great collateral of the spleen?*

DR. WANG: This has long been a subject of debate in Chinese medicine. When I first began practicing, I really didn't know what it meant. It was always said to treat 'pain throughout the body' (一身之痛 *yī shēn zhī tòng)* or 'softness and weakness' (鬆軟無力 *sōng ruǎn wú lì)* and most doctors left it at that. I originally tried to use the associated point SP-21 *(dà bāo)* for arthritic conditions, as this certainly seemed to be a type of pain throughout the body. But I didn't get very good results. I had a patient, an older woman, who was extremely thin. She complained of severe pain in her ribs and upper body. At the time, because of the location of her pain, I thought of SP-21. The point was very effective. Afterwards, I began to think that the reason this particular area has a network vessel of its own is to supply the intercostal muscles. This musculature never really gets to rest because breathing never stops. Yet when these muscles become weak and the fatty tissue in the area becomes thin, pain often results. So far, my understanding and experience with the great collateral of the spleen stops there. I do, however, suspect that the point can also be beneficial for other types of problems with breathing and qi movement. After all, the *tài yīn* system involves nourishment of the muscles and it involves the lung. This needs to be further confirmed with more clinical application.

Q: *This discussion of point categories brings to mind the alarm (collecting) points on the abdomen. How do these points fit into your understanding of the channels?*

DR. WANG: The alarm points (募穴 *mù xué)* are collection points for organ excess. Remember that the character 募 means to accumulate or collect, and the points do just that. Most simply, they should be thought of as reactive points to be checked in cases where excess is suspected in a particular yin or yang organ. If one suspects stomach heat, for example, check CV-12 *(zhōng wǎn)* for tenderness or a sense of tightness.

The alarm points are used to diagnose (and sometimes to treat) conditions of excess. Similarly, the back transport points can be examined and used for treatment in cases of deficiency. Especially when there is a lack of yang qi, the back transport points are helpful. Once again, notice how the back transport points are generally used to treat conditions involving organs in the area near the point. Like the alarm points, the back transport points are used less often for treating conditions far from their locations. When I say this, I understand that one might obviously benefit the tendons of the leg, for example, by stimulating the liver points on the back to benefit liver blood. However, this is still a different idea than that of using distal points to affect the qi dynamic.

Q: *After all of this discussion about five-transport point theory and the role of source qi, I feel like I have a much clearer understanding of how the mechanisms of acupuncture are understood in classical Chinese physiology. How do you respond to the assertion that acupuncture involves nothing more than stimulating nerves?*

DR. WANG: When we talk about the mechanisms of acupuncture, we aren't talking about nerves, but rather about the role of the so-called 'empty spaces' that I associate with the channels. The ability of acupuncture to affect the nerves stems from changes brought about in the environment surrounding the nerves and not from direct stimulation of the nerves themselves. Therefore, while acupuncture certainly affects the nerves, that is only part of the picture. There are also changes in muscle tone and vessel permeability. My opinion is that it all comes down to the fluids and not to the nerves. By changing the circulation patterns of the interstitial fluids, systemic effects seem to follow.

I remember that this same subject came up when the earliest foreign students of Chinese medicine came from the Soviet Union in the 1950s. In fact, that first group of Soviet students attended a series of classes with us at the Beijing University of Chinese Medicine. They were older than us but stayed in our dorms and ate in the cafeteria with the Chinese students. The members of this group were all trained in Western medicine. As a result, they immediately drew conclusions about the similarity of acupuncture channels to nerve pathways. Because many of the Chinese teachers assisting these early groups were also trained more in Western medicine than classical Chinese medicine, it led to a kind of sub-category of acupuncture. In the years that followed, the Russians developed an acupuncture style that relies heavily on nerve stimulation. They did develop some interesting treatment styles that are effective for treating certain conditions, particularly pain. Nevertheless, this is different from classical Chinese acupuncture because it begins from a different premise. Channel theory doesn't really enter into the picture in this style of acupuncture, although I'm sure that it also has adherents in other countries.

Q: *Finally, can you say something about your understanding of the category of 'ghost points' that are associated with Sun Si Miao (孫思邈 7th century A.D.)?[9]*

DR. WANG: I do think of the 'ghost points' in the clinic—especially in psychological conditions such as depression, hysteria, or mania. All of these conditions may have looked, to ancient physicians, like instances of possession by ghosts or spirits. When I needle these points, I usually follow a particular order (listed below). Because there are so many points, and because some are quite painful, I rarely get beyond the sixth or seventh point. There are the 13 ghost points and then there are two additional points that are sometimes listed as ghost points. Each of the 13 points actually has a different name that refers to its function as a ghost point. The point order and alternate names are as follows:

GV-26 *(rén zhōng)*: 'ghost palace' (鬼宫 *guǐ gōng*)

LU-11 *(shào shāng)*: 'ghost communication' (鬼信 *guǐ xìn*)
 Remember that the lung governs the qi of the entire body.

SP-1 *(yǐn bái)*: 'ghost hutch' (鬼壘 *guǐ lěi*)
 This is like another home for the ghost, literally a pile of stones.

PC-7 *(dà líng)*: 'ghost heart' (鬼心 *guǐ xīn*)
 Now you've found the heart of the ghost.

BL-62 *(shēn mài)*: 'ghost road' (鬼路 *guǐ lù*)
 This will hopefully get the ghost walking.

GV-16 *(fēng fǔ)*: 'ghost pillow' (鬼枕 *guǐ zhěn*)
 This point is located where the head should rest.

ST-6 *(jiá chē)*: 'ghost bed' (鬼床 *guǐ chuáng*)
　　More images of resting.

CV-24 *(chéng jiāng)*: 'ghost market' (鬼市 *guǐ shì*)
　　Here one thinks of the manic, chaotic speech that is sometimes
　　heard in a bustling market.

PC-8 *(láo gōng)*: 'ghost cave' (鬼窟 *guǐ kū*)
　　Another place a ghost might hide.

GV-23 *(shàng xīng)*: 'ghost hall' (鬼堂 *guǐ táng*)
　　Another place the ghost might reside in the head (as opposed to
　　the palace).

CV-1 *(huì yīn)*: 'ghost storage' (鬼藏 *guǐ cáng*)

LI-11 *(qū chí)*: 'ghost legs' (鬼腿 *guǐ tuǐ*)
　　Used if the condition has affected the ability of the patient to
　　walk.

M-HN-38 (舌柱 *shé zhù)*: 'ghost closing/seal' (鬼封 *guǐ fēng*)
　　This point, located at the intersection of the frenum linguae and
　　sublingual fold on the underside of the tongue, helps stop raving
　　speech.

The two additional points, sometimes considered to be extra ghost
points, are PC-5 *(jiān shǐ)* and SI-3 *(hòu xī)*.

Besides needling the points in the order set out above, one may
choose points based on their secondary names. For example, a patient with raving, manic speech might be a good candidate for CV-24
('ghost market'). Others may have problems walking, or may walk
constantly, in which case LI-11 ('ghost legs') may be best. I think of
these points creatively, but do consider their secondary names when
I'm putting together a point prescription where emotional imbalance
is obvious.

　　If emotional disorders can be treated in the first six months or
so, acupuncture can be quite helpful. Later, such disorders tend to
go into the collaterals and involve harder-to-treat accumulations of
phlegm.

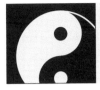

CHAPTER 18

A Brief Discussion of
Classical Technique

THIS CHAPTER WILL evaluate three chapters in the *Classic of Difficulties* which address the concept of acupuncture technique. Obviously, these chapters can in no way summarize the entirety of classical discussion on the subject. In fact, the *Classic of Difficulties* alone mentions the subject of technique in at least thirteen separate chapters. To provide some depth, the following section will focus on the single concept of tonification and draining. While technique is the subject at hand, the goal is also to provide a comparative discussion of these three chapters to give the reader insight into the kind of thinking engaged by a scholar-physician when approaching the classics. These particular chapters were chosen because they summarize concepts that are repeated in different ways in other parts of the *Classic of Difficulties*.[1]

Chapter 78

Chapter 78 of the *Classic of Difficulties* addresses the most commonly discussed subject of acupuncture technique: tonification and draining. As is often the case, the *Classic of Difficulties* is striving to clarify a concept introduced earlier in the *Inner Classic*. Getting right to the point, it asks, "How do you explain this idea that needling involves tonifying and draining?" The answer that follows has spawned a discussion that has lasted nearly two-thousand years. The very first line sets the stage by stating what tonifying and draining *are not*, thus differentiating itself from earlier statements in the *Inner Classic* on the same subject:

"It is not inserting and withdrawing the needle in accordance with the patient's breathing."

This would seem to be a direct response to Chapter 27 of the *Divine Pivot,* which discusses needle technique where there is an invasion of the exterior. The *Inner Classic* asserts that tonification involves inserting the needle while the patient exhales while draining involves inserting the needle during inhalation.[2] Likewise, when removing a needle, tonification involves removing the needle while the patient inhales (with the movement of qi into the body) while draining involves removing during exhalation (creating a draining counterflow to normal qi movement). Simply put, the *Inner Classic* asserts that draining a point involves moving the needle in the direction opposite that of the patient's breathing (the chest is lifting and expanding while needle insertion moves into the point against the flow).

In the clinic, the *Inner Classic* approach to needling with consideration to the breath is particularly appropriate when needling on the abdomen. While the *Classic of Difficulties* seems to downplay this approach, it is still quite important clinically—especially as a means of focusing the practitioner's mind on the task at hand (Table 18.1).

Technique	Patient Inhales	Patient Exhales
Tonification	Needle is removed as qi expands; this is with the qi	Qi sinking inward; needle inserted with the qi
Draining	Needle is inserted as qi expands; this is against the qi	Remove needle against the inward movement of qi

Table 18.1
Tonifying and draining according to *Divine Pivot,* Chapter 27

Returning to Chapter 78, the next line initiates another often cited discussion on the importance of the left hand (assuming that all acupuncturists insert with the right hand):

"Those who know how to needle place faith in the left hand, those who do not place faith in the right."

This is a statement about palpation of the point and preparation of the area for insertion. Generations of acupuncturists have placed greater or lesser emphasis on the admonitions in this line of text, depending on their personal inclinations or the technical style of their teachers. Some traditions emphasize extremely careful determination not only of point location, but also of the nature of the flesh at and around the points as a diagnostic indicator (the left hand). Other traditions focus training on the complex techniques of needle manipulation (the right hand). In the *Classic of Difficulties*, it is clear that the left hand is of primary importance. This means that, according to this text, palpation of the points is as important as (or possibly even more important than) the movement of the needle once inserted.

Chapter 78 then proceeds to discuss the importance of pressing firmly in the area to find the point, and that after one feels "the coming of the qi [which] is like the movement in the vessels," one can insert the needle. The "movement in the vessels" may be a pulsing beneath the finger or it may instead involve the types of changes described in earlier chapters on channel palpation. The main idea here is that the left hand should feel the area until a change or irregularity is found; this is where the point is. In other words, an acupuncture point can actually be felt with the hands if one searches the area and waits for the proper sensation.

Next, the *Classic of Difficulties* describes the basics of tonification and draining:

> "After getting qi, if one pushes toward the interior, this is tonification. If one stretches the needle upward after getting qi, this is draining."

"Stretching the needle upward" is commonly thought to be a description of the technique of lifting the needle from a deeper (nutritive) to a more shallow (protective) level. From there, the chapter concludes by emphasizing the importance of getting qi (得氣 *dé qì*) to effective treatment. (This concept will be discussed more in Chapter 19.) Finally, it asserts that "if one does not get the qi, this is referred to [as a situation in which] ten [out of ten] die and cannot be treated." In other words, if the practitioner is unable to get qi, the treatment is unlikely to be effective.

There are two especially important ideas presented in this chapter:

1. It is important to palpate the area around the point before inserting the needle. This aids diagnosis, prepares the area for insertion (brings qi to the point), and helps the practitioner to find the exact location of the point. Recalling that the first chapter of the *Inner Classic* insists that acupuncture points are not "skin, flesh, tendons, and bones", the fingers should be searching for an opening or separation. The mind should be focused.

2. Tonification includes 'pushing toward the interior' with retention at a relatively deep level, while draining involves first getting qi and then bringing the needle back to a more superficial location.

Chapter 72

The concept of tonification and draining is further refined in Chapter 72 of the *Classic of Difficulties*. There, the text introduces another commonly discussed concept, that of needling with or against the flow of channel qi in the twelve channel circuit model. This question arises from an attempt to clarify a section in the first chapter of the *Divine Pivot* which introduces the idea of 'going against vs. following' the qi (迎隨 *yíng suí*).[3] Thus the *Inner Classic* touches upon the subject and the *Classic of Difficulties* now attempts to clarify:

> That which is referred to as going against or following means that one has to know the courses of the flow of the nutritive and protective and the comings and goings [of the qi] in the channels and vessels. One accesses [the qi] by following [either] the contrary or the normal flow, so one speaks of going against or following. One says that the method of regulating the qi must be located in [the] yin or yang [aspect].

Note that here the *Classic of Difficulties* has also introduced the concept of 'regulating qi' (調氣 *tiáo qi*) with acupuncture. This is an often underutilized treatment approach in the modern clinic. With both acupuncture and Chinese herbal medicine, one is often not striving to 'add or subtract' something from the body. Instead, the techniques translated in English as tonifying and draining are actually describing a fairly subtle alteration of movement which involves changing the qi dynamic. By altering the movement of qi in the channels, a chain reaction is initiated which alters the qi dynamic and eventually leads to noticeable physiological change.

This idea is sometimes difficult to appreciate. Part of the problem may be due to the English terminology. 'Tonify and drain' is just one of many options for translating the Chinese terms 補 *(bǔ)* and 瀉 *(xiè)*. Sometimes, the English terms may lead practitioners to envision that they are literally adding or taking away something from the channel in the course of treatment. While this may be true in a sense when, for example, using source points to guide source qi into the channel, it is often just as important to regulate.

Thus, while Chapter 78 introduces the concept that one might tonify or drain in general, Chapter 72 points out that acupuncture can also regulate. Basically, Chapter 72 is elaborating on the concepts presented in Chapter 78 to include the actual results of tonifying or draining channel flow. When one changes the flow, the net effect might be called 'regulation'. This is especially important to keep in mind when thinking about how acupuncture affects physiology.

Q: *I have to stop and ask you a question at this point. I rarely see you use the method of needling with or against the channel in the clinic. It seems instead that you tend to retain most points perpendicular to the patient's skin. How does this section of the Classic of Difficulties influence your work in the clinic?*

DR. WANG: I'm going to discuss my own clinical approach to technique later, but I should say a few things about how I've come to understand Chapter 72 of that text. I do, in fact, sometimes needle with or against the channel in the clinic, but it is, admittedly, rare. I mainly use this technique when I want to get very strong qi sensation in a particular direction. I've found that most of the time I can do this without changing the direction of the needle.

I don't, by the way, think that Chapter 72 presents an understanding of channel flow that conflicts with the five transport point model described earlier. Remember that (to me, at least) the twelve channel circuit flow, first described in the *Inner Classic*, is occurring at the same time that the channel qi is growing along the five transport points. The two circuits are separate and complimentary (see the summary paragraph at the end of Chapter 17).

Chapter 76

In the course of discussing another aspect of technique, an answer is provided in this chapter to one of the most obvious questions about tonification and draining, namely, where is the qi coming from when we tonify and where does it go when we drain? Before delving into the implications of these questions, it will be helpful to look first at the original text. The perceptive question posed here sounds like one that might be asked by a patient in a modern clinic:

> "What is tonification and draining? When you are tonifying, from where do you get qi? When you drain, how is it that qi is put aside?"

The answer to this question has been another seed for discussion on technique, which has lasted for nearly two-thousand years:

> In tonification, one draws qi from the protective [aspect]. When draining, qi is put aside from the nutritive [aspect]. If there is not enough yang and too much yin, one should tonify the yang before draining the yin. If there is not enough yin and too much yang, one should tonify the yin before draining the yang. The main purpose is to keep the flow of nutritive-protective open.

This statement is one that touches upon both clinical practice and theory. Practically speaking, the protective aspect is thought to be more on the surface of the body, while the nutritive aspect is deeper. Thus, based on the concept described here, most techniques designed to tonify emphasize the more shallow levels (protective) of the acupuncture points first and then finish at the deeper levels (nutritive). As described in the *Classic of Difficulties*, one is drawing qi from the protective aspect to tonify. The reverse is generally true of draining techniques: When draining, one draws qi from the nutritive aspect.

For example, the concept of tonifying the three levels of 'heaven, earth, and humankind', commonly called 'lighting the fire of the mountain' (燒山火 *shāo shān huǒ)*, involves progressive stimulation that begins at the most shallow (protective) of three levels and finishes at the deepest. A similar draining technique, called 'heaven-penetrating coolness' (透天凉 *tòu tiān liáng)*, involves doing the reverse: a quick insertion to the deepest (nutritive) of the three levels is followed by progressive stimulation at more and more shallow levels. Again, tonification begins with the protective aspect while draining begins with the nutritive. There are other, similar techniques that also find their original impetus in this chapter of the *Classic of Difficulties*.

What are the theoretical implications of this chapter? Interestingly, by considering some classical concepts regarding the nature of the nutritive-protective aspects, one can gain insight into how the authors of the *Classic of Difficulties* may have understood the mechanisms of acupuncture. Remember that the protective aspect is thought to be active and defensive while the nutritive aspect is calm, quiet, and supportive. The protective aspect moves outside the vessels while the nutritive aspect is thought of as the substantial core of the blood itself. One might be tempted at first to think that, to tonify, one should simply needle the area where nutrition is most abundant, and that to drain, one should clear from the area with the greatest proclivity for movement. In other words, at first glance it might seem that the best way to tonify would be to needle deeply to the substantive nutritive level, while draining would simply involve clearing from the active protective level at the skin surface.

However, the concept of interdependence of yin and yang requires using one to motivate the other. When yin is diseased, choose yang. When there is a yang condition, choose yin. Considering that excess is primarily a yang condition, the acupuncturist first goes to the nutritive (yin) level to generate material support, which then facilitates a lifting up and out. As deficiency has a yin nature, tonification draws stimulus from the active movement of protective qi to stimulate nutrition at the deeper level. When draining, the needles are retained at a very shallow level (yang) to emphasize the direction of treatment. When tonifying, after stimulating at the protective level initially to generate movement, the needles are retained at a greater depth (yin). When tonifying, retention at a greater depth stimulates the vessels to release the nutritive into the area around the point. In short, classical physicians brought the concept of yin-yang interplay into every aspect of their treatment. Many seemingly arbitrary techniques from these sources make more sense when considering yin-yang theory and how it affects the movement of qi in the channels (Fig. 18.1).

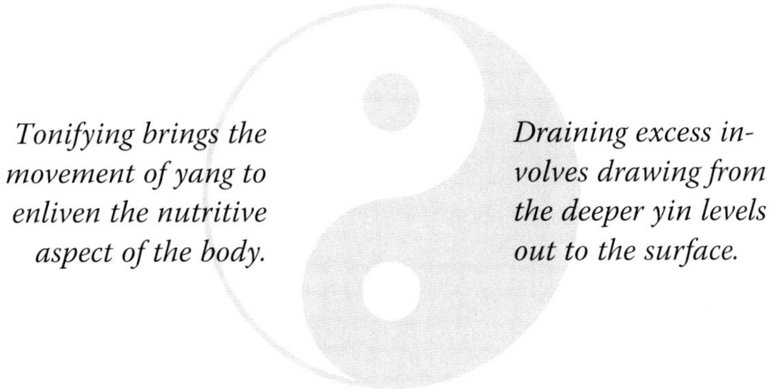

Tonifying brings the movement of yang to enliven the nutritive aspect of the body.

Draining excess involves drawing from the deeper yin levels out to the surface.

Fig. 18.1
Yin-yang theory is helpful for understanding
traditional tonifying and draining techniques.

To conclude this brief discussion of the *Classic of Difficulties* and the concept of tonification and draining, a few summary points should be emphasized:

Chapter 78

Points should be palpated before needling to prepare the area and to aid in diagnosis.

Tonification involves pushing toward the interior while draining involves bringing the needle back to the surface after getting qi.

Chapter 72

Often, when tonifying and draining, the net effect of acupuncture is to regulate the qi dynamic (as opposed to actually 'adding' or 'subtracting').

Needling 'with channel flow' tonifies while 'going to the qi' against channel flow drains. This is subject to various interpretations.

Chapter 76

Tonification involves bringing the chaotic movement of protective qi deeply inward to the nutritive aspect. Draining, by contrast, involves first stimulating the nutritive then 'putting aside' accumulation at the more shallow protective aspect.

Many of the manual techniques developed over the intervening centuries have drawn from Chapter 76.

A Modern Perspective on Acupuncture Technique: Seven Steps

HAVING BRIEFLY CONSIDERED some classical concepts regarding acupuncture technique, the question arises as to what this means for the modern clinician. What is acupuncture technique? Before answering this question, the meaning of basic terms should be clarified. Technique (針法 zhēn fǎ) should be contrasted with a similar concept translated here as manipulation (手法 shǒu fǎ). Acupuncture technique is a broader subject within which manipulation is but one part. Technique involves the subjects of:

- channel selection
- point combination
- needle choice
- angle of insertion
- number of needles used
- manipulation

Many modern discussions of technique tend to emphasize the final aspect at the expense of the other five. Although channel and point selection have been presented as discrete subjects in other chapters of this book, before proceeding the reader should note that, strictly speaking, they actually fall under the broad category of technique. Anything that affects the outcome of an acupuncture treatment is part of a practitioner's technique. While perceptive students may strive to watch the hands of a great acupuncturist, they might still forget to watch his or her mind. In other words, long before the needle is in the hand, much of the technique has already occurred. To that end, this entire book may be thought of as a multi-faceted analysis of technique.

Up to this point, we have been slowly building an edifice from the prehistoric roots of yin-yang and six-stage theory through the solid trunk of channel and organ theory to the branches of channel and point selection. Now we will turn to the final discussion of the manipulation techniques of needle insertion, moving qi (行氣 *xíng qì)*, and getting or obtaining qi (得 氣 *dé qì*).[1] It is important to remember that without the roots provided in the earlier chapters of this text, the ability to achieve superior results with needle manipulation may well be compromised. There are always moments where spontaneity or 'secret' points prove to be miraculously effective, but consistency requires structure. The following pages rest upon the structure of the chapters that have come before.

Early discussions of needle manipulation were often unorganized. The *Inner Classic*, for example, contains many references to manipulation dispersed throughout both of its two extant parts, the *Divine Pivot* and *Basic Questions*. Although the text seems to acknowledge the importance of manipulation in acupuncture by virtue of the sheer number of lines devoted to the subject, there is no systematic discussion. This may reflect the fact that chapters have been lost, or possibly the haphazard reorganization of earlier versions of the text during the Han dynasty (206 B.C.–220 A.D.). Later, the *Classic of Difficulties* organized and clarified many fundamental concepts, but again, the subject of manipulation is spread throughout the text. Of the eighty-one chapters in the *Classic of Difficulties*, no fewer than thirteen touch upon the subject of manipulation. In some chapters, manipulation is a major subject, while in others it is only a small piece of a larger discussion. Nevertheless, while organization and commentary have been the work of later centuries, many fundamental concepts in use today can be traced to the scrolls written at the dawn of the first millennium.

An early organizer of information about acupuncture technique and channel theory is Huang-Fu Mi (215–282 A.D.). Living less than a hundred years after the time that the *Classic of Difficulties* was likely compiled, he authored the famous *Systematic Classic of Acupuncture and Moxibustion* (針灸甲乙經 *Zhēn jiǔ jiǎ yǐ jīng)*. That work became the basic text on the subject of acupuncture during the Tang dynasty (618–907) and continues to exert its influence in the modern classroom. After Huang-Fu Mi, generations of physicians continued the work of systematizing and codifying point locations, needling depths, and indicated pathodynamics for the points that are generally used today. Of note is the *Classic of Nourishing Life with Acupuncture and Moxibustion* (針灸資生經 *Zhēn jiǔ zī shēng jīng)*, written during the Jin dynasty (1115–1234) by Wang Zhi-Zhong (王執中). This work built upon the writings of Huang-Fu Mi and dedicated the majority of its text to discussions of technique (point selection, location, and needling depth) broken down into categories defined by pathodynamics. Many of the ideas about pathodynamics and the nature of the channels in this book owe a debt to this great Jin dynasty physician. Just as Wang Zhi-Zhong acknowledged his intellectual debt to the classics, a modern discussion of technique should likewise pay its respects to the *Classic of Difficulties* and its answers to 'difficult questions' from the *Inner Classic*.

A Modern Clinical Perspective: Seven Steps

STEP 1: OPENING THE POINT TO GUIDE THE QI (導氣開穴 *dǎo qì kāi xué*)

Chapter 78 of the *Classic of Difficulties* emphasizes the importance of palpating the point before insertion. Specifically, it describes the techniques of pressing the area with the fingers (壓按 *yā àn*) and flicking the skin (彈 *tán*). The goal is to bring qi to the area of insertion so that the point is awakened and prepared for what is to come. Many practitioners rush ahead to needle insertion and forget the importance of this simple step in the treatment process. You may be surprised at how much easier it is to get qi if the time is taken to open the point before bringing the right hand to the skin. Once the point has been opened and followed by a careful needle insertion into the open space, the patient will more likely feel the sensation along the pathway of the channel that the *Inner Classic* likens to "moving within a narrow alley" (*Divine Pivot*, Chapter 4)[2] This preliminary technique has two basic aspects:

Opening the point   The practitioner uses the left hand to carefully locate the point by pressing and feeling around the area specified in textbooks as the proper location. Remember that you are feeling for the opening between muscles, tendons, bones, and vessels.

Guiding the qi   This involves tapping along the channel to be needled, both above and below the point (Fig. 19.1).

STEP 2: INSERTION OF THE NEEDLE (進針 *jìn zhēn*)

Sources differ on whether the needle should be inserted quickly or slowly. At some points, such as BL-1 (*jīng míng*), a slow insertion is obviously required while at others, such as KI-1 (*yōng quán*), a quick insertion is

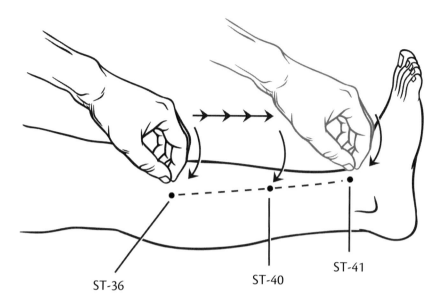

Fig. 19.1
Guiding the qi by tapping along the channel

best. Slow insertion helps prevent the puncturing of veins and small vessels by giving them a chance to slide out of the way. For example, source points are often near larger veins and thus require a relatively slower insertion. In general, the most important thing to keep in mind during insertion is to cause as little pain as possible to the patient. Insert the needle through the outer layer of the skin (epidermis) to a point where the tip of the needle is beyond the surface nerves. Here, not quite into the fascia, the needle will be loose and painless if the practitioner lets go. There is no qi around the needle at this point (Fig. 19.2).

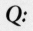 *In schools in the West there is sometimes a debate about the importance of using a guide tube for insertion. You never use a guide tube to help insert the needle. How important is it that we try to learn to insert without the tube?*

DR. WANG: Actually, I don't think it's necessarily that important. I use a fairly traditional insertion style during which I first lay the middle finger of my right hand on the patient's skin then use that finger to help support the needle while guiding it into the point. Nevertheless, I don't personally believe that insertion style is going to make or

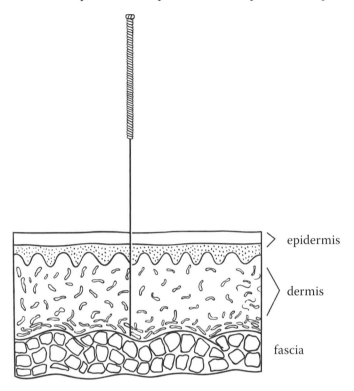

Fig. 19.2
Insertion involves getting the needle through the skin but not into the fascia.

break a treatment. Rather, as was just said, it is most important that the patient experience as little pain as possible. If a practitioner can insert the needle without a tube and cause little pain, then maybe this will give them more control. On the other hand, if one causes the patient so much pain during insertion that their muscles get tense and wrap around the needle, it is often more difficult to get qi. To be honest, when I am in other countries, I sometimes use a guide tube myself on very sensitive patients. The goal is to get the needle in place so that you can go on to the next step.

STEP 3: GETTING QI (得氣 *dé qì*)

After inserting the needle, the next step is to get qi (得氣 *dé qì*). Note that here the sensation of 'getting qi' is one that is felt by the patient. There is also the concept of the 'arrival of qi' (氣至 *qì zhì*) that involves a sensation felt by the practitioner. The late Jin dynasty text *Guide to Acupuncture and Moxibustion* (針灸指南 *Zhēn jiǔ zhǐ nán*) compares the sensation that a practitioner feels when qi has arrived at the needle as being like "a fish on a hook." And for those of us who have fished, the sensation is actually quite similar. There is a feeling under the practitioner's fingers that may also be likened to a small twitch or a slight 'grabbing' by the body of the needle shaft. It is often subtle, however, and is sometimes missed in the rush to move along to the next stage of treatment. Yet before beginning other manipulation, it is important to first let the patient's qi come to the needle. Sometimes this may involve waiting a moment, and sometimes further manipulation may be required. A noticeable muscle spasm is not always indicative of the arrival of qi. For the practitioner, the sensation is often much more subtle.[3]

In order to feel whether qi has arrived, the practitioner must remain as steady and calm as possible. Be aware of every change and sensation, not just with your fingers, but with all of your senses at once. While the patient will often feel radiation or a slight aching sensation when one has got qi (dé qì), this does not always mean that the qi has completely arrived (qì zhì). The primary arbiter of the arrival of qi (as opposed to getting qi) is the practitioner. Sometimes the patient's awareness may be so scattered, or the threshold for sensation so high, that they don't feel much at all around the needle. This does not necessarily mean that the results will be more difficult. If the practitioner can feel that qi has arrived at the needle, the patient may yet be surprised by the results. Nevertheless, whenever possible, it is most important for the patient to actually get a qi sensation at each needle during treatment.

When getting qi at points around the wrists and ankles and other areas without large muscles, it is best for the patient to feel sensation at a fairly shallow depth. While one might get qi at the surface at almost any point, it is sometimes better to focus on deeper levels at points where there is more muscle. At ST-36 (zú sān lǐ), for example, it is best to get qi at a depth of between 0.8–1 inches. GB-30 (huán tiào), another commonly used point, is sometimes needled to a depth of 3–4 inches before adequate qi is obtained. The subject of proper needling depth for getting qi varies with each region of the body (and with each individual patient) and thus a few general principles must suffice here:

Every point has an optimum depth for getting qi on a particular patient. For the practitioner, understanding is best gained from experience. Over time, one begins to know the points better and better.

Different depths are appropriate for the same point at different times, depending on the desired result. In general, deeper needling is used for more serious conditions.

The best place to get qi is at the proper point location for the individual patient. This is a statement about the importance of careful palpation. Remember again that acupuncture points are found in the spaces between muscles, tendons, bones, vessels, and nerves (see Chapter 14). If you are not getting qi and/or there is no sensation of the arrival of qi, you may not be in the proper space. Note that the actual location of any point is not necessarily where that point is located by techniques of proportional measurement. Rather, the point is the place where one can best get qi and facilitate the arrival of qi. It is not fixed.

Manipulation to help get qi

Sometimes, one finds it difficult to get qi. In such cases there are techniques for helping to bring about a sense of radiation from the point. The technique can influence whether the net effect is tonification or draining. There are two general techniques used to help bring about the qi sensation, the choice of which depends on the desired net effect. Relatively strong techniques are said to 'guide' (or hasten) the arrival of qi (導氣 *dǎo qì*) while gentle, slow manual techniques are said to 'await' the arrival of qi (候氣 *hòu qì*). In fact, it is actually possible to await the arrival of qi by simply holding the needle firmly in place. Awaiting the qi is generally thought to be tonifying, while guiding the qi can have a sedating effect. In reality, the two methods sometimes overlap and the difference is thus usually one of intensity. The following manipulative techniques are most often used to help get qi. Depending on the strength used to perform the manipulation, the effect may be to either guide or to await the qi.

Flicking (彈 *tán*)   This involves flicking the needle handle with the index finger off the thumb. It is the most commonly used approach (Fig. 19.3).

Flying (飛 *fēi*)   This slightly more complicated technique requires that the hand first grasp the needle handle and then release with a sudden 'flying' motion. This technique is particularly useful for the stronger technique of guiding the qi (Fig. 19.4).

Scratching (颳 *guā*)   Here, the practitioner scratches the handle of the needle with the nail of the thumb to create vibration at the needle tip (Fig. 19.5).

Pressing (壓 *yā*)   In this case, the needle is grasped very firmly by the practitioner between the thumb and index finger, then turned clockwise, slowly but with conviction, and then held in place. Note that the needle is turned in only one direction; it is not twirled. This technique is particularly useful to facilitate the process of qi arrival (Fig. 19.6).

A.

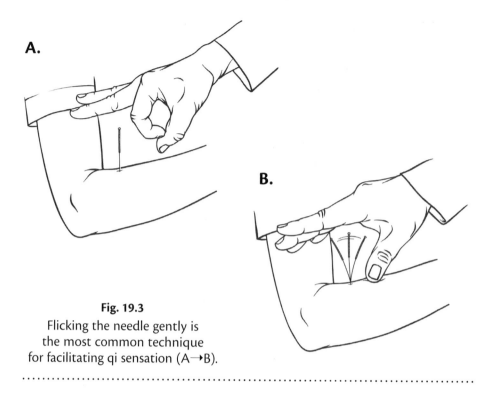

B.

Fig. 19.3
Flicking the needle gently is
the most common technique
for facilitating qi sensation (A→B).

A.

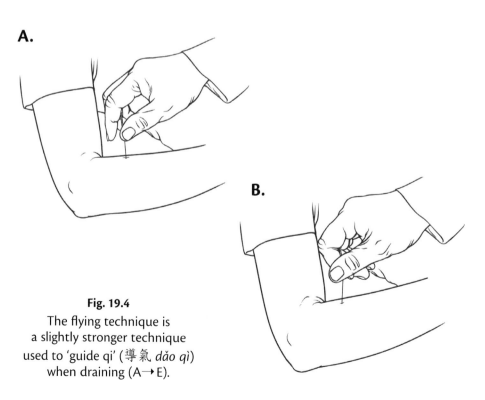

B.

Fig. 19.4
The flying technique is
a slightly stronger technique
used to 'guide qi' (導氣 dǎo qì)
when draining (A→E).

[536]

C.

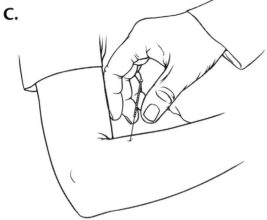

D.

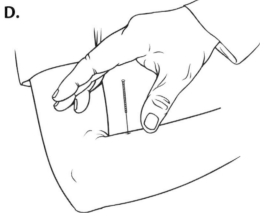

E.

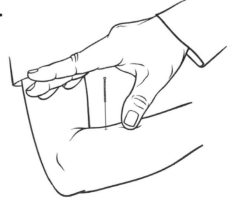

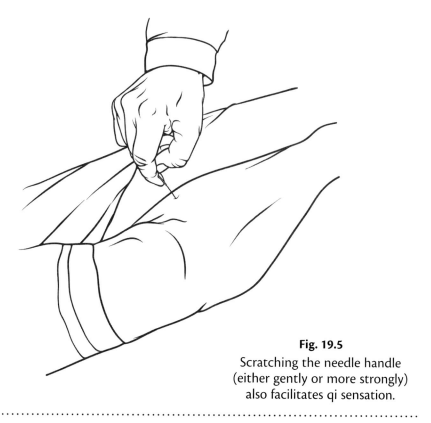

Fig. 19.5
Scratching the needle handle
(either gently or more strongly)
also facilitates qi sensation.

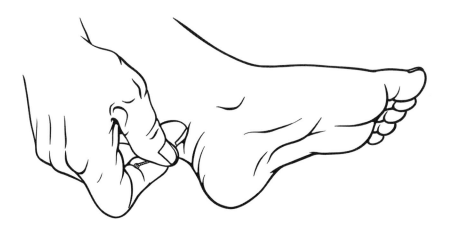

Fig. 19.6
Grasping and gently turning the needle is often best
for facilitating 'qi arrival' (侯氣 *hòu qì*) in tonification.

STEP 4: MOVING QI (行氣 *xíng qì*)

Moving the qi broadens the effect. To the patient, this might involve a widening ache of sensation (酸 *suān*) or a lengthening (extension) along the line of the channel (串 *chuàn*). If possible, the sensation should involve a lengthening along the channel. At this point, the practitioner has already got qi and now wants to gently build. The concept of gentle building is important. Moving the qi does not involve strong, vigorous stimulation of the point (more likely to cause an uncomfortable ache) but should be focused on obtaining a gentle but constant sensation whenever possible. Sometimes, especially when the goal is to drain, there may be a moment of strong sensation that necessarily precedes the onset of lengthening.

Optimal manipulation for moving the qi creates a sensation like that of skipping stones along the surface of a pond. It can be likened to using a flat, round, smooth stone that skips gently along the surface—gentle waves are created far away from the initial impact. This is in contrast to using a rough stone, or simply tossing a heavy rock into the water (Fig. 19.7).

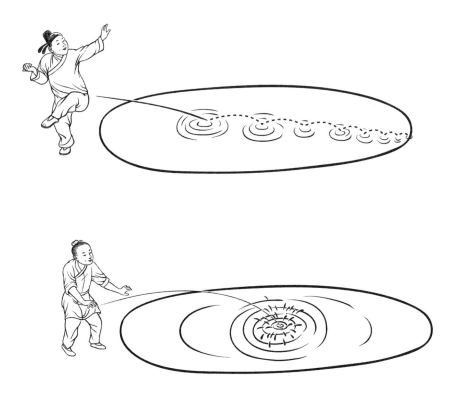

Fig. 19.7
Optimal qi sensation is like skipping a small stone along the surface of a pond.

Methods for moving the qi are similar to those described above for getting qi. However, because qi has already arrived in the area, the manipulation may be even slightly stronger or the needle angle may be changed. As above, one might flick, scratch, press, or use the flying technique. If a particular technique was used to good effect to help obtain the initial qi sensation, that same technique will likely help move the qi as well. In addition:

The practitioner might move the qi by using high frequency twirling of the needle between the thumb and index finger. At source points in particular, the twirling technique is most commonly used to create a gentle radiation along the channel (Fig. 19.8).

Relatively gentle lifting and thrusting might also be used to expand the qi sensation.

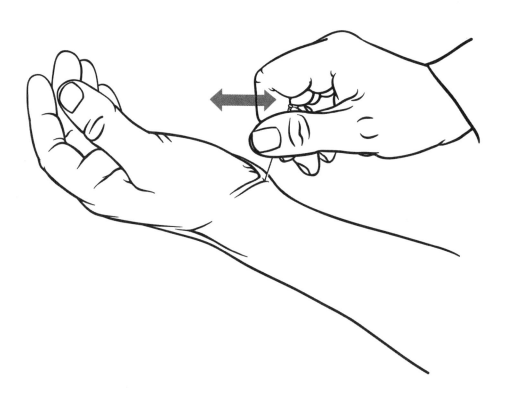

Fig. 19.8
Rapid twirling is often used at source points to facilitate a gentle
radiating sensation down the channel. When twirling, the thumb
stays still while the index finger moves back and forth rapidly.

Q: *In general, do you always move the qi with every patient?*

DR. WANG: Yes. I think that it is important that the patient have a sense of movement in the channels in order to get the very best results. In my experience, the further away from the needle that radiation is felt, the better the result. I do want to emphasize once again, however, that I'm not talking about strong, vigorous stimulation of the points. If, after a few minutes of relatively gentle manipulation, you cannot get the qi to move, then leave the point alone. Sometimes if you come back later the patient will feel the qi better, or you might gently stimulate it to move the qi further. I have seen other doctors who are absolutely determined to get a radiating sensation as far as possible and therefore stimulate the needles with an unnerving intensity. You can see that it is really quite strong for the patient. This is not my approach. In fact, it seems to me that if you are stimulating a point very, very strongly, the patient will eventually tell you that it is radiating just to get you to stop!

When thinking about stimulating a channel, a helpful image is that of water movement. An acupuncture point is a place of interaction where the fluids, qi, and blood gather together in a particular way. Stimulating the point with a needle changes the movement of those fluids and thus the nature of qi/blood interaction in the area. When moving the qi, I am creating a kind of chain reaction of fluid movement down the channel. This is very different than stimulating a nerve, for example.

Sometimes it might take a few treatments with a patient to begin to build qi in the channels. You shouldn't keep switching points around if you are reasonably confident of your diagnosis. Instead, give it three to four treatments to take effect and, often enough, things will begin to change just before you are about to give up and try something else.[4]

In general, for all points, the practitioner should have a clear picture of:

- What the functions of the point are—how does stimulating the point affect qi transformation?

- Exactly where the point is located and the nature of that area of the body. If a practitioner has some doubt about the location of a particular point, they should close their eyes and 'put their heart in their fingertips'. Palpate in the area defined by point location texts and move

[541]

around until an opening or separation is found—this is the actual location of the point on that patient.

• The best technique for getting qi at that particular point.

STEP 5: TONIFICATION AND DRAINING (補瀉 *bǔ xiè*)

As explained in the discussion of tonification and draining in Chapter 18, this is a complex subject. However, Dr. Wang's experience would indicate that the subject can be simplified a great deal. In fact, if the practitioner can become adept at locating the point (with palpation), getting qi, and moving qi, then seventy percent of the time the desired result can be achieved. In other words, if qi sensation can be obtained at a properly chosen point, then the body will take care of tonification and draining on its own. This is largely due to the concept, discussed in Chapter 72 of the *Classic of Difficulties*, that the effects of acupuncture often fall under the category of regulation. Even when one is 'tonifying' or 'draining' a particular channel, the end result is regulation of the nutritive-protective aspect in the channel, and eventually, regulation of the qi dynamic in the organs.

That being said, there is always room for improvement in any practitioner's clinical results. There are times when the concepts of tonification and draining are quite important. In Chapter 18 we touched upon the views of just one classical text, the *Classic of Difficulties*, regarding the concept of tonification and draining. Countless other texts throughout the history of Chinese medicine have also weighed in on the subject. While the vast majority of discussion in later eras continues to at least allude to the original pre-Han dynasty concepts synthesized in the *Inner Classic* and *Classic of Difficulties*, a considerable variety of manipulative techniques were later developed. Most confusing for the scholar and modern student is the fact that some of these approaches to manipulation quite clearly contradict one another. An author in one dynasty might assert, for example, that their reading of the *Inner Classic* indicates that tonification involves retention of the needle at a deep level, while another author four-hundred years later might come to the opposite conclusion.

The short answer to all of this conflict is that tonification and draining are rarely within the full control of the practitioner. Rather, the determining factor is the patient and the pathodynamic at hand. To be more specific, the most important factor is the quality of qi and blood in the patient's channels. If, for example, a patient is weak and channel flow is slow, then it is very difficult to achieve 'draining'. In this type of patient, the results of properly administered acupuncture will tend toward tonification. On the other hand, if a patient truly suffers from a condition of excess, then draining is the natural result *when the proper points are chosen*. Note the emphasis placed here on proper methodology. Once again, technique does not refer only to manual manipulation, but to a clear understanding of classical physiology, diagnosis, channel selection, and choice of points. If the practitioner is headed in the right direction, the body will respond.

How, then, should the vast literature on the subject be understood? Some general statements about tonification and draining can be made:

Any technique that leads to net excitement and movement within the channel at hand can be said to tonify that channel. In general, a net result of excitement and movement in the channel is obtained through gentle building techniques.

Any technique that results in a calming and slowing of qi and blood movement can drain. Thus, while draining techniques often involve stronger stimulation, the net result is relaxation. Think, for example, of the feeling one has after vigorous exercise.

If one keeps these two simple principles in mind, the vast majority of classical approaches to the subject become much easier to digest.

The various manipulative techniques for tonification and draining can be narrowed down to the following three aspects:

1. Overall intensity of stimulation A large stimulus will actually have a net effect of calming the flow of qi and blood in the channel while a properly administered small stimulus has a more gradual but exciting effect. Again, while draining may be compared to the feeling one gets after vigorous exercise, tonification is more like the feeling one gets after restful meditative breathing.

2. Specific nature of the stimulus The nature of the manipulation can modify the more basic tendencies of large vs. small stimulus. Many traditions place a great deal of emphasis on special techniques to be used once the needle is in place and the qi sensation has been obtained. In general, these techniques are variations on the themes of lifting-thrusting, twirling, scratching, and 'wagging' the needle. In addition, *qì gōng* (氣功) techniques, by which the practitioner moves the qi with the breath, fall into this category as well. The nature of the stimulus required at each point to obtain the best results will vary. In general, such techniques are important, but not as crucial as careful location and getting qi.

3. Rhythm of the entire treatment Acupuncture treatments have a rhythm. Sometimes needles are inserted quickly, stimulated fairly strongly, and left to rest for a few minutes, followed by another fairly strong stimulus. In other cases, the insertion may proceed slowly and be followed by gentle and gradual manipulation that builds over time.

Tonification and draining can generally be achieved by working within the parameters of the three aspects of manipulation just outlined. Next, the two techniques will be considered in more detail.

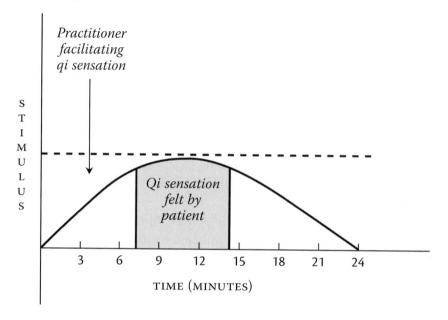

Fig. 19.9
Tonification involves a gradual growth of qi sensation that is maintained for a longer period of time, followed by a slow fade.

Tonification

The graph above (Fig. 19.9) illustrates the general concept of tonification. The vertical line represents intensity of stimulus by the practitioner, as perceived by the patient, and might vary because of everything from thickness and length of needle and angle of insertion to the strength of lifting-thrusting and/or twirling. The horizontal line represents time. The curve within the graph thus describes the growth and strength of qi sensation as felt by the patient over time.

For tonification, one can see that the qi sensation grows slowly but constantly over time, with a fairly long period of maximum intensity (shaded area). This effect is generally achieved by using a gentle insertion with a reasonably thin needle, followed by gentle but continuous lifting-thrusting or twirling of the needle until an even sense of radiation is achieved.

The result is an even excitation of the channel that can be characterized as tonification.

Therefore, from the perspective of the three aspects of manipulation described above, tonification involves:

- small intensity of stimulation

- gradual and constant stimulation that gently radiates from the point

- a rhythm to the treatment that focuses on obtaining a sensation that grows slowly, peaks for some time, and then slowly fades, but may not disappear altogether throughout the treatment.

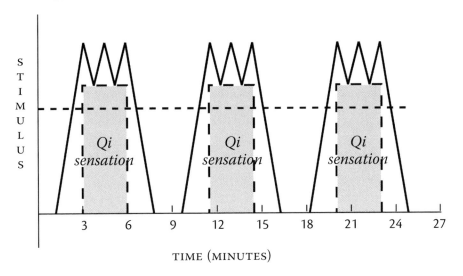

Fig. 19.10
When draining, a slightly more intense qi sensation which comes on more rapidly then drops off is used multiple times in a single treatment.

....

Draining

Remember that the goal of draining is to have a net calming effect on the channel. To that end, a fairly strong treatment that leaves the patient with a sensation of loosening and relaxation is the goal. As illustrated in the graph above (Fig. 19.10), treatments focused on draining generally involve periods of strong stimulation followed by an almost complete disappearance of all qi sensation. To the patient, the stimulation will be relatively strong and may briefly be quite intense. Manipulative techniques are consequently stronger and often involve more vigorous lifting-thrusting and twirling. Of course, even here, the goal is not to stimulate so strongly that the patient cannot endure the treatment. The strength of a draining treatment should be gauged by contrasting it with the gentle, even nature of tonification. Neither should be so far from the other that they no longer seem to be coming from the same person.

To break this process down into the three aspects listed above, draining should involve:

- relatively large intensity of stimulation

- strong and relatively sudden stimulation

- a rhythm to the treatment that involves short periods of strong qi sensation followed by a relatively quick drop in sensation, and then a period of almost no sensation. This process may be initiated multiple times in the course of one treatment.

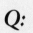 **Q:** *What do you think about the concept described in some texts as 'first draining, then tonifying' during an acupuncture treatment?*[5]

DR. WANG: I think of patient treatment as something that occurs over multiple sessions. Therefore, while I may use both 'tonifying' and 'draining' points in a single treatment, there is still a tendency for that day. Over the course of multiple treatments, I will generally spend the first few treatments clearing away excess, and then begin tonification. I don't think that it is effective to try to do both on a single day.

Once again, tonification and draining manipulation cannot substitute for technique in the more general sense. That is to say, if the practitioner's diagnosis, treatment principle, channel and point selections are inaccurate, even the most elegant manipulation will not ensure the best results.

STEP 6: RETAINING THE NEEDLES (留針 *liú zhēn*)

Once all needle manipulation has been completed, the needles should be retained. The patient should be left to rest peacefully while retaining the needles so that qi and blood can move naturally and respond to the stimulation just provided. In most cases, 20–30 minutes is enough time to obtain the best results. If the patient is sitting in a chair, the needles should be retained a bit longer.

While the patient is on the treatment table, he or she should be encouraged to breathe deeply and regularly. The room should be as quiet as possible. If music is played in the room with the patient, it should be peaceful and not too loud. If one is in doubt about whether the needles have been retained long enough, gently hold the needles to see if they are loose. If the body is still gripping the needle, treatment should probably continue a bit longer.

Step 7: Removal of needles (起針 *qǐ zhēn*)

Like insertion, removing the needles should be done in such a way as to cause the least amount of pain or surprise to the patient. One could cover and press the point to emphasize tonification, or simply remove the needle without covering for draining.

Which manipulative techniques do you use most often in the clinic?

DR. WANG: In general, I place the greatest emphasis on getting and moving qi. Just as important is that there be a proper angle and depth for each point in a particular patient for that particular pathodynamic. I spend a lot of time thinking about angles and depth of insertion so as to obtain a radiating sensation of a particular type. In the end, this is what the classical techniques are trying to do as well. Over time, many of the classical titles for this or that technique have become fixtures in the textbooks. We mentioned earlier [Chapter 18] the technique of 'setting the mountain on fire'. There is also 'shaking the white tiger's tail' and many, many others. Almost all of the classical techniques eventually lead to either a net stimulus or net calming of channel flow.

I'm not trying to oversimplify what is admittedly an extremely complex and subtle subject. I hope instead to sketch the broad outlines within which each practitioner can develop. Many students become so overwhelmed by the apparent complexity of manual technique that they decide that it's beyond them and thus use none at all. They might just insert the needles and leave it at that. As I mentioned earlier, if one has done everything else right, then this approach will quite often still get good results. However, one can increase one's average by incorporating the basic concepts of getting qi, moving qi, and tonification/draining. I would like to encourage students to initially focus on the first four steps that I've outlined here for manipulation. Open the point before insertion, then get and move the qi after insertion as often as possible. Over time, you can begin to work on tonifying and draining, beginning first with a few points that you are very familiar with, like ST-36 *(zú sān lǐ)*, for example. After you have become comfortable with these more advanced manipulative techniques at a particular point, you can begin to broaden your applications. Just remember that there is always more to learn and plenty of room for improvement.

There is one other related thing I'd like to point out about technique and doctors of Chinese medicine. Namely, throughout the history of acupuncture, there have always been those who cloak themselves in mystery so as to create a sense of wondrous skill for their students and patients. These are usually doctors who have 'secret' points or techniques. I do not like this approach to medicine at all. I've also seen other doctors who pride themselves in the very strength of their treatments and use extremely strong techniques that actually cause pain to patients. Thirty years ago, I even saw one quite famous acupuncturist who would sometimes remove the needle and occasionally find small bits of flesh attached to the needle shaft. This is not proper healing. The best side of our field lies in the direction of sensitivity and carefully cultivated skill.

In fact, below the surface of the best treatments is a complexity of technique not unlike that learned by professional musicians. Think of the movements of the hand during acupuncture as being somewhat like those of a violinist. There are a wide variety of sounds that a violin can make. You can move the bow with greater or lesser frequency and strength. One might bow loudly or softly with harmonic notes, or instead create a cacophony of contrasting sounds. Sometimes, one might not use the bow at all and instead pluck the strings to get the desired sound. An acupuncturist 'plays' the channel system in a similar manner.

Of course, the channels of the body are more complex than the strings of a violin—they are part of an even greater whole. In a larger sense, the organs of the body are like the instruments in an orchestra. There is the constant, even beating of the heart, the slow bass thrum of the lungs, and the pervasive hum of the liver. The stomach and intestines constrict with a rhythm of their own. When healthy, the process of life is a symphony. As a doctor, when one treats a patient, that person's channels should be treated delicately and with respect. One should create effects in the channel system that are like the music of an experienced musician. Don't beat on the strings or play indiscriminately. A successful treatment should be like conducting a piece of beautiful music.

Summary of the Seven Steps

1. Open the point by pressing, massaging, and tapping along the channel.

2. Insert the needle through the skin to just above the fascia, causing as little pain as possible.

3. Facilitate the sensation of 'arrival of qi'; a variety of techniques might be used.

4. Broaden the qi sensation by moving qi.

5. Refine the effects of the treatment using techniques for tonifying and draining.

6. Retain the needles.

7. Remove the needles.

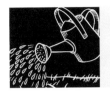

POINT PAIRS
(配穴 *pèi xué*)

THE TERM 'POINT PAIRS' refers to two points often used together in an acupuncture treatment. Each pair can be thought of as having a specific effect on qi transformation which, when properly chosen, helps to transform a pathodynamic in a way that might be likened to turning a key in a lock. Point pairs should not be thought of in the context of treating a particular symptom or even disease, but should always be considered in the context of their effects on the physiological system as a whole. This is a very important point. When considering the information below, the practitioner should always keep in mind that these pairs are understood as having specific effects on the qi transformation of the channel system. They are not used to 'treat headache' or even for basic TCM functions such as 'resolving dampness'. Each pair has a specific effect on the qi transformation of one or more of the six channels, as described in earlier chapters.

Incidentally, the term 'qi transformation' (氣化 *qì huà*) is a concept fundamental to a clear understanding of classical physiology.[1] Although there is some risk in using the English term 'physiology' in this context, as it implies an understanding borrowed from modern science, it does provide a helpful starting point. Qi transformation is both the movement within and the functions of the channel and organ systems. It is therefore the primary functional principle of classical Chinese physiology. Acupuncture and herbal therapies can always be thought of as having one effect or another on qi transformation and therefore 'physiology' insofar as it is understood in Chinese medicine. When using the point pairs described below, keep the channels and their physiological functions in mind.

Many of the point pairs discussed below can be found in classical texts. The particular understanding of those pairs is largely drawn from the clinical experience of Dr. Wang. The inclusion of a pair in the following pages implies that it has been used extensively by him.

Benefits of Using Points in Pairs

There are three reasons why thinking of points in pairs can help clinical results:

1. Concise formulation

In acupuncture therapy, the best treatments are often those which do not use too many needles. Point pairs help reduce the number of needles in a given treatment, as the pair alone might be an acceptable prescription. For many patients, a treatment will consist of the point pair needled bilaterally (four needles). Although one or two other points may be added, the pair serves as the primary manifestation of the treatment principle.

2. Clear understanding of the distinct effects of the points used

This use of point pairs facilitates a clear understanding of the effects a particular treatment will have on qi transformation. This helps the practitioner to clearly understand why a particular treatment is (or is not) effective. Effective treatments can then be more easily replicated while ineffective treatments can be more easily modified.

3. Synergy

By using points with complementary and coordinated effects, better results can be achieved. This differs from the more common approach to point selection in which various points are chosen based on their individual 'functions'. In the case of point pairs, the pair itself has an effect that is greater than the sum of its parts.

Types of Point Pairs

Point pairs on the same-name channel

Pairs of this type involve combining points from the upper and lower aspects of one of the six main channels. For example, a *tài yīn* point pair would include a point from the lung *tài yīn* channel and the spleen *tài yīn* channel.

Internal-external point pairs

Pairs of this type involve the selection of points on channels associated with organs traditionally considered to have an internal-external (yin-yang) relationship. An example would be a pair involving points on the lung *tài yīn* with points on the large intestine *yáng míng* channel.

Mother-child point pairs

This involves points chosen from channels having a mother-child relationship in five-phase theory. In the case of the following point pairs, the approach utilizes the generative (生 *shēng)* cycle of wood-fire-earth-metal-water. For example, a pair may include points from the kidney *shào yīn* and liver *jué yīn* channels, as water generates wood in five-phase theory. This may or may not involve a further consideration of the five-phase association of the particular points along each channel (five-transport point theory).

Eight extraordinary vessel point pairs

These are combined points chosen from among the eight extraordinary vessel command points. Combinations are not limited to those traditionally paired (such as SP-4 *[gōng sūn]* and PC-6 *[nèi guān]*) and may actually involve the combined use of the extraordinary vessels with other channels.

Experiential point pairs

Some point pairs are difficult to categorize but nonetheless have proven to be very effective in the clinic. There are only a few of these and, because they defy traditional classification, they are more difficult to analyze physiologically.

One important broad concept should be outlined regarding point pair selection and the evolution of disease conditions in the Chinese model. One way to think about the ways in which a given pathodynamic might change involves considering how the condition evolves according to five-phase theory. Experience has shown that conditions which are primarily acute or in the channels themselves tend to move along the same channel lines, internal-external paired channel lines (同名/表裡關係 *tóng míng/biāo lǐ guān xi),* or in the circular generating cycle. On the other hand, more chronic conditions that involve internal organ dysfunction tend to move and be treated with considerations of mutual control five-phase channel/organ relationships (相生/相克 *xiāng shēng/xiāng kè).* This is a fairly large concept that should be considered over and over when trying to get a grip on the nature of complex conditions where the pathodynamic seems to involve more than one of the six main channels (Fig. 20.1).

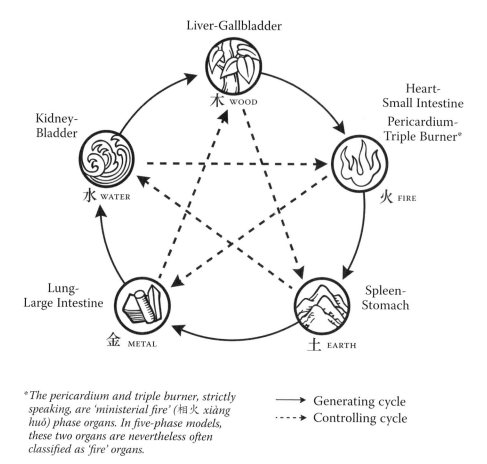

*The pericardium and triple burner, strictly speaking, are 'ministerial fire' (相火 xiàng huǒ) phase organs. In five-phase models, these two organs are nevertheless often classified as 'fire' organs.

⟶ Generating cycle
----➤ Controlling cycle

Fig. 20.1

In more acute and less serious conditions, disease often moves in the circular generating cycle, while more serious or chronic conditions tend to affect other organs through the controlling cycle.

Point Pairs

PAIRS FOR TREATING DYSFUNCTION OF *Jué yīn-shào yáng*

LR-5 *(lǐ gōu)* and PC-6 *(nèi guān)*

This same-name channel pair has the function of dredging and unblocking the *jué yīn* channels and collaterals (疏通厥陰經絡 *shū tōng jué yīn jīng luò)*. This action is likened to shaking out a fold in a piece of cloth or stretching out a string that has become twisted or wrapped upon itself. Clinically, this pathodynamic often includes irregular menses associated with qi stagnation, including symptoms involving a generalized lack of motivation. In this case, there is a lack of movement in *jué yīn* but little heat. This collateral point pair unblocks the *jué yīn* collaterals and stimulates circulation down to the smallest levels along the *jué yīn* pathway.

PC-7 (*dà líng*) and LR-2 (*xíng jiān*)

This same-name channel pair clears and transforms in the *jué yīn* (清化 厥陰 *qīng huà jué yīn*). This pair, which has a stronger heat-clearing function than the LR-5 and PC-6 pair above, is used to clear heat and transform stagnant qi and/or blood. Specifically, this often involves qi constraint in the liver and blood stagnation in the pericardium. The effect of this pair can be likened to relaxing and expanding the channel so that stagnation and heat can move smoothly out of the channel and organs.

In five-phase acupuncture styles, the PC-7 and LR-2 pair is the classic pair for using child points to drain the mother channel: PC-7 is the earth point on a fire channel while LR-2 is the fire point on a wood channel.

In menstrual regulation, this point pair is better for irregular menses and PMS associated with irritability, restlessness, and other heat signs. In cases where the patient has been affected by external wind evils that have been driven into the yin collaterals, this pair is also helpful because it can also extinguish wind to some degree by improving blood circulation. Uses for this pair include *jué yīn* heat-type patterns with such symptoms as insomnia, vascular headaches, menopause syndrome, irregular menstruation, and even attention deficit disorder (ADD) in children. In general, emotional conditions in relatively young patients due to excessive stress often cause stagnation that leads to heat in the *jué yīn*. This point pair can also be appropriate in those conditions.

TB-5 (*wài guān*) and GB-41 (*zú lín qì*)

This pair is both a *shào yáng* same-name channel and an extraordinary vessel pair. It is used to clear and drain *shào yáng* (清瀉少陽 *qīng xiè shào yáng*). Specifically, this refers to the ability of the pair to clear and drain excess heat from the channel. In this case, counterflow of liver/gallbladder fire has led to wind-fire rising upward with such symptoms as vomiting, headaches, red eyes, nasal congestion, ear ringing, tooth pain and/or a sense of tightness in the throat. In the clinic this pair is often used for conditions such as tinnitus, conjunctivitis, dry-itchy eyes, dizziness, or high blood pressure due to heat rising. TB-5 is the command point of the *yáng wéi* extraordinary vessel while GB-41 is the command point of the *dài* vessel. The pair can therefore not only clear heat from the head but the lower body as well *(dài* vessel conditions). Finally, this pair is also often used for pain that occurs along the path of the *shào yáng* channel.

TB-6 *(zhī gōu)* and GB-34 *(yáng líng quán)*

This same-name channel pair is used to dredge and drain the *shào yáng* (疏瀉少陽 *shū xiè shào yáng).* In this case, the *shào yáng* function of dredging and draining at the pivot of the three yang channels has been compromised. The effects of this pair tend to strongly move *shào yáng* stagnation but have less of a heat-clearing effect than the previous pair (TB-5 and GB-41). The pair is useful for constipation or abdominal distention, intercostal pain, sciatic nerve pain, some types of shingles, premenstrual syndrome involving breast tenderness/irritability, and dysmenorrhea. In all of these cases, there should be an underlying pathodynamic of compromised movement in the *shào yáng* due to stagnation. Coursing and draining the *shào yáng* pivot can also have an effect of releasing upward toward *tài yáng* above. This means that this pair can sometimes be used in the case of excess *external* (not *shào yáng* channel type) heat that is threatening to drop into *shào yáng.* The defining symptom that might indicate the appropriateness of this pair would be abdominal, hypochondriac, or intercostal pain and/or tightness in conjunction with an external pattern.

The previous four pairs have similar but distinct functions. There are two pairs on the *jué yīn* channel and two pairs on the *shào yáng* channel. On both the yin and yang channels, one pair is more useful for clearing heat while the other is more helpful for moving stagnation. In the case of the *jué yīn* channel, the LR-5 and PC-6 pair is more moving while the LR-2 and PC-7 pair is more useful for clearing heat. Similarly, on the *shào yáng* channel, the pair TB-6 and GB-34 is more moving while the pair TB-5 and GB-41 is more helpful for clearing heat.

Of course, the *jué yīn* and *shào yáng* channels have a yin-yang relationship as well. It is helpful to remember that pairs on yin channels will always have a slight tonifying effect while those on yang channels are generally more draining. Yin channels tend to deficiency while yang channels tend to excess. In addition, yin channel heat tends to transfer to the yang channels. In this light, compare the clinical application of the LR-2 and PC-7 pair with that of the TB-5 and GB-41 pair. A person with signs of heat in the *jué yīn-shào yáng* channels can be compared to a tree dried and browned in the summer sun. Use of the yang channel pair can be thought of as quickly clearing out the heat, much like dousing a tree with cool water. Use of the yin channel pair is more like watering the roots so that the tree can be cooled from the inside out. Both can be appropriate treatment methods for excess heat in different situations. The relative excess and deficiency of the patient should be considered (Fig. 20.2).

The LR-2 and PC-7 pair and the TB-5 and GB-41 pair can be thought of as two ends of a spectrum of *jué yīn-shào yáng* treatment. In one case, heat is cleared off the top (TB-5 and GB-41) while in the other, the yin channel is relaxed so that qi and blood stagnation can be cleared and transformed, thus reestablishing the normal nourishing function. In both cases, the net result is the removal of heat.

Next, in the case of stagnation without heat, one can compare the PC-6 and LR-5 pair with the TB-6 and GB-34 pair. The functions of both pairs begin with the Chinese character 疏 *(shū)*, meaning 'to dredge' (strongly open circulation, like dredging a ditch). Their effects are to open their respective channels in a way that Dr. Wang likens to shaking wrinkles out of fabric. The yang pair also has a slight draining effect, while the yin pair dredges and opens, but also has a regulating effect on liver and pericardium function. The yang pair has a strong clearing function that might be too much for some patients.

One final consideration for these four pairs should be mentioned. If a patient presents with a clear case of both heat and stagnation involving *shào yáng*, a helpful approach would be to use the TB-5 and GB-41 pair until heat symptoms recede, followed in later treatments with the more moving TB-6 and GB-34 pair. If the heat and stasis involve both the *shào yáng* and *jué yīn*, one might first clear the yang channel, followed later by clearing the yin channel.

PAIRS FOR TREATING PATTERNS THAT INVOLVE DIGESTIVE COMPLAINTS

PC-7 (*dà líng*) and LU-5 (*chǐ zé*)

This pair is used to clear and drain static heat (清瀉瘀熱 *qīng xiè yū rè*) from the pericardium, lung, and stomach. The pair is a variant on the mother-child pair concept. PC-7 is the source point of the pericardium *jué yīn* channel and, among the five transport points, is associated with earth. Its ability to clear and drain static heat from the pericardium can be under-

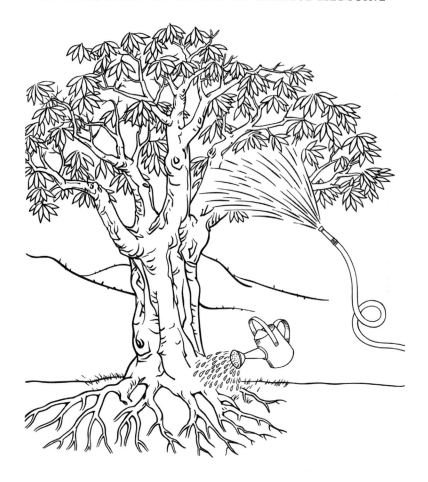

Fig. 20.2
The LR-2 and PC-7 point pair cools *jué yīn* / *shào yáng* by loosening and opening
deep blood circulation and might be likened to watering the roots of a tree.
In contrast, the TB-5 and GB-41 pair cools the same system by releasing heat
upward and outward, like hosing off the leaves.

stood as an earth point draining a fire channel. The very clear tendency of
PC-7 to clear heat makes it a bit of an anomaly among the source points of
the yin channels. LU-5 is the uniting, water point of the lung *tài yīn* channel
(a metal channel) and has a similar mother-child five-phase sedating effect.
One of the effects on qi transformation that comes from stimulating LU-5
involves the clearing of heat and moistening of the lungs. Together, these
points reinforce and broaden each other's heat-clearing effects so as to drain
fire from the upper burner. Symptoms of the pattern for which this pair
would be appropriate include dry throat, mouth, and nose; loss of voice;

chest pain with a bitter taste in the mouth; red tongue; sores in the mouth or nose; constipation; and/or dark urine and cough with purulent phlegm.

As noted above, this pair is also used to clear heat from the stomach. This is not the same as what is normally thought of as 'stomach heat'. In this case, the pair is still clearing static (i.e., trapped) heat from the upper burner (lung and pericardium). This type of heat can often descend to the stomach causing nausea and/or vomiting. Again, this is most commonly seen in situations where an invasion of external heat has become trapped in the upper burner.

PC-6 (*nèi guān*) and SP-4 (*gōng sūn*)

This pair alleviates pain and regulates qi (止痛理氣 *zhǐ tòng lǐ qì*). A careful analysis of exactly how these effects are achieved provides an interesting window into physiology. The pair is best understood as an extraordinary vessel pair but can also be understood by considering the qi transformation relationship of the pericardium and spleen organs.

First, consider the extraordinary vessel relationship. PC-6 is the command point of the *yīn wéi* vessel. The *yīn wéi* links and inter-regulates the yin channels (維系調理陰經 *wéi xì tiáo lǐ yīn jīng*). In some ways, it may be likened to the parasympathetic nervous system in that it is responsible for nourishing the internal organs. SP-4 is the command point of the *chōng* vessel. The *chōng* vessel, the 'sea of blood', is also associated with the nourishment of the internal organs. Classical texts point out that the *chōng* vessel flows upward along the middle of the abdomen. Many modern texts have speculated about the association of the *chōng* vessel with the pulsing felt as the abdominal aorta descends through the abdomen. In any case, it is clinically helpful to think of bringing the *chōng* vessel into treatment in cases where blood needs to be brought toward the internal organs.

At the same time, consideration of the relationship between the qi transformation of the pericardium *jué yīn* and spleen *tài yīn* channels and organs is also interesting. *Jué yīn* 'closes to the inside' and is regarded as being the most internal of the six main channels. It is the quiet center where yin and blood are stored. By contrast, *tài yīn* 'opens to the outside' and is the most external of the three yin channels. *Jué yīn* holds and nourishes blood at the deepest level of the body while *tài yīn* governs the blood. Most readers are familiar with the concept that the liver organ stores blood. The *tài yīn* spleen, on the other hand, through its association with fluids, can be thought of as being responsible for the maintenance of the nutritive quality of the interstitial fluids around the cells as well as the reabsorption of blood cells and other components into the blood at the capillary level. This is one aspect of what is meant when one says that *tài yīn* 'opens to the outside'. *Tài yīn* function is opening to the outside of the *internal* environment—the capillary intersections where blood is reabsorbed into the venous system. As described in Chapter 5, this is one way of understanding the association of the spleen with bruising.

Finally, both PC-6 and SP-4 are collateral points on their respective channels and thus have a particularly close relationship with the microcirculation and small vessel connections of their respective channels. That the collateral points affect small vessel circulation in areas associated with the channel suggest their use as command points for the eight extraordinary vessels. Recall from Chapter 11 that the extraordinary vessels are thought to be areas of influence just beyond the level of this collateral point microcirculation. In any case, collateral points have particularly broad effects on the circulation.

In conclusion, one can see from a variety of angles how the PC-6 and SP-4 pair has an effect on the appropriate distribution of healthy blood to the organs. This opens a window for understanding how this point pair can alleviate pain and regulate qi. The pathodynamic for which the pair is designed involves pain and qi disorders that are caused by a lack of adequate, healthy blood—a condition often associated with blood stasis. This condition often involves the heart, stomach, and intestinal tract with symptoms such as atrophy of the stomach, palpitations, and gastrointestinal disorders. The concept of 'regulating qi' suggests the ability of this pair to treat emotional conditions such as irritability, stifling sensation in the chest, or even a combined focal distention and stifling sensation in both the abdomen and chest (胸腹痞悶 *xiōng fù pǐ mèn*).

PC-6 (*nèi guān*) and ST-44 (*nèi tíng*)

This pair is used to stop vomiting and reverse upward counterflow (止嘔 降逆 *zhǐ ǒu jiàng nì*). The *yīn wéi* vessel command point PC-6 is combined with the spring point of the stomach channel to facilitate the clearing of acute *yáng míng* heat that has led to counterflow. Together, the pair acts to regulate the qi and direct counterflow downward. This is a case where peristaltic rhythm has been compromised. Relevant presentations may include acute vomiting and diarrhea or even acute colitis. The pair is also often used in cases where there is an acute invasion of summerheat leading to severe nausea and vomiting and an inability to keep down either food or liquids. The hands and feet of the patient will often be cold due to counterflow qi. This pair is useful in cases where children affected by summerheat are unable to eat or take any medication. Experience has shown in many cases that this pair can help to stabilize the stomach so that medication and fluids can be kept down.

LI-4 *(hé gǔ)* and ST-43 *(xiàn gǔ)*

This pair is similar in application to the previous pair, but is more appropriate in cases of stomach deficiency leading to nausea.[2] Symptoms may be similar to those for which the PC-6 and ST-44 pair was indicated—belching, distention, and sounds in the intestines—but there will be a history indicating more chronic stomach qi deficiency. The primary difference in the condition is the absence of vomiting (counterflow).

CV-11 *(jiàn lǐ)* and ST-36 *(zú sān lǐ)*

This is an experiential pair (often seen in classical texts) with synergistic effects. The pair has the function of warming and strengthening the spleen and stomach (溫健脾胃 *wēn jiàn pí wèi*). It is helpful in situations where spleen-stomach deficiency has led to abdominal pain, diarrhea, low appetite, spontaneous sweating, and/or fatigue. CV-11 strengthens the middle, raises the yang, and reverses counterflow, while ST-36 has its familiar tonifying effects. Together, the pair can reestablish proper qi transformation (CV-11) while tonifying (ST-36). Often, LI-10 *(shǒu sān lǐ)* is combined with this pair in a trio that is known as the 'three *lǐ*' treatment. Finally, the CV-11 and ST-36 pair is often combined with CV-12 in cases where a slight draining effect is desired to facilitate the clearing of food stasis, dampness, and/or phlegm.

CV-12 *(zhōng wǎn)* and ST-36 *(zú sān lǐ)*

This experiential pair is used to regulate the spleen and stomach (調理脾胃 *tiáo lǐ pí wèi*). It has less of a tonifying action than the previous pair, and may even be used in treating excess conditions where qi transformation is not moving properly.

CV-12 *(zhōng wǎn)* and ST-40 *(fēng lóng)*

This is an experiential pair that is used very often in conjunction with other points. The pair is used to transform phlegm and benefit the spleen (化痰健脾 *huà tán jiàn pí*). It is used when damp pathogens block the middle burner and cause abdominal distention, stifling sensation in the chest, vomiting, diarrhea, cough, and/or fatigue. In the clinic, the pair is combined with other points to strengthen the spleen, disperse wind, or benefit the qi depending on differential diagnosis. Recall that CV-12 is a point where the small intestine, triple burner, and stomach channels meet with the *rèn* vessel, thus expanding its effects.

All of the seven pairs in this group are used for conditions that involve digestive disorders to some degree. The first, PC-7 and LU-5, is used for static heat in the upper burner due to an external invasion which has dropped downward to the stomach, causing nausea and vomiting. The pair is also sometimes used for other types of external invasion which have become trapped in the *yáng míng/jué yīn* channels. The second pair, PC-6 and SP-4, is used when the supply of healthy blood to the organs is insufficient and has led to pain, discomfort, or dysfunction. The third pair, PC-6 and ST-44, is used when counterflow and/or summerheat has led to nausea and vomiting. The fourth pair, LI-4 and ST-43, is appropriate for nausea due to stomach qi deficiency. By contrast, CV-11 and ST-36 are used to warm and fortify the spleen and stomach in classic cases of middle burner qi deficiency. The sixth pair, CV-12 and ST-36, has a more regulating effect than the preceding pair in cases of problems with middle burner qi transformation that can involve stasis. The final pair, CV-12 and ST-40, is used to transform phlegm and benefit the spleen in cases where dampness and phlegm predominate. When deciding whether to include CV-11 or CV-12 in any of the above treatments, it is always helpful to palpate the abdomen and look for any noticeable changes along the *rèn* vessel pathway (Table 20.1).

THREE *Yáng míng* PAIRS WITH BROAD CLINICAL APPLICATION

ST-36 (*zú sān lǐ*) and LI-11 (*qū chí*)

This same-name channel combination can also be used for digestive conditions, but it has broader applications. When used for digestive disorders, the pair regulates and strengthens *yáng míng* function in cases where there is insufficient absorption of nutrition from food.

The pair is also commonly used to reestablish proper qi transformation in the *yáng míng* channel in the case of 'channel exhaustion', which may occur due to long-term, unsuccessful treatment which causes the whole channel to become unresponsive. For example, this sea-point pair is used clinically in *yáng míng* facial paralysis that hasn't responded to long-term treatment. It may also be considered for chronic pain that is affecting the pathway of the *yáng míng* channel including, of course, local knee and elbow pain, but also pain in the shoulders and throughout the legs.

Point Pair	Effect on Qi Transformation	Common Pathodynamic
PC-7 *(dà líng)* & LU-5 *(chǐ zé)*	Clears and drains static heat	Heat (often external) trapped in the upper and middle burners
PC-6 *(nèi guān)* & SP-4 *(gōng sūn)*	Regulates qi and circulates blood	Improper blood circulation to internal organs, causing pain and dysfunction
PC-6 *(nèi guān)* & ST-44 *(nèi tíng)*	Causes counterflow to descend	Vomiting due to acute counterflow; often caused by external invasion
LI-4 *(hé gǔ)* & ST-43 *(xiàn gǔ)*	Regulates qi	Nausea combined with chronic stomach deficiency
CV-11 *(jiàn lǐ)* & ST-36 *(zú sān lǐ)*	Warm/strengthens the spleen-stomach	Spleen-stomach deficiency
CV-12 *(zhōng wǎn)* & ST-36 *(zú sān lǐ)*	Regulates the spleen-stomach	Compromised or irregular middle burner qi transformation
CV-12 *(zhōng wǎn)* & ST-40 *(fēng lóng)*	Transforms phlegm and benefits the spleen	Condition of excess involving phlegm/dampness in the middle burner

Table 20.1
Commonly used point pairs for gastrointestinal disorders

LI-1 *(shāng yáng)* and ST-45 *(lì duì)*

This same-name channel pair is used to clear and drain the *yáng míng* channel (清瀉陽明經 *qīng xìe yáng míng jīng*). Fire-toxin stagnation in the *yáng míng* channel can lead to symptoms such as toothache, hemorrhoids, or sleep disorders characterized by restlessness and sweating. These points may also be bled in the case of painful eczema due to excessive heat trapped in the blood, or for teeth grinding at night due to stomach fire.

LI-4 *(hé gǔ)* and LR-3 *(tài chōng)*

Much has been said about this popular 'four gates' (四關 *sì guān*) pair. It is helpful first to consider the name 'four gates' and what it implies. The four gates are the gates of qi on the *yáng míng* channel and the gates of blood on the *jué yīn* channel. This pair moves both qi and blood, and, although both are source points on their respective channels, they are not used for toni-fication. Instead, the benefit of using source points in this case is derived from their ability to move qi and blood throughout the body due to the association of source points with the triple burner. The *yáng míng* channel is said to have 'more qi and more blood' while the *jué yīn* channel is said to have 'less qi and more blood'.[3] By combining the source points of both channels, a synergistic and wide-ranging effect on blood circulation can be achieved. Also remember that the *yáng míng* channel is the most internal of the three yang channels, while the *jué yīn* channel is the most internal of the three yin channels. They are both said to 'close to the inside'. This tendency of the channels facilitates the ability of the *yáng míng* and *jué yīn* source points to affect qi transformation so deeply. There are four primary functions of this pair:

1. Scatters external wind (散外風 *sàn wài fēng*)

By systemically moving qi and blood, the pair can direct wind out of the body. This is most helpful in the case of an external excess condition where there may be some fever but no significant sweating. The pair does not, however, clear heat and therefore the addition of GV-14 *(dà zhuī)* is often helpful. This aspect of the four gates explains its use in cases of recent wind invasion into the joints, which causes pain.

2. Extinguishes internal wind (熄內風 *xī nèi fēng*)

This is due to the ability of the combined pair to both open the gate of blood at the *jué yīn* level and also to move blood throughout the body by opening the gate of qi. Areas of the body that have been experiencing blood deficiency leading to twitching, spasms, or other wind signs may thereby be nourished and pacified. SP-6 *(sān yīn jiāo)* is often added in these cases. Acute epilepsy might also fall under this category.

3. Tracks wind in the hundred joints (搜一身百節之風 *sōu yī shēn bǎi jié zhī fēng*)

This is a less appreciated application of the four gates. When a patient has symptoms of pain moving from one area of the body to another in the course of treatment, the condition is said to have a wind-like nature. In this case, the pair can track and stabilize wind. Chronic arthritic conditions which come and go (sometimes affecting one joint, then later affecting an-other) may be of this type.

4. Regulates the channels and collaterals (調和經絡 *tiáo hé jīng luò*)

For this application, the pair is used in situations where a patient is not responding normally to acupuncture treatment. These might be conditions that have defied treatment by other practitioners. Often, repeated unsuccessful treatment can lead to 'channel exhaustion' or 'channel confusion', in which the channel system is like a violin out of tune. In these cases, the four gates can be helpful to reset the patient's channel qi transformation. For this purpose, the four gates are often combined with SP-6 *(sān yīn jiāo)*. The uniting points on affected channels can also be used in a similar way (in particular, the qi/blood abundant *yáng míng* channel uniting points, LI-11 and ST-36, described above). After one or two treatments using only these regulating points, normal point selection can resume, often with much better results.

Stimulation of the four-gate points should be with 1-inch needles using a gentle insertion followed by a strong arrival of qi. The more distant the sensation radiates, the better the effect.

> Because the *yáng míng* channel contains an abundance of qi and blood, stimulating the channel can have broad systemic effects. In the case of the first pair (ST-36 and LI-11), besides helping to reestablish proper absorption, this can also invigorate the *yáng míng* when the channels are exhausted due to a chronic condition. Often, patients who have had a stroke exhibit this type of channel deficiency, which causes them to be less responsive to acupuncture treatment. The second pair (LI-1 and ST-45) uses the abundance of qi and blood in *yáng míng* to help clear systemic heat to benefit a wide variety of conditions involving excess heat affecting the upper body. The third pair (LI-4 and LR-3), while not strictly a *yáng míng* pair, also has a broad systemic effect derived from its ability to dredge the pathways of qi and blood throughout the body.

Pairs for treating *Tài yīn*

LU-5 *(chǐ zé)* and SP-9 *(yīn líng quán)*

This is both a mother-child and a same-name channel pair. Its effects are to reverse counterflow and to raise clear qi (降逆升清 *jiàng nì shēng qīng*). Its functions are best understood by thinking of these as paired uniting points on a same-name channel. The points are broadly used in the presence of a wide variety of counterflow qi affecting *tài yīn* (recall that all uniting points treat counterflow qi). Together, they also have a strong ability to facilitate the transformation of dampness by stimulating the movement of qi. Note that their functions derive from their ability to regulate *tài yīn* qi transformation—which is not the same as tonification. When this pair is applied, there is a regulation of the ascending/descending (升降 *shēng/jiàng*) movement within the lung and a stimulation of the movement of clear qi upward from the spleen.

The net result of this resetting of qi transformation in *tài yīn* has systemic benefits that exceed the parameters of just the lung and spleen. Because the lung 'commands the whole body's qi' (主一身之氣 *zhǔ yī shēn zhī qì*), this pair can also be used as a general qi regulator. Counterflow qi in the *tài yīn* can lead to a wide variety of conditions including high blood pressure, chest fullness, asthma, cough, abdominal distention (due to damp accumulation), edema, constipation (spleen-type over assimilation of fluids), damp accumulation skin problems (including eczema), leucorrhea, and a variety of digestive disorders due to qi stagnation or dampness. This pair is used by Dr. Wang very often in treating a wide variety of cases.

LU-9 *(tài yuān)* and SP-3 *(tài bái)*

This is also a same-name channel pair. LU-9 is the source point of the lung and also the earth point of the channel. Likewise, SP-3 is both a source and an earth point for the spleen. This pair has the effect of tonifying the *tài yīn* qi by warming and strengthening the lung and spleen (溫健肺脾 *wēn jiàn fèi pí*). It should again be recalled that the source points of all channels are thought to have a particular affinity for the warming and tonifying qi that comes from the triple burner. This pair can be used for qi deficiency in either the lung or the spleen (or both). The appropriate pathodynamic might include symptoms such as lowered lung capacity, shortness of breath, asthma, chest tightness, cough, diarrhea, abdominal distention, abnormal uterine bleeding (light spotting between periods—漏 *lòu*), or sudden facial edema (due to head wind 頭風 *tóu fēng*). The pair can also be used to treat incontinence, especially when the problem is more pronounced during the day. In the case of daytime incontinence, the lung function of raising qi is often compromised, which affects the ability of the bladder qi to properly hold (lift up) the urine. Note that HT-7 *(shén mén)* is often added to treatments where nighttime incontinence is more predominant—this includes bedwetting.

Manipulation at LU-9 should be gentle and tonifying, with a light twirling motion and no lifting and thrusting. Many practitioners will use the pressing hand to gently move the radial artery out of the way here. However, this is not wise, as it generally results in an insertion that misses the true point. Instead, insertion should be gentle and slow so as to slip to the radial side of the artery. Sensation should include a gentle radiating sensation down to the thumb. Technique at SP-3 *(tài bái)* should be similarly gentle and tonifying.

LU-8 *(jīng qú)* and SP-2 *(dà dū)*

This is also a *tài yīn* same-name channel pair. It is an interesting pair for releasing exterior conditions when there is significant underlying deficiency. This pattern is similar to the one for which Cinnamon Twig Decoction *(guì zhī tāng)* is indicated in the *Discussion of Cold Damage* (傷寒論 *Shāng hán lùn)*. The effects of these two points can be considered in the light of the functions of that formula. LU-8, the river point, moves qi circulation to open the lung. SP-2 is the fire point on an earth channel and thus has a mother-child warming/tonifying effect. SP-2 is also the spring point on the channel and clears heat from deficiency. Together, the pair opens the exterior through the lung while warming the interior by tonifying the spleen. The net effect is a release of the exterior facilitated by an outward movement of fluids from *tài yīn* that can bring about gentle sweating. Again analogous to the Cinnamon Twig Decoction pattern is the presence here of an exterior condition that the body is unable to release through sweating. One difference is that the condition could have originally been due to either cold or heat. Sensation at LU-8, like that at LU-9, should involve a gentle radiating sensation down to the thumb. Without significant sensation, the effectiveness of this treatment will be less.

All three of the previous pairs are on the *tài yīn* channel. The LU-9 and SP-3 pair is used to tonify and warm in cases of deficiency, while LU-5 and SP-9 regulate and reestablish normal qi transformation in the *tài yīn*. A condition such as damp accumulation involving the spleen might be approached with either of these pairs. Careful differentiation of excess and deficiency is paramount. If there is concurrent excess and deficiency, a helpful approach would be to first regulate qi transformation to remove damp stagnation (LU-5 and SP-9) followed by strengthening the *tài yīn* organ function (LU-9 and SP-3). Again, the general clinical goal is to first clear excess before beginning tonification. Finally, the LU-8 and SP-2 pair has a more specific application, with the goal of reestablishing the healthy diffusion of lung qi when it is blocked by an exterior condition.

Three lung-kidney pairs

LU-7 (liè quē) and KI-6 (zhào hǎi)

This extraordinary vessel pair is often used clinically for problems affecting the throat (especially sore throat). Both the *rèn* vessel (LU-7) and the *yīn qiáo* vessel (KI-6) travel through the throat. The *yīn qiáo* vessel is often involved in problems where a lack of nourishment to the throat has led to dysfunction or pain. The *rèn* vessel provides 'sea of yin' nourishment while the lung is an organ involved in the metabolism (and provision of) fluids. Together, the pair powerfully affects and nourishes the fluids of the throat and upper respiratory tract. Interestingly, this pair is also often effective for problems with urination including painful urination and some types of lung-kidney type edema. When trying to understand these functions, one should think more about the relationship between the lung and kidney organs in the metabolism of fluids.

LU-5 (chǐ zé) and KI-6 (zhào hǎi)

This is a mother-child channel pair. It is often used in acute conditions (both externally- and internally-generated) where the lung is not receiving enough fluids, often due to an accumulation of heat. Common symptom patterns involve loss of voice following an external wind-heat, wind-dry pattern, or extreme fatigue. Remember that KI-6 is also the command point of the *yīn qiáo* vessel. The *yīn qiáo*, besides the more commonly described function of regulating the muscles of the inner leg, is also responsible for coordinating the muscle movements in and around groups of internal organs (including the vocal chords). Where there is loss of voice, have the patient talk while stimulating KI-6.

LU-5 (chǐ zé) and KI-7 (fù liū)

This is a mother-child channel pair. LU-5 is the uniting point of the lung channel and is helpful for regulating the ascending/descending movement of the lung. KI-7 is the mother (metal) point on the kidney *shào yīn* (water) channel, and, as a tonification point, is most helpful for nourishing yin. As might be expected, the pair is often used to foster the yin and regulate the lung (育陰調肺 *yù yīn tiáo fèi*). It is used for chronic issues due to lung dysfunction with associated lack of kidney nourishment. Clinically, this pair is often appropriate for patients with chronic allergies and asthma. It has proven particularly effective in treating chronic seasonal allergies, especially those that have been treated with steroid inhalers and other pharmaceuticals that may have damaged the kidney yin. The pair is also helpful for chronic scratchiness of the voice.

Note that both the LU-5 and KI-6 and the LU-5 and KI-7 pairs treat problems with the throat and voice. The important difference is that LU-5 and KI-6 treat acute problems (often due to heat) while LU-5 and KI-7 are used in more chronic conditions with underlying kidney deficiency. In the first instance, the *yīn qiáo* is able to relax and nourish the muscles around the throat, while in the second, there is a stronger, generalized yin-tonifying effect that acts more broadly. The first pair in this group (LU-7 and KI-6) is also a classic point pair used to benefit the throat for both interior and exterior type patterns due to either deficiency or excess. In general, the LU-7 and KI-6 pair is used in cases where throat pain is more severe.

Shào yīn PAIRS TO BENEFIT THE YIN AND BLOOD

KI-7 *(fù liū)* and LR-2 *(xíng jiān)*

This is another mother-child pair. Here the mother (kidney) is used to regulate the child (liver). This pair is especially helpful for cases of kidney yin deficiency with concurrent liver yang counterflow leading to symptoms such as dizziness, tinnitus, red face, dry mouth, and red tongue. These symptoms often arise in cases of high blood pressure (deficiency type) and diabetic conditions. Dr. Wang uses this pair more often than the KI-3 *(tài xī)* and LR-3 *(tài chōng)* pair (which follows) when there is obvious liver excess.

KI-3 *(tài xī)* and LR-3 *(tài chōng)*

This is another mother-child pair and, in contrast to the previous one, is a case where the mother (kidney) benefits from regulation of the child (liver). It is similar to the KI-7 and LR-2 pair, but tends to be used when the symptom pattern is more one of kidney deficiency than liver excess. The pair is used to secure the source (固原 *gù yuán)*, calm the liver, and extinguish wind. Proper technique for this treatment principle involves a tonification technique at KI-3 and an even technique at LR-3. The pathodynamic involves noticeable kidney deficiency with possible concurrent ascendant liver yang. Symptoms would include high blood pressure, dizziness, insomnia, tinnitus, seminal emission, vomiting, and other conditions related to excess above and deficiency below. This pair also has a spirit-calming effect.

HT-7 (shén mén) and SP-6 (sān yīn jiāo)

This is another mother-child channel pair. Because HT-7 is the source point for the heart and SP-6 the meeting point of the three leg yin channels, the two points have a beneficial effect on the production and movement of blood. Together, they are used to tonify the heart and spleen, foster blood, and calm the spirit. The related pathodynamic is most often dual deficiency of heart and spleen leading to lack of blood nourishment to the heart. Associated symptoms may include palpitations caused by emotional stress from the environment (驚悸 jīng jì), and palpitations caused by internal disharmony which may, in turn, cause emotional instability (also known as 'panicky throbbing' 怔忡 zhēng chōng). Among the two types of palpitations, the second, zhēng chōng, is thought to involve more severe deficiency of the heart and spleen while the first is often more acute and less likely to be caused by severe internal disharmony. Both may be treated with the HT-7 and SP-6 pair as a core point prescription. Another associated pattern would be due to the spirit's inability to be calm in its abode (神不寧捨 shén bù níng shè), leading to insomnia combined with excessive dreaming when the patient is finally able to sleep. This pair often serves as a foundation for this pattern as well. Additional points and/or herbal prescriptions can be used to fine-tune the effects.

HT-5 (tōng lǐ) and KI-6 (zhào hǎi)

This is a same-name channel pair used to stimulate the shào yīn function of opening the yin collaterals. The pair is used to address problems in microcirculation of the brain and heart leading to cognition or speech difficulties. In the *Inner Classic*, deficiency of circulation in the heart collaterals is associated with speech problems.[4] Clinically, this might also include brain development. The pair is commonly used for developmental problems in children involving difficulties with cognition or speech. These two points are also especially effective for speech problems or esophageal insufficiency (choking easily) resulting from stroke. In the case of stroke, treatment should begin as soon as possible, as the benefit is considerably reduced after six months. 'Problems with speech' can also refer to dementia or the early stages of Alzheimer's. In these cases, the points can be beneficial at any stage during the progression of the disease.

HT-5 is the collateral point of the heart channel and helps to open collateral circulation not only in the heart and brain, but throughout the body. KI-6 is the command point of the yin qiáo. As noted above, the yin qiáo helps to harmonize the function of involuntary (smooth) muscle tissue in the body and also more internal muscles, such as the tongue or heart. This particular pair is helpful in cases where insufficiency of kidney water leads to rising heart fire with such symptoms as insomnia and irritability. The pair also quiets the spirit and calms the emotions (安神寧志 *ān shén níng zhì*). Thus it is also used clinically in some types of emotional conditions, especially in the elderly. For example, the pair is used in the treatment of elderly patients who have trouble controlling their emotions and find that they cry or laugh inappropriately. This should be contrasted with the more excess-type emotional conditions that often affect younger patients. In general, excess-type emotional conditions tend to affect the *jué yīn* channel (see PC-7 and LR-2 pair above) while deficiency-type often affect the *shào yīn*. Because of the wide variety of pathodynamics that can result from problems with the yin collaterals, this pair is used very broadly in the clinic.

HT-5 (*tōng lǐ*) and KI-4 (*dà zhōng*)

This is very similar to the HT-5 and KI-6 pair and likewise has an effect on the *shào yīn* collaterals. Here, both points are *shào yīn* collateral points and thus have a particularly strong effect on the collaterals along the pathway of the *shào yīn* channel itself. In other words, the effects of this pair aren't thought to have as broad an effect on brain microcirculation as the previous pair—there is no corresponding effect on the *yīn qiáo* in this case. When considering which pair to use, one must evaluate the symptom pattern at hand. If there are problems with cognition or speech, the pattern more likely involves the yin collaterals of the brain and heart. On the other hand, patterns along the *shào yīn* pathway are varied but can even include problems with hearing. Note that the name of KI-4 in Chinese (大鐘 *dà zhōng*) means 'great bell' and thus brings to mind its effect on the ears.

HT-6 (*yīn xī*) and KI-7 (*fù liū*)

Like the previous two combinations, this is also a *shào yīn* channel pair. HT-6, the cleft point on the heart channel, is used to move and benefit heart qi, especially in cases of deficiency. When combined with the mother point on the kidney channel (KI-7 is the metal point on a water channel), the effect is to use heart qi to facilitate restraint on the kidney yin. This pair is often used clinically in cases where children have organ imbalances that manifest as heart-kidney yin deficiency. In the case of children, actual yin deficiency is often not severe. The apparent symptoms of heart-kidney yin deficiency in children are actually more often caused by an *imbalance* in *shào yīn* qi transformation. Unlike older patients, the signs of yin deficiency can disappear rather quickly, especially if the balancing presence of heart qi can be facilitated. A common symptom pattern of this type is attention deficit disorder (ADD/ADHD).

Finally, it should be pointed out that the HT-6 and KI-7 pair is often effective for sweating due to heart qi deficiency. Many sources list KI-7 in a variety of patterns that involve abnormal sweating (either too much or too little).

The previous six pairs all affect the *shào yīn* qi dynamic and yin/blood metabolism. Both the KI-7 and LR-2 and the KI-3 and LR-3 pairs are used in patterns involving dual kidney and liver yin deficiency. The first pair is more often used to pacify the liver by benefiting kidney yin, while the second pair benefits the kidney by strengthening the liver. The difference is one of emphasis: KI-7 and LR-2 have more of a yin-tonifying effect while KI-3 and LR-3 have more of a moving effect that leads to kidney tonification. The third *shào yīn* pair—HT-7 and SP-6—also calms the spirit but has more of an effect on the generation of blood through the heart and spleen. The next two pairs have an effect on *shào yīn* collateral circulation. HT-5 and KI-6 affects microcirculation in the brain to benefit cognition, speech, and brain function in both the elderly and developing children. By contrast, the HT-5 and KI-4 pair is used to stimulate circulation in the collaterals along the pathway of the *shào yīn* channel, especially in the ears. The final *shào yīn* pair, HT-6 and KI-7, like the first two, is used to foster yin, but, in this case, has and effect on the pivotal relationship between the heart and kidney organs when they are 'not communicating'.

Pairs for treating *Tài yáng*

HT-6 *(yīn xī)* and SI-3 *(hòu xī)*

In contrast to the HT-6 and KI-7 pair described above, this pair is used in cases involving spontaneous sweating. Primarily it is used in cases where defensive qi is not rooted. Sweating disorders of this type might also include an inability to sweat. Here, there is a deficiency of yang qi at *tài yáng*. SI-3, a *tài yáng* point and also the command point of the *dū* vessel, helps to stimulate circulation of warming yang qi on the surface of the body. HT-6, the cleft point of the heart channel, regulates the heart qi to help stabilize sweating.

SI-3 *(hòu xī)* and BL-62 *(shēn mài)*

This is a classic extraordinary vessel pair. It is usually thought of in the clinic as a treatment for both chronic and acute lumbar pain. This is primarily due to the fact that SI-3, as noted above, is the command point of the *dū* vessel while BL-62 is the command point of the *yáng qiáo* vessel (associated with coordinated muscle functioning).

The pair can also be thought of as helping to open and regulate the kidney channel while clearing the heart and calming the spirit. With respect to these functions, one should note that both points are on the yang-paired channels of the heart and kidney *shào yīn*. Once again, one sees the familiar pattern of using yang channels to clear excess accumulation from its paired yin channel.

In addition to its traditional use in treating lumbar issues, this pair is also used to treat numbness in the extremities due to neurological problems (often associated with the *dū* vessel), hysterical paralysis (sudden paralysis/ muscle weakness due to emotional shock), epilepsy, mania, and pain patterns that tend to move around the body. The pair is often used clinically for epilepsy, spinal problems leading to neurological syndromes (numbness in the extremities), and problems with motor skills. It is also often used for developmental problems in children where the primary difficulty is with movement—unbalanced walking or inconsistent muscle tone. In these types of cases, GB-30 *(huán tiào)*, GB-34 *(yáng líng quán)*, and GB-39 *(xuán zhōng)*, the influential point for marrow, are often added to help improve difficulties with walking.

BL-63 *(jīn mén)* and SI-5 *(yáng gǔ)*

The combination of the cleft point of the bladder channel with the river point of the small intestine channel reduces acute pain along the vast pathway of *tài yáng*. Specifically, the pair is often a first-line treatment for patients who present with relatively acute low back pain. In these patients, the pain will often be more of an excess type (relatively sharp, worse in the morning, doesn't like too much pressure). Similarly, *tài yáng* channel neck pain also responds well to this pair, especially in cases where the cervical joints have some degeneration or displacement leading to fairly sharp, acute pain.

BL-64 *(jīng gǔ)* and SI-4 *(wàn gǔ)*

In contrast to the previous pair, the two source points of the *tài yáng* channel are used in cases of chronic, deficient-type back or *tài yáng* channel neck pain. When considering neck pain, it is important to clearly determine the channel which is most affected. Neck pain also affects the *shào yáng* and (to a lesser degree) the *yáng míng* channels. In cases of relatively severe deficiency, these points might even be treated with moxa.

Before comparing the *tài yáng* pairs with each other, another contrast should be highlighted, namely, that between the SI-3 and BL-62 pair and the HT-5 and KI-6 pair in the treatment of developmental problems in children. HT-5 and KI-6, as noted above, is most often used in cases where microcirculation in the brain may be involved. This would include problems with speech development, cognition, or certain types of problems where the brain itself seems to be developing too slowly. The SI-3 and BL-62 pair, on the other hand, is found on the corresponding yang channels and its use involves more distal (from the brain) considerations. This includes situations where problems are more focused on communication between the spine and the peripheral muscles. Of course, many cases are hard to differentiate and thus both pairs may seem appropriate. In this case, treatment can involve a short course with one pair followed by a short course (3 to 5 treatments) with the other. *Dū* vessel points are very often combined with either of these pairs.

Turning to the *tài yáng* channel pairs, the first (HT-6 and SI-3) pair is used in cases were there is a lack of warming defensive qi at the surface of the body, especially in cases where one of the primary symptoms involves spontaneous sweating. The next three *tài yáng* pairs are all used to treat pain along the pathway of the channel. SI-3 and BL-62 warm the surface and harmonize the muscles of multiple muscle channels along the yang areas of the body *(yáng qiáo* vessel function). BL-63 and SI-5 are often used as a lead point pair in cases of acute low-back and neck pain, while the BL-64 and SI-4 are used more in chronic, deficient pain patterns.

Rèn (CONCEPTION) VESSEL AND *Dū* (GOVERNING) VESSEL PAIRS

CV-6 *(qì hǎi)* and KI-2 *(rán gǔ)*

This is an experiential pair that opens and warms the collaterals of the lower burner in cases of yang deficiency. The pair can also tonify kidney qi. The associated pathodynamic is lower source (下原 *xià yuán)* insufficiency leading to coldness and/or pain in the lower abdomen. KI-2, the fire point on the kidney channel, can actually have either a cooling or a warming effect. In this case, symptoms of the pattern include urinary incontinence, impotence, leucorrhea, and cold/qi deficiency-type infertility. In the clinic, moxa is often used at CV-6 and a tonifying needling technique at KI-2.

CV-6 (*qì hǎi*) and KI-3 (*tài xī*)

This pair is also used to strengthen kidney deficiency. It is appropriate for generalized kidney deficiency and most often involves deficiency without clear signs of yin-yang deficiency or a combination of both.

> The previous two pairs are both used in the case of kidney deficiency. Dr. Wang notes that separating the two can often be problematic. When there is a predominance of cold stagnation, the CV-6 and KI-2 pair may be better. Of course, palpation of the kidney channel may also provide clues as to which points are more appropriate.

CV-21 (*xuán jī*) and CV-14 (*jù què*)

This pair diffuses and guides gathering qi (宣導宗氣 *xuān dǎo zōng qì*). Gathering qi (also known as ancestral qi) is the qi that converges and concentrates in the chest. Its health is reflected in normal, deep, and even breathing and a strong voice. This pair helps to reestablish healthy diffusion of the gathering qi when dysfunction has led to symptoms such as asthma, phlegm cough, pain/fullness/stuffiness in the chest, counterflow vomiting, or even epilepsy. The pair is also used clinically for spasms of the diaphragm, spasms of the cardiac sphincter of the stomach, or other neurological problems in the chest and diaphragm associated with gathering qi disharmony.

GV-26 (*rén zhōng*) and BL-40 (*wěi zhōng*)

This is a commonly cited pair used to dredge and open the *tài yáng* channel qi to control pain. The problem is due to either wrenching and contusion (閃挫 *shǎn cuò*) or wind-cold that has damaged the collaterals leading to stagnation in the *tài yáng* channel and lumbar stiffness and/or pain. Consequently, the pair is also commonly used for acute lumbar sprain. In these types of cases, Dr. Wang often uses GV-19 *(hòu dǐng)* with strong stimulation while the patient is seated before treatment begins on the table.

ALTERNATIVE EIGHT EXTRAORDINARY VESSEL POINT PAIRS

LU-7 (*liè quē*) and SP-4 (*gōng sūn*)

This *rèn* and *chōng* pairing can be effective for regulating menstruation when the length of the time between periods is irregular. For example, the patient may have a 15-day cycle one month followed by a 35-day cycle the next. It is less effective for treating menorrhagia, lack of menses, or painful menstruation.

PC-6 (nèi guān) and KI-6 (zhào hǎi)

This is *yīn wéi* paired with *yīn qiāo*. As noted in earlier chapters, the *yīn wéi* can be thought of as an overall regulator of metabolism for the internal organs and may roughly be likened to the function of parasympathetic nervous system. The *yīn qiāo*, on the other hand, is associated with the coordination of muscle movement on the inside of the body—the muscles of the internal organs. This pair is often used in neurological problems which affect the internal organs. Symptoms often include palpitations or other heart functional irregularities that defy modern cardiovascular diagnosis. Another type of neurological organ condition might be stomach pain or vomiting without discernible organic disorder, or discomfort in the throat without observable changes (including plum-pit qi).

TB-5 (wài guān) and BL-62 (shēn mài)

This is a pairing of the command points associated with the *yáng wéi* and *yáng qiāo* vessels. It is useful in the very specific instance of sudden paralysis (either partial or total) due to severe emotional/psychological strain. This is obviously not a condition that is encountered often, but two cases in 40 years justifies considering this approach (see the narrative following Chapter 11).

SI-3 (hòu xī) and LU-7 (liè quē)

The *rèn* and the *dū* vessels can be paired for another very specific condition that is not often seen. In this case, a difficult case led to the pairing. A patient, in the course of *qì gōng* practice, had developed a severe occipital headache which did not respond to other treatment. In discussing the case history with the patient, he reported that the headaches began after practicing a technique designed to circulate qi around the abdomen and back, known as the microcosmic orbit. The pathways of the *rèn* and *dū* vessels obviously came to mind, and this treatment was used. The results were very good and, in fact, for awhile many *qì gōng* practitioners who were so afflicted began to come for treatment. The results were most often quite good. One might also consider this pair for similar conditions that seem to involve a blockage of circulation around the *rèn-dū* axis (e.g., headaches, back pain, fixed low abdominal pain).

Conclusion

Having now explored a number of point pairs, the next step involves innovation. As one might imagine, the possible combinations of points and their effects on physiology are quite varied. When considering this information, it is important to imagine the effects on a living, dynamic system. Not only in this chapter, but throughout the text, what is described is a system that actually defies strict classification. As soon as something is defined or observed, it returns to its rightful place within the unnerving complexity of an actual human body.

The point pairs are but snapshots of practitioners and patients interacting in the face of disharmony. These pairs, and the acupuncture treatments they help define, are but points of brief interaction before the body returns to the business of self-regulation. The goal of treatment, then, is to intercede briefly, suggest a change, then step back to watch the dominos of qi dynamic drop in a spreading arc. The possibilities for point pairs are limited only by the ability of the practitioner to carefully consider the body as a dynamic system.

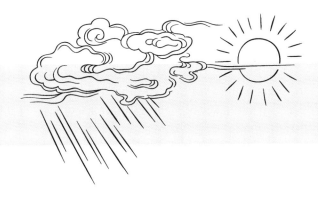

Postscript

The Greatest Walk in Beijing

B EIJING IS A city best seen on foot. Of course, other types of transportation abound. The ubiquitous cabs and buses are good for skipping over small distances, while the growing subway system covers long-distance treks. Bicycles, for the time being, continue to ply the far right-hand lane of the city's largest thoroughfares. Nevertheless, even bicycles don't allow for the ambling pace that best reveals this city of subtle contrasts. Theoretically at least, a bicycle would seem to be a perfect form of conveyance. Beijing is in fact much more amenable to bicycle travel than many of the other huge cities of Asia. However, those who have ridden in Beijing would probably agree that constant vigilance is still required to avoid being crushed by buses, cabs, cars, and other bicycles. On foot, one can slow down to the pace of the older residents of the city who walk down leafy avenues with hands clasped behind their backs. Moving at this pace, it is still possible to experience 'Old Beijing' even in the midst of the upheaval that characterizes so much of the modern city.

In writing this book, the goal has always been to provide context for the teachings of Dr. Wang. Various devices have been used to that end. The clinic where he works, the experiences of his life, the cadence of his thought, and even the shape of his home have all been brought to the page. The reader has surely noted that the city of Beijing itself has also been crucial to shaping the person that Dr. Wang has become. In the evenings and weekends between my studies with Dr. Wang, I would explore the city that he describes with such animation. To him, Beijing is the only home he could ever imagine. Once he showed me on a map all of the places that he had lived. Besides a few trips abroad to teach and lecture, Dr. Wang has spent his entire life living within the ten square miles that comprise central Beijing. I wanted to know as much about the place as I could—and so I walked.

Much of the time I walked with my wife Tracy, who was working and traveling while I studied. At other times, when she was busy, I walked alone. The best thing about walking alone was that I could go quite far without either stopping or speaking and was therefore free to spend my time observing. Eventually, my wanderings coalesced into a favorite hike that came to be known to visiting friends and students as The Greatest Walk in Beijing. A statement like this might reek of hubris if it weren't for the fact that Beijing itself aspires these days to be one of the greatest cities on earth. A city with great aspirations should contain walks of equal stature (Fig. P1.1).

The walk is a long one and thus requires a fine pair of shoes. A visitor to Beijing these days doesn't have to actually bring good shoes as they can be had for a song at one of literally thousands of small shoe stores sprinkled throughout the city. If one wants name brands, they too can be found at rock-bottom prices at the 'Silk Market' next to the Yong An Li subway stop. This postscript is not about shopping, however. In fact, an entire book would be required to cover the myriad buying opportunities in this schizophrenic capital of a nominally communist nation. For now, it is assumed that shoes have been bought and the legs properly prepared for a 3–5 hour, 10 kilometer stroll. Let us assume that it is now one of a string of sunny days during Beijing's long, mild spring.

The walk begins in the small alleys to the south of Tiananmen Square. Here, just outside the former south-facing gates of the imperial city, merchants have bought and sold products from all over China for centuries. Many afternoons, I would take the subway to the He Ping Men subway stop and walk south to the alleys of the Liu Li Chang market. Officially, the walk begins here on Nan Xin Hua Jie at the China Books store. This store, and others like it, are the remnants of the dynastic literati. Even today, window after window is filled with heavy writing paper, brushes, ink, and thousands of scrolls. Now there are also antique stores for tourists, but the memory of past centuries remains. The walk heads east past shops once filled with bearded Confucians and top-knotted Taoist teachers haggling over the tools of their scholarly trade.

Because context for Chinese medicine is the goal, the reader should think of the written Chinese characters that are the vehicles upon which the ideas of ancient China travel to the present day. In writing these ideas, the medium was brush and ink, and the raw material was a long paper scroll. To write with ink, one must first grind the black inkstone and then

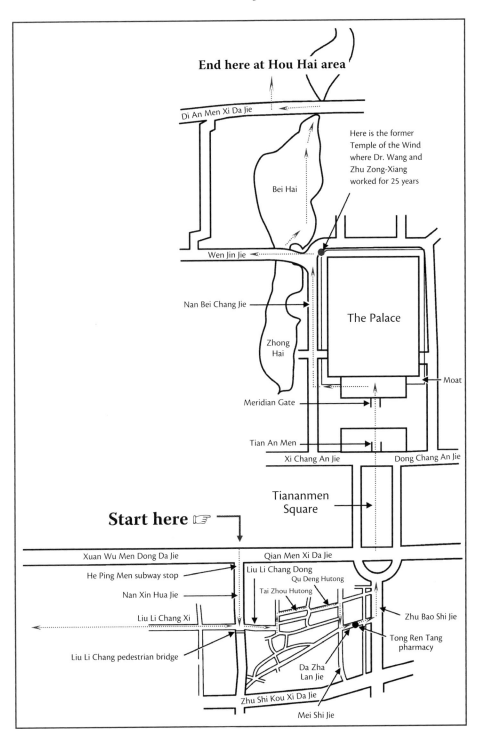

Fig. P1.1

The greatest walk in Beijing

mix just the right amount of water. Watery ink leads to bleeding while ink that is too thick can congest the brush and leave whiskers on the characters due to errant bristles. The streets of Liu Li Chang were, and continue to be, filled with some of China's greatest experts on the subtle art of calligraphy. The street eventually ends though, and, after a dog-leg to the left, there is a stretch of twentieth-century poverty which is quickly being renovated and cleaned in preparation for the waves of wandering tourists.

The next little alley, while poor, is not at all dangerous. Because this area is between the fairly famous Liu Li Chang and the ancient shopping street Da Shi Lan, it seems likely that the *hutongs* here will survive when many others nearby are torn down for modernization. As mentioned in earlier chapters, these alleys are picturesque for the tourist but actually quite miserable for some of the residents. This is mainly due to a lack of modern plumbing in the small courtyard houses. Residents use shared public facilities. Couple this fact with a lack of central heating that necessitates small coal-burning stoves on long winter nights and one can understand why at least some are not so sad to see them go. For Dr. Wang, the people in these crowded brick homes were often the majority of his patients. Although he now treats many of the air-conditioned denizens of 'New China', he spent decades in a large hospital treating those who could barely pay as part of a now-fading national health care system. Walking through these alleys where the frying of meals and the dialogue of family life can be plainly heard brings to mind the real differences between the patients of twentieth-century China and those seen in the West today. Chinese medicine practiced outside of China must adapt to different needs. When I think of adaptation, I can hear Dr. Wang reminding me that this will require an adept familiarity with fundamental concepts in their original context. Everything keeps coming back to understanding context and interrelationships—appreciating the patterns of health and disease and how environment matters.

After ten minutes or so in this residential alley, the street begins to widen and the buildings grow taller and are better built. The walk now enters the shopping street of Da Shi Lan. This street is almost directly in front of the old Front Gate. Now, as in ages past, commerce is heady along this road. There is an abundance of modern knock-off clothing among some remnants of proud trading companies from centuries past. I look up to see the intricate amalgam of Chinese and European architecture in the upper floors of the former offices of Qing dynasty commercial players. Today, a few remain, including Beijing's oldest Chinese herbal pharmacy, the Tong Ren Tang. Tong Ren Tang has actually adapted quite well to the twenty-first century. The family that has run the business for centuries is still involved and products have grown to include a huge variety of patent herbal pills, tinctures, and granules for export. There are also Tong Ren Tang pharmacies all over China. For the student of Chinese medicine, the four large floors of the Tong Ren Tang building are a feast for the eyes. The bottom floors contain mostly patent formulas, but the top two floors are filled with high quality raw herbs and a bustling raw herb pharmacy. Patients flow in holding the tissue-thin green papers that every doctor in China seems to use for writing herbal prescriptions. As patients wait on blue benches, the air is filled with the smell of cooking herbs.

Outside the Tong Ren Tang, the walk continues east to the crowded Qian Men Da Jie and then heads north along that street toward the vastness of Tiananmen Square. I heard somewhere that the square once held a million people at the time of Mao Ze Dong's death in 1976. Now, the former chairman rests in waxy splendor at the very center of modern China in a huge marble mausoleum ('Maosoleum'). The ambitious tourist can verify this by waiting in line during the rather unpredictable times that the mausoleum opens to the public. When it is open, the masses are allowed to pass (quickly) by the carefully preserved body of the founder of the People's Republic. For the student of Chinese medicine, credit should at least be given to Mao Ze Dong for having the foresight to preserve Chinese medicine against the tide of scientism that threatened it during the first half of the last century. While the former government of the Republic of China had actively pursued policies to eliminate Chinese medicine from the mainstream, the communists tried to integrate proven therapies for the benefit of a people mostly without health care of any kind. Although the so-called 'barefoot doctors' trained in the early years of nationalized Chinese medicine only had the most basic understanding of acupuncture and herbal medicine, they were still able to bring relief to hundreds of thousands of patients. Our applause is significantly dampened, however, by the all-out assaults carried out during the Cultural Revolution on Chinese scholars across all disciplines. Chinese medicine was not exempt from this harassment, but it managed not only to survive, but eventually to thrive. Over time, the system that Mao allowed to develop has grown to become the modern schools of traditional Chinese medicine (TCM). For better or for worse, these schools continue to play a vital role in preserving the field for the future. Today, they are spending more and more time reflecting upon how best to play that role in the coming decades.

Crossing Tiananmen Square can take quite awhile and, depending on the weather, can be quite grueling because of a conspicuous lack of trees or shelter of any kind. On the north side of the square, the famous painting of Mao hangs above the gates to the Forbidden City. The huge open space of Tiananmen Square provides a cross section of the Chinese people. Here, in the political center of the nation, people come together from all over to pay their respects to both the new and old China. Any self-respecting Chinese tourist from one of China's twenty-one provinces would consider a trip to both Tiananmen Square and the Forbidden City a must. As a result, walking through the square gives the ambling foreigner a window to all of China. Unlike other parts of Beijing that are generally filled with locals, the center of the city is filled with out-of-town families taking pictures and rural visitors gawking at the sheer size of the architecture. Of course, the millions of Chinese who live today on less than fifty U.S. cents a day are rarely represented in the square, even though they have certainly heard of its existence.

Having crossed Tiananmen Square, the walk now enters the Gate of Heavenly Peace itself. The square is named for this gate that served for at least four-hundred years as the final barrier between the emperor and his people. Only those qualified to enter the outer sanctum of the imperial city were permitted to enter here. Today, hordes of tourists from every nation cross under the red gate into the first of the many large open courtyards that were the ritual space for the imperial political cult. Dr. Wang described to me how these gates and the entire palace within lay open to the people of Beijing in the 1940s and 50s. He described how, as a child, he and his friends had played in the giant public park that the former palace became. As one can imagine, he said it made for the most amazing games of hide and seek. He described coming upon rooms in which old clocks still hung— possibly gifts from European missions a hundred years past. As unlikely as this story might sound at first, it should be remembered that the Forbidden City is huge, covering six full city blocks with hundreds of buildings. Today, less than half of the palace is open to the public as the authorities struggle to maintain row upon row of ancient edifice.

For the modern student of Chinese medicine, the Forbidden City represents the continuity of a culture. The culture of China managed to preserve and modify an ancient healing art through 2,000 years of constant appraisal. For Dr. Wang, the practice of Chinese medicine is not a sterile reapplication of ancient techniques, but involves the embodiment of a living, growing cultural system. That system is still evolving and has the malleability to jump to other cultures, as proven by the Koreans, Japanese, Vietnamese, and others. However, in the places where it most successfully adapted, care was always taken to study the culture from which it grew. For many years, the Forbidden City was one of the major hubs of that culture.

At this point in the walk, instead of going into the Forbidden City itself, the path turns to the east and out a side gate to a small road that traces the ancient moat just outside the fifty-foot walls of the inner sanctum. For anyone visiting Beijing, the Forbidden City is a must-see, but its very impressiveness makes it less amenable to a brisk city walk. One is often drawn to the details of the inner buildings in such a way that the pace of the walk is broken. Even the drainage systems of the Forbidden City are distracting, with their huge dragon and tiger heads that spew water into giant bronze cauldrons during a heavy downpour. Instead, I usually head north along the tree-lined Bei Chi Zi with its high metal gates on the left guarding the homes of Politburo members.

At the north end of Bei Chi Zi, on the opposite side of the street from the moat of the Forbidden City, is a small metal gate blocking the entrance to an ancient temple (#2 Bei Chi Zi). The sign on the wall reads "The Senior Cadre Club of Beijing Bureau of Public Health." If one steps back a bit, it is quite easy to see the rooftop of the former Temple of the Wind where, until 2003, Dr. Zhu Zong-Xiang conducted his research (see narrative on pages 429–435). In earlier decades, Dr. Wang also worked in this former temple complex, seeing up to eighty patients a day and sleeping in a small on-site room. He once described to me how he and other doctors would heat up their meals in the courtyard while rehashing the cases of the day. The core of doctors who practiced here in the 1960s eventually became the faculty backbone of the huge Xuan Wu Hospital of Chinese Medicine that was built in the late 60s and early 70s. During the few visits we made to the former temple during my stay there, Dr. Wang would look at the crumbling buildings with the humor of someone remembering years long past. Today, the 90-year-old Dr. Zhu has finally retired and the entire temple complex has recently been renovated for tourists. The sign for the Senior Cadre Club is slated for removal.

At this point, the walk veers slightly west and travels through the two most impressive public parks in Beijing. The walk first crosses busy Jing Shan Qian Jie and enters the south gate of Jing Shan park. For those whose legs still have plenty of energy, a climb to the top of the large hill in the center of the park is worth the effort. The 'mountain' in the park is the highest point in central Beijing and provides a commanding view of the city on a clear day. Looking south, one can see the hundreds of roofs of the Forbidden City and Tiananmen Square in the distance. As the mountain is located on the north-south axis of the city, going to the other side provides a view directly up Di An Da Jie to the huge drum tower that marked the north gate of the former city wall. Both this park and Bei Hai Park next door comprised the imperial gardens in former times. It is truly amazing to contemplate the scale of everything imperial. Imagine having a gigantic city park as one's backyard. During the Qing dynasty, the parks were full of rare trees and live animals from all over the country. Today, the trees are still there, but the animals have been replaced by old men practicing *tài jí quán* (tai qi) and crowds of laughing children.

The walk then leaves Jing Shan park and travels to Bei Hai park next door. This second imperial garden is dominated by a huge lake with a restaurant in the center serving dishes from the imperial menu (at similarly regal prices). The west side of the lake is lined with some of the best ancient buildings in the city. In particular, there is a giant Ming dynasty Buddhist temple, constructed entirely from a type of dark cypress that still smells of the incense of four-hundred years. Today, very little incense burns inside but a huge rotating pagoda rests on the temple floor filled with tiny, glowing lights. For the student of Chinese medicine, the parks of Beijing are the best place to witness the healing movements of *tài jí quán* and *qì gōng*. I would sometimes wake up early and walk the fifteen minutes from my apartment to these parks to watch retirees practice in groups of over fifty. There would often be a leader with a megaphone calling out the names of the moves as they went through the graceful form. The front of the line invariably contained a cadre of extremely serene octogenarians with supple legs and flowing pants. In the parks, I was reminded that Chinese medicine is more than the practice of acupuncture and herbal therapy. As practitioners, we are required to care for our bodies as well so as to motivate patients to engage in healing movement. For the people of modern Beijing, there is quite a diversity of morning exercise. While some would practice the more recognizable forms of *tài jí quán*, others would join calisthenic groups who waved their arms and shook their legs to the rhythm of modern Chinese pop songs. The parks also contain a strong contingent of morning calligraphers who write poetry with huge broom-sized brushes on the gray cement pathways using nothing but water for ink. The fluid movement of their writing leaves characters on the paths to fade in the growing sun.

The final leg of the Greatest Walk in Beijing begins after leaving the north end of Bei Hai park and loops around another lake called Hou Hai. Ironically, one of the first things that one confronts when crossing Di An Men street to begin the paved loop around Hou Hai is a Starbucks coffee franchise. Beijing, like so many cities worldwide, is host to a growing population of consumers of Western-style food and drink. In the clinic, this has caused old patterns of disease to shift and led to new modifications of old formulas. The aging doctors at the Ping Xin Tang clinic claim that the need to modify old formulas for new times is part of an ancient pattern. The medicine has changed with the culture in successive dynasties, and modern changes in food and lifestyle present a challenge but not a death knell for the medicine.

The loop around Hou Hai lake is my favorite. It isn't far from my apartment in the nearby *hutong* alleys and holds some of the best memories for me. At the northeast end of the lake is a large classical gate that guards the former home of Soong Qing Ling. The former 'Madame Soong' was born the daughter of one of the most powerful men in prerevolutionary Shanghai and died the widow of the founder of modern China, Dr. Sun Yat Sen. Twenty-five years his junior, Madame Soong lived to a ripe age and played an active role in her country's history until her death in 1982. Today, her former home can be toured for a few dollars and draws a slow trickle of mostly local tourists.

On a very cold November morning in 2002, I arranged to meet Dr. Wang in front of Soong Qing Ling's gate to ask if I might study with him. When he arrived, we went to a small restaurant nearby and ate the first of a hundred noodle meals together. As we ate, he asked me what I had come to China to learn. I told him that originally I had thought about studying more herbal medicine so as to build upon work I had done two years before in Chengdu. As the time for my return to China neared, I had begun to think more and more about Beijing. I told him that I had always remembered the lectures he had given when he visited the U.S. during my student years in California. The clarity of his descriptions of physiology had impressed me then, but there was much I didn't understand. Because of that memory, I had asked a teacher in San Francisco to give me his phone number. Amazingly, when I got to Beijing, I dialed the number and found him at home. That phone call had led to lunch that November day. As I sat there eating, I described how I had been thinking in recent months that I would like to learn more about his understanding of the mechanisms of acupuncture. I didn't know at the time that I had unwittingly asked exactly the right question.

Thus the long walk around Beijing ends where my work with Dr. Wang began. There is one final moment from the shores of Hou Hai lake that I would like to describe here. This happened three or four months after that initial visit—after a clinic shift and a meal at a nearby duck restaurant. Dr. Wang and I were taking a break and sitting, for some reason, outside on a park bench on a fairly cold late-winter afternoon. The sun must have been out. I told him that I had been trying to write down and organize my notes from the lectures that he had been giving. After asking a few questions about the subject matter of those lectures, I asked Dr. Wang what he thought about making a book about all of this. Characteristically, he paused for a moment in thought and then said, "Well, it sounds like a good idea, but it certainly shouldn't be another boring textbook!" I sincerely hope that we have succeeded.

Pathways of the Channels

Introduction

T HE FOLLOWING PAGES show the pathways of the twelve primary channels and the *dū* and *rèn* vessels. The darker red lines in the images represent the internal pathways of the primary channels as well as the trajectories of the collateral vessels (絡脈 *luò mài*) and channel divergences (經別 *jīng bíe*). The lighter red lines represent the more familiar external pathways of the channels, upon which the points are found.

Readers should also take note of the graphics in the lower corners of the illustrations. These show the organs and structures that are traditionally said to be enlivened by each of the channels. More specifically, classical sources have multiple terms to describe the ways that channels pass through or over the structures of the body. Channels are seen to 'collateralize' (絡 *luò*), 'go along' (循 *xún*), 'enter' (入 *rù*), 'move' (行 *xíng*), 'encircle' (環 *huán*), and 'scatter' (散 *sǎn*) around the body. While the small graphics on these pages do not show these distinctions, it is important to remember that the relationship that a channel has with a particular body structure can be better understood by considering the way that the channel is thought to interact with it. 'Entering' the stomach, for example, is quite different from 'going along' its surface. Chinese sources provide the best place to explore these finer distinctions of 'connective physiology'. The images on the following pages are adapted from one such source, *Diagrams of the Channels and Collaterals* (經絡圖解 *Jīng luò tú jiě*), edited by Lin Yun-Gui (蔺雲桂). Fuzhou: Fujian Science and Technology Publishing House, 1991.

For some of the channels, no mention is made in the classics of significant organs or structures that are reached by the collateral vessels. In other words, sometimes the collateral vessels are described as connecting more to areas right around the collateral points of the channel. In those cases, the graphics here do not list the collateral vessels. Nonetheless, the reader should remember the concept, discussed in Chapter 17, that the term 'collaterals' encompasses not just the internal collateral pathways, but also small vessel microcirculation along the entire pathway of each of the primary channels.

The ultimate source of channel pathway information is the *Inner Classic*. In fact, most of the information comes from a single chapter, "Channels and Vessels" (經脈篇 *jīng mài piān),* found in the *Divine Pivot.* The channel divergences are discussed separately in the next chapter, which is appropriately titled 經別 *(jīng bié),* or "The Divergences." However, there are other sections of the *Inner Classic* which add detail (and occasional controversy) about the exact trajectory of a few of the channels. There are also very important additions to our understanding of classical channel pathways in other texts, most notably from the *Systematic Classic of Acupuncture and Moxibustion* (針灸甲乙經 *Zhēn jiǔ jiǎ yǐ jīng),* written by Huang-Fu Mi sometime around 282 A.D.

Finally, it should be noted that the 'sinew channels' (筋經 *jīn jīng),* also described in the *Inner Classic,* are not shown on the following pages. These pathways tend to follow the trajectories of the external aspects of the regular channels, while broadening to include a swath of musculature in areas adjacent to the more narrowly-defined regular channels. Most acupuncture textbooks have illustrations of the sinew channels, which the reader is encouraged to consult.

An important goal of this appendix is to provide a different prism through which to view the relationships among the organs. Simply put, when considering the channel system as a whole, it is important to remember that there are both organs and channels. The connections imply functional relationship. Thus, when palpating the channels, one should keep in mind the trajectory and connections of the entire channel, both internally and on the surface of the body. By fixing one's mind on the pathway, it will be easier to think about the significance of palpated change.

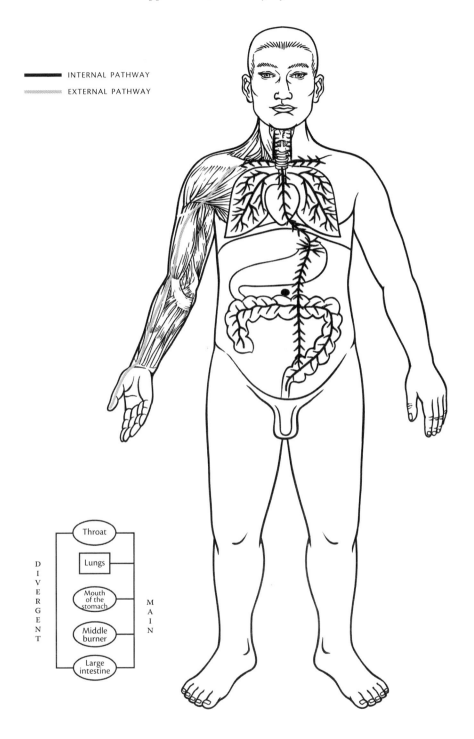

INTERNAL PATHWAY
EXTERNAL PATHWAY

D I V E R G E N T

Throat
Lungs
Mouth of the stomach
Middle burner
Large intestine

M A I N

Arm *tài yīn* lung channel
(手太陰肺經 *shǒu tài yīn fèi jīng*)

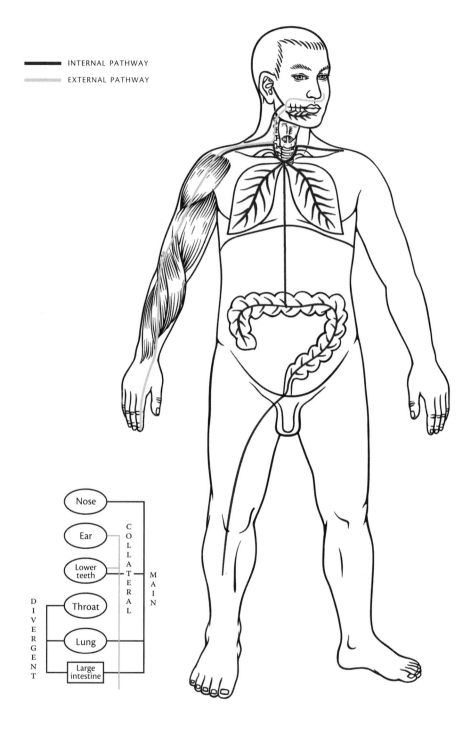

INTERNAL PATHWAY

EXTERNAL PATHWAY

Nose

Ear

Lower teeth

Throat

Lung

Large intestine

COLLATERAL

MAIN

DIVERGENT

Arm *yáng míng* large intestine channel
(手陽明大腸經 *shǒu yáng míng dà cháng jīng*)

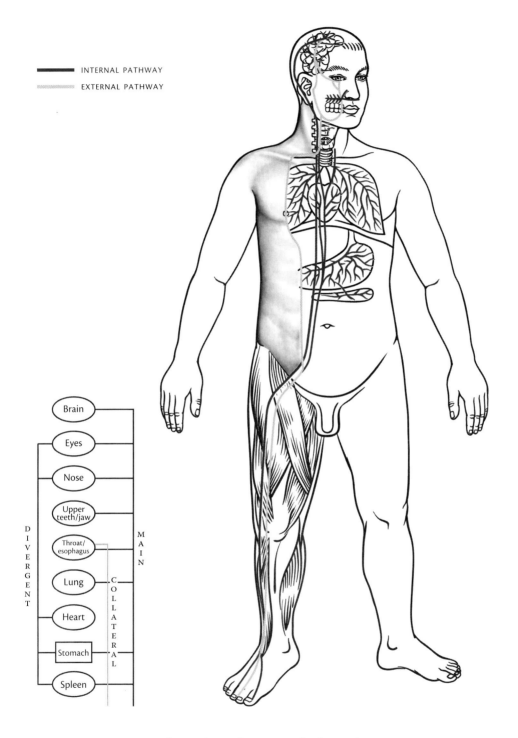

INTERNAL PATHWAY
EXTERNAL PATHWAY

Brain

Eyes

Nose

Upper teeth/jaw

Throat/ esophagus

Lung

Heart

Stomach

Spleen

D I V E R G E N T

M A I N

C O L L A T E R A L

Leg *yáng míng* stomach channel
(足陽明胃經 *zú yáng míng wèi jing*)

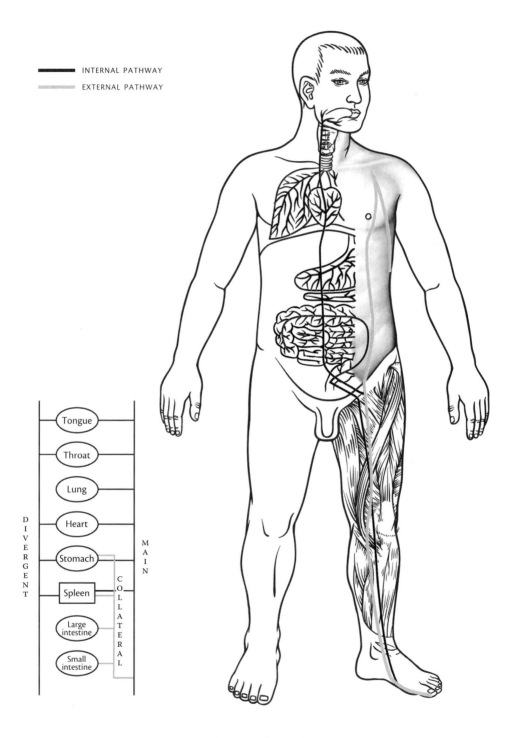

Leg *tài yīn* spleen channel
(足太陰脾經 *zú tài yīn pí jīng*)

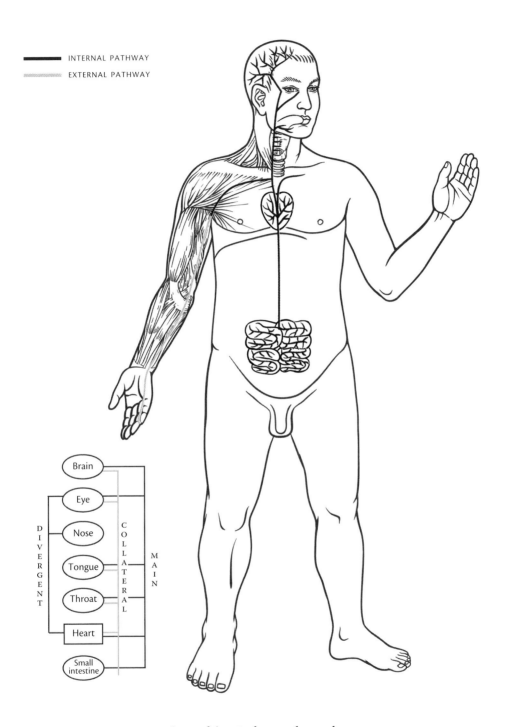

INTERNAL PATHWAY
EXTERNAL PATHWAY

Arm *shào yīn* heart channel
(手少陰心經 *shǒu shào yīn xīn jīng*)

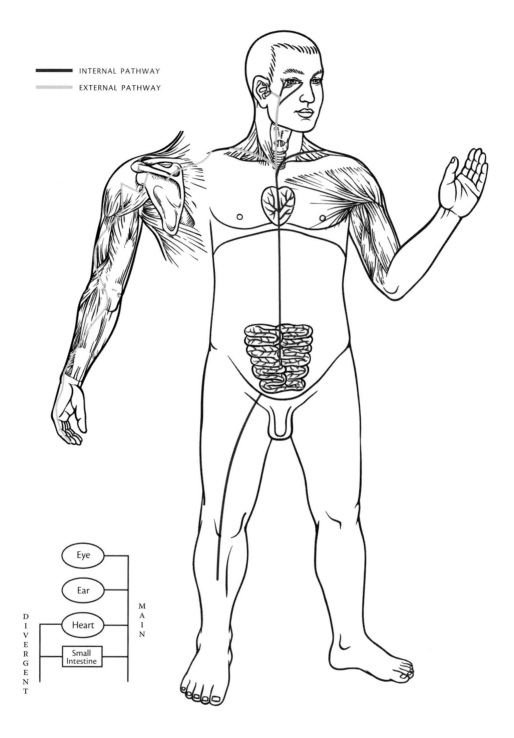

INTERNAL PATHWAY
EXTERNAL PATHWAY

Eye

Ear

Heart

Small Intestine

DIVERGENT

MAIN

Arm *tài yáng* small intestine channel
(手太陽小腸經 *shǒu tài yáng xiǎo cháng jīng*)

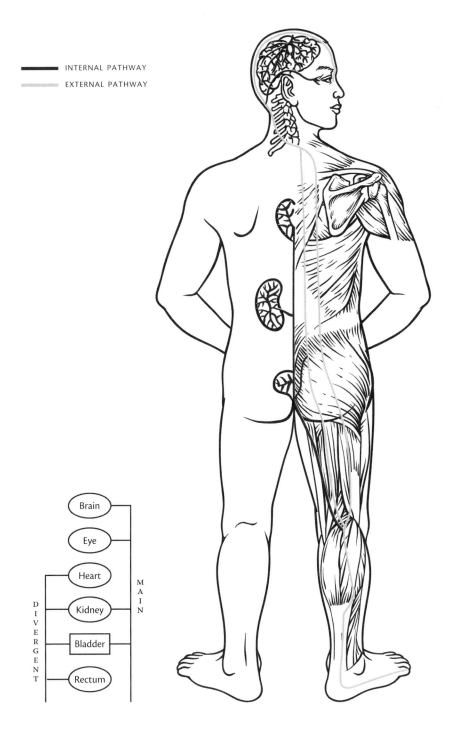

INTERNAL PATHWAY
EXTERNAL PATHWAY

Brain
Eye
Heart
Kidney
Bladder
Rectum

MAIN

DIVERGENT

Leg *tài yáng* bladder channel
(足太陽膀胱經 *zú tài yáng páng guāng jīng*)

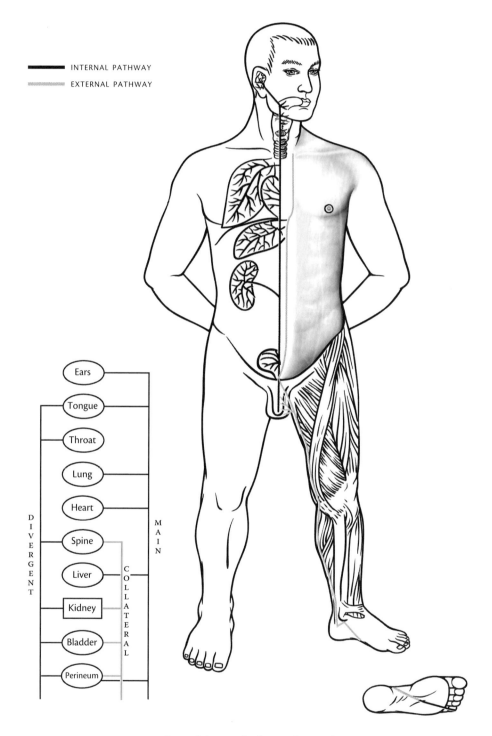

INTERNAL PATHWAY
EXTERNAL PATHWAY

Ears
Tongue
Throat
Lung
Heart
Spine
Liver
Kidney
Bladder
Perineum

DIVERGENT

MAIN

COLLATERAL

Leg *shào yīn* kidney channel
(足少陰腎經 *zú shào yīn shèn jīng*)

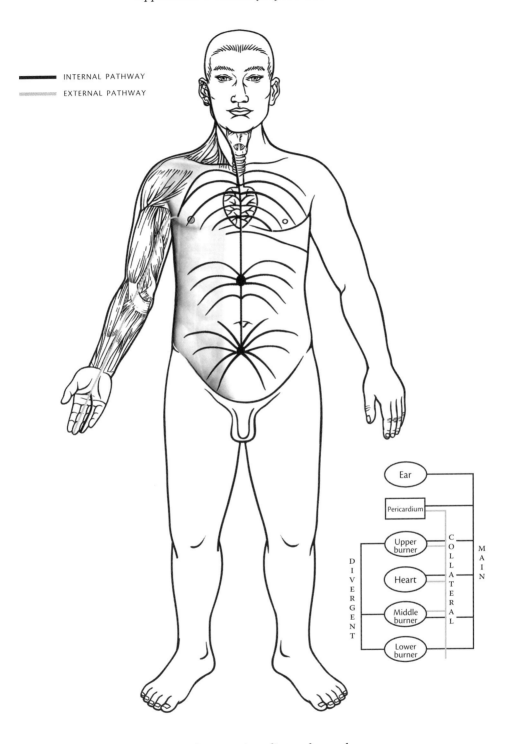

INTERNAL PATHWAY
EXTERNAL PATHWAY

Ear

Pericardium

Upper burner

Heart

Middle burner

Lower burner

DIVERGENT

COLLATERAL

MAIN

Arm *jué yīn* pericardium channel
(手厥陰心包經 *shǒu jué yīn xīn bāo jīng*)

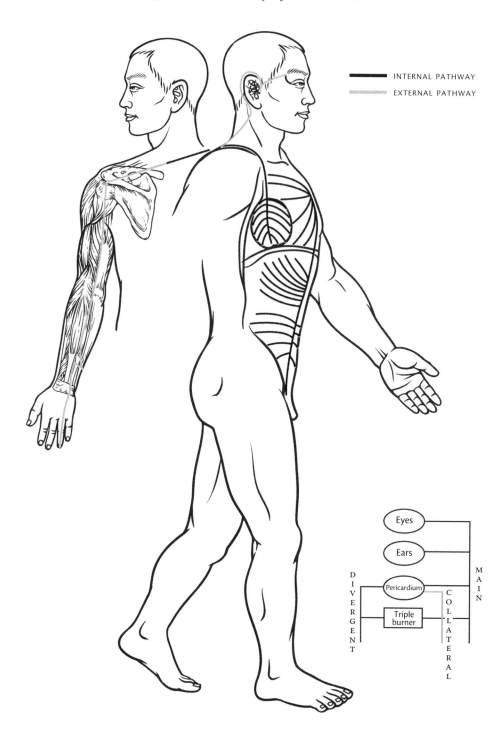

INTERNAL PATHWAY
EXTERNAL PATHWAY

Arm *shào yáng* triple burner channel
(手少陽三焦經 *shŏu shào yáng sān jiāo jīng*)

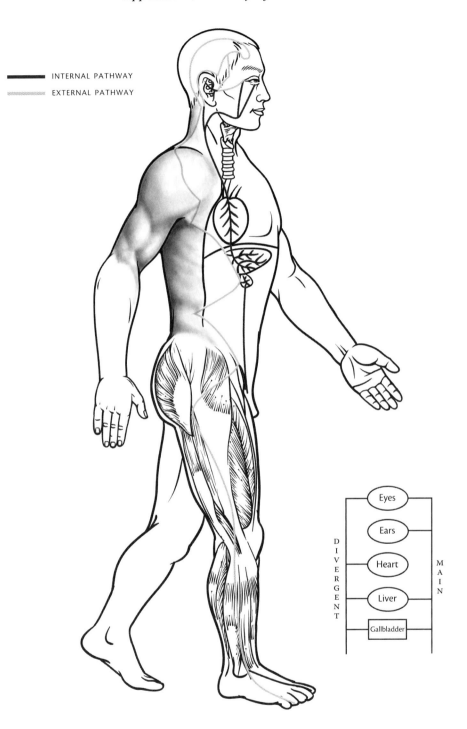

INTERNAL PATHWAY
EXTERNAL PATHWAY

Eyes
Ears
Heart
Liver
Gallbladder

DIVERGENT

MAIN

Leg *shào yáng* gallbladder channel
(足少陽膽經 *zú shào yáng dǎn jīng*)

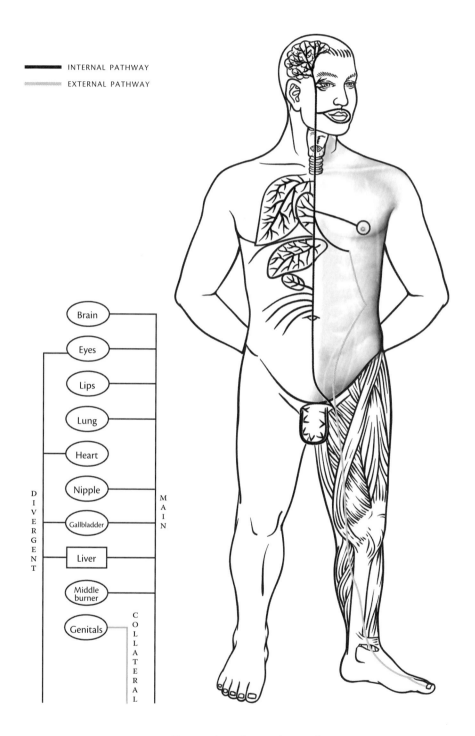

INTERNAL PATHWAY
EXTERNAL PATHWAY

Brain
Eyes
Lips
Lung
Heart
Nipple
Gallbladder
Liver
Middle burner
Genitals

DIVERGENT

MAIN

COLLATERAL

Leg *jué yīn* liver channel
(足厥陰肝經 *zú jué yīn gān jīng*)

INTERNAL PATHWAY
EXTERNAL PATHWAY

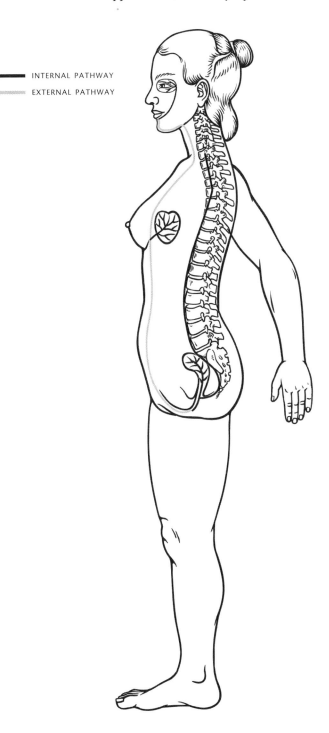

The *rèn* (conception) vessel
(妊脈 *rèn mài*)

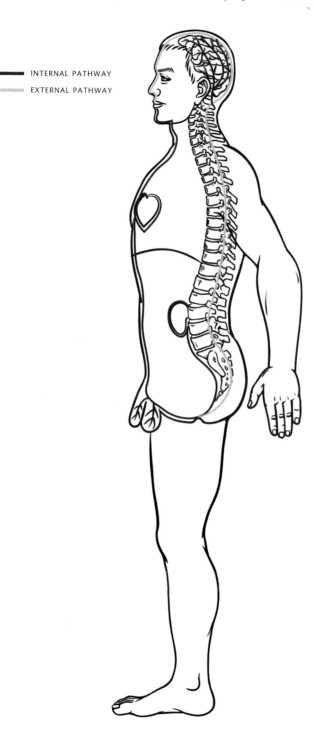

INTERNAL PATHWAY
EXTERNAL PATHWAY

The *dū* (governing) vessel
(督脈 *dū mài*)

The Sensory Organs

CLASSICAL TEXTS OFTEN list seven orifices (七竅 *qī qiào)* on the head by including each nostril and ear as an individual orifice plus the two eyes and the mouth. In modern parlance, the concept is often narrowed to the 'five senses' (五官 *wǔ guān)* and includes the nose, ears, eyes, mouth, and tongue. From the earliest stages of Chinese medicine, an important clinical goal has been to understand how the internal organs relate to the senses. At its most useful, these debates have tended to focus on different opinions about the selection of points or herbs, and on technique. However, the association of specific organs with each of the orifices has also often involved rather inflexible classification along five-phase lines. One often hears, for example, that since the liver is associated with the eyes in five-phase theory, then most eye conditions must involve liver imbalance. In reality, a useful clinical approach requires a nuanced understanding of the systemic roles of each of the organs and the relationship of organ function to the five senses.

The following pages will summarize some modern clinical experience with the five senses by exploring within the traditional categories of the five yin organs. The description of the five orifices provided in Chapter 37 of the *Classic of Difficulties* will be used as a starting point. That chapter describes the relationship of the five yin organs to the senses as follows:

- The qi of the lung opens through [通 *tōng*] the nose. If the nose [functions] harmoniously, then one knows both good and bad odors.

- The qi of the liver opens through the eyes. If the eyes [function] harmoniously, then one can know light from darkness [lit. "white from black"].

- The qi of the spleen opens through the mouth. If the mouth [functions] harmoniously, then one can know the flavor of grains.

- The heart opens through the tongue. If the tongue [functions] harmoniously, then one can know the five flavors.

- The kidney opens through the ears. If the ears [function] harmoniously, then one can know the five sounds.

- If the five yin organs are not harmonious, then the nine orifices will be blocked [不通 *bù tōng*]. If the five yang organs are not harmonious, then flow will become knotted leading to abscesses [癰 *yōng*].

Besides what are likely to be familiar associations of the internal organs with the sensory organs for most students of Chinese medicine, it is interesting to think about the final line from the passage excerpted above. The *Classic of Difficulties* notes that harmonious function of the yin organs keeps the senses open. This is yin nourishment giving rise to yang function. On the other hand, if the yang organs do not function harmoniously, there is knotting and the growth of abscesses or sores. Here, lack of yang movement may cause the orifices to become blocked. Thus, when considering all of the senses in the discussion below, it is important to keep in mind that fundamental need for all of the sensory organs to receive both yin nourishment and the warm movement of yang.

The Liver Opens through the Eyes

While the *Classic of Difficulties* states that "the liver opens through the eyes," there are actually a variety of other organs and channels which can affect eye function. Altogether, classical sources describe sixteen different channels, collaterals, and vessels which are said to connect to the eyes.[1] Among them are seven regular channels and five collateral vessels from the regular channels. Furthermore, the extraordinary vessels *yīn qiáo, yáng qiáo, rèn,* and *dū* are also said to travel to the eyes. In short, the relationship of the liver to the eyes, while special, is mediated by the relationship of the eyes to many other channels and organs.

Most often, in cases of liver-type eye problems, the diagnosis will involve either liver blood deficiency or liver heat. The association of qi transformation of the liver with the eyes has three primary theoretical underpinnings: structural, physiological, and psychological.

Structural   The classical structural connection involves the pathways of the liver channel and its divergent channel, both of which are said to reach the 'root' of the eyes. In modern anatomical terms, this most often involves a relationship between liver pathomechanisms and problems with the optic nerve and retina at the back of the eyes.

Physiological   The liver function of storing blood is also related to the eyes. In its role as a determiner of blood distribution, the organ is linked to eye problems due to changes in vascular circulation. These types of problems can come on quickly and be due to a relatively sudden change in blood flow to the area. Often, these are cases in which modern evaluations reveal little or no physical change in the organ itself. These types of changes may lead to problems with the optic nerve.

Psychological   The liver is said to hold the ethereal soul. If a patient reports hallucinations, this is often traditionally viewed to be a symptom of a problem associated with this aspect of liver function.

Common liver points for treating the eyes

LR-2 *(xíng jiān)* and BL-18 *(gān shū)* are often used in treating liver-type eye conditions that involve redness and itching in the eyes or night blindness. Less often, LR-1 *(dà dūn)*, LR-3 *(tài chōng),* and LR-8 *(qū quán)* are also used, depending on the pathodynamic. As the paired yang channel, gallbladder channel points are also often used in liver-type eye problems, especially when excess is clearly involved.

CLINICAL APPROACH TO EYE CONDITIONS

Acupuncture can be quite effective in treating eye conditions. The types of conditions treated may be broken down into the following five general categories (Fig. A2.1):

1. Retina and optic nerve

As noted above, problems in this area are often related to *jué yīn.* This includes degenerative diseases of the retina and optic nerve as well as more acute cases of inflammation in and around the nerve. The *jué yīn* area also extends behind and around the eyeball to include issues of blood circulation to the entire area; this often includes circulatory problems, such as glaucoma. However, differentiation is still recommended as sometimes the *shào yīn* kidney channel may also be involved with problems in this area. Check for corresponding kidney patterns, often involving deficiency and heat, as seen in the Lycium Fruit, Chrysanthemum, and Rehmannia Pill (*qǐ*

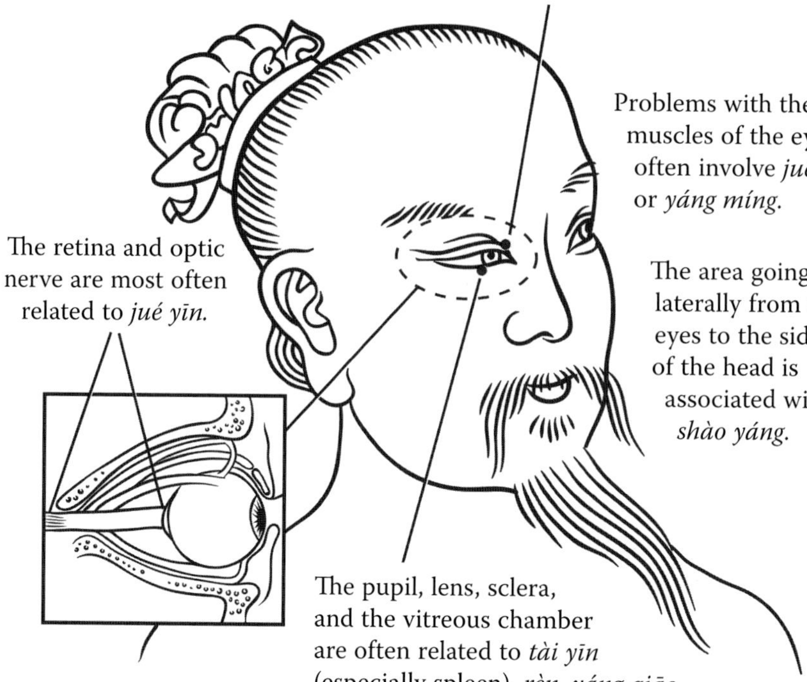

The 'borders' of the eyes, especially the lacrimal ducts and conjunctiva, are associated with *yáng míng, yáng qiāo, tài yáng,* and *tài yīn.*

Problems with the muscles of the eyes often involve *jué yīn* or *yáng míng.*

The retina and optic nerve are most often related to *jué yīn.*

The area going laterally from the eyes to the side of the head is associated with *shào yáng.*

The pupil, lens, sclera, and the vitreous chamber are often related to *tài yīn* (especially spleen), *rèn, yáng qiāo,* and *yáng míng* (especially stomach).

Fig. A2.1
Acupuncture can be quite effective in treating eye conditions.

· ·

jú dì huáng wán) pattern. *Jué yīn* eye problems are often treated with GB-20 *(fēng chí)* to facilitate circulation in the paired *shào yáng* channel, along with BL-18 *(gān shū)* and LR-3 *(tài chōng).* In cases of clear excess and/or heat affecting *jué yīn,* an effective point prescription would also include GB-41 *(zú lín qì).* For *shào yīn* types, KI-3 *(tài xī)* and BL-1 *(jīng míng)* are more appropriate.

2. Pupil, lens, sclera, and the vitreous chamber

Structural problems related to the eyeball itself are more often associated with the *tài yīn* (especially spleen), *rèn, yáng qiāo,* and *yáng míng* (especially stomach) channels. Patients who present with the various types of refractive errors or inflammation in the area respond better to treatment with these channels. In the clinic, the spleen channel is particularly helpful as this area of the body is full of fluids. Points like SP-9 *(yīn líng quán)* and SP-4 *(gōng sūn)* are almost always used to treat problems with this part of the eye. Palpation along the spleen channel can be helpful in point selection. It should also be pointed out that swelling in the area below the eye is related to the spleen.

3. Borders of the eye

This includes the conjunctiva, the lacrimal (tear) glands, and the eyelid. These areas are more associated with the *yáng míng, yáng qiāo, tài yáng,* and *tài yīn* channels. In particular, the conjunctiva are often related to the *yáng míng* and *tài yīn* channels. Conjunctivitis, for example, often responds to treatment with LI-11 *(qū chí)*, SP-4, and SP-9.

4. Muscles of the eye

Problems with moving the eyes often involve either *jué yīn* (bringing blood to nourish these 'tendons') or the *yáng míng* channel, which has a collateral vessel in the area. When *jué yīn* is causative, there is often a chronic degenerative condition that involves twitching of the muscles (wind) or a lack of proper quickness and responsiveness (blood deficiency). *Yáng míng* is often chosen in more acute cases. For example, if the eyes are not moving due to stroke, external invasion, or infection, they require a strong burst of qi and blood. A very effective technique involves threading a 3-inch needle up the large intestine channel from LI-14 *(bì nào)*; needling should be subcutaneous. LI-4 *(hé gǔ)* might be added as well. Finally, the muscles of the eye may suffer from developmental disorders in children (lazy eye). This is caused by a lack of clear yang qi to the head and responds best to treatment using GV-20 *(bǎi huì)*, CV-12 *(zhōng wǎn)*, CV-6 *(qì hǎi)*, and ST-36 *(zú sān lǐ)*.

5. Area lateral to the eyes

The area lateral to the eyes extending to the side of the head is generally associated with the *shào yáng* channel. Headaches in this area that affect eye function may involve excess in that channel. Distal *shào yáng* points such as GB-37 *(guāng míng)* and GB-41 *(zú lín qì)* can be helpful.

■ CASE STUDY

52-year-old female

Chief complaint   Blurry vision in the left eye for six months

History of present illness   The patient had been slowly losing visual acuity in the left eye for the previous six months (eventually having vision of 20/80) but experienced a sudden deterioration in vision to 20/200 in the three weeks prior to her first visit. She had also experienced a narrowed range of vision and a sense of radiating light (aura) in recent weeks—all signs of retinal problems. Direct ophthalmoscopy revealed bleeding in the vessels in and around the retina and signs of blood clotting in the area. On presentation, the patient complained of pain in the left eye accompanied by headache and watering from the eye. She also had little appetite, abdominal distention, a history of hepatitis, and chronic kidney inflammation. She experienced intense dreams at night.

The tongue was swollen with scallops and dry cracks along the edge. The pulse was fast and wiry.

Channel palpation Palpation around the eyes showed significant tenderness but there were no nodules along the gallbladder channel on the head. There was a pronounced softness and weakness at both KI-3 *(tài xī)* and KI-16 *(huāng shū)*. There was also tenderness at BL-18 *(gān shū)*, especially on the left side.

Diagnosis Kidney yin deficiency leading to liver yang rising

Treatment The treatment principle in this case was to clear heat from the *jué yīn* liver while opening the collaterals of both *jué yīn* and *shào yáng*. Later stages involved strengthening kidney yin.

Treatment was broken down into the following stages. In general, the patient was treated twice weekly.

Stage 1 The first three treatments focused on clearing excess from the collaterals. To that end, BL-18 was bled using a three-star needle followed by cupping. In addition, GB-20 *(fēng chí)* and TB-5 *(wài guān)* were needled on the left side only. After three treatments, the pain and headache subsided, but the blurry vision remained.

Stage 2 The next ten treatments involved a combination of moving and draining with underlying support of the kidney deficiency. Gentle support of *shào yīn* was achieved by using the source point KI-3 with very light stimulation. At the same time, the overall goal of each treatment was still to gently move and drain. Thus *jué yīn* was drained (gently) using the point pair KI-7 *(fù liū)* and LR-2 *(xíng jiān)*. More supporting movement was achieved by using the *yáng míng* channel point pair LI-10 *(shǒu sān lǐ)* and ST-36 *(zú sān lǐ)*.

Stage 3 Following the ten treatments in stage 2, the patient's vision had improved to 20/80 but she still complained of a limited field of vision. The treatment was then modified to include BL-1 *(jīng míng)* and GB-37 *(guāng míng)*. BL-1 is obviously a local point that can help increase circulation in the area. GB-37, often treated for eye issues, is also the collateral point of the gallbladder channel and is thus associated with problems in microcirculation throughout the *shào yáng* channel. After two more weeks of treatment, the patient's vision returned to 20/50 in the left eye. At that point, vision in the right eye was tested at 20/40.

Analysis   This is a fairly typical case of using *jué yīn* to treat eye problems involving the retina. In the clinic, one must consider *jué yīn* and all the other channels that relate to its physiology. Note that the treatment included considerations of both the internally-externally paired *shào yáng* and the 'mother' kidney channel.

The general arc of treatment moved from strong clearing in the initial stage to a gradual shift to more moving and even treatments that had some elements of tonification. Altogether there were approximately eighteen treatments given over a nine-week period. Note as well that local needling at BL-1 was not used until later, after some of the initial excess had been cleared away.

The Heart Opens through the Tongue

Before discussing the relationship of the heart to the tongue, the traditional Chinese medical understanding of the tongue should be briefly summarized. In general, the tongue is associated with the following functions.

1. Speech

In conjunction with the mouth and the teeth, the tongue obviously plays a vital role in the verbalization of language. There are two aspects of tongue function as it relates to speech. The first is the actual movement of the muscles of the tongue. The second is the ability of a person to verbalize one's thoughts. While the second function is generally related to the brain in modern medicine, classical Chinese medicine associates both types of speech problems with the tongue. This will be discussed further below.

2. Knowing the five flavors (知五味 *zhī wǔ wèi*)

An important tongue function is the ability to clearly discern the flavors of food. This is similar to the concept, also associated with the heart, that the spirit must clearly 'recognize' (認 *rèn*) the nature of one's surroundings. A healthy spirit, supported by the fullness of heart-blood, can better discern the qualities of a given situation or environment. The tongue has a similar function of discerning, through taste, the quality of food. Pathomechanisms involving the heart may lead to an inability to properly discern whether a particular food is good for the body.

3. Swallowing

The ability to move fluids from the mouth down the throat is associated with tongue function in Chinese medicine.

In the clinic, problems with any of these functions may indicate dysfunction of *shào yīn*. The heart channel connects to the tongue through a collateral vessel. Remember from earlier discussions that the collateral vessels are often associated with microcirculation. This concept plays a part in steering one's clinical approach. The heart channel is not the only one that affects the area, however. For example, while the heart connects to the tongue through a collateral vessel, the spleen channel travels directly to the tongue body. In addition, the spleen has a divergent channel that reaches this area. Similarly, both the primary and a divergent channel of the kidney 'spread' through the 'root' of the tongue (舌本 *shé běn)*. The *yīn wéi* vessel, following the path of the kidney channel, also spreads out at the root of the tongue to provide yin nourishment. Consequently, not only the heart, but also the spleen and kidney in particular are associated with tongue function. These channel connections also play an important part in determining one's clinical approach (Fig. A2.2).

How, then, is the heart involved in tongue function? As noted earlier, the association of the heart with the tongue is in many ways related to its function of holding the spirit. Spirit function involves the ability of a person to clearly recognize the nature of the world at large. This is both similar to and greater than the idea of 'consciousness'. A person is conscious if they are awake but may not necessarily be able to clearly recognize things. In the case of a stroke, for example, a patient may appear completely conscious but often seems unable to recognize the world around them in the same way. This is a case in which the qi transformation of the *shào yīn* channel has been affected. In this type of stroke patient, the ability to speak is often also compromised. More specifically, this type of patient may have relatively normal tongue movement, but nevertheless be unable to properly vocalize ideas because of changes in the brain itself. This involves the concept of microcirculation and the collateral vessels, in particular, the collateral vessels of *shào yīn*.

In the clinic, then, the most common type of 'tongue condition' treated with the heart channel involves cases where cognition problems have af-

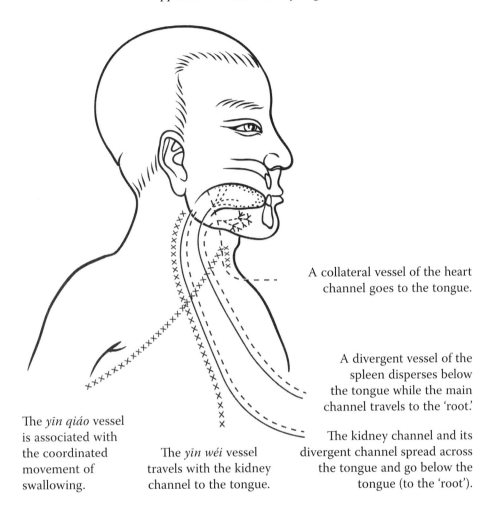

A collateral vessel of the heart channel goes to the tongue.

A divergent vessel of the spleen disperses below the tongue while the main channel travels to the 'root.'

The kidney channel and its divergent channel spread across the tongue and go below the tongue (to the 'root').

The *yīn qiáo* vessel is associated with the coordinated movement of swallowing.

The *yīn wéi* vessel travels with the kidney channel to the tongue.

Fig. A2.2
Multiple channels and collaterals travel to the tongue.

fected speech. Nevertheless, because of the relationship of the *shào yīn* channel to the yin collaterals, blood nourishment of the tongue body itself is also related to the heart to some degree. As noted elsewhere, the point pair HT-5 *(tōng lǐ)* and KI-6 *(zhào hǎi)* is often used to improve circulation in the yin collaterals, especially those which nourish the tongue. This useful point pair is discussed at some length in Chapter 20. Also, as a fire-type channel, *shào yīn* is often involved in pathomechanisms involving heat, especially those that have a psychological aspect. Thus the heart channel is most likely involved in cases where sores on the tongue coincide with emotional imbalance.

Problems involving an inability to taste may also be related to spleen *tài yīn*. While differentiating tastes (辨味 *biàn wèi*) is more of a heart function, the tongue requires adequate moisture and a healthy appetite to stimulate the sense and desire for taste—the urge for postnatal nourishment. When the tongue is dry because of spleen-stomach yin deficiency, for example, taste will be affected. Similarly, a lack of interest in food due to spleen qi deficiency can also cloud the perceptive ability of the tongue.

The act of swallowing, while related to the heart, also involves the co-ordination of integrated movement in the area associated with the *yīn qiāo* (see Chapter 11). Consequently, because the *yīn qiāo* vessel is particularly associated with the throat, one often uses KI-6, the command point of the *yīn qiāo*, for speech and throat problems, instead of the collateral point of the kidney, KI-4 (*dà zhōng*).

CLINICAL APPROACH TO TONGUE CONDITIONS

On the heart channel, HT-5 (*tōng lǐ*), HT-7 (*shén mén*), and HT-8 (*shào fǔ*) are most commonly used to treat the tongue. The use of HT-5 was de-scribed above and primarily involves deficiency of circulation at the level of the yin collaterals. HT-7, the source point of the channel, is used more for problems with development and aging that affect speech. Mental retarda-tion, developmental problems in children, or senility and Alzheimer's dis-ease in the aged, for example, fall into this category. HT-8, the fire point of the channel, is often used with GV-15 (*yǎ mén*) when the patient describes a sense of hardening and/or thickness in the tongue. This point is also used

Point	Pattern/Disorder
HT-5 (*tōng lǐ*)	Blocked collaterals of the tongue: speech problems
HT-7 (*shén mén*)	Developmental problems affecting speech
HT-8 (*shào fǔ*)	Heat leading to hardness/thickening of the tongue
KI-1 (*yōng quán*)	Qi deficiency leading to weak voice
KI-2 (*rán gǔ*)	Qi deficiency leading to weak, soft tongue
KI-4 (*dà zhōng*)	Assists HT-5 in cognition problems in the elderly
KI-6 (*zhào hǎi*)	Assists HT-5 in facilitating movement of throat/tongue
HT-3 (*shào hǎi*)	Hyperactive tongue: spleen-stomach qi deficiency

Table A2.1

Shào yīn points for treating tongue conditions

when heart heat flares upward to cause mouth sores or tenderness. Finally, HT-8 may also be used for problems with speech that are related to fear (a type of kidney *shào yīn* condition).

Continuing with the theme of *shào yīn*, kidney channel points are also used to treat tongue problems. Specifically, KI-1 *(yōng quán)* is used when a patient's voice is too weak to be clearly heard. KI-2 *(rán gǔ)* is used sometimes in the specific case of a weak, soft tongue that has trouble moving. KI-4 *(dà zhōng)*, the collateral point, is used in combination with HT-7 or HT-5 to help slow the effects of Alzheimer's. KI-6, noted above, should also be considered in cases where a patient doesn't speak because of depression, that is, an unwillingness to speak.

In addition to *shào yīn*, the *tài yīn* channel not only travels to the tongue, but, as described below, is also said to "open through the mouth." In reality, the two sometimes overlap. Consequently, the *shào yīn* channel may also be helpful for conditions elsewhere in the mouth, especially the sores and boils that often arise from digestive complaints (not limited to heart fire).

In general, the *shào yīn* heart channel (in conjunction with the kidney channel) is most often used for problems with the tongue where there is some involvement of microcirculation. This may include cognition problems, developmental disorders, problems in the elderly, or the sequelae of strokes. Treatment of problems with movement of the tongue muscles in particular can often involve the addition of other channels and vessels which may not travel directly to the tongue, specifically the *rèn*, *dū*, and *yáng míng*. When considering conditions that affect tongue function, the overriding concern should be a determination of the primary channels involved. Without clear diagnosis of the channels and organs, treatment of these conditions can be difficult.

Other tongue problems related to the *shào yīn* channel include the following:

Tongue swelling If there is heart heat, use HT-8 *(shào fǔ)*. In the case of heart qi deficiency, use the pair HT-5 *(tōng lǐ)* and KI-6 *(zhào hǎi)*.

Lack of sensation in tongue (numbness) This also falls within the domain of microcirculation and is therefore also best treated with the pair HT-5 and KI-6. In these cases, the pair is often combined with ST-24 *(huá ròu mén)*. ST-24 is a point on the *yáng míng* channel (full of qi and blood) that is classically prescribed to help with tongue problems involving deficiency.

Withered tongue This is most often due to heart fire blocked inside the upper burner. Bleeding TB-1 *(guān chōng)* can help clear upper burner heat and thus allow normal nourishment to return to the tongue.

Lolling tongue Here, the tongue hangs weakly out of the mouth; the condition is related more to kidney *shào yīn*. The uniting point of the kidney channel, KI-10 *(yīn gǔ)*, is often used for this condition in combination with CV-23 *(lián quán)*.

Difficult tongue movement When movement of the tongue is possible but not smooth, the point pair HT-5 and KI-6 is once again helpful. As noted above, if the tongue feels hard and thick, HT-8 is more appropriate.

Hyperactive tongue This is often seen in young children who are constantly moving their tongue in and out of the mouth. Often, this is seen in cases of spleen-stomach qi deficiency. In these cases, ST-24 and HT-3 *(shào hǎi)* are often helpful.

The Spleen Opens through the Mouth

Before considering the relationship of the spleen to the mouth, it is important to clearly define the concept of mouth in the context of traditional Chinese medicine. In general, and depending on the text, references to the inner cheeks, gums, lips, and, to some degree, the tongue all fall into the category of mouth. There are three primary functions of the mouth:

1. Discerning the flavor of foods

In describing the sense of taste, there is some overlap between the heart association with the tongue and the spleen association with the mouth. With regard to taste, the *Classic of Difficulties* (Chapter 37) differentiates the tongue and mouth by noting that the tongue "knows the five flavors" while the mouth "knows the flavor of grains" (知穀味 *zhī gǔ wèi*), which means that of foods. Both are obviously related to the sense of taste. As noted above, not only taste but also hunger is related to the spleen and mouth. In other words, if the appetite is weak, a patient will often be uninspired to appreciate the tastes of food. The heart, on the other hand, is involved more in conditions where the appetite may be relatively strong, but the tongue simply cannot discern flavor or the person is unable to clearly recognize appropriate foods for their body.

2. Speech

Once again, there is some overlap here with the heart and its connection to the tongue. In this case, the spleen is associated with the movements and health of the lips in particular. The musculature of (and around) the mouth, and its movements to form words in speech, depends on nourishment from the spleen.

3. Holding in qi and fluids

The ability of the mouth to 'hold qi' is also a function of the musculature around the mouth. If the muscles of the lips aren't properly nourished, not only air but also fluids may escape from the mouth. Thus one often encounters texts which associate the spleen with drooling or excess saliva.

Besides the spleen channel and its divergent channel, the stomach, liver, *rèn*, *chōng*, and *yīn wéi* vessels also travel to the mouth and its surroundings. Of these, the spleen and stomach channels are the most important as the health of the mouth and lips very often reflects the quality of spleen-stomach qi transformation. Note that the coating of the tongue also reflects the health of stomach qi.

When observing a patient in the clinic, one way to assess spleen function is to note the quality of the lips. While the gums and inner surface of the cheeks also very often reflect the health of the spleen and stomach, it is the lips that can be most easily observed.

The spleen function of governing blood and nourishing the muscles is thus woven into its relationship with the mouth. The mouth and lips are nourished by the fullness of nutritive and protective aspects of the blood and are often one of the first areas to show changes in the presence of *tài yīn* deficiency. The practitioner should take note of lips that seem to hang away from the mouth, or fail to properly shut, thus allowing loss of fluids; or lips that are dry and malnourished. These are both signs that the transformative function of spleen qi is likely affected.

CLINICAL APPROACH TO TREATING
CONDITIONS OF THE MOUTH

In general, what the spleen shows on the mouth is a reflection of digestive health. Thus, when considering points that affect the 'mouth', it is most important to have a clear diagnosis of the pathodynamic and how it affects *tài yīn* qi transformation. On the spleen channel itself, all the points below the knees have various effects on spleen qi transformation and, consequently, on the mouth as well.

Some specific mouth conditions include:

Sores and swelling In the case of mouth sores due to dampness and/or heat in the *tài yīn*, SP-5 *(shāng qiū)* can be very effective. The area around SP-5 may also be tender in cases of gum swelling related to *tài yīn*. Most often, however, swelling in the gums is related to the *yáng míng* and may therefore respond better to treatment with LI-7 *(wēn liū)*.

Point	Pattern/Disorder
SP-5 *(shāng qiū)*	Spleen dampness: hot mouth sores
LI-7 *(wēn liū)*	Hot-type gum swelling
SP-3 *(tài bái)*	Deficiency-type drooling (especially in children)
LI-3 *(sān jiān)*	Bad breath: *yáng míng* fire
PC-8 *(láo gōng)*	Assists other points in clearing heat from upper burner
GB-34 *(yáng líng quán)*	*Shào yáng* stasis leading to bitter taste

Table A2.2
Common points for treating the mouth

Drooling In case of excess drooling, especially in children, the combination of SP-3 *(tài bái)*, ST-36 *(zú sān lǐ)*, and CV-24 *(chéng jiāng)* is helpful. This condition was often seen in China decades ago in cases of malnutrition and responds very well to acupuncture.

Other conditions that may be associated with the mouth can involve the qi transformation of other channels. Among other examples are the following:

Bad breath and bitter taste This is often a reflection of *yáng míng* heat trapped in the upper burner. It might be treated by clearing fire from the *yáng míng* and the upper burner by combining LI-3 *(sān jiān)* with a fire-clearing point like PC-8 *(láo gōng)*. On the other hand, a more pronounced bitter taste is often a sign of heat trapped in the *shào yáng* pivot, which responds better to regulation of the pivot with the *shào yáng* uniting point, GB-34 *(yáng líng quán)*.

The Lung Opens through the Nose

The relationship of the lung to the nose is slightly different than the relationship of the spleen to the mouth or the heart to the tongue, for example. It is less often the case that actual nose problems like nasal polyps or problems with the sense of smell can be treated with points from lung *tài yīn*. Instead, the relationship of the lung to the nose is woven into the anatomy of breathing and the physiology of immunity.

If the lung organ is having problems breathing due to exterior invasion or protective qi deficiency, symptoms may present as nasal congestion. Treatment, however, usually involves opening the nasal passages with more local points like GV-23 *(shàng xīng)*, GB-20 *(fēng chí)*, or LI-20 *(yíng xiāng)*.

This clinical approach reflects the traditional channel pathways. In fact, classical sources show that neither the lung channel nor any of its collateral or divergent channels travel to the nose. Instead, both of the *yáng míng* channels (stomach and large intestine) and both of the *tài yáng* channels (bladder and small intestine) reach the nose and surrounding area. In addition, the *dū* and *yīn qiāo* vessels, as well as a divergent channel of the heart, travel to the nose.

Consequently, when there are problems with the nose, one must consider the health of the body's protective qi. This might mean considering the lung *tài yīn*, but could just as easily include the spleen *tài yīn*, bladder *tài yáng*, or even kidney *shào yīn*. The key to treating nasal disorders lies in stepping out of the box that rigidly associates the nose exclusively with the lung. Furthermore, one should consider all of the complex physiology which gives rise to protective qi. Although protective qi is often associated with the lung, it also travels to the surface of the body at the level of *tài yáng*. As noted in Chapter 5, protective qi is produced by the harmonized qi transformation of the *tài yīn* spleen and lung but depends on the beating of the heart for its movement around the body to areas just outside the vessels. The kidney is also involved as the purveyor of source qi that stimulates the entire process via its pathway in the triple burner. Thinking in these broad physiological patterns is a much more useful way to approach symptoms that manifest in the nose than falling back on a rigid association of that orifice with the lung.

CLINICAL APPROACH TO TREATING NASAL CONDITIONS

In general, nasal problems are most often treated with the *yáng míng* and *dū* channels and can be broken down into the following categories:

Sinusitis, blocked nasal passages   When the nasal passages are blocked due to sinus infection, the most common points used are GV-23 *(shàng xīng)*, LI-20 *(yíng xiāng)*, GB-20 *(fēng chí)*, LI-4 *(hé gǔ)*, and GV-16 *(fēng fǔ)*. In cases of chronic sinusitis, GV-23 and/or ST-36 *(zú sān lǐ)* are often treated with moxa.

Sneezing, runny nose, allergies   In these cases, one might regulate the lung *tài yīn* by using the uniting point LU-5 *(chǐ zé)* in combination with KI-7 *(fù liū)*, a point pair discussed in Chapter 20. In addition, the nasal pathways can be opened up with LI-20 and GB-20, as described above. One should also palpate the *dū* vessel between GV-24 *(shén tíng)* and GV-22 *(xìn huì)*, and the

Point	Appropriate Indications
GV-22 *(xìn huì)*	Adult allergies (use moxa)
GV-23 *(shàng xīng)*	Chronic, deficiency-type allergies and/or nasal polyps
GV-24 *(shén tíng)*	Deficiency-type allergies: check around this point for softness, then needle
GV-25 *(sù liáo)*	Chronic phlegm accumulation in nose and sinuses
BL-5 *(wǔ chù)*	For defensive qi deficiency, check the area around and between these two points; needle soft-weak areas
BL-7 *(tōng tiān)*	
LI-4 *(hé gǔ)*	Command point for the head and face
LI-20 *(yíng xiāng)*	*Yáng míng* heat stasis in the nasal passageways
GB-20 *(fēng chí)*	*Shào yáng* phlegm-heat stasis
GB-39 *(xuán zhōng)*	Dry nasal passages (use moxa)
LU-3 *(tiān fǔ)*	Nosebleed: press to stop
LU-5 *(chǐ zé)*	Regulates the *tài yīn* to stimulate production of nutritive-protective aspect
KI-7 *(fù liū)*	Strengthens kidney yin (with LU-5 *[chǐ zé]*) for deficiency-type allergies

Table A2.3
Common points for treating the nose

bladder channel between BL-5 *(wǔ chù)* and BL-7 *(tōng tiān),* for other active points or areas of softness. In adults, GV-22 may also be treated with moxa.

Nasal polyps In these cases, the nose is completely occluded by benign nasal tumors. Often associated with chronic sinusitis, this condition often responds to strong moxa treatment at GV-23. Also consider BL-4 *(qū chāi)* and GV-25 *(sù liáo).* If polyps are larger and more advanced, the use of acupuncture and moxa can help reduce the symptoms, but is rarely curative. In some cases, surgery is the best option.

Dry nasal passageways, nosebleed Classical sources describe using moxa at GB-39 *(xuán zhōng)* for dry nasal passageways. If dryness leads to nosebleed, there is often a very tender spot around LU-3 *(tiān fǔ).* This area can be pressed to help stop an acute nosebleed or needled preventatively.

The Kidney Opens through the Ears

The relationship of the kidney to the ears is often misunderstood and sometimes leads to ineffective clinical treatment. Classical references that link the kidney to the ears should be placed in the context of the kidney as an organ involved in the grand arc of growth, development, and decline through the stages of life. In short, the kidney is most often related to hearing problems in the elderly, when the kidney essence is thought to wane.

The relationship of the kidney to the ears is thus a systemic one. If bones throughout the body are weakening with age, the bones of the ear may be weakening as well. In fact, like the nose and the lung described above, classical sources mention no direct channel connections of the kidney to the ear. Instead, both *tài yáng* channels (bladder and small intestine), both *shào yáng* channels (triple burner and gallbladder), and both *yáng míng* channels (large intestine collateral and stomach main channel) connect to the ears. In other words, the ears are effused with all of the yang channels. Because of the anatomy of the inner ear, an area filled with fluids that do not circulate well, there is a need for the constant stimulus of yang movement.

Consider ear anatomy a bit further. This organ is divided into an outer, middle, and inner ear. It is helpful to realize that each section of the ear is affected by different aspects of classical Chinese physiology. The outer ear is basically a conveyor of sound inward; it is made of cartilage connected by ligaments to the head. Problems in this area largely fall within the purview of dermatology in both Western and Chinese medicine. The middle ear is an open area that contains three bones (malleus, incus, and stapes) that convert the sound waves bouncing off the eardrum into movement that is then conveyed to the fluid-filled passageways of the inner ear. Eventually, small hairs within the curved membrane-lined passageways of the inner ear convert the movement of sound waves in liquid into a nerve impulse that is relayed to the brain. Thus a general system exists that involves membranes, bones, fluids, hair, and nerves. Each of these structures may be associated with the physiology of different organs in the Chinese physiological system, as shown in Fig. A2.3. This is obviously a simplification of a very complex process, but one that can help guide the practitioner of Chinese medicine.

As with any case in Chinese medicine, an ear-related complaint should be categorized as involving either excess or deficiency. If due to excess, it will largely involve problems with dampness or heat in the fluids of the ear. If due to deficiency, it often involves the movement of bones and the tendons that hold those bones in place. In classical physiology, one might then generally place excess-related ear problems within the purview of *tài yīn* and *shào yáng* (dampness and heat). Because of internal channel con-

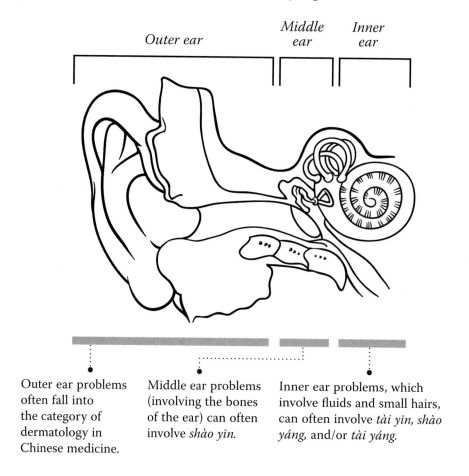

Outer ear problems often fall into the category of dermatology in Chinese medicine.

Middle ear problems (involving the bones of the ear) can often involve *shào yīn*.

Inner ear problems, which involve fluids and small hairs, can often involve *tài yīn, shào yáng,* and/or *tài yáng*.

Fig. A2.3
Each section of the ear is affected by
different aspects of classical Chinese physiology.

nections, the *tài yáng* small intestine is also helpful in treating excess. Deficiency-related ear problems are often systemic and usually involve the *shào yīn* kidney or *jué yīn* channels (bones, blood distribution, and tendons).

CLINICAL APPROACH TO TREATING EAR CONDITIONS

Ear problems, especially those associated with deficiency, can be difficult to treat. Relatively acute cases of excess dampness and heat are by far the easiest to treat with Chinese medicine. This includes problems with balance due to inner-ear abnormalities. In cases of deficiency, improvement is gradual at best. Ear problems may be broken down into the following categories:

Tinnitus

Deficiency-type tinnitus This is low-pitched tinnitus that is often worse in the afternoon or if the patient is tired. Treatment should include stimulation of yang circulation through the use of the channels which travel to the area. TB-21 *(ěr mén)*, GB-3 *(shàng guān)*, SI-4 *(wàn gǔ)*, and GV-20 *(bǎi huì)* can be useful in such cases. Often, these patients may have coexisting dampness and thus SP-9 *(yīn líng quán)* might be added. In these cases, herbs that transform dampness should also be included in the formula that is prescribed.

Excess-type tinnitus This is high-pitched and often more acute. The point pair TB-5 *(wài guān)* and GB-41 *(zú lín qì)* can dredge and drain *shào yáng* in such cases and might be combined with TB-2 *(yè mén)*. One should also palpate the *shào yáng* points around the ears, TB-21 and GB-2 *(tīng huì)*, to check for local qi and blood stasis.

Deafness

Deafness is extremely difficult to treat. If there is no hearing at all, then Chinese medicine cannot treat the condition. In general, the term 'deafness' in Chinese literature refers to diminished hearing. In that context, some types of deafness are easier to treat than others:

Diminished hearing As noted above, this refers to a condition in which hearing acuity is reduced. Simply put, sounds are less loud than before. This should be differentiated from a problem in discerning sounds, discussed below. Cases of this type are often treated with SI-3 *(hòu xī)* and BL-65 *(shù gǔ)*, both of which are stream points, to invigorate the channel qi in their respective channels. BL-23 *(shèn shū)* can also be used to strengthen the kidney, while TB-7 *(huì zōng)*, the cleft point of the triple burner, can be used if excess stasis is suspected.

	Often involves	Affected channels
Deficiency	Problems with smooth movement of the bones of the ear, or with blood circulation in the ligaments which hold these bones in place	*Shào yīn* (especially kidney) and *jué yīn*
Excess	Dampness and heat affecting the fluids of the ear	*Tài yīn, shào yáng,* and/or *tài yáng*

Table A2.4
Excess and deficiency in the ear

Gradual deafness that begins with tinnitus This is a condition of excess that has transformed into deficiency. It rarely responds to treatment with either acupuncture or herbs.

Sudden deafness This is the type of deafness that comes on suddenly as a result of exterior invasion, high fever, or stress. In such cases, GB-31 *(fēng shì)* should be stimulated very strongly while the patient holds the ears and blows out. Once again, the goal is to strongly move the *shào yáng*.

Problems with discerning sounds This is the type of ear problem most clearly associated with the qi transformation of the kidney. In Chinese medicine, this form of impaired hearing is called 'heavy hearing' (重聽 *zhòng tīng)* and is often a complaint in aging patients. Physiologically, it involves a lack of clear yang qi in the head due to the gradual decline of the fire at the gate of vitality. Treatment is thus systemic and involves points like KI-3 *(tài xī)*, ST-36 *(zú sān lǐ)*, CV-6 *(qì hǎi)*, GV-4 *(mìng mén)*, and GV-14 *(dà zhuī)*. Moxa is often used on these points.

Ear pain

Pain in the ears should be evaluated by an ear specialist. If, after examination, no treatable cause is found, then acupuncture can help reduce the symptoms. Treatment may include moxa at GB-3 *(shàng guān)*, and needling at GB-20 *(fēng chí)* and TB-21 *(ěr mén)*.

Conclusion

The most important thing to keep in mind when treating problems with the senses, as with everything else in Chinese medicine, is to consider the entire physiological system. When working in the clinic, one should avoid the type of thinking that says, "Ah, this patient has problems with her eyes; it must be a liver condition" and the like. By considering the channel pathways and channel theory, one can begin to get a picture of how problems with the sensory organs reflect imbalances in the internal organs.

The practitioner should also keep in mind that, even when a problem with one of the five orifices is not itself the chief complaint, one can gain important diagnostic information by asking careful questions about the patient's perception of their world and the ways that perception is affected by the openness (通 *tōng)* of the orifices.

CASE STUDIES

THE FOLLOWING ARE representative case studies from the private practices of two of Dr. Wang's students in North America. Case numbers 1 to 3 are from C.T. Holman, L.Ac. and case numbers 4 to 6 are from Jason Robertson, L.Ac. These cases represent the creative application of the treatment approach described in this text.

■ Case No. 1

36-year-old female

Chief complaint   Significant loss of both smell and taste for three years

History of present illness   The condition began three years earlier after using significant amounts of a weed-killing agent in her yard. Following exposure to the strong smell of this agent, she lost much of her sense of smell. Over time, the condition worsened until it now also affects her sense of taste. Upon presentation, the patient was able to smell only strong chemicals such as cleaning and gardening agents. She was unable to smell more delicate scents such as flowers, food, or perfume. Visits to specialists led to no conclusive diagnosis or treatment.

The patient also reported low energy, constipation, difficulty in both falling and staying asleep, and depression.

Her pulse was thin. Her tongue was pale purple with a thick, white coating.

Channel palpation   There were a series of small soft nodules all along the lung channel. On the spleen channel, the patient reported tenderness around SP-9 *(yīn líng quán)* while a small, firm nodule could be palpated at SP-4

(gōng sūn). The triple burner channel had an overall roughness that felt like an ungraded road. There was also tenderness at LR-3 *(tài chōng)*

Diagnosis Blockage of *tài yīn* collaterals with concurrent qi stagnation affecting *shào yáng*

Treatment The following points were needled on the right side: LU-5 *(chǐ zé)*, ST-36 *(zú sān lǐ)*, ST-40 *(fēng lóng)*, and GB-41 *(zú lín qì)*. At the same time, LI-4 *(hé gǔ)*, SP-9 *(yīn líng quán)*, and SP-4 *(gōng sūn)* were needled on the left. GV-20 *(bǎi huì)* was also needled.

Technique involved first needling the collateral points ST-40 and SP-4 with a strong draining technique to open microcirculation in the areas associated with *tài yīn*. To clear *shào yáng*, a draining technique was also used on GB-41. Next, LU-5 and SP-9 were needled and then stimulated with an even technique. Because of some underlying deficiency, a tonifying technique was used on ST-36.

Results Results were fairly dramatic in this case. The patient reported that, after one treatment, there was significant improvement in both her sense of smell and taste. During the five days following the first treatment, smell and taste returned to a level she described as normal. She was able to discern the smells of both syrup and flowers, for example. On follow-up two years later, the condition had not returned.

Analysis Upon initial presentation, the patient's primary symptom pattern appeared to be stagnation in the collaterals of *tài yīn*. In particular, the sense of smell was affected by a lack of microcirculation in the collaterals of the nose. This is a case where a strong, aromatic (toxic) external pathogen had literally burned the collaterals of the nose. The patient may have had a pre-existing tendency to *tài yīn* deficiency with concurrent fluid accumulation, as reflected in the thin pulse and thick, white tongue coating.

At the same time, there was qi stagnation affecting the *shào yáng*. She mentioned that both before and since the onset of the condition, she experienced a great deal of stress. It might also be surmised that the toxic external pathogen had affected other parts of the body, possibly becoming trapped in the pathways of the triple burner. Channel palpation revealed bumpiness all along the path of the triple burner channel, which is often seen in cases of chronic, systemic inflammation.

Acupuncture treatment focused on both reversing the counterflow and opening the collateral vessels of *tài yīn*. The lead point pair in this case was ST-40 and SP-4, as collateral points affecting the *tài yīn* (internal-external pair). Of course, one might also have used the lung channel collateral point

LU-7 *(liè quē)*, but, in this case, the association of ST-40 with the clearing of phlegm accumulation made it a more appropriate choice.

Next, three uniting points (ST-36, LU-5 and SP-9) were used to reverse counterflow so as to strongly reestablish proper movement in the *tài yīn*. Finally, GB-41 was used to help clear and drain the *shào yáng* stasis, while LI-4, the command point of the face and head, was used to guide the effects of the treatment toward the nose.

It is interesting to note that this case provides an example of a slight modification of the bilateral needling approach. Here, an effective treatment was devised which involved using point pairs on opposing internal-external channels crossways on opposite limbs. The points on the left and right sides of the body were different. This is a common and very effective approach which can help the practitioner affect more channels without using too many needles.

The results in this case were surprising in that they were almost immediate and sustained. This illustrates one of those cases where, by facilitating qi and blood circulation to the affected area, the body quickly reestablishes normal function.

■ Case No. 2

55-year-old female

Chief complaint   Lower left quadrant abdominal pain

History of present illness   Upon presentation, the patient reported having a strong, sharp pain and ache in her lower left quadrant which had persisted for three days. The symptoms varied throughout the day, increasing with both stress and fatigue. One month before, experiencing a similar pain, the patient visited her doctor and underwent a CT scan which revealed a series of small cysts on the upper pole of her left kidney. Her urologist suggested that the abdominal pain may be due to referred pain from the cysts on her kidney. A gynecological cause was ruled out given that the patient underwent a complete hysterectomy twenty years previously. The patient came to the clinic in the past for treatment of significant epigastric pain, which had responded favorably to acupuncture, herbs, and occasional use of over-the-counter antacids. Upon presentation for the current complaint, she also complained of fatigue, stress and constipation.

At this time, she had neither low back pain nor fever.

Her pulse was thready and particularly weak in the proximal positions on both sides. Her tongue was slightly pale and swollen, but generally appeared normal.

Channel palpation   In channel palpation, the most notable changes were found on the kidney channel and *rèn* vessel. There was discernible softness and lack of muscle tone in the area between KI-3 *(tài xī)* and KI-7 *(fù liū)*. There was also severe tenderness in the medial knee around KI-10 *(yīn gǔ)*. On the abdomen, strong pulsations could be palpated at both the CV-6 *(qì hǎi)* and CV-9 *(shuǐ fēn)* points. In addition, both KI-16 *(huāng shū)* points were extremely tender when pressed. When treated in the past, the patient had always had significant palpatory changes along the spleen channel. Upon presentation for this complaint, however, although the spleen channel continued to exhibit tenderness and some nodules, they were less significant than those found on the kidney channel. It is noteworthy that, while the spleen channel changes had improved over time, there was a marked increase in the above-described changes along the kidney channel.

Diagnosis   *Shào yīn* disharmony: impairment of fluid metabolism

Treatment   As in the previous case, treatment utilized different channels on the right and left sides. On the right, HT-7 *(shén mén)*, BL-39 *(wěi yáng)*, and ST-36 *(zú sān lǐ)* were needled, while on the left side, SI-3 *(hòu xī)*, KI-10 *(yīn gǔ)* and KI-3 *(tài xī)* were used. In addition, GV-21 *(qián dǐng)* was needled and both KI-16 *(huāng shū)* and ST-28 *(shuǐ dào)* were needled bilaterally on the abdomen. Finally, an *a-shi* point was needled very gently on the left side, lateral to ST-28. The kidney and *shén mén* (neurogate) points were also needled on the right ear. Tonifying technique was used at HT-7, KI-3, and ST-36 while an even technique was used at KI-10 and KI-16. The yang channel (stomach and bladder) points were treated with a draining technique.

Results   The patient reported a significant reduction in pain on the night following the first treatment. She came again for treatment three days later and, after that, reported that the pain had completely resolved. She had two follow-up treatments over the next few weeks. These treatments continued the use of KI-10 and KI-16, but added CV-9 *(shuǐ fēn)* and *tài yīn* points in view of her history of epigastric pain and the palpated condition along her spleen channel. During the months following the first visit, she had one minor recurrence of low abdominal pain, which also resolved following a treatment similar to that described above.

   During the two weeks following the initial treatment, the condition of her abdomen improved significantly. Following the first two treatments, the pulsing palpated at CV-6 and CV-9 diminished. Of particular gratification to the patient, the extreme tenderness at KI-16 had also quickly abated and could be pressed with little discomfort.

Analysis   This case provides another interesting example of the use of channel palpation to help refine diagnosis and treatment. While abdominal palpation in cases such as this is relatively common, the use of distal channel palpation helped to refine channel selection. In particular, given the involvement of fluid metabolism and the patient's history of epigastric pain, it might have also been tempting to include spleen or stomach channel points in this treatment. However, because the kidney channel had significant, newly-developed changes while the spleen channel remained relatively unchanged, treatment was able to focus on *shào yīn*. One might have used spleen channel points, but the effects may have been slower and/or less complete.

It is interesting to note that, on visits two months prior for epigastric pain, weakness had been noted at both KI-3 and KI-7. However, when asked about the presence of kidney type symptoms (low back pain, urinary irregularity) she reported that she had none. Consequently, early treatment focused more on *tài yīn*. In retrospect, it might have been appropriate to consider those early changes as predictive of an underlying condition that should also have been addressed.

Consideration of the points chosen for treatment is also interesting. The lead point pairs in this case included both the HT-7 and KI-3 source points and the BL-39 and KI-10 uniting point pair. As source points on the *shào yīn* pivot, the HT-7 and KI-3 pair acts to warm and stimulate source qi and the ultimate root of fluid transformation. The addition of SI-3, stream point on the paired *tài yáng* channel, helps to further accentuate *movement* at *shào yīn* to help reduce pain. At the same time, because there is significant impairment of the qi dynamic due to fluid accumulation, the strong regulating effects of uniting points are also called for. BL-39 is the lower uniting point of the triple burner. The movement of fluids throughout the body can be harmonized by using this point. In a synergistic way, the kidneys were regulated with the kidney uniting point (KI-10).

Note as well the use of GV-21 *(qián dǐng)* in this case. Dr. Wang often uses this point to facilitate the rising of clear yang qi to the head. This approach is appropriate in cases where fluid (phlegm) accumulation has begun to mist upward and affect cognition. In this case, it provides a nice upper balancing point for the prescription. ST-36 was used to create general stimulus from the fullness of *yáng míng* qi and blood. Finally, local points on the abdomen were used (KI-16, ST-28 and a left-side *a-shi* point) to direct the treatment to the location of the disease.

In this case, a chronic build-up of fluids led to a diminished qi dynamic in the lower abdomen. In this area, when there is deficiency and fluid accumulation, the bladder organ and channel must obviously be considered as well. Long term herbal and acupuncture treatment would focus on regulating the function of both the *shào yīn* and *tài yáng* so as to help the kidney cysts gradually resolve.

■ Case No. 3

58-year-old female

Chief complaint   Heart throbbing/palpitations

History of present illness   The patient described both an acute awareness of her heart beat and a sense of irregularity in its rhythm that had been ongoing for a month. The sensation tended to occur mainly at night and often coincided with an acute sense of anxiety. Her blood pressure was normal (120/75).

The patient had come to the clinic in the past for the treatment of tooth pain and symptoms associated with menopause. Those symptoms included a general sense of increased warmth, occasional night sweats, frequent urination in the evenings, and dry skin. These symptoms preceded the onset of the throbbing and palpitations.

In general, the patient tended to be anxious, often becoming very focused on health complaints, and was therefore quite aware of the irregular sensations in her heart beat.

The patient's tongue body appeared small and red with a thin, white coating. In the past, the tongue coating exhibited a tendency to occasionally have a thicker, yellowish coating in the center and back. The pulse was thready and rapid-irregular (促脈 *cù mài*).

Channel palpation   Because of confidence in the diagnosis given her symptoms, pulse, tongue, and peri-menopausal status, channel palpation was skipped during the first few visits for this case.

Diagnosis   Heart-kidney *(shào yīn)* yin deficiency with heat

Treatment   Points were chosen to facilitate the connection between the heart and kidney. For three, once-weekly treatments, *shào yīn* points were used in combination with points on the *yáng míng* channel to address a concurrent *yáng míng* channel tooth pain. The *yáng míng* points included LI-4 *(hé gǔ)* and LI-11 *(qū chí)* on the right side ipsilateral to the tooth pain. On the *shào yīn* channel, either HT-7 *(shén mén)* or HT-5 *(tōng lǐ)* were needled on the left side, combined with either KI-7 *(fù liū)* or KI-6 *(zhào hǎi)* respectively on the right leg.

Herbs

A variation of Prepared Licorice Decoction *(zhì gān cǎo tāng)* was given in granules with the following dosage:

Rehmanniae Radix *(shēng dì huáng)*—12g
Glycyrrhizae Radix preparata *(zhì gān cǎo)*—9g
Ginseng Radix *(rén shēn)*—6g
Cinnamomi Ramulus *(guì zhī)*—7g
Ophiopogonis Radix *(mài mén dōng)*—7g
Asini Corii Colla *(ē jiāo)*—5g
Cannabis Semen *(huǒ má rén)*—6g
Gardeniae Fructus *(zhī zǐ)*—5g
Polygoni multiflori Caulis *(yè jiāo téng)*—7g
Citri reticulatae Pericarpium *(chén pí)*—5g
Zingiberis Rhizoma recens *(shēng jiāng)*—3g
Jujubae Fructus *(dà zǎo)*—3g

Results   By the third treatment, the patient reported improvement in the sense of throbbing (palpitations) but could still feel an irregular heart beat when she palpated her pulse. At this point, the patient decided to see a cardiologist. Using an electrocardiogram (EKG), the cardiologist confirmed that she did, in fact, have a mild irregularity of her heart beat but felt the condition to be so mild as to not require medication. The patient therefore returned for her fourth visit.

Reevaluation   Given the patient's obvious concern, careful channel palpation was undertaken to look for confirmation or adjustment of the original diagnosis. Interestingly, upon palpation, the heart, pericardium, and kidney channels exhibited relatively few notable changes. On the other hand, the lung channel presented with diffuse nodules throughout the forearm while the spleen channel was generally extremely tender and had increased muscle tone (tightness), especially at SP-9 *(yīn líng quán)*. On the *rèn* vessel, the areas around both CV-9 *(shuǐ fēn)* and CV-12 *(zhōng wǎn)* were both tight and tender.

Because of the new information provided by channel palpation, other signs and symptoms were also reconsidered. In particular, the patient claimed to have had quite a bit of difficulty loosing weight in recent years and often complained of swelling in her fingers. Despite the fact that her digestion (including appetite and bowel movements) were normal, a new diagnosis was made of *tài yīn* disharmony with fluid accumulation.

Second round of treatment   For the second round of treatment, a paired *tài yīn / yáng míng* approach was used. Specifically, on the left, LU-5 *(chǐ zé)* and ST-36 *(zú sān lǐ)* were used, and on the right, LI-11 *(qū chí)* and SP-9 *(yīn líng quán)*.

LI-4 *(hé gǔ)* was also chosen on the right in view of the continued, occasional tooth pain on that side. (It was later revealed that the patient had an abscess in her gums below a tooth, and the affected tooth was removed by her dentist.)

Herbs

The patient continued taking the same herbal formula as above.

Results   After three (once weekly) treatments using the above approach, the patient reported a noticeable improvement in the irregular heart beat. The irregularity slowly disappeared over a series of months (treatments eventually became twice monthly). Two years after the initial visit, the patient reported no occurrence of either irregular heart beat or palpitations for six months.

Analysis   This case provides a clear example of how channel palpation will sometimes differ from an initial diagnosis made by eight-parameter and radial pulse diagnosis. In these situations, it is often important to return to the asking of questions so as to reevaluate the initial hypothesis. Menopausal women often exhibit complex patterns that go beyond the typical kidney yin and yang deficiency types. Because of the decline in stimulus from the gate of vitality, the spleen in particular can be affected in women of this age. When in doubt as to which type of pattern is presenting, channel palpation will often provide the necessary clues for making a correct diagnosis.

Also, as all of us who have studied with Dr. Wang have found, sometimes in the clinic one gets too busy to do careful palpatory diagnosis, especially in situations where the diagnosis seems to be clear given the symptom-pattern. Sometimes, one can get away with quick channel palpation to confirm or deny one's initial hypothesis. Often, however, in the hurry to move on to treatment, one sees what one expects to see and sometimes misses other clues. This case provides an example of how what might at first appear to be a case that is not responding well to acupuncture can be turned around.

■ Case No. 4

48-year-old female

Chief complaint   Severe low abdominal pain and urinary discomfort

History of present illness   Upon presentation, the patient reported frequent, stabbing, and often debilitating lower abdominal pain off and on for the previous six months. The pain was associated with difficult urination. Specifically, she complains of a sense of incomplete urination that is difficult and painful to initiate, along with stress incontinence. Although the pain and urinary symptoms were originally rather infrequent, they had recently occurred almost daily. On days when the pain was less obvious, her urination was also more normal. The abdominal pain was particularly noticeable as a sharp pain to the right of the umbilicus at ST-28 *(shuǐ dào),* which tended to radiate downward toward the groin. All of the symptoms were significantly worse with fatigue or physical exertion—lifting is particularly difficult. When severe, her entire body became extremely cold and she had an acute sense of exhaustion, which was only relieved by bed rest. The symptoms were improved with rest and a low-acid diet. Her biomedical physician diagnosed interstitial cystitis.

The patient had a history of frequent urinary tract infections, painful menstruation, and an irregular heart beat. Ten years before, the patient had a hysterectomy during which her ovaries were not removed. Recently, she experienced what she described as peri-menopausal depression and night sweats. Her temperature fluctuated somewhat between feeling very warm in the mornings and evenings to suddenly feeling cold when the symptoms became severe. She reported that her sleep was restless and that she could get to sleep but woke throughout the night "for no reason." On the first visit, the patient complained of a tendency to get laryngitis quite easily and sounded hoarse. Her digestion, appetite, and bowel movements were normal (however she did have a history of occasional bouts of constipation).

Her pulse was thready-wiry overall and particularly deep and weak at the proximal positions. Her tongue body was small and pale with a dry, white coating and a reddish tip. The patient appeared quite healthy with a robust body type, good facial skin tone, and a normal gait.

Channel palpation On the *tài yīn* channel, a small, firm, movable nodule was palpated below LU-5 *(chǐ zé)* while skin in the area around SP-9 *(yīn líng quán)* felt extremely tight and was quite tender to the touch. The *shào yīn* channel, by contrast, presented with a general sense of deficiency. There was a series of very small, soft nodules around HT-6 *(yīn xī)* while the kidney channel was slightly swollen, but soft and cold to the touch, around KI-7 *(fù liū).* On the *shào yáng* channel there was a very clear, broad line of diffuse soft nodules along the triple burner channel which felt like an "ungraded road." On the gallbladder channel, GB-34 *(yáng líng quán)* was also a bit tender. Finally, the lower abdomen was cold to the touch.

Diagnosis *Shào yáng* source qi deficiency with cold accumulation affecting the pathways of the triple burner

Treatment In this case, treatment involved a combination of contralateral same-name channel pair needling and bilateral needling. LU-5 *(chǐ zé)* on the right was combined with SP-9 *(yīn líng quán)* on the left, while TB-6 *(zhī gōu)*

on the left was combined with GB-34 *(yáng líng quán)* on the right. KI-7 *(fù liū)* was needled bilaterally, and a heat lamp was placed over the abdomen, focused on CV-6 *(qì hǎi)*.

Results At the next visit, the symptoms had not changed. In fact, the patient now had a fairly severe cold with congestion in her sinuses. The same treatment was continued, but followed this time with GV-14 *(dà zhuī)* and BL-13 *(fèi shū)* bilaterally to help release the exterior condition.

At her third visit, there was a reduction in the intensity of the abdominal pain and urinary difficulty. For this treatment, points were added at ST-28 *(shuǐ dào)*, CV-9 *(shuǐ fēn)*, and BL-7 *(tōng tiān,* discussed below) after which the condition continued to improve. At each treatment, a heat lamp was also used on the lower abdomen. Altogether, a series of twelve treatments were used over a period of ten weeks, generally using the points described above. Three months after the first visit, the patient reported no abdominal pain and normal urination. She found that she was able to re-introduce certain high-acid foods in controlled amounts. Also, she was able to resume more active physical activities without any recurrence of pain, fatigue, or cold.

Analysis This is an instance where what appeared to be a fairly complex case responded to a reasonably simple treatment generated by integrating the eight-principle and channel palpation diagnostic approaches.

The initial diagnostic hypothesis (before palpation) was of kidney yang qi deficiency. That diagnosis was modified based on the palpated findings. The kidney deficiency was confirmed somewhat by the puffy softness on the kidney channel. However, palpation pointed to the importance of a concurrent excess fluid accumulation. Specifically, nodules and tenderness along the *tài yīn* channel suggested involvement of not only the kidney, but also the fluid transformation functions of the spleen.

At the same time, there was the important diagnostic indicator of diffuse bumpiness along the triple burner channel. What was one to make of this? This is a case of multiple channels being involved in what is still, primarily, a case of *shào yīn* deficiency. Because of the complex interrelationship of fluid metabolism (see Fig. 8.6 in Chapter 8), it is quite easy for the physiology of other organs to become affected in cases of kidney yang qi deficiency. In this case, underlying kidney deficiency was failing not only to adequately support the transformations of the spleen, but also to properly diffuse the source qi through the pathways of the triple burner. Fundamentally, it was the systemic source qi deficiency which led to the more recent presentation. The frequent, difficult urination was of a deficient type, while the tendency to a complete collapse of yang (cold, sudden, severe fatigue) indicated a lack of connection between prenatal and postnatal qi.

The palpated changes on the triple burner channel were thus crucial to a further refinement of the initial diagnosis. They directly influenced the choice of treatment strategy, not only because *shào yáng* points were used, but also because the new information influenced the specific point choices on the *tài yīn* channel as well. Specifically, the LU-5 and SP-9 point pair was chosen because of its broad qi- and fluid-regulating actions (as opposed to the qi-building actions of the LU-9 *(tài yuān)* and SP-3 *(tài bái)* pair, for example).

As for the chosen *shào yáng* pair (TB-6 and GB-34), this strongly-moving pair was used in initial treatments to clear the passageways of the triple burner. Later treatments also alternated with the more tonifying source point pair of TB-4 *(yáng chí)* and GB-40 *(qiū xū)*.

Finally, the use of BL-7 *(tōng tiān)* is noteworthy. Dr. Wang often refers to the area around this point either as 'lung palace' (肺殿 *fèi diàn)* or 'gate of vitality point' (命門穴 *mìng mén xué)*. His understanding and use of this point seems to have evolved in recent years. It is most often used in cases of chronic, difficult-to-treat cough, but has also been used, as the name implies, in cases where there is a kind of deficiency in the provision of source qi from the gate of vitality. If you're thinking of using this point, it is very important to palpate the area. Dr. Wang believes that the point is most often found on the right side, but occasionally, when the same area on the left feels tender or 'squishy' to the touch, he will use the one on the left. The point is needled subcutaneously with a 1.5-inch needle. Once the needle is in place, it is held with the right hand and the skin on top of the needle is stimulated with the left hand. Dr. Wang describes the resulting effect as being like rubbing two pieces of cloth together so as to generate static electricity. Once this technique has been completed, the needle is retained for the rest of the treatment.

■ Case No. 5

40-year-old male

Chief complaint Severe shoulder pain for three months

History of present illness The patient complained of severe left-sided shoulder pain resulting from an injury sustained during a bar fight three months earlier. During the fight (which spilled out onto the street), the patient was thrown to the ground and landed with all of his weight on his extended left hand (arm locked). The full shock of the fall was absorbed by his shoulder. Repeated visits to the doctor revealed no broken bones or significant muscle or tendon tears, and he was diagnosed as having severe tendinitis. A chiropractor did note a displaced tendon in the rotator cuff that was repeatedly put back into place over the previous six weeks; when the tendon was in place, he felt much better. However, the tendon kept coming back out of place, which caused severe pain and a very limited range of motion.

For eight weeks prior to his visit, the patient had suffered from nausea, with increasing sensitivity to most foods. At the time of his first visit, he had been eating nothing but peanut butter and chocolate for the previous two days. The patient reported a fuzzy sensation in the head and a sense of muddled thinking. He described the arm pain as radiating from the shoulder (large intestine channel focus) down through the lateral forearm (lung channel).

The pulse was generally slippery, but wiry in the middle position on both sides. The tongue was normal in both size and color, and had a thin, noticeably yellow coating.

Channel palpation   Palpation revealed points of sensitivity at both LI-14 *(bì nào)* and LI-15 *(jiān yú)*. There was also a soft, tender nodule at LI-10 *(shǒu sān lǐ)*. In addition, very clear, small, purplish vessels could be seen in the area around ST-40 *(fēng lóng)* on the right side, with accompanying tenderness throughout the stomach channel on the lateral right leg (which was also swollen).

Diagnosis   Qi and blood stasis in the collaterals of the *yáng míng*

Treatment   The lead point pair for this case was LI-6 *(piān lì)* and ST-40 *(fēng lóng)*, which was combined with SP-9 *(yīn líng quán)*, LU-5 *(chǐ zé)*, and LI-11 *(qū chí)*. All points were needled bilaterally. For the first two treatments, the visible collaterals at ST-40 on the right were bled before needling using a lancet (15–20 drops removed). In addition, a 2-inch needle was used to connect LI-14 to LI-15 on the unaffected (right) side.

Results   The patient reported a reduction in both pain and radiation down the channel after the first treatment, which lasted roughly twenty-four hours. The same points were used for three subsequent treatments, during which the pain abated for longer and longer periods of time. At the fifth treatment, LI-14 and LI-15 were needled on the affected (left) side. After eight treatments the shoulder pain had resolved and, encouragingly, the chiropractor's repositioning of the tendon stayed in place. Interestingly, the veins that were visible at ST-40 slowly became less and less noticeable. During the course of treatment, the sense of nausea gradually abated, and the patient was able to return to a more normal eating routine.

Analysis   This case provides a very clear illustration of a condition affecting yin-yang paired channels. It seems that the initial injury on the large intestine *yáng míng* channel (shoulder), likely because of a congenital weakness, later affected the paired (lung *tài yīn*) channel. As a result, what began as a relatively minor physical injury gradually affected the qi transformation of the internal organs. By the time the patient arrived for his first visit, digestive function had been significantly compromised. As the condition in the channels improved, normal function of the organs ensued.

Besides the quite obvious visible collateral vessels observed at ST-40 in this patient, other signs and symptoms suggest the involvement of these vessels as well. The tendency of the condition to radiate from the yang (large intestine) to the yin (lung) channel highlights the involvement of paired channels (often treated by using the collateral or 'connecting' points). In addition, it should be recalled that collateral points such as LI-6 can be used for conditions affecting microcirculation along the pathway of the associated channel. The difficulty experienced by the chiropractor in getting the adjustments to 'stick' may have been caused by a lack of vigorous blood circulation throughout the small spaces in the sinew channels (筋經 *jīn jīng*) of the large intestine. The slippery pulse and swelling in the lower right leg indicated a rising accumulation of dampness due to compromise of *tài yīn* qi transformation.

The use of a 2-inch needle connecting LI-14 to LI-15 on the *opposite* side from the injury during the initial treatments is an example of 'odd needling' (奇刺 *qí cì*). This is the traditional term used to describe the often-seen practice of needling a point on the opposite side from the injury during the initial stages of treatment. This is particularly applicable in cases where more severe inflammation (or deficiency) is suspected that might respond negatively to a more direct attack. By using a point on the channel on the opposite side of the body, more gradual qi and blood movement in the affected area can be initiated.

■ Case No. 6

48-year-old female

Chief complaint   Severe right-sided arm/hand/shoulder pain accompanied by an extreme sensation of heat in the palms

History of present illness   On her initial visit, the patient presented with severe pain in the right arm and hand which had been constant and worsening over the previous month. The pain radiated down the posterior arm to the third digit (middle finger). The pain began four months earlier during a sailing competition when she overexerted herself and injured her mid-back.

The patient had a history of chronic off and on mid-low back pain following a skiing injury at age sixteen. In addition, X-ray exams revealed narrowed cervical foramina in the C5–C7 area.

She was also diagnosed five years before with Sjogren's syndrome, and had used two courses of steroids three years previously to help with the rheumatoid-like symptoms. The Sjogren's symptoms had been in remission for the past two years, but she feared that the current injury seemed to be causing a flare-up (she had swelling and some redness in the third, fourth, and fifth fingers on her right hand). She often experienced acid regurgitation with many foods (wine, spicy, greasy) and complained of frequent bloating and constipation. Despite complaints of recent depression and irritability, her demeanor was calm and pleasant. Her skin color was normal.

The most obvious swelling was observed on the initial visit in the area of SI-4 *(wàn gǔ)*/SI-5 *(yáng gǔ)*.

The tongue body was pale and the coating was dry and yellow. The pulse was thready overall and noticeably more slippery in the spleen and liver positions.

Channel palpation The most obvious palpated channel changes were on the *tài yáng, shào yáng,* and *yáng míng* channels. A series of grainy, sand-like changes could be palpated around SI-4/SI-5 bilaterally, with a similar sensation found around BL-63 *(jīn mén)* and BL-64 *(jīng gǔ)*. On the arm, the *yáng míng* channel was puffy and tender, with severe tenderness at LI-10 *(shǒu sān lǐ)*. On the leg, there was a sense of hypertonicity (tightness) in the fascia all along the stomach channel. On the arm, the triple burner had a very clear sense of being like an 'ungraded road.'

Diagnosis Yin channel excess affecting the yang channels *(tài yīn/jué yīn* excess).

Treatment Treatment in this case evolved over time, but began by clearing heat from the *shào yáng* and *yáng míng*. Thus, in the early treatments, the point pairs TB-5 *(wài guān)* and GB-41 *(zú lín qì)*, and LI-11 *(qū chí)* and ST-44 *(nèi tíng)*, were primary. Following twenty-five minutes with the lead pairs, points more local to the injury, such as SI-4, SI-10 *(nào shū)*, and GB-21 *(jiān jǐng)*, were then needled, and the needles were retained for a further twenty minutes.

Over time, the lead pairs shifted first to the more strongly-moving (but less heat-clearing) pair TB-6 *(zhī gōu)* and GB-34 *(yáng líng quán)*, combined with LI-10 and ST-36 *(zú sān lǐ)*. Eventually, the treatment focus shifted to clearing the underlying yin channel excess stagnation and heat, using the pairs PC-7 *(dà líng)* and LR-2 *(xíng jiān)* and LU-5 *(chǐ zé)* and SP-9 *(yīn líng quán)*. In every treatment over a course of fifteen, the lead point pairs were needled and left in place for twenty-five minutes, followed by removal of the needles from those points and needling of the more local points, as described above.

Herbs

A modified Bupleurum Powder to Dredge the Liver *(chái hú shū gān sǎn)* was used in the initial stages, followed about two months later by a modification of Six-Gentleman Decoction with Aucklandiae and Amomum *(xiāng shā liù jūn zǐ tāng)*, which was taken for two more months. Eventually, the dosage of herbs in the second formula was gradually reduced to a total dosage of 2g/day.

• Modified Bupleurum Powder to Dredge the Liver *(chái hú shū gān sǎn)*

    Bupleuri Radix *(chái hú)*—8g
    Citri reticulatae Pericarpium *(chén pí)*—6g
    Aurantii Fructus *(zhǐ ké)*—6g
    Paeoniae Radix alba *(bái sháo)*—7g
    Chuanxiong Rhizoma *(chuān xiōng)*—6g
    Cyperi Rhizoma *(xiāng fù)*—7g
    Scutellariae Radix *(huáng qín)*—9g
    Glehniae/Adenophorae Radix *(shā shēn)*—7g
    Ophiopogonis Radix *(mài mén dōng)*—7g
    (63g/week—9g/day taken in three 3g doses with warm water)

• Modified Six-Gentleman Decoction with Aucklandia and Amomum
  (xiāng shā liù jūn zǐ tāng)

    Aucklandiae Radix *(mù xiāng)*—6g
    Tsaoko Fructus *(cǎo guǒ)*—6g
    Magnoliae officinalis Cortex *(hòu pò)*—6g
    Pinelliae Rhizoma preparatum *(zhì bàn xià)*—7g
    Codonopsis Radix *(dǎng shēn)*—9g
    Atractylodis macrocephalae Rhizoma *(bái zhú)*—6g
    Poria *(fú líng)*—6g
    Glycyrrhizae Radix *(gān cǎo)*—4g
    Polygonati Rhizoma *(huáng jīng)*—6g
    Coptidis Rhizoma *(huáng lián)*—7g
    (63g/week—9g/day taken in three 3g doses with warm water)

Results After the first two weeks of treatment the pain moved, with the same intensity, to the opposite (left) shoulder. Then, after two more weeks, the pain moved to the right. Finally, over time, the pain slowly dissipated, continuing to occasionally alternate between the left and right shoulders before completely abating three months after treatment began.

During this same period of time, the patient's sense of heat in the palms slowly faded and her digestion improved dramatically. In fact, her digestion improved quite quickly while the shoulder complaint had a slower (but relatively constant) rate of improvement. During the first few weeks after switching from Bupleurum Powder to Dredge the Liver *(chái hú shū gān sǎn)* to Six-Gentleman Decoction with Aucklandia and Amomum *(xiāng shā liù jūn zǐ tāng)* she experienced a brief return of the heat sensation in the palms, which abated by temporarily lowering the daily herb dosage to 6g/day for two weeks.

Four months after the first visit, the patient returned for a refill of herbs. Having had no treatment for a month, she reported that her shoulder, palms, and digestion were all back to normal, but that she continued to take 2g of herbs/day without which she gets some indigestion after eating greasy foods.

Analysis This case provides an interesting example of using channel palpation to help determine not only acupuncture treatment, but also to help guide herbal strategy. Dr. Wang also often uses his findings from channel palpation to help determine his herbal treatment approaches.

In this case, the treatment approach is strongly influenced by the palpated finding on the triple burner channel, described here and elsewhere in this text as feeling like an 'ungraded road'. Experience in the U.S. would indicate that many patients present with this type of change, with fewer noted by Dr. Wang in China.

When the sense of bumpiness on the triple burner channel is combined with puffy tenderness noted on both aspects of the *yáng míng* channel, a picture emerges of an excess pattern affecting multiple yang channels. In addition, many of the signs reported by the patient (bloating/gas, depression/irritability), combined with the slippery nature of the spleen and liver pulses, describe a concurrent yin channel excess. Finally, graininess around both source points on the *tài yáng* channel indicates a chronic, underlying deficiency affecting that channel. These changes are very often found in cases involving degenerative cervical vertebrae.

The general treatment approach involved first clearing heat and moving the *shào yáng* and *yáng míng* channels. This was followed by harmonizing and clearing the paired *tài yīn* and *jué yīn* channels. Throughout the acupuncture treatments, the *tài yáng* channel was included as the 'branch' of the underlying pattern. The location of the patient's fundamental disharmony, however, seems to be more clearly understood by considering the nature of the triple burner organ, as described in this text.

In Chapter 9 we described the triple burner organ as constituting the 'spaces', not only around the internal organs, but also those which make up the channels throughout the entire body. When there is chronic heat in the body, it seems to sometimes lead to a kind of congealing of the fluids within the triple burner organ. Clinically, this is often seen in auto-immune conditions. In Chapter 9, we discussed the possibility of considering a formula like Reach the Membrane Source Decoction *(dá yuán yǐn)*, which relies on warm, aromatic, and moving lead herbs like Tsaoko Fructus *(cǎo guǒ)*, Magnoliae officinalis Cortex *(hòu pò)*, and Arecae Semen *(bīng láng)*, to activate circulation in the triple burner when one suspects this systemic stagnation. The modification of Six-Gentleman Decoction with Aucklandia and Amomum *(xiāng shā liù jūn zǐ tāng)* described above was inspired by this idea.

In conclusion, this is a case where careful channel palpation, combined with other diagnostic tools, provided a clear picture of the underlying pathodynamic. Instead of treating only the triple burner and small intestine channels based on the described location of the chief complaint, a more systemic treatment approach was devised. The approach regarded the patient's presenting shoulder problem as but a piece of a larger, systemic tendency to inflammation in both the *yáng míng* and *shào yáng* channels that is rooted in paired yin channels *(tài yīn* and *jué yīn)*. Consequently, acupuncture treatment evolved from first clearing heat from the yang with the initial point pairs, to clearing and regulating the yin channels in later treatments. In tandem, the herbal formulas gradually moved from clearing at the surface to regulating and tonifying in the final months.

One might also view the case as being one where stagnant heat in the 'deeper' yang channels *(shào yáng* and *yáng míng)* led to a lack of radiating warmth upward and outward to the surface *tài yáng*. As a result, a chronic cervical issue had worsened, leading to the pain in the upper body.

OTHER DIAGNOSTIC TOOLS: OBSERVATION AND PALPATION OF ALTERNATE PULSES

THIS APPENDIX IS an excerpted section from lectures summarized in Chapter 12. The following pages summarize some of Dr. Wang's experience with observation of the body surface and palpation of alternate pulses. The section on pulse palpation does not focus on the radial (LU-9 [tài yuān]) pulse, but provides instead a general overview of other pulses that are traditionally palpated in other areas of the body.

Observation (審 *shěn*)

Observation means looking at the color of the skin, shape of the body, and condition of surface vessels. This is similar to the concept described within the 'four examinations' (四診 *sì zhěn*), of which 'observation' (望 *wàng*) is also a part. Variations on this diagnostic technique can be found in many modern texts. Here, however, our observation will focus on the channel pathways. The general approach is to observe changes in the vasculature and skin quality along the course of the channels. Each person's channel system is unique to their anatomy and thus careful observation can often provide helpful overall impressions about the condition of particular channels or groups of channels. Careful attention should therefore be paid to the location of change. In general, observation falls into two broad categories. The first is observation of the collaterals (络 *luò*) and the second is observation of changes on the skin. Here, the term 'collaterals' refers to capillaries that can be seen on the surface of the body.

Observing the collaterals

Changes on the collaterals may be observed anywhere on the body, but there are a few areas that are stressed repeatedly in classical texts. The first involves the two large vessels that can be seen beneath the tongue. These are particularly important collaterals because they can be consistently observed in nearly any patient. The tongue is most often associated with the collaterals of the heart, pericardium, spleen, stomach, and kidney channels. Clinically, if the vessels under the tongue are expanded, purple, or deep red, this generally indicates heat, fire, or toxins in the heart *shào yīn*, pericardium *jué yīn*, or stomach *yáng míng* channels. The tongue vessels are also often distended and purplish in the presence of summerheat. Fire toxin in the heart or pericardium may also present as hot painful sores in other areas of the body. Observation of distended, purplish vessels under the tongue serves to verify this diagnosis where these types of sores are present.

Fire toxin in the heart and pericardium is often treated by bleeding the two extra (miscellaneous) points located at the vessels beneath the tongue (金津 *jīn jīn* and 玉液 *yù yè*). If the vessels beneath the tongue are distended but have more of a deep, dull, purplish tone, this is indicative of blood stasis and is thus different from a diagnosis of heat toxin. On the other hand, vessels that are thin, dry, pale, or light purple generally indicate blood stasis with cold. This most often indicates yang deficiency of the kidney and/or spleen.

Collateral vessels can also often be observed behind the elbows and knees. Most commonly, changes here can be seen in the presence of low back pain. Often, patients with back pain will have distended purplish veins around BL-40 *(wěi zhōng)*. These vessels can be differentiated from normal veins by palpating. If the vessels feel hard and tight, they are likely involved in pathology. Bleeding these vessels is often an important part of treatment. The practitioner should be aware that pressure often builds in these small veins because of compromised venous return through the low back, and, as a result, bleeding the points occasionally involves an initial spurt of blood. Care should be taken to keep the face at a safe distance from the veins when doing this procedure. It should also be noted that 'collateral vessels' are not the same thing as varicose veins. Many patients will present with varicose veins that are not indicative of channel pathology. These should not be bled.

Observation of changes on the skin

The second major type of observable change includes changes that can be seen on the surface of the skin. These may be raised red areas known as papules (丘疹 *qiū zhěn*), fluid-filled sacs known as vesicles (濕疹 *shī zhěn*), or discolorations below the skin surface known as dormant papules (癮疹 *yǐn zhěn*). Changes on the skin that meet the following preconditions are significant to channel diagnosis:

- in a clear line along channel pathways
- concurrent with disease symptoms; come and go as the condition ebbs and flows
- located bilaterally.

If skin changes do not meet at least two of these three conditions, they fall instead under the category of dermatological conditions and are better treated in that context. If the changes do meet these conditions, they deserve further observation. If pressing the surface of a papule results in blanching (the area turns white, then becomes red again), there is strong heat or toxin in the channel. The presence of vesicles often indicates heat or dampness. Dormant papules usually correspond to the presence of blood stasis in the channel on which they appear.

Observation of the skin in all areas on the body can be relevant. The area lateral to the spine is particularly helpful. When observing this area, keep in mind the bladder transport points and the organs with which they are associated. Specifically, changes in the area between T3 and T5 usually indicate lung *tài yīn* or possibly heart *shào yīn* issues. Changes between T5 and T9 generally indicate spleen *tài yīn* and stomach *yáng míng* issues, while those seen below T11 are usually related to kidney *shào yīn* or liver *jué yīn*. Changes around the sacrum are often indicative of large intestine *yáng míng* conditions (such as hemorrhoids), gynecological issues, or even some types of epilepsy. If raised papules are observed in this area in the presence of such conditions, it is often helpful to release a few drops of blood from the papules.

■ Case Study No. 1

33-year-old female

Chief complaint   Painful facial boils

History of present illness   The patient complained of painful boils on the face that had come and gone for over a month. Boils were generally found around the jaw line and cheeks. The patient had been under a great deal of emotional pressure recently. Observation revealed the presence of deep-red tender papules around the lung, pericardium, heart, and liver transport points (BL-13 ~ BL-18, lateral to the third to the ninth thoracic vertebrae). There was also severe tenderness beneath the fifth and sixth thoracic vertebrae (GV-11 [*shén dào*] and GV-10 [*líng tái*].

Diagnosis   Heat in the pericardium and chest due to emotional excess

Treatment   Seven-star needling, bleeding, and cupping at GV-10

Stimulation   During cupping, deep-red blood was drawn.

Results   The patient noticed no change for the first few days after initial treatment. The same treatment was repeated three days later. A few days after the second treatment, the boils began to clear, and four days later were markedly improved. The symptoms eventually disappeared and did not return. The area around GV-10 is often bled in cases of heat in the blood. As a reservoir of yang qi, draining the *dū* vessel in cases of excess heat is often appropriate (remember as well the use of GV-14 [*dà zhuī*] in cases of exterior excess).

Another case also highlights the importance of careful observation of channel pathways:

■ Case Study No. 2

36-year-old female

Chief complaint   Sacral pain due to injury

History of present illness   The patient had recently made a trip to Beijing and visited the Forbidden City on a cold, snowy day. Due to slippery conditions, she fell and injured her sacrum. X-rays showed no breaks or bone chips. Two weeks later, upon returning to the United States, she still had severe tenderness at the coccyx. She complained of pain radiating down the leg and cramping in the calf. Upon observation, there were noticeable papules in a line 5cm long and 2cm wide around BL-57 *(chéng shān)* and BL-58 *(fēi yáng)*. These papules were accompanied by a burning sensation in the area.

Diagnosis   Cold stasis (turning to heat) in the bladder channel

Treatment   BL-40 *(wěi zhōng)* and BL-7 *(tōng tiān)*

Stimulation   BL-40 was bled and strong stimulation with a 1.5-inch needle was used at BL-7.

Results   The burning sensation decreased during the treatment. On follow-up two days later, the patient reported no pain when resting, but still had some pain on exertion. The same regimen was used for three treatments, after which the pain completely subsided.

Pulse Palpation (切 *qiē*)

The concept of using the pulse as a diagnostic tool goes back to the most ancient literature in Chinese medicine. Myriad approaches to this complex subject have been proposed. As noted earlier in this text, due to a combination of cultural, clinical, and intellectual trends, radial pulse palpation has become most common. However, there are many other areas on the body where the pulse can be felt or even seen. While most large vessels in the body are held safely within the folds of muscles or protected by fatty tissue, there are certain areas where the vascular system seems to come up to the surface.

These areas might be thought of as places where the blood system interacts with and 'takes the pulse' of the external environment at large. Because the system of blood circulation rises in these areas, they have been used for centuries as a means for doctors to gain insight into the condition of the internal organs. Note that the pulses that rise to the surface at certain points of the body reflect not only the blood pressure in general, but also the relative tension of the muscles and fascia in the immediately surrounding area. Consequently, pulses on the surface of the body can also be helpful indicators of the relative state of muscles and connective tissue in various areas. In other words, when one of the surface pulses becomes especially strong and flooding, the muscles in that entire area are likely to be in a state of increased tension. On the other hand, pulses that are weak and difficult to find may reflect local qi and blood deficiency.

In sum, palpation of the pulse in Chinese diagnosis may be thought of as a complex system for ascertaining the condition of blood flow and the tone of muscles and connective tissue in the area. The 'twenty-eight pulses' that are described in modern textbooks as occurring at the radial artery are the most commonly definable patterns of change. The more one palpates, the more one may discern beyond this basic level. Similarly, information can also be gleaned by checking pulses in other parts of the body.

Classically, the locations of palpable pulses on the body were divided into three general areas. The names of the areas correspond to the three fundamental levels of existence in Chinese thought, namely heaven (天 *tiān*), humankind (人 *rén*), and earth (地 *dì*). There are three pulses at each of these levels for a total of nine classical pulses. The earliest description of these nine pulses can be found in Chapter 20 of the *Divine Pivot* (靈樞 *Líng shū*). In the two millennia that have passed since the writing of the *Divine Pivot*, debates about the diagnostic significance of pulses found in areas other than at the radial artery have gradually subsided. In most modern clinics, pulse diagnosis focuses entirely on the radial pulse. Nevertheless, there are still some benefits to be gained from developing a familiarity with the other traditional pulses and the information that might present at these locations.

Heaven pulses

The head is associated with heaven in Chinese physical cosmology. The first pulse to consider in this part of the body is that found on the forehead inferior and anterior to ST-8 *(tóu wéi)*. It is at this point that the 'qi of the head' (頭氣 *tóu qì*) is said to gather. This area is most clearly associated with *yáng míng* and *shào yáng*, although divergent vessels of the *tài yáng* channel also go through here. While there is no direct anatomical connection of the vasculature at this point with the cerebral circulation beneath, clinical experience suggests a diagnostic link. Patients with irregular blood pressure, blood sugar levels, or even unusual intracranial pressure may have changes in this pulse. When they are elevated, the pulse will feel flooding and large, while vessels in the area may be distended or show increased vascularization (extra vessels). Conversely, lowered blood pressure, blood sugar or intracranial pressure may sometimes lead to pale or withered vessels around ST-8 and a deep, thready, weak pulse. Signs associated with 'weak qi in the head' include dizziness, blurring eyes, or even nausea, all of which are possible symptoms of lowered blood pressure or blood sugar.

The second point in the upper portion of the body is found at ST-7 *(xià guān)* where the 'qi of the face' (面氣 *miàn qì*) is said to gather. The qi of the face refers to circulation in the eyes, nose, and jaw. In the clinic, ST-7 is in fact very useful for treating a broad spectrum of facial conditions. Because of both vascular and lymphatic passageways below the zygomatic arch, acupuncture at ST-7 can increase healthy circulation throughout the face. If palpation of the area reveals a pulse that is flooding, large, and/or wiry, the qi of the face is said to be rising up or even blocked. A thready, fine pulse is indicative of a lack of abundant qi to the face. The point is particularly useful for differentiating excess and deficiency in cases of Bell's palsy or trigeminal neuralgia.

Finally, the 'qi of the teeth' (齒氣 *chǐ qì*) is found on another stomach channel point, ST-5 *(dà yíng)*. Diagnosis of the severity of oral/dental conditions can therefore include evaluation of the condition of the pulse around this point.

Humankind pulses

The 'humankind' level of the body includes the neck and abdomen. The uppermost pulse in this region is found at ST-9 *(rén yíng)*, on the carotid artery. Modern physiologists recognize that the body has baroreceptors in this area which inform the brain of changes in blood pressure. In Chinese medicine, the carotid artery pulse was classically thought of as being a palpable reflection of the general condition of postnatal qi. Clinical experience has shown that checking this pulse is of particular importance when differentiating the final stages of life. During what Chinese medicine terms the 'separation of yin and yang' (陰陽分解 *yīn yáng fēn jiě*) just before death, the pulse at ST-9 can be seen quite clearly on the skin surface. Palpation of the carotid pulse at this time often reveals a pulse 'without root'—one with very little strength when pressed firmly. Therefore, a general prognosis for the ability of a very sick patient to survive might be gained by following changes in the ST-9 pulse. As long as a patient has ample postnatal qi, some strength and 'root' will remain at the carotid pulse.

A second diagnostic pulse at this middle level of the body is found at CV-12 *(zhōng wǎn)* above the umbilicus. Deep to this point, one can find the descending aorta. When palpating this area, the pulse should generally be difficult to find. Strong pulsing at CV-12, known classically as 'pulsing beneath the heart' (心下動脈 *xīn xià dòng mài)*, is indicative of excess-type problems in the spleen and stomach.

Alternatively, some texts consider the second pulse in the humankind level to be the commonly discussed radial pulse found at LU-9 *(tài yuān)*. One reason why the LU-9 pulse carries such significance in diagnosis is because of the designation of the lung organ as 'commander of the hundred vessels'. As the ruler of all the vessels in the body through its function of commanding qi, the lung has a special ability to represent the general condition of the qi of all the internal organs. Located at the source point of the channel, the radial pulse is therefore a unifying location at which to discern the status of the 'hundred vessels' of the body. Consequently, while some texts place the radial pulse here at the center of the humankind level within the nine pulses, others place it in a category of its own.

The third pulse of diagnostic significance at the humankind level can be found at CV-6 *(qì hǎi)* below the umbilicus. This pulse should not be felt at all on the surface and should be flexible at the middle and deep levels. If the CV-6 pulse is hard with a strong pulsation, this generally indicates cold or stagnation in the lower burner. Softness of the CV-6 pulse often indicates kidney deficiency.

Earth pulses

In the lower body, the first classical diagnostic pulse is found at SP-12 *(chōng mén)*. It is not often used in the modern clinic due to its location in the groin area, but it was used classically to ascertain the condition of qi and blood in the lower abdomen. The second pulse can be found at ST-42 *(chōng yáng),* which reflects the strength of the stomach (organ) qi. This should be contrasted with the pulse found at ST-9 *(rén yíng),* which, because of its association with postnatal qi, is also reflective of the stomach. However, ST-9 is said to reflect the nutritive qi of the *yáng míng* channel, the final result of the digestive process, as opposed to the strength of the stomach organ itself. The ST-9 pulse is therefore more of a broad indicator of the general state of postnatal qi in the patient.

The third and final diagnostic pulse can be found at KI-3 *(tài xī)* and is associated with the source qi of the kidney. Strength of the pulse at KI-3 indicates the health of prenatal qi. It is interesting to note that the pulse at KI-3 will often be weak in cases of tooth and gum pain due to kidney deficiency. This is often a type of pain that is exacerbated by cold foods or air on the teeth and gums. Tooth pain of this type can be treated with moxa just below KI-3, as moxa on the vein itself might damage the vessel.

Because there is a wealth of information in other texts regarding radial pulse diagnosis, the subject will not be covered here. However, as noted earlier, the radial pulse is a vital part of classical diagnosis. As anyone who has studied pulse diagnosis will surely concede, there is a great variability in how each doctor will describe the condition of a particular patient's pulse. It is therefore helpful for many practitioners to have other methods at hand to verify or refine a particular pulse diagnosis. For some, the methods described here for palpating change along channel pathways are actually easier to learn and transmit than many of the radial pulse approaches. The techniques outlined here are a synthesis of what is still quite a large body of material on channel diagnosis in extant classical sources, and there is still much work to be done.

ATTENTION DEFICIT HYPERACTIVITY DISORDER (ADHD)

THE FOLLOWING SECTION is a short discussion of concepts surrounding ADD/ADHD. The reader should note a few broad themes in the diagnostic approach described below. The condition is generally categorized by organ diagnosis and symptom patterns, as is done in most texts. However, another diagnostic tool is provided by including a discussion of the palpated channel changes most commonly seen in connection with particular organ diagnoses. Reports of palpable changes in the channels have been a part of all case studies provided thus far, and hopefully at this point in the text, it is becoming clear how these changes can be used in the clinic to refine the diagnosis. In the discussion below, channel palpation (and thus channel theory) is included as part of differential diagnosis. This discussion provides a window into how an understanding of channel physiology (including organ theory) can facilitate the understanding of an all-too-common problem in modern society.

This syndrome is most commonly seen in children between the ages of 5 and 15 and is characterized by distractibility, short attention span, impulsive behavior, hyperactivity, and learning and behavior disabilities. In biomedicine, improper functioning of neurotransmitter systems has been proposed as a possible cause. Pharmaceutical treatment most commonly involves central nervous system stimulants such as amphetamine, dextroamphetamine, and methamphetamine, or similar drugs such as methylphenidate (Ritalin). These tend to allow the child to focus while also, paradoxically, calming hyperactivity. Most children, however, are not cured by pharmaceutical treatment.

Perspective of Chinese medicine

Chinese medicine views the pattern to be rooted in a generalized imbalance in the inter-regulation of the organs. Although the pattern might be broken down into ascendant liver yang, liver-kidney yin deficiency, and spleen qi deficiency types, there will likely be fairly rapid changes from one to another symptom-pattern during the course of treatment. The internal organs of children are delicate and thus easily disturbed by irregularities in diet, environment, or emotional situation. Therefore, this pattern in children is not the same as it might be in adults, where a particular pathodynamic (e.g., spleen qi deficiency) may be fairly stable throughout the course of treatment. In children, because the cause is fundamentally one of imbalance and not a case of pure deficiency, manifestations are changeable.

In all of its forms, the condition is ultimately rooted in a deficiency of prenatal qi and is generally not caused by any of the six externally-contracted excesses (wind, cold, summerheat, dampness, dryness, and fire).

Etiology

Children with congenital deficiencies of prenatal qi do not necessarily develop this pattern. Children with prenatal qi deficiency who go on to develop this pattern generally also experience one of the following:

- Emotional stressors such as increased pressure in school or socially. This also includes emotional issues related to family life.

- Severe fear or traumatic experiences.

- Irregular diet, especially one where the child eats only certain foods without sufficient variety (especially an excess of sweets).

Symptomatology

There are five basic symptom categories. A child experiencing this pattern may not necessarily have all of the symptoms below:

1. Difficulty concentrating

   The child is easily distracted, has problems in school, wants to move about, tries to do too many things at once and/or has difficulties with memory.

2. Emotional problems

   Affected children are often irritable and difficult to control. They are often unconcerned about the results of their actions or their effects on others. They may also be easily angered.

3. Sleep disorders

Symptoms may include waking easily, sleepwalking, or talking during sleep.

4. Muscular changes

These may include twitching or tightness of the muscles, usually in the neck or face.

5. Difficulties with balance

The child may be clumsier than others and may fall often or have an unusual gait.

Channel diagnosis

The pattern most often includes palpable changes on the *jué yīn* liver channel, *jué yīn* pericardium channel, *tài yīn* spleen channel, or *tài yīn* lung channel. There may also be changes along the *shào yīn* channel or the *dū* vessel. Palpation of these channels is helpful in differential diagnosis.

Differentiation

In most cases, patterns will involve an intermingling of yin deficiency, phlegm, and fire.

Exuberant liver fire/liver fire harassing and stirring (肝火擾動 *gān huǒ rǎo dòng*)

In this pattern, irritability and constant movement will be most obvious. The child may talk excessively and will have difficulty getting to sleep (yin deficiency). Palpation may reveal small nodules along the *jué yīn* pericardium channel, especially in the area between PC-3 *(qū zé)* and PC-4 *(xī mén)*.

The treatment principle in this case is to clear heat, transform phlegm stasis, calm the liver, and extinguish wind.

Acupuncture

A helpful point pair for this pattern is PC-7 *(dà líng)* and LR-2 *(xíng jiān)*, which clears and transforms heat from the *jué yīn* channel. KI-7 *(fù liū)* may also be added to benefit the yin (mother point of the kidney channel).

Herbs

Gastrodia and Uncaria Drink *(tiān má gōu téng yǐn)*, with modifications

Gastrodiae Rhizoma *(tiān má)*

Uncariae Ramulus cum Uncis *(gōu téng)*

Paeoniae Radix alba *(bái sháo)*—with a higher dose of up to 30g

Perillae Folium *(zǐ sū yè)*

Lonicerae Flos *(jīn yín huā)*

Ziziphi spinosae Semen *(suān zǎo rén)*

Anemarrhenae Rhizoma *(zhī mǔ)*

Angelicae sinensis Radix *(dāng guī)*

Rehmanniae Radix *(shēng dì huáng)*

Fossilia Dentis Mastodi *(lóng chǐ)*—if sleep problems are pronounced

Puerariae Radix *(gé gēn)*—if neck stiffness is pronounced

Elements of Warm the Gallbladder Decoction *(wēn dǎn tāng)* may be added as well to transform phlegm and open the collaterals.

Liver and kidney yin deficiency Attention problems are often most pronounced is this pattern. The child may also have dry eyes, warm palms and/or abdomen (five-center heat), a red tongue, and a thin, rapid, or frail pulse. The child will often wake easily during the night. Palpation may reveal changes along the *shào yīn* channel, especially the area around HT-5 *(tōng lǐ)* to HT-7 *(shén mén)* and KI-6 *(zhào hǎi)*. Palpable channel changes in children are often very small, and differentiation is a skill that will only be gained with practice over time. In this type of case, the changes may feel like very small, crunchy thickening along the *shào yīn* channel.

The treatment principle is to benefit the kidney and liver yin.

Acupuncture

The point pair HT-6 *(yīn xī)* and KI-7 *(fù liū)* is most often used in combination with LR-3 *(tài chōng)*. This pair benefits the kidney yin, as HT-6 *(yīn xī)*, the cleft point of the heart channel, provides qi from the heart to facilitate the yin-strengthening action of KI-7 *(fù liū)*. This is an instance of regulating the *shào yīn* qi transformation to facilitate communication between the heart and kidney. LR-3 *(tài chōng)*, the source point of the liver channel, benefits the liver yin.

Herbs

Six-Ingredient Pill with Rehmannia *(liù wèi dì huáng wán)*, with modifications

Consider adding Anemarrhenae Rhizoma *(zhī mǔ)*, Nelumbinis Semen *(lián zǐ)*, Platycladi Semen *(bǎi zǐ rén)*, and/or Testudinis Plastrum *(guī bǎn)*.

Heart and spleen deficiency A child with this pattern will likely present as more generally deficient, as there is a coexisting deficiency of both heart and spleen qi. In the case of the spleen, however, the pattern will also include what may be termed spleen yin deficiency. This can be understood as *yáng míng* yin deficiency affecting the spleen, thus leading to the common complaint of constipation. The child will also often be tired, have a low appetite, excessive dreams, and will be easily scared. The pulse will often be slow, and the tongue pale with a dry coating. Palpation often reveals soft nodules or a decrease in muscle tone along both the lung and spleen *tài yīn* channels, and occasionally on the *shào yīn* channels as well.

The treatment principle is to benefit the qi.

Acupuncture

The point pair LU-9 *(tài yuān)* and SP-3 *(tài bái)* is most commonly used together with the pair CV-11 *(jiàn lǐ)* and ST-36 *(zú sān lǐ)*. Both pairs are used to benefit the qi throughout the body. Source points on the *tài yīn* channel stimulate the production of postnatal qi. The CV-11 *(jiàn lǐ)* and ST-36 *(zú sān lǐ)* pair fortifies the spleen-stomach, primarily by stimulating yang movement.

Herbs

Emperor of Heaven's Special Pill to Tonify the Heart *(tiān wáng bǔ xīn dān)*, with modifications

Ziziphi spinosae Semen *(suān zǎo rén)*—higher dose

Platycladi Semen *(bǎi zǐ rén)*—higher dose

Asparagi Radix *(tiān mén dōng)*

Ophiopogonis Radix *(mài mén dōng)*

Rehmanniae Radix *(shēng dì huáng)*

Polygalae Radix *(yuǎn zhì)*

with the addition of Four-Gentleman Decoction *(sì jūn zǐ tāng)* to support the spleen

Conclusion

In all ADD/ADHD patients, it should be remembered that wind, phlegm, fire, and qi stasis may always be part of the presentation. Because the pattern may change fairly quickly during a course of treatment, the diagnosis should often be reevaluated. The operative concept for these patients is a general loss of inter-regulation among the organs.

Other acupuncture points that may be considered include GB-20 *(fēng chí)*, TB-18 *(qì mài)*, and BL-10 *(tiān zhù)* if neck complaints are present. Also *dū* vessel points such as GV-21 *(qián dǐng)* and GV-24 *(shén tíng)* can be used to bring clear yang qi up to the head/brain. Finally, the spleen, liver, and heart back transporting points (BL-20 *[pí shū]*, BL-18, and BL-15 *[xīn shū]*) as well as the point pair CV-12 *(zhōng wǎn)* and ST-40 *(fēng lóng)* can also be used to facilitate phlegm transformation.

Because of the tendency of these patients to also present with phlegm (sometimes 'formless' or unseen phlegm), formulas should often include variations of Warm the Gallbladder Decoction *(wēn dǎn tāng)* and Two-Cured Decoction *(èr chén tāng)*. These formulas can open *shào yáng/jué yīn*, transform phlegm, and unblock the collaterals of the brain.

If the patient is older and the condition more long-standing, it may be advisable to consider herbs that more strongly calm wind and transform phlegm, such as Bombyx batryticatus *(bái jiāng cán)* and Scolopendra *(wú gōng)*; or herbs that strongly move blood, such as Carthami Flos *(hóng huā)*.

In general, the Liver is an important part of most ADHD patterns in the sense that inter-regulation is compromised. Many of the treatment principles outlined above involve clearing and regulating to facilitate *jué yīn* function (via not only the *jué yīn* channel, but also by using *tài yīn* and *shào yīn* to clear and stimulate). Only in the case of a more 'pure' deficiency of postnatal qi does the liver play a less important role in treatment. In the most commonly seen patterns, the liver function of dredging and draining the pathways of qi is at the center of this syndrome (Fig. A5.1).

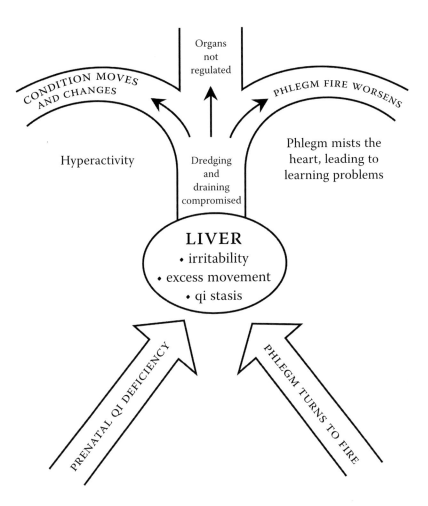

Fig. A5.1
The involvement of the liver in ADHD
(excess-movement syndrome)

Notes

Introduction

1. The version of the *Inner Classic* studied and used today is likely a compilation put together by scholars over many centuries. While the first text of that name can be traced to 23 A.D., the currently used versions are likely multilayered reworkings of a later date. The current *Inner Classic* is composed of two main parts, *Basic Questions* (素問 *Sù wèn*) and *Divine Pivot* (靈樞 *Líng shū*).

Ch. 1 / Channel Theory and the Pillars of Chinese Medicine

1. To be precise, Dr. Wang said that "Chinese medical theory has within it three principal aspects." (中醫理論裡面有三個主要內容 *Zhōng yī lǐ lùn lǐ miàn yǒu sān gè zhǔ yào nèi róng.*)

2. There is some debate within the field regarding the best translation for the Chinese term *jīng luò* (經絡). The term 'meridian' is obviously a reference to the longitudinal and latitudinal meridians used to mark degrees east-west and north-south of the prime meridian and equator respectively. While helpful as a metaphor for unseen, interconnected lines on the body surface, the term 'meridian' is not broad enough to encompass the Chinese term. Another popular English translation has been 'warp and woof', a reference to the interwoven threads on a weaver's loom. This term conveys nicely the concept implied by the original Chinese that there are both larger pathways (*jīng*) and secondary pathways (*luò*) woven together. Yet, while there is no exact equivalent in English, the concept of 'channels' in the body, with all that this term implies about a complex and changeable water system in the natural environment, seems to be the most appropriate choice. One drawback to the use of this word, however, is that the reader must remember that the original Chinese term is actually 'channel-collateral', a very

[659]

descriptive but awkward construction. Another drawback is the common association of the word 'channel', in modern English, with telecommunication—a more narrow construct than that implied by dynamic water channels.

3. The Chinese term for analysis is 分析 *fēn xi* and for categorization/unification is 分類 *fēn lèi* / 聯繫 *lián xi*.

4. Counterbalance (制約 *zhì yuē*), interdependence (相互依存 *xiāng hù yī cún*), mutual convertibility (相互轉化 *xiāng hù zhuǎn huà*) and waxing-waning (消長 *xiāo zhǎng*).

5. In this and the previous paragraph, Dr. Wang is reflecting a commonly-held belief of practitioners in both China and other countries that channel-style acupuncture suffered when forced to fit the mold of organ theory. He thinks that this was not so much a matter of official policy to eliminate channel theory, but instead a gradual de-emphasis in the process of trying to make Chinese medicine more 'scientific' during the last century. Dr. Wang makes this assertion based on his own experience as a student, practitioner, and educator during the very time when early twentieth-century-style Chinese medicine evolved into what is now called 'TCM'. It is important to point out that he never mentioned an ideological witch hunt designed to eviscerate channel theory. It is interesting to note that Dr. Wang, like some other senior practitioners of his generation whom I encountered while preparing this text, would often contrast his own approach to Chinese medicine with the 'textbook' TCM that many of us in the West assume to be the norm in China. For an examination of how Chinese medicine has fared during the past century from the perspective of a medical anthropologist who is also a practitioner of Chinese medicine, see Volker Scheid's *Chinese Medicine in Contemporary China: Plurality and Synthesis* (Durham, NC: Duke University Press, 2002) and *Currents of Tradition in Chinese Medicine 1626–2006* (Seattle: Eastland Press, 2007).

6. See, for example, Chapter 45 of the *Classic of Difficulties*, which discusses weights and measurements in detail.

7. For a fascinating parallel to this concept of channels as connective tissue pathways, see the article "Relationship of Acupuncture Points and Meridians to Connective Tissue Planes" by Helene M. Langevin and Jason A. Yandow in *The Anatomical Record* (*New Anat.*) 269:257–265, 2002. In this article, the authors, using ultrasound imaging of interstitial connective tissue, propose that acupuncture channels might be equivalent to connective tissue planes. When this article was described to Dr. Wang, he replied: "It's pretty amazing that we both came to such similar conclusions from different angles. I came to this conclusion after years of treating and palpating patients; they came to it through modern imaging. There must truly be something here!"

Ch. 2 / **Fundamentals of Channel Theory**

1. The concept of opening, closing, and pivoting among the six levels is mentioned not only in Chapter 5 of the *Divine Pivot* but also in Chapter 6 of *Basic Questions*. The concept is further discussed in the *Classified Classic* (類經 *Lèi jīng*) by Zhang Jie-Bin (張介賓), written in 1624 during the Ming dynasty. In that text, a passage in Chapter 29 of the 9th scroll (卷 *juǎn*) comments on the meaning of Chapter 6 of *Basic Questions*. Zhang writes: "The opener rules exiting, the closer rules entering, and the pivot rules the spaces between entering and exiting" (開者主出.闔者主入.樞者主出入之間 *Kāi zhě zhǔ chū, hé zhě zhǔ rù, shū zhě zhǔ chū rù zhī jiān*). Dr. Wang also cites the Qing dynasty text *Essential Meaning of the Medical Classics [Approached] through the Convergence and Assimilation of Chinese and Western [Knowledge]* (中西匯通醫經精義 *Zhōng xī huì tōng yī jīng jīng yì*), written by Tang Zong-Hai (唐宗海 1847–1897), as influencing his understanding of this and other key concepts.

2. The concept of 'outside of the inside' is summarized in the *Classified Classic* section cited in note 1. There it says that "*tài yīn* opens, it resides in the external aspect of yin" (太陰為開.居陰分之表也 *Tài yīn wéi kāi, jū yīn fēn zhī biǎo yě*).

Ch. 3 / **An Introduction to Channel Diagnosis**

1. There is lively debate in the field about the use and meaning of the term 'TCM' (Traditional Chinese Medicine). It is most clearly associated with the so-called eight-principle (eight-paradigm) style of diagnosis and treatment advocated by modern institutions of Chinese medicine in the People's Republic of China. Certainly, this style of Chinese medicine has had a very large impact on the understanding and development of Chinese medicine outside of China. For the purposes of accuracy, the term might also be thought of as 'textbook Chinese medicine,' in contrast to the varied forms that theory and practice take once real patients are encountered. It is interesting to note that, in 2003, the Beijing University of Traditional Chinese Medicine (北京中医药大学) shortened its English name to Beijing University of Chinese Medicine.

Ch. 4 / *Basic Questions,* **Chapter 8**

1. The title of *Basic Questions*, Chapter 8 (靈蘭秘典 *Líng lán mì diǎn*) might be translated in English as "The Secret Treatise of the Divine Orchid." This rather mysterious title, according to Dr. Wang, is utilized to draw the

reader's attention to the fact that something significant is being said here. Who hasn't found that, when something is called a secret, one feels that it is all the more important to know what exactly is going on.

2. The translations of bureaucratic terms were greatly assisted by Charles O. Hucker's *A Dictionary of Official Titles in Imperial China* (Stanford: Stanford University Press, 1985).

3. Rectifiers were local dignitaries who ranked and classified all males in their jurisdictions who were considered eligible for office.

4. The original term translated here as 'pericardium' is 膻中 (*tán zhōng*) and might literally mean 'center of the chest'. It is also the name of the modern acupuncture point CV-17, considered to be the alarm (*mù*) point of the pericardium. Also, the term translated here as 'happiness' (樂 *lè*) might also be pronounced *yuè*, meaning music. To complicate the matter a bit more, another archaic pronunciation of the same character is *yào*, meaning 'to take pleasure in,' as in the famous line in the *Analects of Confucius*, "The good find pleasure in the mountains while the wise find pleasure in water." (仁者樂山.知者樂水。 *Rén zhě lè shān, zhī zhě lè shuǐ*). In the end, music and pleasure seem to also denote happiness, hence the translational choice.

Ch. 5 / The *Tài Yīn* (Greater Yin) System

1. This oft-quoted summary of the natures of the yin and yang organs is from Chapter 11 of *Basic Questions*. The modern understanding of the original text also draws from the commentary of classical scholars such as Wang Bing (王冰 710–805 A.D.) who may be the first extant commentator to point out that, when the *Inner Classic* says that the yin organs should be 'replete' (滿 *mǎn*), it is a reference to an abundance of essence. Essence, in this case, is likely the prenatal essence stored by the kidney and the postnatal essence that is the result of normal yin-organ function. Wang Bing also pointed out that the reference to the yang organs as normally being 'full' (實 *shí*) means that they don't store essence, but are receivers and conveyors of the less refined food and grains (and their dregs).

2. The locations of each organ here and in the following chapters, as well as the *dū* (governing) vessel points that they group around, are Dr. Wang's personal amalgamation of locations from a variety of premodern sources.

3. In this case, the character 經 (*jīng*) is translated as 'level' instead of 'channel'. For the purposes of this text, the term will be translated as channel when discussing the lung channel, and as level when discussing the broader six levels of *tài yáng, shào yáng, yáng míng, tài yīn, shào yīn,* and *jué yīn.* For the broader concept, 經 (*jīng*) is also often translated as 'warp'.

4. The term 悍 (*hàn*) is used to describe defensive qi in *Basic Questions*, Chapter 43 and in the *Divine Pivot*, Chapter 71.

5. Chapter 13 of the *Classic of Difficulties* describes the weights and measurements of the organs and includes the five psychic aspects in juxtaposition to these very concrete observations of organ structure.

6. *Divine Pivot*, Chapter 8. The original passage is 隨神往來者謂之魂,並精而出入者謂之魄 *Suí shén wǎng lái zhě wèi zhī hún, bìng jīng ér chū rù zhě wèi zhī pò.*

7. The term 'corporeal soul', the English translation of the Chinese term 魄 *pò,* serves to emphasize the relationship of the soul with the earth and human form, while the term 'ethereal soul', for 魂 *hún,* emphasizes the relationship of the soul to heaven or the world at large.

Ch. 6 / The *Shào Yīn* (Lesser Yin) System

1. This function, and other familiar organ associations, originates in *Basic Questions*, Chapter 44: "The lungs govern the skin and hairs, the heart governs the vessels of the body, the liver governs the tendons, the spleen governs the muscles, and the kidneys govern the bones and marrow."

2. See, e.g., Giovanni Maciocia, *Fundamentals of Chinese Medicine* (London: Churchill Livingstone, 2005), 107. Here it is asserted that blood is "created" in the heart. I am unfamiliar with any modern Chinese source that makes this statement.

3. The character 行 (*xíng*) carries a meaning of regulated, normal movement along a preset path as the character originally was a pictograph for the columns of trees by the side of the main road. The meaning of 'column' was then transformed into substantive buildings that had columns, as in the term for bank (銀行 *yín háng*). Thanks to Dan Bensky for this insight.

4. Dr. Wang did not elaborate on this example, but it is included here because it provides, I think, a helpful window into how he applies physiological concepts when choosing and modifying herbal formulas. By thinking of the opening, pivoting, and closing of the six levels, a feel for the mechanism and location of action can be cultivated. This is the interesting area where physiology (as described by channel theory) serves to provide a link between the mechanisms and practice of acupuncture and Chinese herbal medicine.

5. Quoted, with modification of terminology ("vexation" changed to "irritability"; "downbear" to "direct downwards") from Charles Chace and Zhang Ting Liang, trans., *A Qin Bowei Anthology* (Brookline, MA: Paradigm Publications, 1997), 88.

Ch. 7 / The *Jué Yīn* (Terminal Yin) System

1. See discussion in Chapter 2 of the classical antecedent for the concept that the channels "open, pivot, and close."

2. The term *xū* (虛) is translated in this text as 'deficiency' while the term *bù zú* (不足) is translated as 'insufficiency.' After some discussion with Dr. Wang, he agreed that, for many modern practitioners, the two terms are interchangeable. In his mind, however, they are along a spectrum with insufficiency involving a less-serious form of deficiency.

Ch. 8 / The *Tài Yáng* (Greater Yang) System

1. Dr. Wang would often point out that his understanding of the tendency of the channels to "open, pivot, and close" was informed by the work of the Ming dynasty physician Zhang Jie-Bin (張介賓). In Chapter 29 of Zhang's *Classified Classic* (1624), he comments on *Plain Questions*, Chapter 6. The *Plain Questions* chapter contains the earliest reference to the concept that the channels open, pivot, and close. Zhang further elaborates that *tài yīn* is the "exterior of the yin [levels]" (陰分之表 *yīn fēn zhī biǎo*) while *yáng míng* is the "exterior of the yang [levels]."

2. An original reference to the concept of 'transformation to red' can be found in Chapter 81 of the *Divine Pivot* where it describes the production of blood from the middle burner and dissemination of blood into the small collateral vessels (孫絡 *sūn luò*). Regarding the relationship of the small intestine to blood production, Dr. Wang would point out that it serves as a kind of assistant to the spleen-stomach, initiating the first steps in separating food from waste.

3. When asked about this association of the 'thick' secretions in the body with the small intestine, Dr. Wang cited *Divine Pivot*, Chapter 1. There, not only is 液 (*yè*) mentioned in association with the small intestine, but also 津 (*jīn*—thin fluids) in association with the large intestine. Chapter 10 of our book discusses the concept of thin fluids and the large intestine.

Ch. 9 / The *Shào Yáng* (Lesser Yang) System

1. Dr. Wang uses the slightly idiosyncratic term 'sinew-bones' 筋骨 (*jīn gǔ*) to denote the area of influence for *shào yáng*. Traditionally, the sinews (筋 *jīn*) are associated with the liver while the bones (骨 *gǔ*) are associated with the kidney. Here we see the pivot of *shào yáng* moving in the area between liver and kidney—in the fluids of the joints. The chosen term underlines this fact.

2. *Divine Pivot,* Chapter 8.

3. The current Qing dynasty formulation of Warm the Gallbladder Decoction *(wēn dǎn tāng)* has a decidedly cool nature. Thus, in the case of true gallbladder qi deficiency, it is advisable to increase the dosage of Zingiberis Rhizoma recens *(shēng jiāng)* to the 12g advocated by Sun Si-Miao in his *Important Formulas Worth a Thousand Gold Pieces.*

4. An excellent modern Chinese resource for introducing the *Classic of Difficulties* is *Solutions to the Classic of Difficulties* (難經通解 *Nàn jīng tōng jiě*) (Xi'an: Santai Publishing House, 2001). This is the basic textbook used by Dr. Wang for his classes on the subject.

5. 三焦者.原氣之別使也.主通行三氣.經歷於五藏六府 *(sān jiāo zhě. yuán qì zhī bié shǐ yě. zhǔ tōng xíng sān qì. jīng lì yú wǔ zàng liù fǔ)*

6. Qu Li-Fang and Mary Garvey come to similar conclusions about the nature and form of the triple burner in an article in the *Journal of Chinese Medicine* (JCM:65, February 2001, 26–32). One interesting difference of opinion regards the role of the interstices (腠理 *còu lǐ*). Qu and Garvey seem to assert that the transformations of the triple burner also involve the interstices. In other words, they discern a link between the 'corridors' of the triple burner and the interstices. Dr. Wang's opinion is that the interstices are more involved in the interplay of the nutritive-protective aspects at the surface of the body (closer to the *tài yáng* level) while the pathways of the triple burner are somehow deeper, in the fluids below that level.

7. There is an interesting discussion in English of the concept (and classical antecedents) of the 'membrane source' in Kiiko Matsumoto and Stephen Birch's text *Hara Diagnosis: Reflections on the Sea* (Brookline: Paradigm Publications, 1988). The discussion begins on page 141, but is interspersed throughout the text.

8. This and the similar quotations that follow are from Chapter 31 of the *Classic of Difficulties.*

9. This and the metaphors that follow for the three burners are from Chapter 18 of the *Divine Pivot.*

10. *Commentary and Notes from the Inner Classic, Basic Questions* (黃帝內經素問譯註 *Huáng dì nèi jīng sù wèn yì zhù*) (Beijing: Ancient Chinese Medical Works Publishing Company, 2003), 79.

11. Qin Bo-Wei (秦伯未) was an important personage in twentieth-century Chinese medicine. The teacher of many great practitioners of the next generation, Dr. Qin's writings continue to be very popular today. An excellent translation of a series of Dr. Qin's lectures can be found in *A Qin Bowei Anthology,* trans. Charles Chace and Zhang Ting Liang (Brookline, MA: Paradigm Publications, 1997).

12. The ghost points of Sun Si-Miao are discussed in some detail at the end of Chapter 17.

Ch. 10 / The *Yáng Míng* (Yang Brightness) System

1. Dr. Wang considers the collateral points to be places at which circulation in the collaterals (small vessels) throughout the channel can be affected. An example was provided in Chapter 6 on the *shào yīn*, where the collateral point HT-5 (*tōng lǐ*) was used to stimulate microcirculation in the collaterals of the brain (the heart is related to consciousness). Another example involves the use of the collateral point ST-40 (*fēng lóng*) or LI-6 (*piān lì*) to affect the *yáng míng* collaterals on the face in cases of stroke, paralysis, or Bell's palsy. The collateral point on any channel should be considered when there is a condition that seems to be affecting microcirculation along the path of that channel.

Ch. 11 / The Extraordinary Vessels

1. The extraordinary vessels are mentioned, but not described with the same thoroughness as in the *Classic of Difficulties*, in *Basic Questions*, Chapters 41 and 60, and *Divine Pivot,* Chapter 65. The first chapter of *Basic Questions* also mentions the *chōng* and *rèn* vessels in conjunction with fertility in females.

2. The "27 vessels" refer to the 12 regular channels and the collateral vessels of those channels plus the collateral vessels of the Governing and Conception vessels and the "great collateral" of the spleen (脾大絡 *pí dà luò*). Thus there are 12 regular vessels and 15 collateral vessels. Note that the collateral vessels are considered to be within the purview of the regular channels. The 15 collateral vessels described here represent the largest of the three categories of collateral vessels described in modern texts. The three categories include the (large) collateral vessels (別絡 *bié luò*), the minute collaterals (孫絡 *sūn luò*), and the floating collaterals (浮絡 *fú luò*). The minute and floating collaterals are what Dr. Wang is referring to when he describes the use of the collateral points to affect "microcirculation." In addition, many modern texts equate the floating collaterals with the small blood vessels often seen on the skin surface (capillaries).

3. Channel divergences should be clearly differentiated from collateral vessels. The channel divergences have a general function of connecting internally-externally paired channels while the collateral vessels are branches of the regular channels. The divergences are said to reinforce the functional relationship of yin-yang paired organs through pathways of connection

while the collaterals represent the classical understanding that the channel system branches into smaller and smaller pathways. To be specific, the channel divergences of the yang channels travel through other structures in the body then return to their original channel. The channel divergences of the yin channels travel through other structures of the body then connect with their paired yang channel. The other structures of the body linked by the channel divergences often explain some of the more idiosyncratic uses of the channels (using them to treat areas not usually associated with the pathway of the regular channel).

4. This passage in the 28th difficulty has been the source of some debate. One can see some parts of this debate in English by consulting the translated commentary in Paul Unschuld's *Nan-Ching The Classic of Difficult Issues* (Berkeley: University of California Press), 330. The crux of the debate revolves around the meaning of the phrase 溢蓄不能環流灌溉諸經者也 (*Yì xù bù néng huán liú guàn gài zhū jīng zhě yě*). Unschuld translates this phrase as "When they are filled to overflowing, [their contents] stagnate; they cannot [return to the] circulating [influences] by drainage into the [main] conduits." Dr. Wang takes a quite different view of this same phrase by interpreting it to mean "overflows to fill [when areas] are not circulated and irrigated by the various [regular] channels." This interpretation of the phrase opens the way to more clearly understanding the next phrase, "the *yáng wéi* begins where the yang meets and the *yīn wéi* begins where yin intersects," as describing the vessels as actors in areas not reached by regular channel circulation, in areas of final destination for yin and yang. The following paragraphs describe what this means functionally and how it influences clinical thinking, especially in the context of why particular points are chosen as the command points for the two *wéi* vessels.

5. Some commentary to the *Classic of Difficulties* takes note of the phrase, translated in note 4 as "the *yáng wéi* begins where the yang meets and the *yīn wéi* begins where yin intersects," to be a description of specific points on the body. Some assert that this phrase refers to BL-63 (*jīn mén*) as the beginning of the *yáng wéi* and KI-9 (*zhú bīn*) as the beginning point of the *yīn wéi*. When one sees these points associated with the *wéi* vessels in modern texts, it is likely from this source.

6. For example, scrolls 6, 8, and 9 of *Case Records as a Guide to Clinical Practice* contain cases where inappropriate treatment or serious conditions caused problems of either excess or deficiency in specific extraordinary vessels. Appropriate herbal treatment strategies are discussed. Thanks to Charles Chace for digging up these references.

7. This concept of layering within historical texts is a crucial component

of classical Chinese scholarship and contrasts quite starkly with the modern scientific approach.

8. An interesting historical and terminological discussion of the terms 'bulging disorder' and 'mobile abdominal masses' (疝 and 瘕) can be found in a footnote in Unschuld's *Nan-Ching The Classic of Difficult Issues*, 338.

9. Dr. Wang often refers to the small intestine as being involved in the "transformation of red to maintain blood" (化赤維血 *huà chì wéi xuè*). This is likely drawn from an interesting connection he makes to discussions of the separation of clear and turbid in connection with blood found in the *Inner Classic* (*Basic Questions*, Chapter 43 and *Divine Pivot*, Chapter 81).

10. An excellent chart of the extraordinary vessel confluent points can be found in Peter Deadman and Mazin Al-Khafaji, *A Manual of Acupuncture* (London: Journal of Chinese Medicine Publications, 1997).

The Terrain So Far

1. The Yellow Emperor is generally believed to be an historical myth utilized by members of a certain school of early Chinese thought to lend particular credence to their writings. Now known as the *Huáng-Lǎo* (黄老) tradition, it represented a kind of innovation in early Daoism which took place during the Han dynasty. The author/compilers of the *Inner Classic* used the literary device of a dialogue between this mythic ancestor and his court physician as a means of both maintaining the spirit of oral teaching while also lending a particular credibility to its authorship. In most portions of the *Inner Classic*, the dialogue is between the Yellow Emperor and his court-physician Qi Bo (岐伯), but questions are also sometimes asked of figures named Lei Gong (雷公) or Shao Shu (少俞).

Ch. 12 / Physiology Under the Fingertips

1. The concept of change in the channels (是動 *shì dòng*), first mentioned in the *Divine Pivot,* Chapter 10, is taken up again and again throughout the centuries by Chinese physicians. In this respect, Dr. Wang is continuing an ancient discussion about the meaning of the *Inner Classic*. The first significant appraisal of the meaning of this term occurred quite soon after the *Inner Classic* in the *Classic of Difficulties* (22nd difficulty). A brief survey of some of the commentary to this particular difficulty can be found in English in Unschuld's *Nan-Ching* (beginning on p. 278) and reflects the fact that physician/scholars over the ages have long debated the meaning of the original classic. In that text, Unschuld translates the Qing dynasty physi-

cian Xu Da-Chun's (徐大椿) assessment of the true meaning of the *Classic of Difficulties* when it refers to change in the channels. Dr. Wang seems to agree most with Xu, and, when discussing this difficulty, asserts that there are certain changes which might be felt along a particular channel which, in the end, are not necessarily best treated on that channel. For example, when one feels small nodules along the liver channel, it might be best to consider other channels in the treatment of that condition. Certain channels show changes (是動 *shì dòng*) in the presence of a particular condition, but, as noted in *Divine Pivot,* Chapter 10, each organ also gives rise to certain diseases (所生病 *suǒ shēng bìng*). Thus, although the channel with palpated changes has 'given rise' to a particular condition, it may now be located in another channel or organ. Dr. Wang asserts that in these cases, one first palpates the channels, then considers qi transformation in the entire system before finally choosing a particular channel for treatment. This concept will be discussed further in Chapter 14.

Ch. 14 / Selecting Channels for Treatment

1. This passage is found in Chapter 1 of the *Divine Pivot,* translated in full on the first page of the introduction to this text. Often, after describing this short passage, Dr. Wang would tell his students that the sentiments described in this particular chapter are at the heart of classical acupuncture and that they have inspired him many times. When there is a difficult case or if other doctors have not succeeded at treating a particular condition, he often resolves to more carefully determine the pattern at hand, repalpating, asking more careful questions, and even carefully considering the Western medical diagnosis and laboratory results. The answer to difficult diseases is often found in this process and may in fact be as easy as pulling out a thorn, if one carefully considers and reconsiders the patterns of disharmony.

2. In some of the more commonly-used styles of five-phase acupuncture, in a case like this, one would be more likely to combine the mother (water) point on the kidney channel (KI-10 *[yīn gǔ]*) with the water point on the liver channel (LR-8 *[qū quán]*).

Ch. 15 / What is an Acupuncture Point?

1. 身形支節者. 藏府之蓋也 *Shēn xíng zhī jié zhě zàng fǔ zhī gài yě.*
2. While the first chapter of the *Divine Pivot* describes 365 of these meetings, in reality the *Inner Classic* only lists just over a hundred acupuncture points. A few centuries later, the *Systematic Classic* (甲乙經 *Jiǎ yǐ jīng*)

listed over 340 points. According to the texts that are now available, it was not until the writing of the *Great Compendium of Acupuncture and Moxibustion* (針灸大成 *Zhēn jiǔ dà chéng*) in the Ming dynasty that over 365 points were finally described in some detail.

3. There are a variety of ways to understand these empirical points. In fact, throughout history, many of them were the guarded secrets of family lineage's of acupuncturists. It is Dr. Wang's opinion that most of these so-called 'secret points' can be found in the clinic by logically considering the mechanisms of channel theory. 'Tong-style acupuncture' (董氏針灸 *Dǒng shì zhēn jiǔ*), which is quite famous in modern Taiwan (and explained in such texts as Miriam Lee's *Master Tong's Acupuncture*), provides many examples of experience points that can also be understood by considering the channels on which they are found and the categories of the major points in the area. Many of these points might actually represent alternate locations for major points, as determined by palpation. Nevertheless, it cannot be denied that although many of these points defy explanation with channel theory, they generate effective results.

Ch. 16 / The Five Transport Points

1. The most thorough discussion in English of the relationship of the cultural, linguistic, and textual traditions which gave rise to significant portions of the modern corpus of the *Inner Classic* can be found in Paul Unschuld's *Huang Di Nei Jing Su Wen: Nature, Knowledge, Imagery in an Ancient Chinese Medical Text* (Berkeley: University of California Press, 2003). This very helpful text introduces the reader to the interesting evolution of ideas that began in the early stages of Chinese medical history and continued through the millennia.

2. To be precise, Chapter 2 of the *Divine Pivot* describes in detail the transport points on eleven channels below the elbows and knees (the heart channel is not described). It describes the beginnings of all the channels on the toes and fingers. It then proceeds to describe points on the yang channels on the head (thus implying that those channels travel to the head) but does not describe yin channel points beyond the uniting points at the elbows and knees. Later chapters of the *Inner Classic* (and later texts) describe other yin channel points on the abdomen and chest. Thus later scholars and practitioners assert that the qi circulation model first outlined in Chapter 2 of the *Divine Pivot* is describing a movement from the hands and feet to the head (yang channels) and chest/abdomen (yin channels).

3. Most of the modern five-element (phase) styles of acupuncture can

trace their development to the meridian therapy (經絡治療 *jīng luò zhì liáo/ keiraku chiryō* [Japanese]) school of acupuncture that was started in Japan in the 1920s. For an excellent discussion of the historical trends that led to the development of Japanese five-element acupuncture, see Shudo Denmei, *Japanese Classical Acupuncture: Introduction to Meridian Therapy* (Seattle: Eastland Press, 1990). A discussion of some of the basic principles of an important five-element acupuncture style can also be found in J.R. Worsley, *The Five Elements and the Officials* (*Classical Five-Element Acupuncture, Volume III*) (Worsley Institute, 1998). This is the most common style of five-element acupuncture practiced in the West, and was developed by J.R. Worsley beginning in the 1960s.

4. Dr. Wang often uses points on the scalp for musculoskeletal and pain conditions. He often locates points along the *dū* vessel or bladder channel line based on palpation, then stimulates these points strongly before moving on to other semi-local and/or local points. He does not seem to use ear acupuncture at all.

5. The discovery of the circuit of blood by William Harvey, first published in 1628 in his small pamphlet, "On the Motion of the Heart and of Blood", is the result of inferences made from the work of a great many researchers at the famous medical school of Padua. Most notable were the observations of Harvey's teacher at Padua, Fabricius, who noted the presence of one-way valves in the venous system during dissection. From these observations, and the work of others who traced the movement of blood in vivisected animals, Harvey was able to describe a system in which blood moves from the heart to the extremities and back again. Before Harvey, the dominant opinion in Western medicine was that blood left the heart and was disseminated to the body and appendages for absorption in the course of metabolic function. Blood creation was thought to depend on the absorption of 'juices' from digested foods.

Many modern texts of Chinese medicine also paint a picture of one-way movement of blood in the body. This is, in fact, at odds with some of the fundamental source material in the Chinese classics. In fact, like Harvey, the ancient anatomists of Han dynasty China perceived that blood moves in a circuit from larger to smaller vessels out to the appendages, then back again into increasingly larger vessels. Chapter 30 of the *Classic of Difficulties* describes the circuitous movement of blood in connection with the movement of nutritive-protective aspects:

> [They] move in a circuit without ceasing. There is a great return after fifty [circuits]. Yin and yang are linked and move like a circle without end. This is why the nutritive and protective [aspects] are said to move together.

Integral sub-components of the blood system, the nutritive and protective aspects are said to move in a circuit that has a measurable rate of return. The exact amount of time that the 'fifty circuits' represents has been a source of some debate over the centuries. The important fact to note is that the blood was thought to move in a circular manner and to return (to the heart?) with predictability.

Ch. 17 / The Source, Cleft, and Collateral Points

1. Chapter 66 of the *Classic of Difficulties* is generally acknowledged to provide the earliest extant listing of the twelve source points used today. Chapter 1 of the *Divine Pivot* omits the modern source point of the heart channel, and instead lists PC-7 (*dà líng*) as the heart source point. While omitting the modern heart channel source point, the *Divine Pivot* does list two more points as source points—both relating to the much debated concept of the fatty-substance *gāo* (膏, also translated as 'vitals'). In the *Divine Pivot*, the two source points associated with *gāo* are CV-15 (*jiū wěi*) and CV-6 (*qì hǎi*).

Dr. Wang often describes his understanding of *gāo* in the context of explaining what he sees as the related concept of *huāng* (肓) spaces. Noting that the two terms are paired, for example, in the name of the point BL-43 (膏肓俞 *gāo huāng shū*), he describes *gāo* as a kind of protective padding in the body that can be found in special types of less-vascularized open spaces (the *huāng* 肓) around vital organs. Note that classical anatomy seems to highlight other spaces that might be associated with *gāo* substance at BL-51 (*huāng mén*), BL-53 (*bāo huāng*), and KI-16 (*huāng shū*). To be precise, Chapter 66 of the *Classic of Difficulties*, like the *Divine Pivot* before, does list PC-7 as the source of the heart, but then goes on to describe the "*shào yīn* source" as being the 兌骨 (*duì gǔ*)—possibly a reference to the styloid process of the ulna near the current source point HT-7 (*shén mén*). Interestingly, the character 兌 (*duì*) is also used to describe the trigram in the *Book of Changes* for lake (or joy), a concept which also alludes to the classical understanding of the heart.

2. Despite this relationship of the source points with the concept of channel qi development outlined in five-transport point theory, most modern texts place the source points in a separate category of their own as places where source qi enters the channel.

3. For a fascinating discussion of ways in which the research of recent decades might be used to understand the role of connective tissues in chan-

nel theory, see J.L. Oschman, *Energy Medicine: The Scientific Basis* (Edinburgh: Churchill Livingstone, 2000).

4. Dr. Wang is quoting from a Chinese translation of a text entitled 針灸精髓 (*Zhēn jiǔ jīng suǐ*). The original text, *Shinkyu Shinzui,* was actually written by a student of Dr. Sawada's, Shiroda Bunsh, and published in Yokosuka, Japan by Ido-no-Nippon Company in 1977.

5. Some believe that it is physiologically impossible to create new essence or fire at the gate of vitality. In fact, one of the main projects of the two-thousand-year tradition of health maintenance in Chinese medicine is the search for methods which minimize unnecessary waste of these fundamental, irreplaceable substances that come into the body in the mysterious process of life creation. As the fundamental substances wane, so does the vitality of life in any living being.

6. It should be noted at this point that each of the collateral vessel pathways described in Chapter 10 of the *Divine Pivot* is rather distinct from the pathways of the regular channels. For this reason, certain regions of the body have traditionally been thought to be irrigated by the collateral vessels. These regions are shown, and the associated areas and symptoms are described, in Shanghai College of Traditional Chinese Medicine, *Acupuncture: A Comprehensive Text,* trans. by John O'Connor and Dan Bensky (Chicago: Eastland Press, 1981): 83–89.

7. Dr. Wang often finds this point in a slightly more medial location, closer to the actual pathway of the lung channel, and 1.5 inches above LU-9 (*tài yuān*). This puts the point more along the pathway of the lung channel and less toward the large intestine channel. Nevertheless, at other times, he finds the point more in the traditional location between the tendons of the styloid process. When deciding which location to use, palpation is an important consideration. Small nodules or tenderness can be helpful. Obviously, when trying to needle the point more deeply so as to treat cervical issues, the more medial location is easier.

8. A standard dosage for Pinellia and Millet Decoction *(bàn xià shú mǐ tāng)* is 15g of treated Pinelliae Rhizoma *(fǎ bàn xià)* with 50g of millet (or husked sorghum). The herbs are then cooked together to make a porridge. The formula harmonizes the stomach to provide restful sleep (和胃安眠 *hé wèi ān mián*) in cases where there is insomnia due to heat in the stomach.

9. The information on the ghost points came about in response to a discussion with Dr. Wang on October 31, 2003. One of the visiting students pointed out that the day was Halloween. Dr. Wang then digressed into this interesting discussion of these points with secondary names.

Ch. 18 / A Brief Discussion of Classical Technique

1. Of course, many of the ideas in the *Classic of Difficulties* find their antecedent in the *Inner Classic*. For those who are interested, Chapters 1, 3, 9, 27, and 75 of the *Divine Pivot* and Chapters 25, 54, and 62 of *Basic Questions* also discuss the concepts of tonification and draining.

2. It is interesting to note that this same chapter of the *Divine Pivot* is often cited as the earliest reference to 'getting qi' (得氣 *dé qì*).

3. 迎 (*yíng*) means to go against and is an early cognate of 逆 (*nì*—counterflow). It has something to do with the idea that going to meet someone is a violation of protocol and is therefore being contrary.

Ch. 19 / A Modern Perspective on Acupuncture Technique: Seven Steps

1. The term 得氣 (*dé qì*) is also often translated as obtaining qi, qi sensation, or needle sensation. The exact meaning of this concept is the subject of some interesting debate. As stated here, for Dr. Wang, this concept describes a noticeable sensation that is felt by the patient—most often one which involves a radiating sensation up or down the channel. This should be contrasted with the arrival of qi (氣至 *qì zhì*), which is a sense by the practitioner that qi has arrived at the needle.

2. 刺比者,必中氣穴,無中肉節,中氣穴則針游於巷 (*Cì bǐ zhě, bì zhòng qì xué, wú zhòng ròu jié, zhòng qì xué zé zhēn yóu yú xiàng*).

3. Thanks to Stephen Brown for asking the question that led to this paragraph. Apparently, there is a greater emphasis in the Japanese acupuncture tradition upon the subtle perception by the practitioner of the arrival of qi (氣至 *qì zhì*). Some Japanese practitioners thus assert that the arrival of qi is actually of equal or even greater importance than the sensation felt by the patient, which we call 'getting qi' (得氣 *dé qì*). From what I can gather, Dr. Wang, like many Chinese acupuncturists, places a great deal of emphasis on getting qi and having the patient feel a radiating sensation down (or up) the channel away from the needle. However, Dr. Wang clearly stops speaking, focuses intently (sometimes even pulling up a chair to sit down), and places all of his concentration on the needle after completing his insertion. When asked what he is doing, he often says that you must "put all of your heart at the needle" (心都要聚在針 *xīn dōu yào jù zài zhēn*). Sometimes, he appears to be waiting, with very little movement of the hands, while at other times he is clearly using one of the techniques described below for moving qi. It is therefore difficult to clearly separate the sensation that he himself feels at

the needle from the manipulations he is using to modify the qi sensation as felt by the patient.

4. Dr. Wang generally asks patients to come in once weekly for treatment. There are many exceptions, however, especially in the early stages of treating a relatively complex case. Like many doctors working in China, he is quite willing to ask a new patient to come twice or even three times a week for the first two to four weeks of treatment. This reflects one significant difference between his practice environment and that of many of us outside of China. Because, for much of the twentieth century, acupuncture in China was very inexpensive at the state-funded hospitals, doctors and patients alike became used to the possibility of using frequent treatment in the early stages. Despite the systemic disincentives, practitioners outside of China should still consider the possibility of encouraging patients to come relatively frequently (at least once a week) for treatment in chronic or more serious cases.

5. For readers of English, a reference to the concept of combining tonifying and draining in a single treatment can be found in Robert Johns, *The Art of Acupuncture Techniques* (Berkeley: North Atlantic Books, 1996), 167–168.

Ch. 20 / Point Pairs

1. In modern Chinese, the term *qì huà* (氣化) refers to 'gasification,' as in the process of transforming a solid to a gaseous state. While this is different than the meaning of the same term in traditional medicine, it does convey a similar sense of transformation in the presence of heat (yang qi).

2. Dr. Wang often uses ST-43 (*xiàn gǔ*) as a kind of stand-in source point on the stomach channel. He often says that he has had trouble getting adequate qi sensation (in fact, he reports that there is often pain) when he needles the actual source point, ST-42 (*chōng yáng*).

3. A passage in Chapter 24 of *Basic Questions* describes the relative amount of qi and blood in each of the six channels: "*Tài yáng* normally has more blood and less qi, *shào yáng* normally has less blood and more qi, *yáng míng* usually has more qi and more blood, *shào yīn* has less blood and more qi, *jué yīn* has more blood and less qi, *tài yīn* has less blood and more qi." From this, one can see again the unique relationship of *tài yīn* and *yáng míng*: while each of the other channels is balanced by the relative amounts of qi and blood in its interior-exterior channel, there is a relative abundance of qi associated with the *tài yīn-yáng míng* pair.

4. *Divine Pivot*, Chapter 10.

Appendix 2 / The Sensory Organs

1. Dr. Wang often uses the modern channel and collateral atlas by Lin Yun-Gui (蘭雲桂), *Diagrams of the Channels and Collaterals* (經絡圖解 *Jing luò tú jiě*). Fuzhou: Fujian Science and Technology Publishing House, 1991. He feels that professor Lin has provided, through very meticulous studies of the classics, a series of clearly drawn, textually accurate renderings of the channel pathways. In that text, next to careful illustrations of various regions of the body with the channel pathways, there are collections of classical excerpts describing what one sees. In this Appendix and in other sections of our book, Dr. Wang often draws from this source as a basis for such statements as "Classical texts list seventeen channels, collaterals, and vessels which travel to the eyes."

Point Index

General Index

— **E** —

U

V